Practice of Osteosynthesis

Practice of Osteosynthesis

Frank Schauwecker

Primary Care
An Accident Surgery Atlas · Ligaments, Joints, Bones

Foreword by S. Weller
2nd Revised Edition, 1018 Illustrations, mostly in two colors

1982
Georg Thieme Verlag
Stuttgart · New York

Thieme-Stratton Inc.
New York

Prof. Dr. FRANK SCHAUWECKER
Chefarzt der Abt. Unfallchirurgie
der Städtischen Kliniken der Landeshauptstadt
Schwalbacher Straße 62, 6200 Wiesbaden

Drawings by JOACHIM HORMANN, Stuttgart

Translator: Dr. G. STIASNY
Van Neyenrodeweg 574
Amsterdam/Nederlande

CIP-Kurztitelaufnahme der Deutschen Bibliothek

Schauwecker, Frank:
Practice of osteosynthesis : primary care ; an accident surgery atlas ; ligaments, joints, bones / Frank Schauwecker. Foreword by S. Weller. [Transl.: G. Stiasny]. – 2., rev. ed. – Stuttgart ; New York : Thieme, 1982
Dt. Ausg. u.d.T.: Schauwecker, Frank: Osteosynthese-Praxis

Important Note: Medicine is an ever-changing science. Research and clinical experience are continually broadening our knowledge, in particular our knowledge of proper treatment and drug therapy. Insofar as this book mentions any dosage or application, readers may rest assured that the authors, editors and publishers have made every effort to ensure that such references are strictly in accordance with the state of knowledge at the time of production of the book. Nevertheless, every user is requested to carefully examine the manufacturers' leaflets accompanying each drug to check on his own responsibility whether the dosage schedules recommended therein or the contraindications stated by the manufacturers differ from the statements made in the present book. Such examination is particularly important with drugs which are either rarely used or have been newly released on the market.

This book is an authorized translation from the 2nd revised German edition published and copyrighted 1981 by Georg Thieme Verlag, Stuttgart, Germany. Title of the German edition: Osteosynthesepraxis.

1. German edition 1972
1. English edition 1974
1. Spanish edition 1974

Typesetting: G. Müller, Heilbronn, gesetzt auf VIP-Comet
Printed in West-Germany by K. Grammlich, Pliezhausen

ISBN 3-13-619202-3 (Georg Thieme Verlag, Stuttgart/New York)
ISBN 0-86577-054-9 (Thieme-Stratton Inc., New York)
LC 81-86374

Foreword

Modern osteosynthesis requires an atraumatic and accurate operating technique. Points particularly worthy of emphasis include the anatomically correct approach to the bone, with careful regard for all the soft structures, especially the blood vessels and nerves, as well as the least possible exposure of the bony segments to be fixed.

As for the osteosynthesis itself, greatest stress must be laid on meticulous adherence to the biomechanical principles ensuring the desired stability.

Practicing the diverse techniques of osteosynthesis on a human skeleton would not take into account the soft structures and the surgical approach. Since adequate practice with cadavers on such a large scale is not feasible, the graphic representation of the routes of approach and the technical performance of osteosynthesis as done here is a welcome contribution and a useful resource. For clarity of presentation the illustrations were limited to the most customary approaches and operations. Thus, this atlas is intended to provide complementary guidance and information for all those who are not regularly engaged in performing osteosyntheses.

Tübingen, Spring 1972

SIEGFRIED WELLER

Preface to the Second German Edition

The present book began with a collection of sketches drew, illustrating operative approaches and preparations for surgical interventions. I particularly recorded those details of which previous atlases of operating technique had thus far taken but little notice. In the course of doing so, I collected and completed a great number of descriptive drawings. Thus it is that the book does not propose to present anything original but rather to illustrate the existing material by readapting it and supplementing it with certain seemingly unimportant details. But a number of difficulties met with in ordinary practice are pointed out.

The selection of the individual procedures was the result of a number of operations in which I acted as the responsible assistant to colleagues who were novices in this branch of surgery; it was their questions and problems I became familiar with. I also dispensed with a detailed bibliography; they are never-ending and still incomplete. The drawings undoubtedly make clear that the procedures presented have been worked out by the A O group for the problems of osteosynthesis.

Experience has shown that technical problems are involved not only in osteosynthesis but also in injuries to ligaments. So I have gone beyond "The Practice of Osteosynthesis" and have attempted to discuss those operative techniques for ligament injuries which have proved their value in the clinical field. That necessitated inserting illustrations from the field of functional anatomy.

I have made an effort to portray the operative sites as they are seen by the surgeon, i.e., often unlike those pictured commonly in anatomy atlases and textbooks of operating surgery. I am indebted to Mr. Hormann for his inexhaustible patience and careful attention devoted to the execution of the anatomical drawings.

A special word of thanks is due to those reviewers who called my attention to a number of important details. I hope that I have taken due account of their suggestions.

Wiesbaden, Summer 1980 FRANK SCHAUWECKER

Preface to the First German Edition

The present atlas is designed to portray the practice of osteosynthesis in traumatic and orthopaedic surgery. It should be of service to surgeons and orthopaedists who are already familiar with the basic principles of osteosynthesis. Everyday experience proves that to successfully perform an osteosynthesis it does not suffice only to master the general principles of the management of fractures. Just as the technically correct performance of the osteosynthesis itself is indispensable for the unimpaired functioning of the parts involved, the successful outcome depends equally on the operative procedure as a whole.

The atlas proposes to offer the possibility of viewing the fracture in connection with the soft structures involved so as to make the course of the operation abundantly clear. I hope that thereby the operator will succeed in determining the correct anatomic approach to the bone and the fracture, without inflicting additional damage on the soft structures, and in performing the osteosynthesis in a technically uncompromising fashion.

By means of individual illustrations I shall present, step by step, the correct positioning, the sterile draping, the approach through the soft tissues and the performance of the osteosynthesis, including local peculiarities of otherwise typical findings, such as have proved their value as guidelines for residents with little experience. Among several techniques which have proved of equal values in the hands of the skilled surgeon, I have selected those which hold the most promise of success.

I am anxious to express my thanks to Professor Weller, my head of department, who introduced me to the wide field of traumatic surgery and who was, moreover, my kindly teacher for many years. It was only he who, through continual critical explanation of the problems involved, made it possible for me to conceive this book. He has given me many valuable suggestions towards its completion.

I am also indebted to Mr. Hormann who, with endless care and patience, has retouched a great many of the drawings, as well as to my wife who has checked over each sketch of the drawings as to its lucidity and conclusiveness.

Last but not least, I have to thank the publishers for the liberality with which, in producing the book, they have complied with my wishes – and those of the readers.

Tübingen, Spring 1972 FRANK SCHAUWECKER

Contents

1. General Aspects

- Traction (with reposition and plaster cast) is used in all cases where there is no guarantee that an operation can be performed within a few hours.
- Because of the danger of infection, wire traction should never be applied to a bone that cannot be operated on under the same general anaesthesia.
- There are three degrees of open fractures:

First degree: Fracture with perforation of the skin *from within.*
Second degree: Fracture with clean injury of skin and muscles by contusion and penetration *from without.*
Third degree: Fracture with extensive local lesions accompanied by destruction of muscular tissue and other concomitant local injuries.

Blood Supply

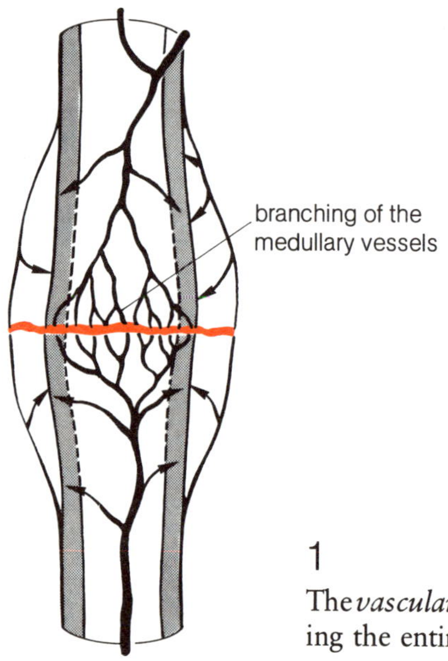

1

The *vascular system of the bone marrow* is capable of supplying the entire nutrition of the bony cortex.

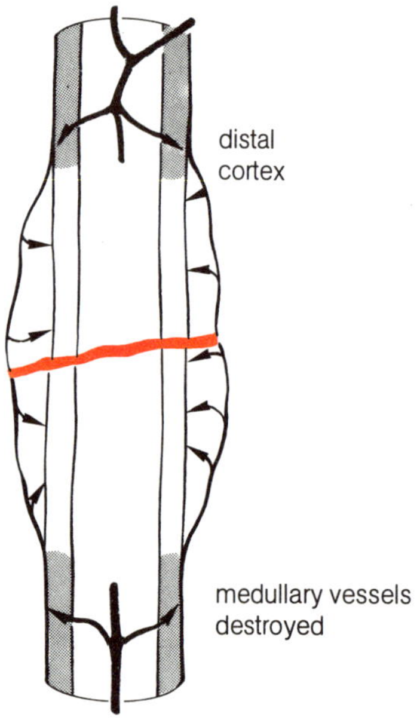

2

The *vascular system of the periosteum* is not, by itself, capable of providing nourishment to the cortex.

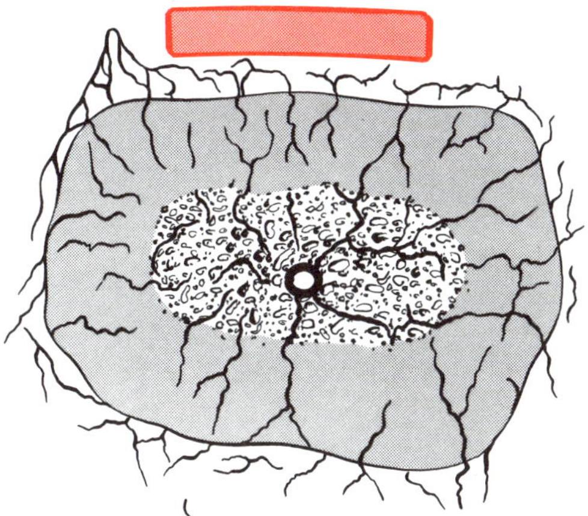

3

Bone plates should, whenever possible, be placed directly *on the periosteum.* Even with extreme tightening of the screws, pressure exerted by the plate on the surface underneath it can never become strong enough to interfere seriously with periosteal circulation.

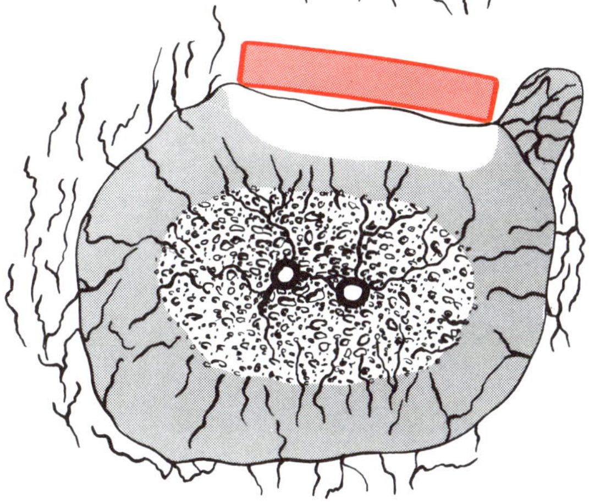

4

Blockage of circulation as a result of pushing the periosteum aside leads to necrosis of the cortical areas lying just underneath the plate. Such necrosis is apt to affect half the thickness of the cortical wall.

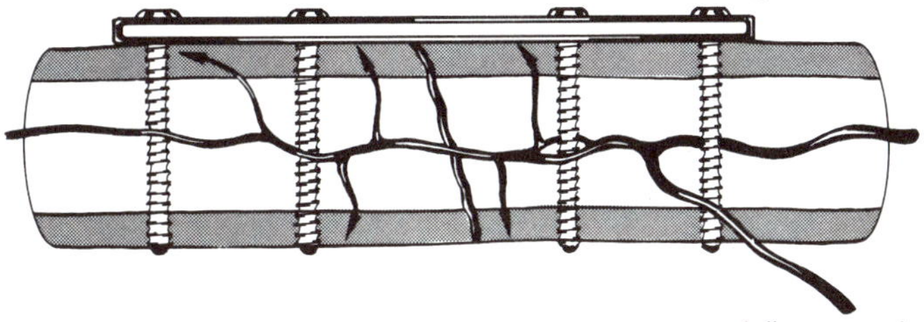

5

With both *plate fixation*...

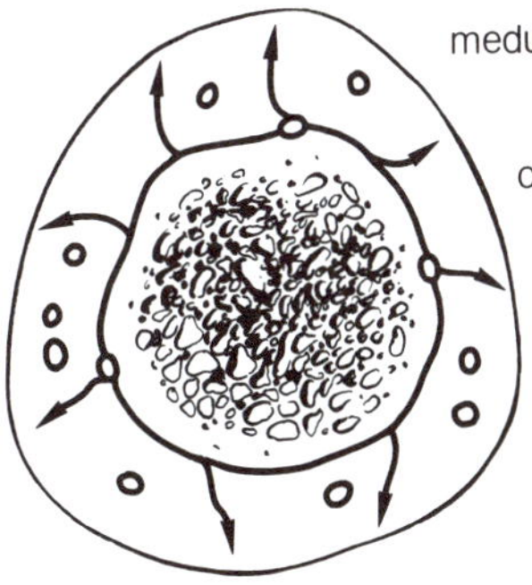

6

... and *nail fixation,* the central vascular system will be restored, under physiologic conditions (including, for instance, a perfectly stable osteosynthesis), via the nutrient vessels within about two weeks.

Retention sutures

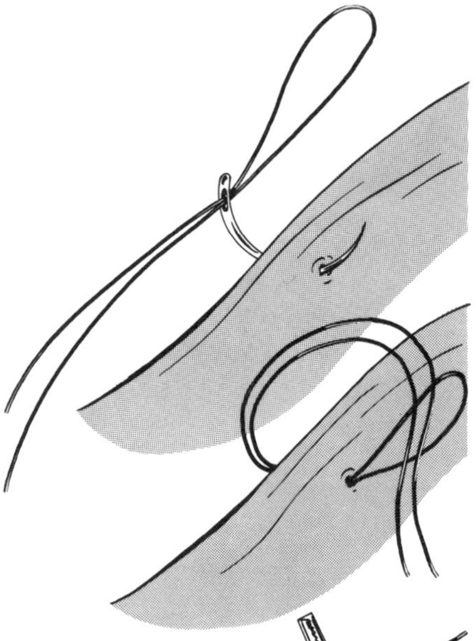

1
The thread is doubled and passed through the eye of the needle, the loop becoming its short end.

2
The ends of the thread are passed through the loop. When the loop is tightened, the thread becomes securely fixed.

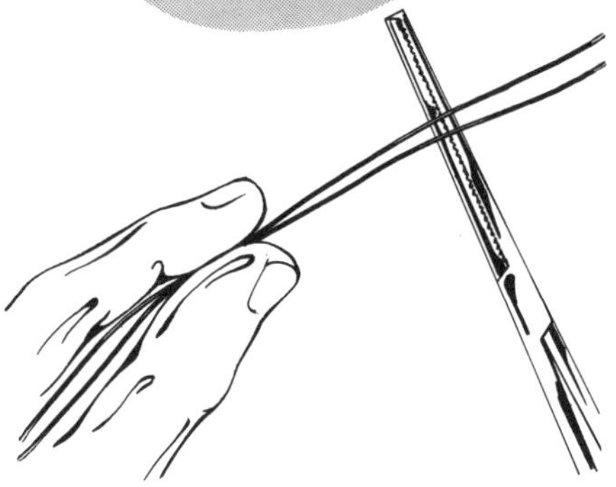

3
The free ends are then fitted with a clamp. The closed clamp is placed on top of the thread.

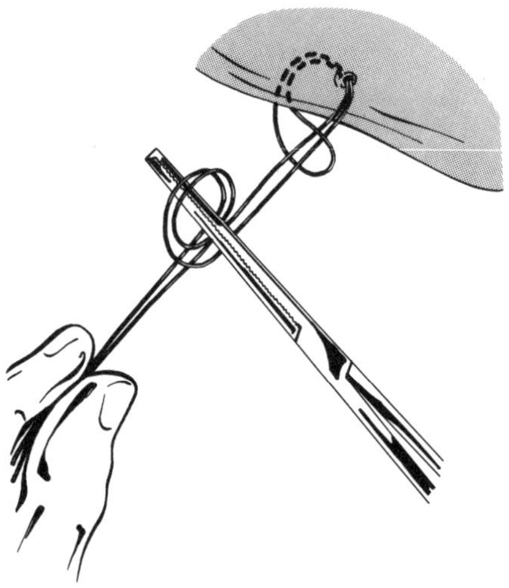

4
A loop is formed around the clamp.

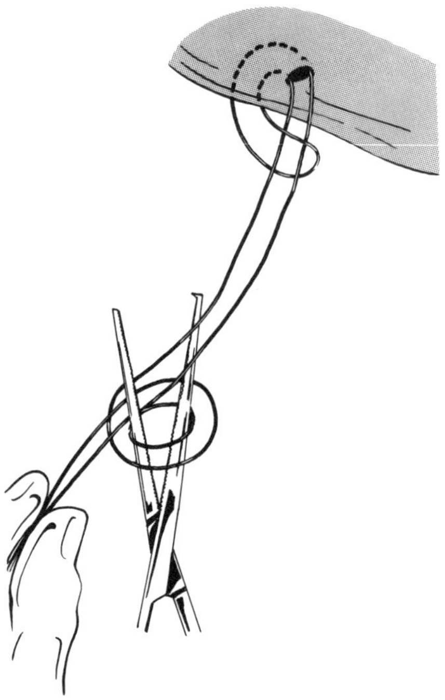

5
The clamp is turned 90°. Then it is opened to grasp the thread coming out of the soft structures and is thus prevented from slipping off the thread.

Handling of the tendon

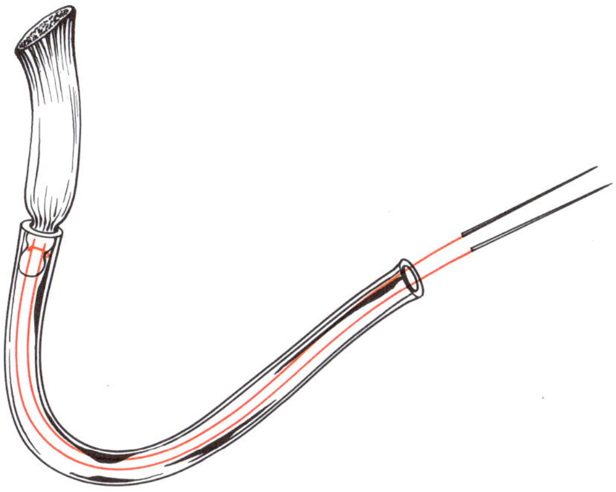

1
Handling the tendon, as in performing a tenoplasty, for example, is facilitated by using a thin-walled plastic tube.

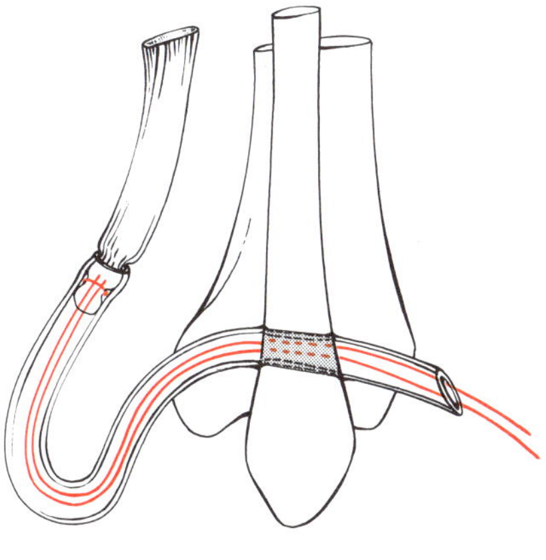

2
The plastic tube prevents the extremity of the tendon from fraying and thereby getting caught.

Open fractures

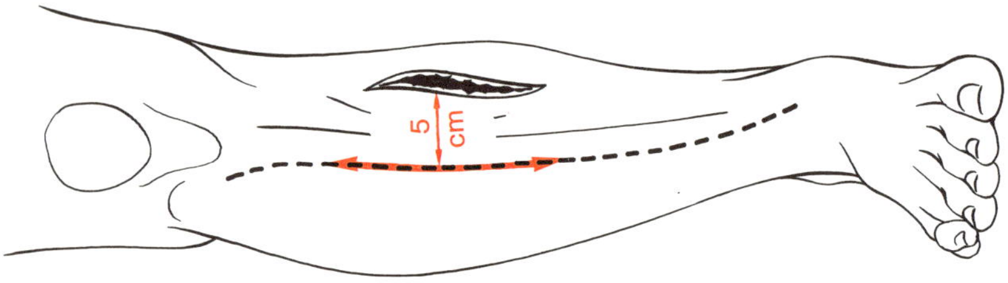

1

When the distance between the wound and a standard incision exceeds 5 cm, access to the fracture should not be sought through the wound.

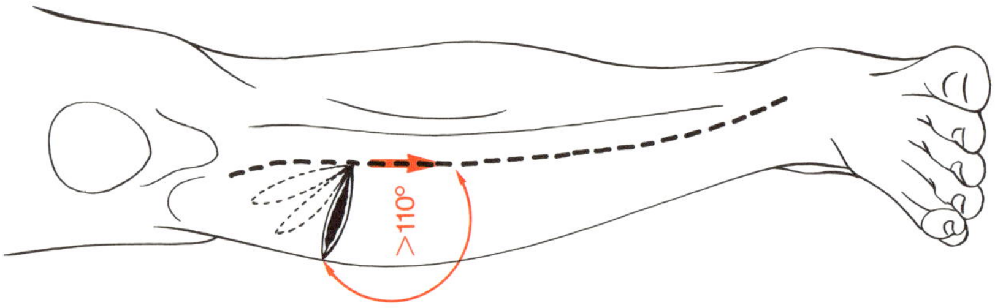

2

Wounds must not open into a standard incision at an angle inferior to 110°.

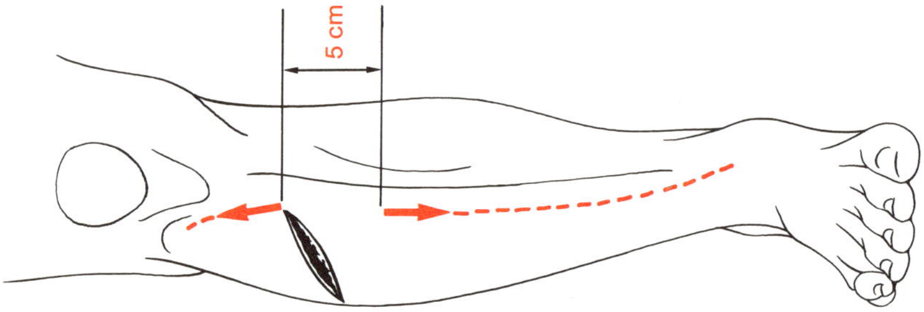

3

Bearing in mind this 110° stricture, when the standard incision does not give sufficient access to the wound, the operator must leave a soft-tissue bridge measuring 5 cm in width in place.

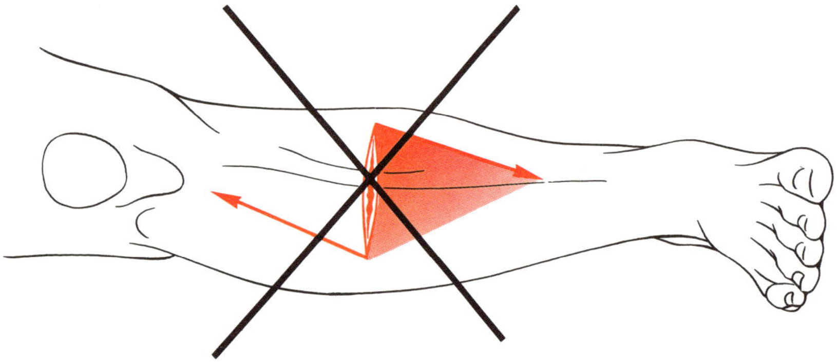

4

To widen a wound in the fashion illustrated inevitably leads to necrosis of soft tissues.

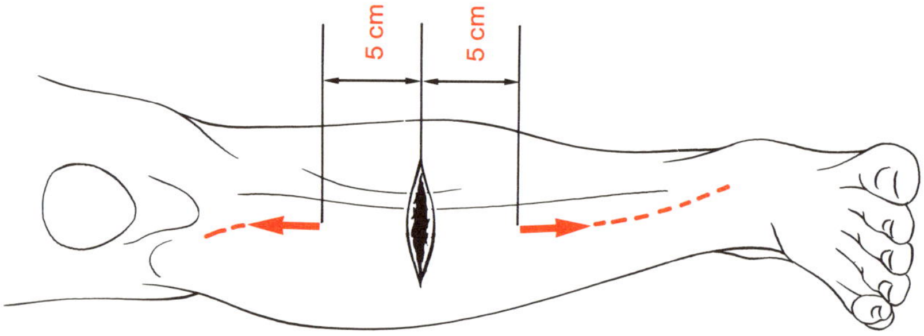

5

Widen the access to the fracture along the standard incision, leaving soft-tissue bridges 5 cm in width.

Sterile draping

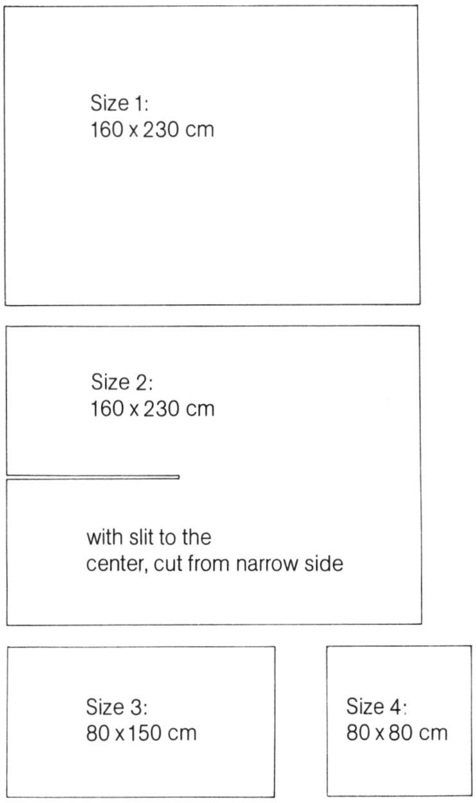

1
Recommended sizes of wound drapes, washed and sewn.

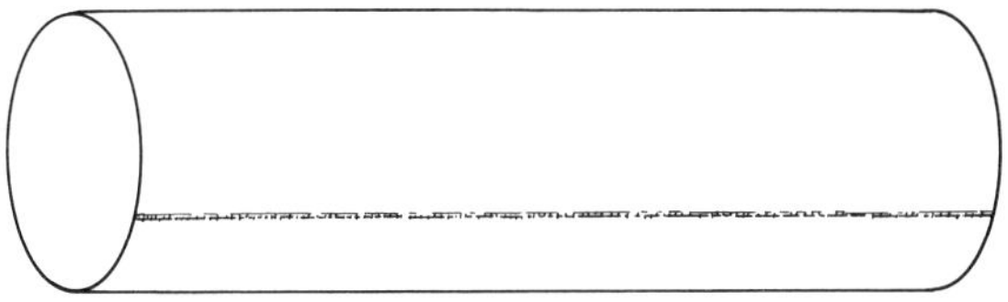

2
Size 1 wound drape, sewn together to form a tube.

Roentgenographic image intensifier

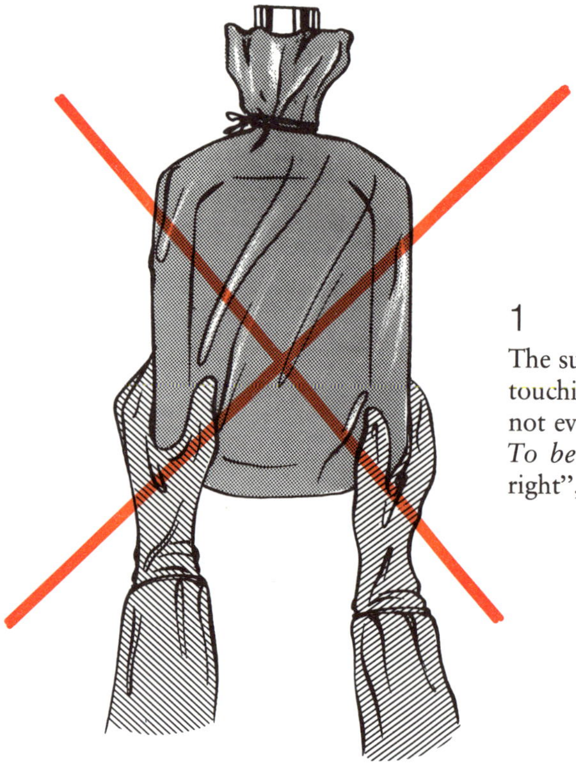

1
The surgeon should accustom himself to giving *precise directions*, since touching the image intensifier is not compatible with the laws of sterility, not even if the device is wrapped in sterile packing.
To be avoided: directions such as "upward", "downward", "to the right", "to the left", or "backward".

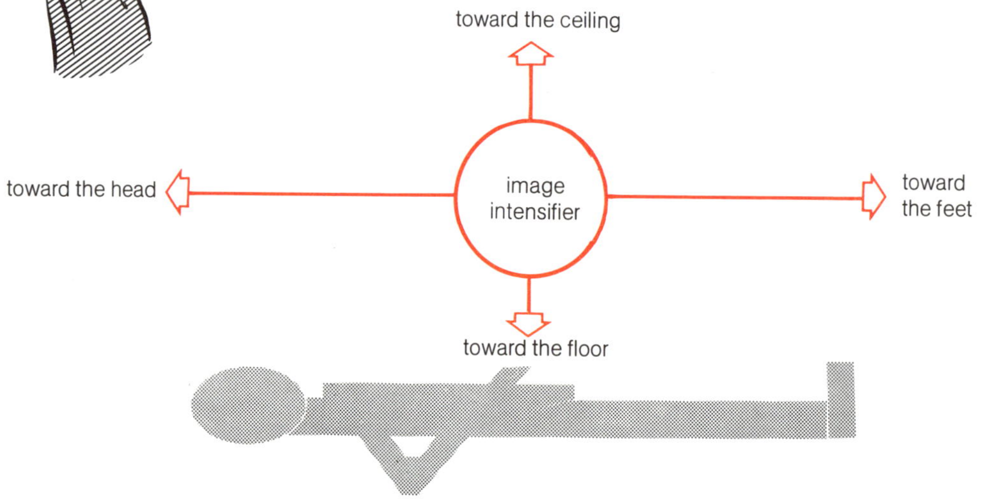

2
Examples of directions to be used for the vertical plane.

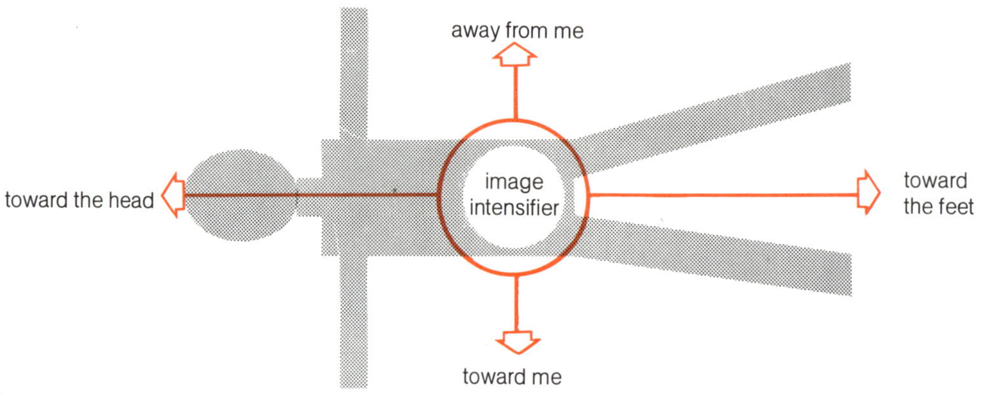

3
Examples of directions to be used for the horizontal plane.

Postoperative care

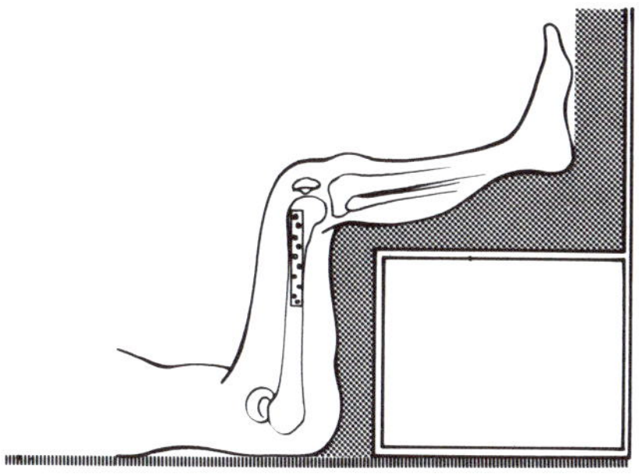

1
Elevation of the leg until swelling subsides, i.e., until the skin begins to shrivel.

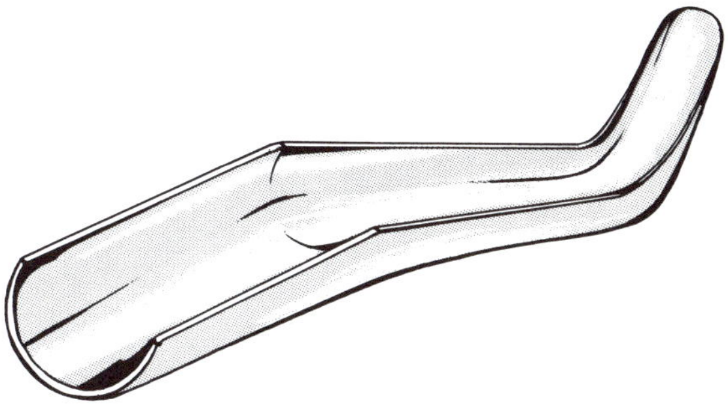

2
Early movement, starting on the first postoperative day, under guidance of the physiotherapist, twice a day.

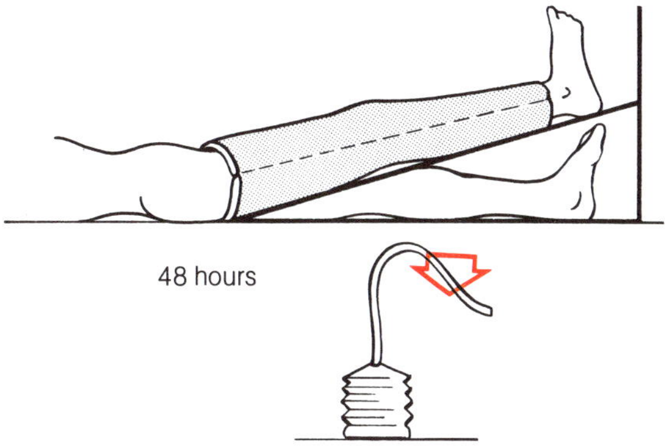

3
The *suction drainage* is loosened on the first day after surgery (by removing the retention suture) and dispensed with on the second day, provided the secretion does not exceed 5 ml.

Dressing changes:
a) Do not allow the dressing to become wet.
b) Change the dressing at least every other day and watch for a hematoma.
c) Between the 4th and 5th day, dressings can be dispensed with and should be replaced by a wound film (Nobecutan®). In this way, the daily control for irritation of the wound or formation of a hematoma can be done visually.

Sutures: Remove sutures on the 11th postoperative day.
Hematomas: These require continual accurate checks and, when encountered, must be immediately removed in the operation room (even when in doubt).
Never squeeze a hematoma. Do not be reluctant to reopen an osteosynthesis when there is suspicion of a hematoma.

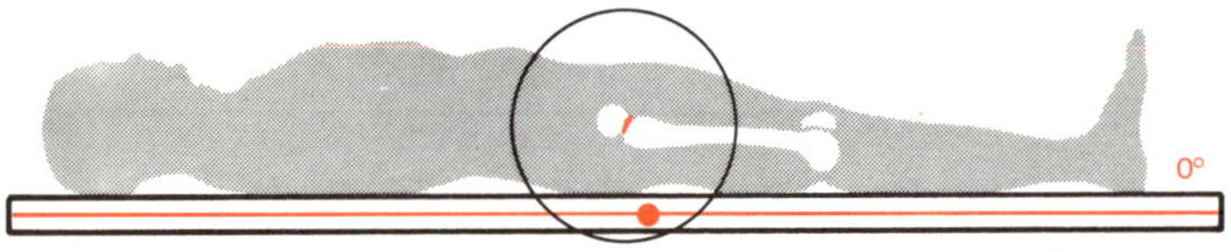

4

Positioning for an injury in the region of the *hip (joint, subtrochanteric area of femur)*.

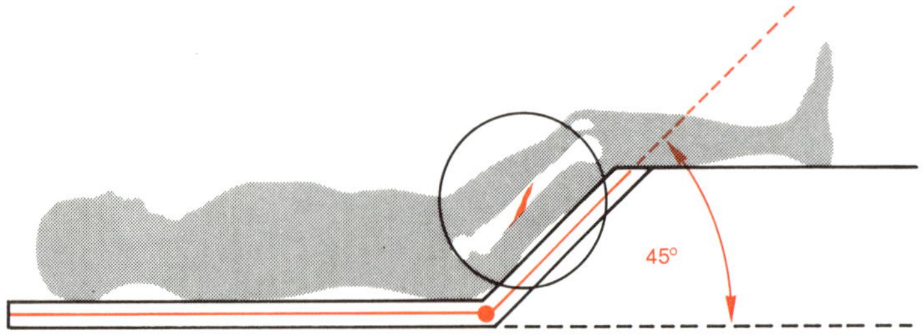

5

Positioning for an injury in the region of the *mid-thigh*.

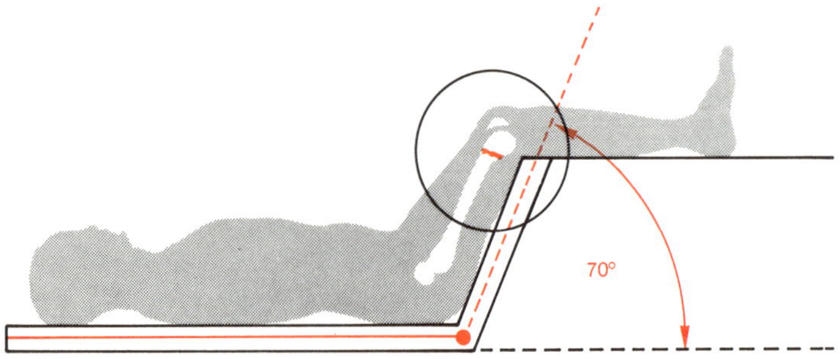

6

Positioning for an injury of the *supracondylar region*, the *knee*, *lower leg* and *foot*.

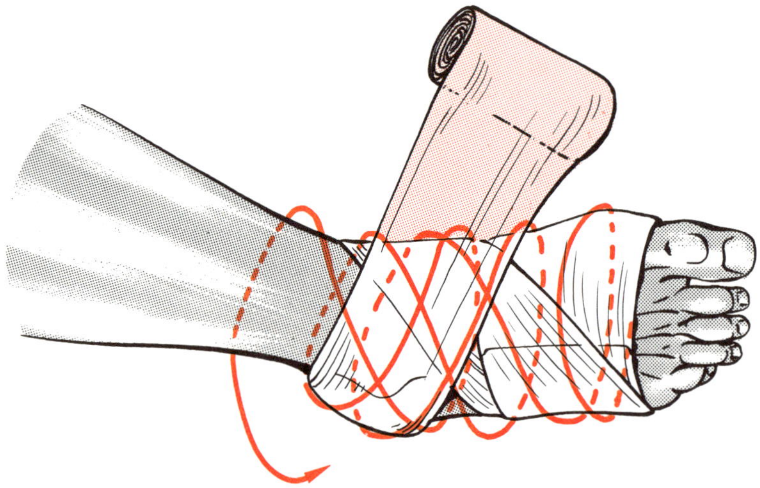

7

When, as frequently happens in the course of treatment, an elastic bandage is used, an effective fit can be achieved only by expert application, avoiding all wrinkles. The ball of the great toe has to be included.

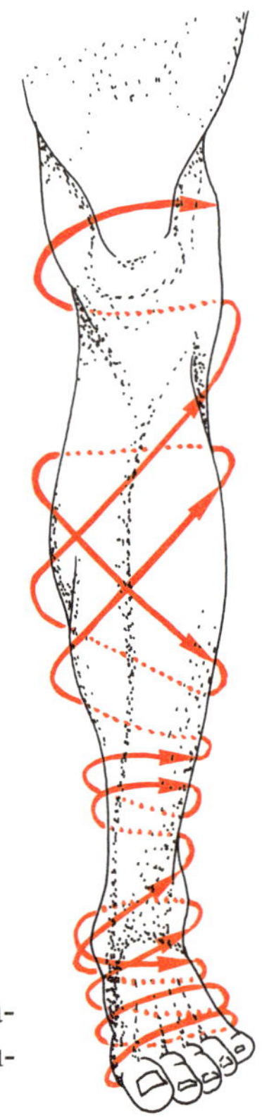

8

The turns of the bandage should run as shown in the diagram; the bandage should not be applied too tightly, particularly when postoperative edema is to be expected.

Cancellous bone grafting

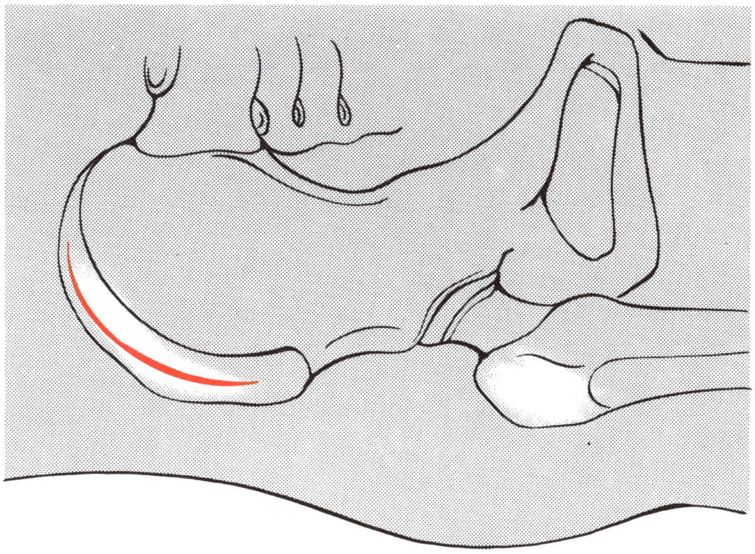

1

Skin incision. With the patient lying on his side or in a prone position, the following techniques can be applied without difficulty, even to the posterior part of the iliac crest as well.

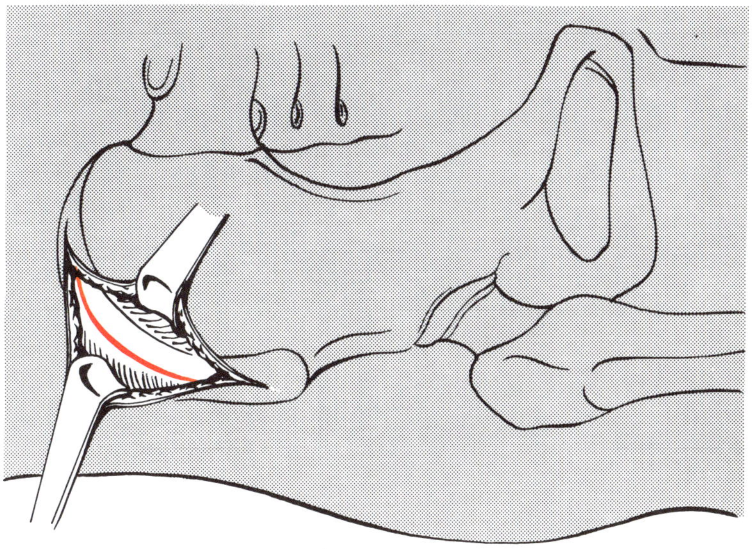

2

Incision of fascia and periosteum down to the bone.

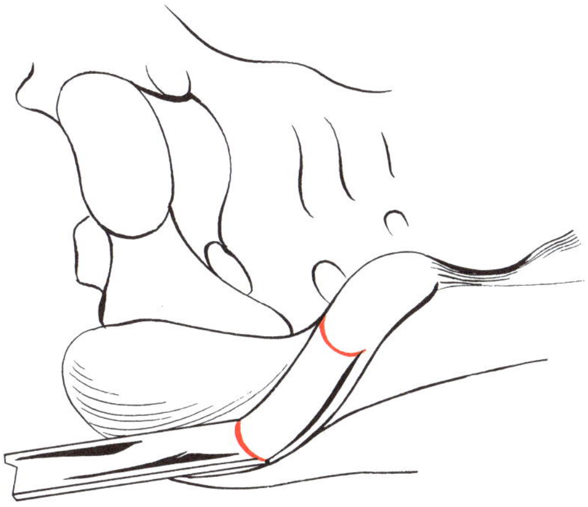

3

To procure *cancellous chips,* the cortical edge of the iliac crest is lifted up like the lid of a chest. First, a lateral nick is made in the bone with a narrow chisel, then…

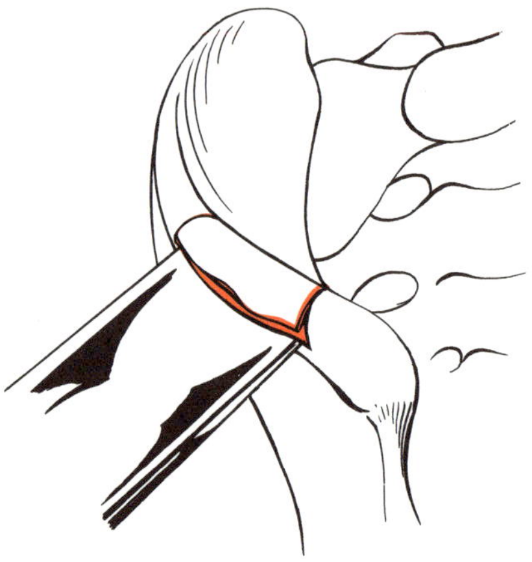

4
... the lid is fashioned with a very wide chisel without sectioning the periosteum on the inner side...

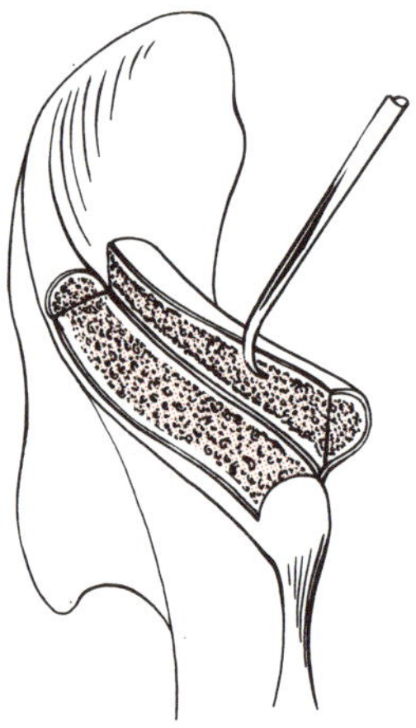

5
... so that the latter forms the "hinge" of the lid.

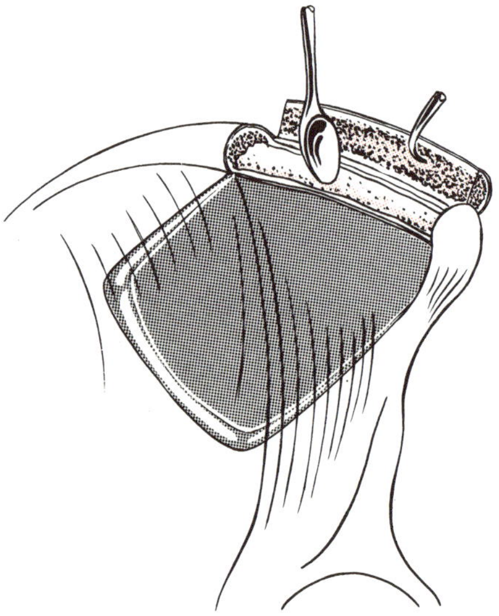

6
Procuring the chips with a spoon.

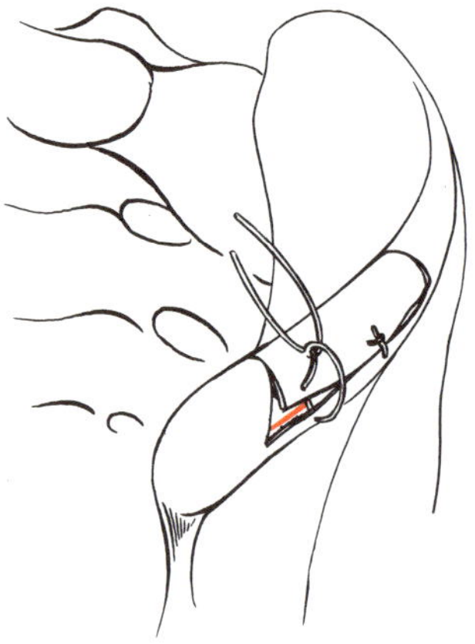

7
By turning the lid back and reuniting the periosteum and fascia with tight stitches, the contour of the iliac crest is preserved and the formation of a hematoma in the soft tissues is prevented.

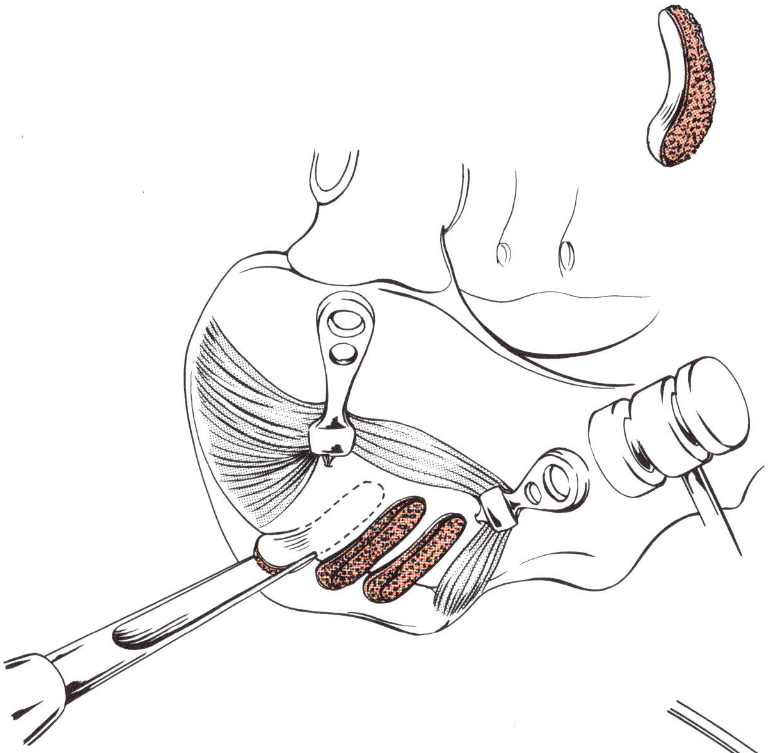

8

Cancellous slivers, which are frequently needed, are obtained from the inner side by use of a grooved chisel that should not be too narrow.

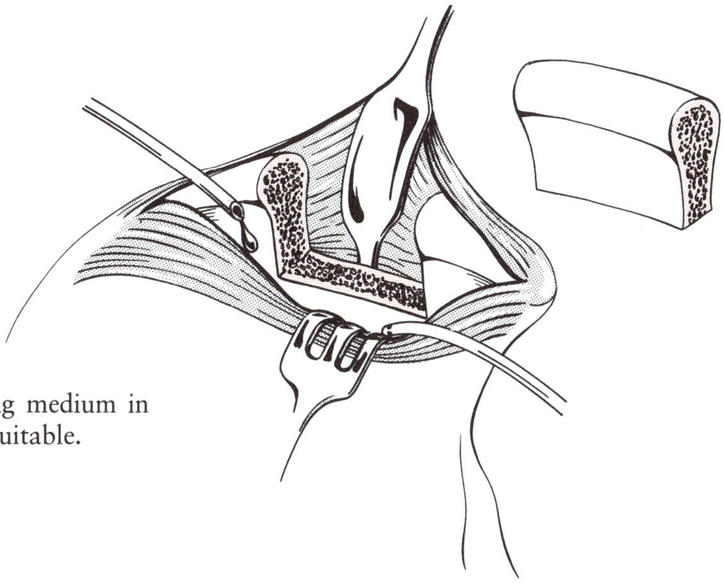

9

For *corticocancellous blocks,* e.g. as an interposing medium in defects of the ulna or fibula, the iliac crest is very suitable.

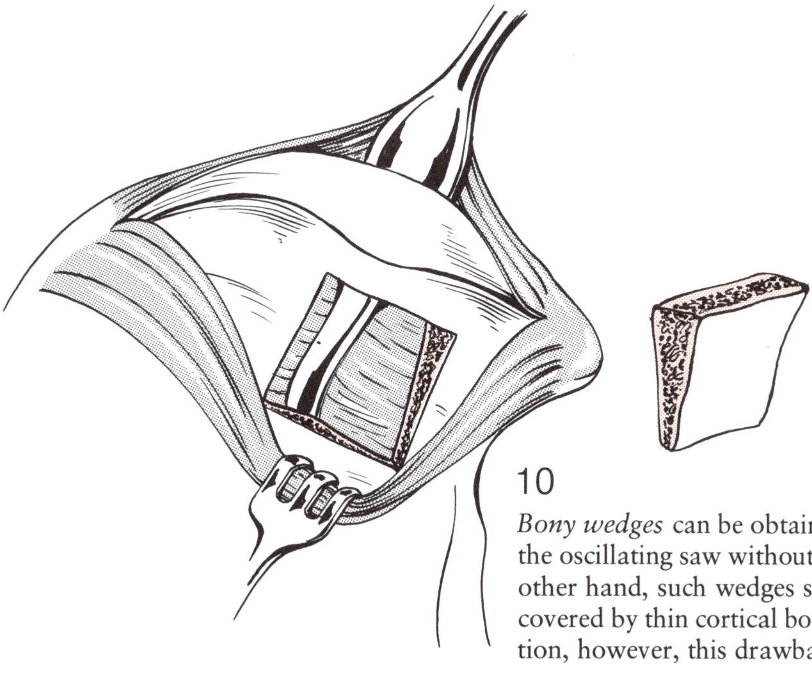

10

Bony wedges can be obtained from the surface of the ilium by means of the oscillating saw without changing the contour of the iliac crest on the other hand, such wedges suffer the disadvantage that their surfaces are covered by thin cortical bone. With regard to the Eden-Hybinette operation, however, this drawback can be accepted in exchange for stability.

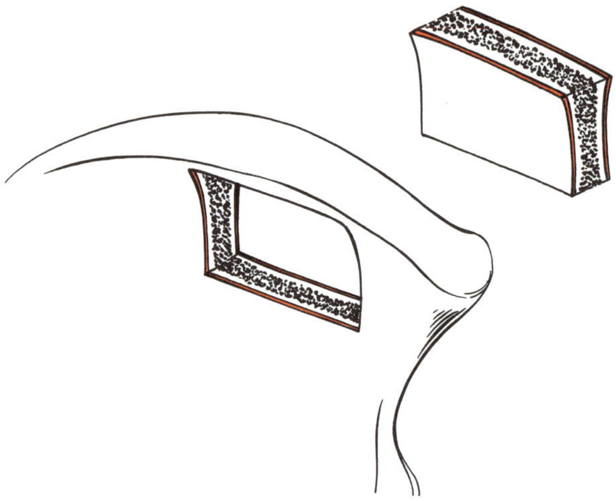

11

Blocks of greater thickness are obtained from the vicinity of the iliac crest.

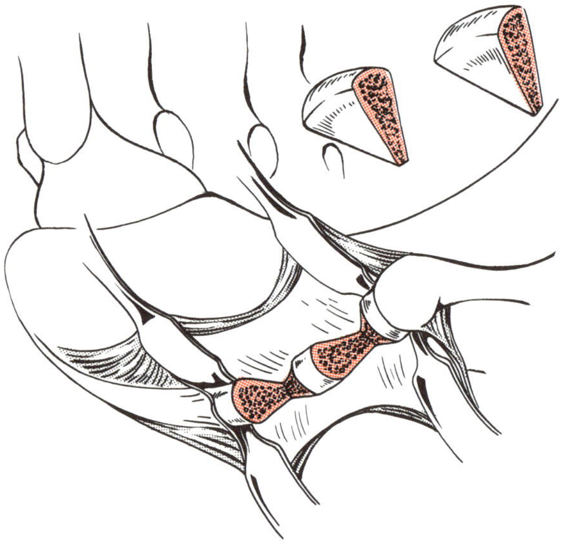

12

In performing an osteotomy one can make very good use of wedges obtained with the oscillating saw in this manner. Mostly, however, two or more wedges are required. In such cases, it is best to leave bony pillars between the sites of removal.

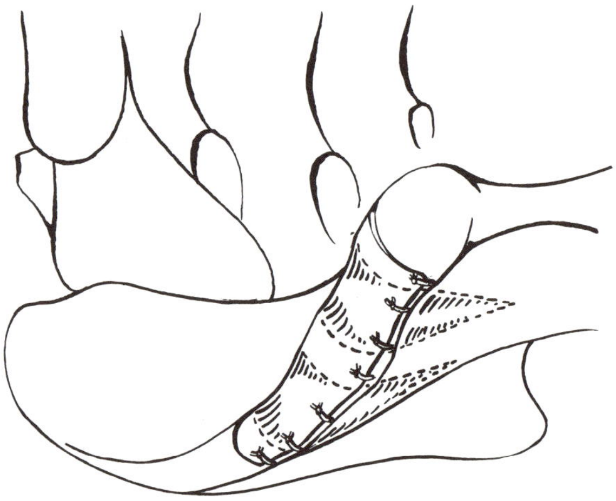

13

Provided the periosteum has been detached with great care, the occluding suture, supported by one or more bony pillars, does not produce any change in the contour of the iliac crest.

Hazards in operations on the iliac crest

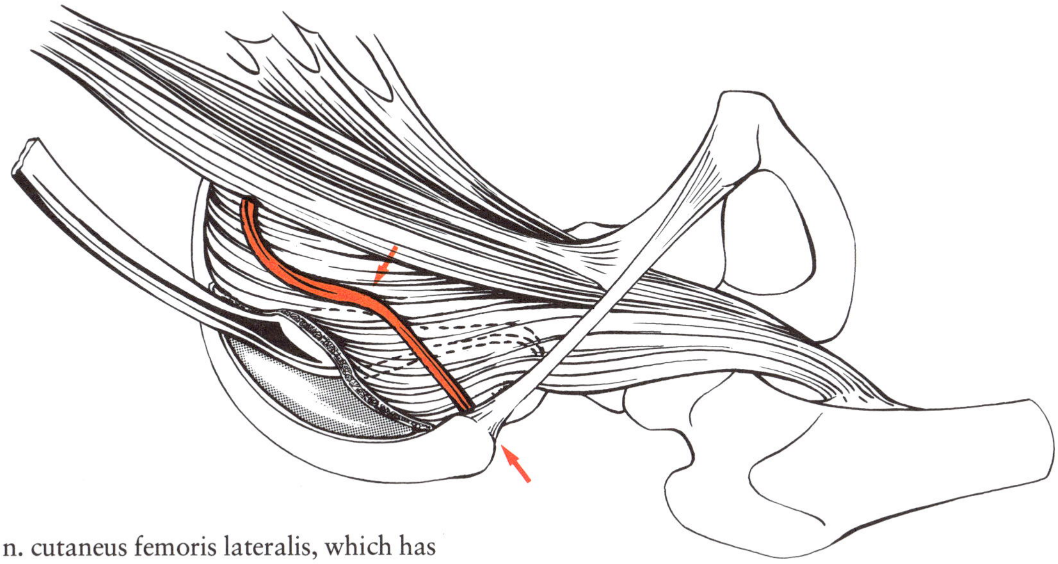

1
In the first place, the n. cutaneus femoris lateralis, which has little freedom of movement, is exposed to damage by Hohmann retractors when these are applied very deeply and when excessive traction is exerted on them.
Prevention: Flex the hip joint and rotate it internally. Do not insert the Hohmann retractors too far ventrally, but insert as far as possible in the direction of the sacrum.

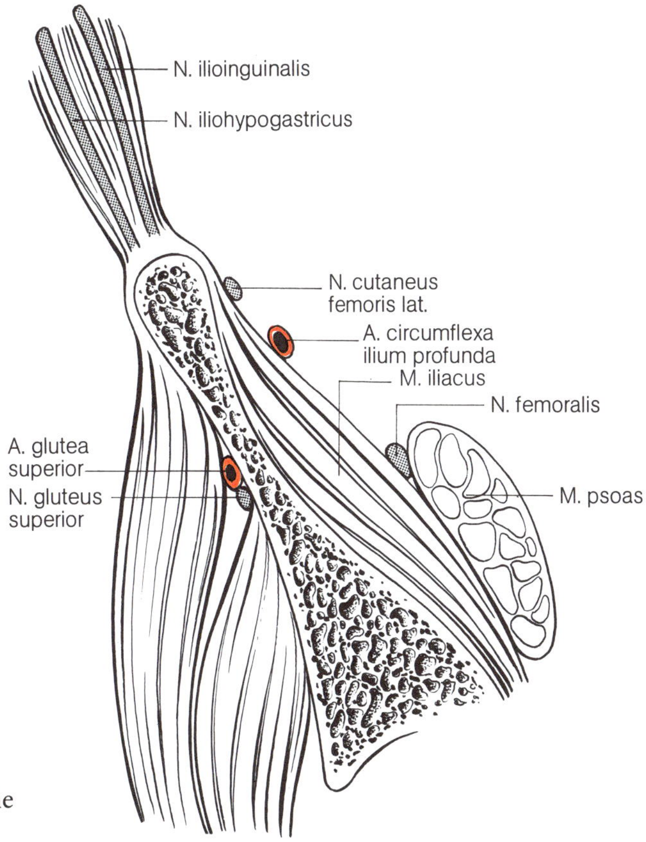

2
Anatomy: Section through the right ilium at the level of the hip joint.

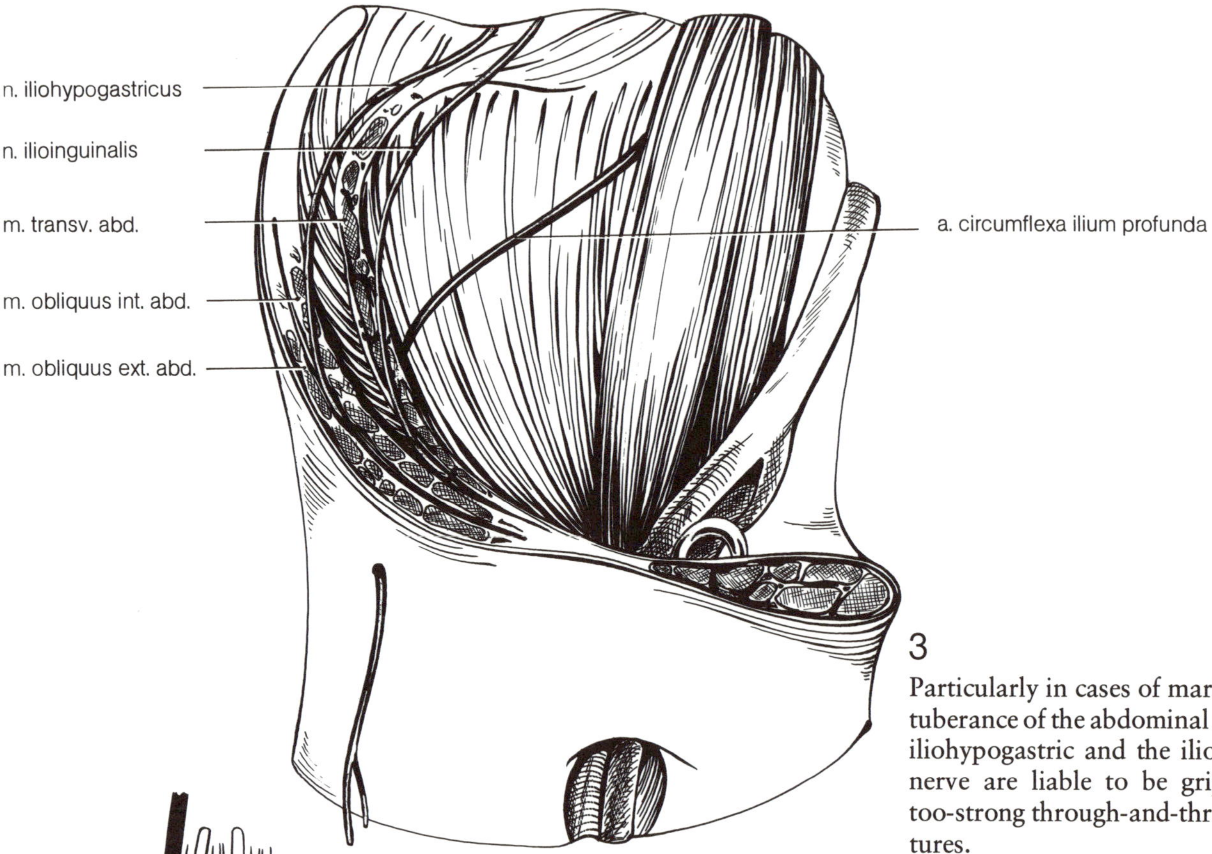

3

Particularly in cases of marked protuberance of the abdominal wall, the iliohypogastric and the ilioinguinal nerve are liable to be gripped by too-strong through-and-through sutures.

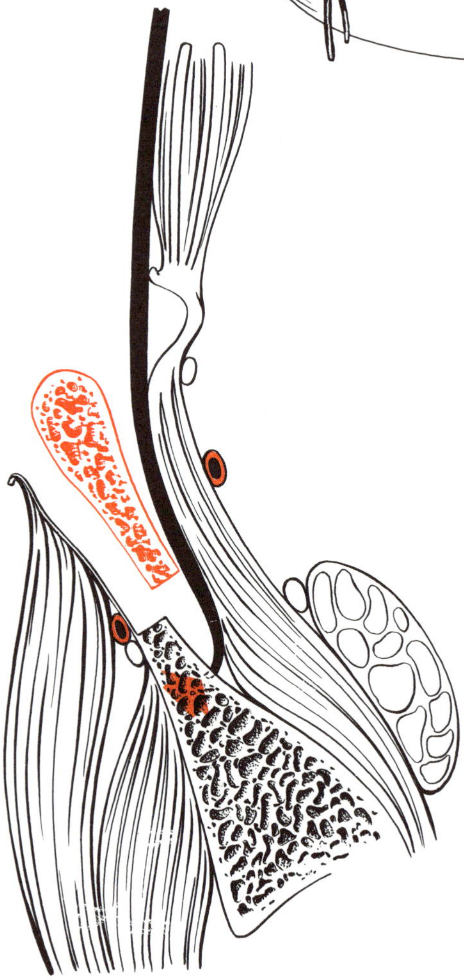

4

A Hohmann retractor presses the iliac muscle, including nerves and vessels medialward. A bone block has been removed. The superior gluteal artery and nerve are exposed and can be directly injured by the tip of the Hohmann retractor.

2. Implants

Screws

1
Initial situation I: Screws with identical body diameter. Neither of them can be screwed into a hole with this body diameter without special preliminaries.

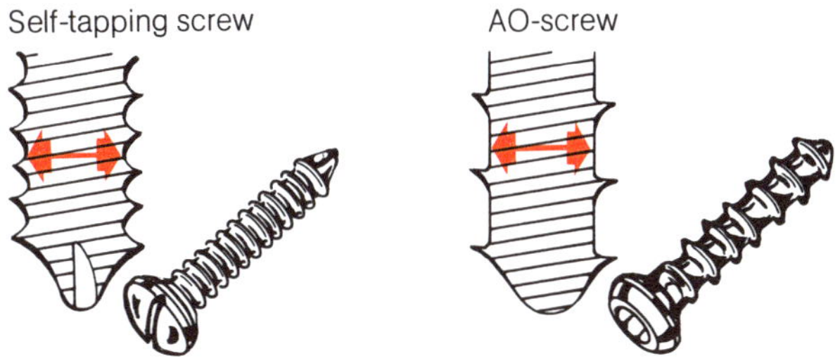

2
Initial situation II: Drill holes of identical diameter, somewhat larger than the body diameter of the screws.

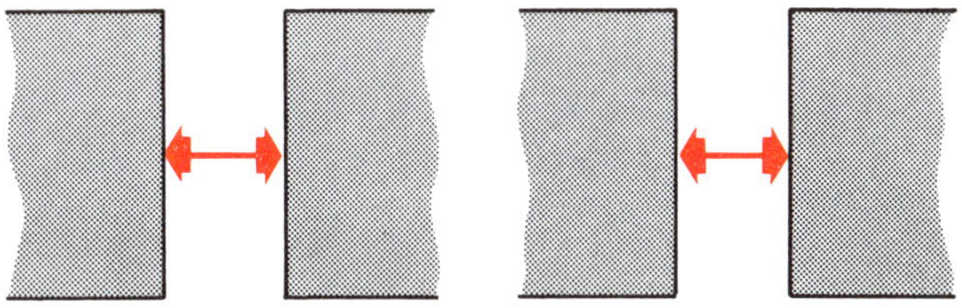

3
For the self-tapping screw, the hole must be widened before the screw can be put in. For inserting the AO screw, a thread must be cut.

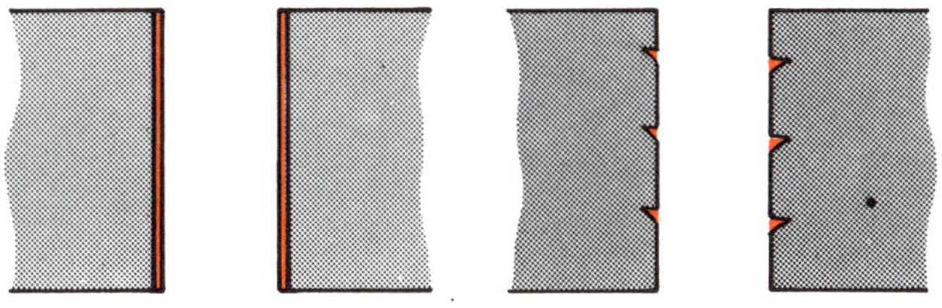

4
The self-tapping screw is fastened in the bone solely by the edges of the thread. At these edges very high pressure is generated. The turns of the AO screw adapt themselves smoothly to the previously created bed of the thread with a broad contact surface and without any pressure from the edges.

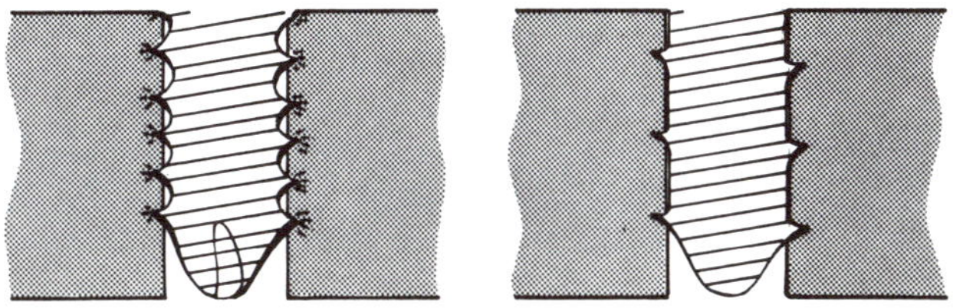

5a
With use of the self-tapping screw, the high pressure produced by the edges of the thread leads to bone resorption at the sides within a few days, so that the screw loses its purchase, whereas the correctly inserted AO screw produces no pressure and no subsequent bone resorption.

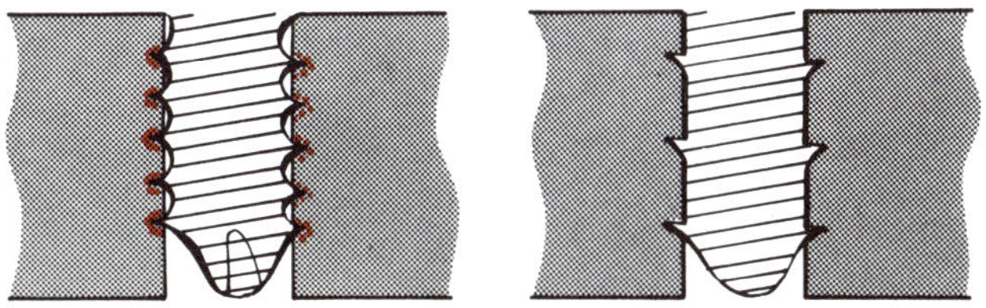

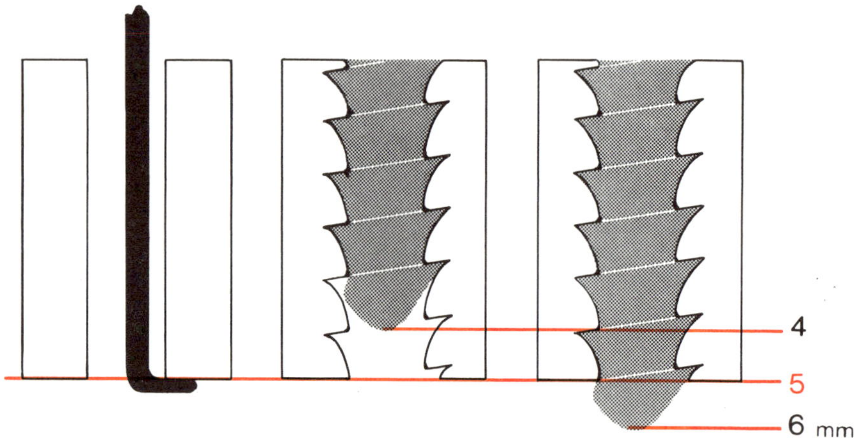

5b

Determining the length of the screws: the gradation of screw lengths is 2 mm. The points of the screws should always project a short distance (1 to 2 mm). This means, for instance, that a measured length of 4 or 5 mm corresponds to an actual screw length of 6 mm. Only in this way can the thread hold fully along the entire opposing cortex.

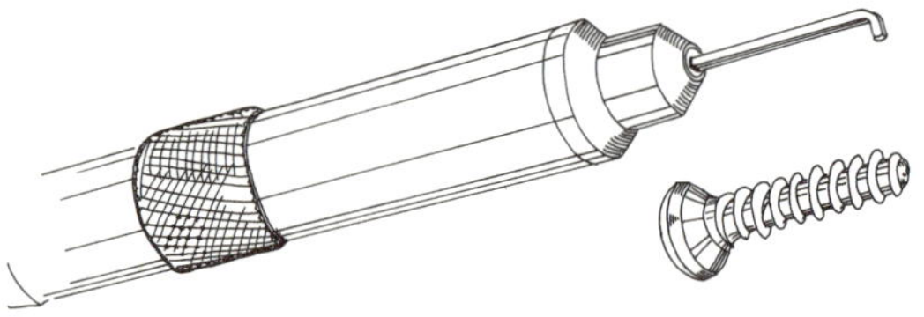

6

The measuring device for screw length also takes into account the bone space which, because of the conical point of the screw, is not usable for its anchorage.

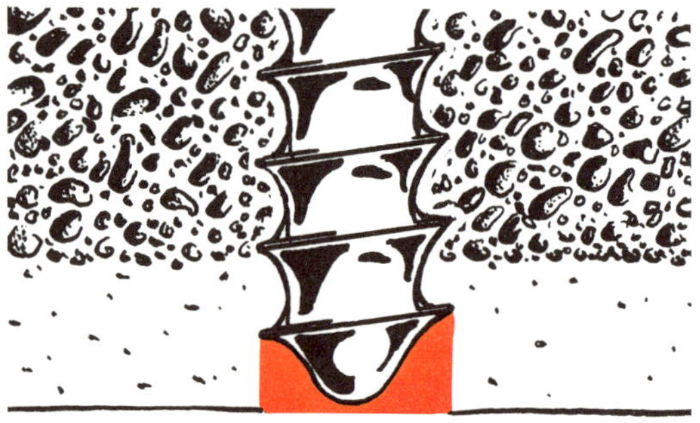

7

Bone space not utilized for anchoring the screw, unless its point is allowed to project 1 to 2 mm.

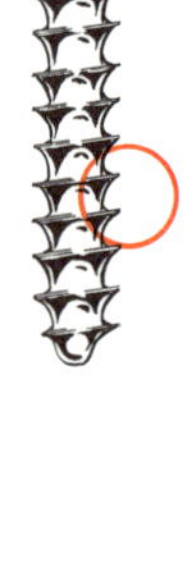

8

4.5 mm cortical screw. For its utilization as traction screw see Figs. 22–1ff. Fitting drill: 3.2 mm.

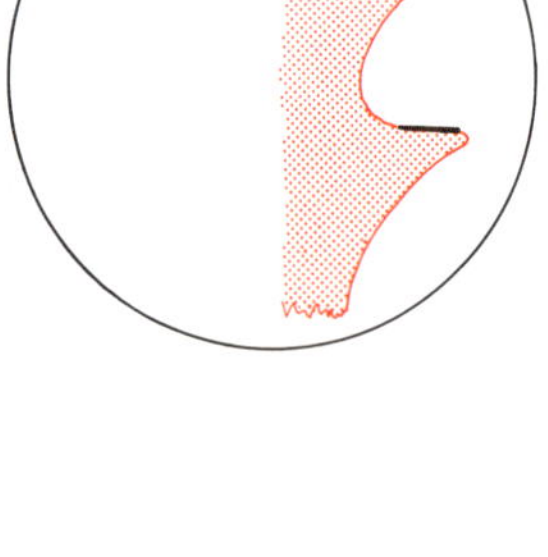

9

The screw is so made that, on tightening, it transmits the pressure which originates in the turns of the thread over broad contact surfaces.

10

Long thread:
There are cancellous screws with long threads and short threads. Whenever possible, screws with long threads should be used.

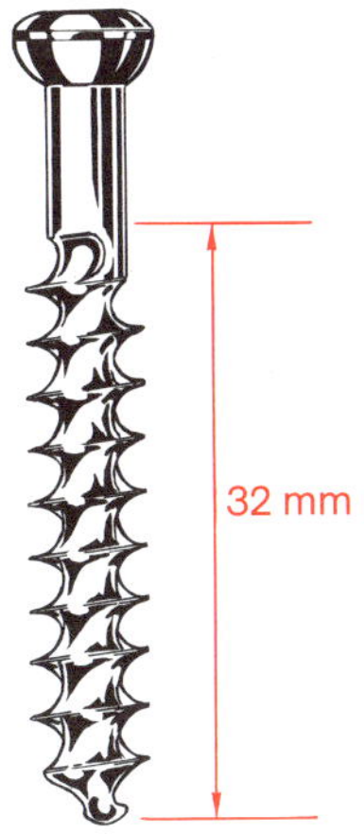

11

Short thread:
These screws may be required for special kinds of fractures with small fragments (Volkmann's triangle in the tibia, transcondylar fractures). The shortest cancellous screw measures 25 mm in length.

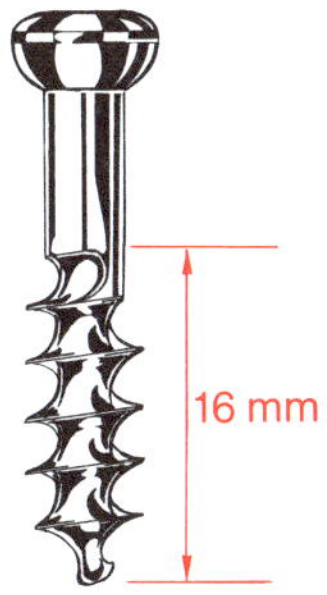

12

4.5 mm malleolar screw. The appropriate drill measures 3.2 mm. Useful only in cancellous bone when no major degree of weightbearing is to be expected. Only practical utility is in the medial malleolus on clear indication.

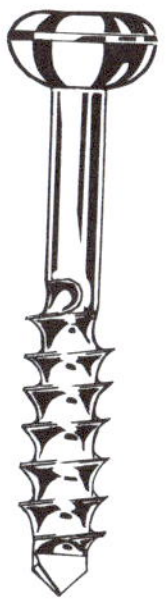

13

Toothed, supporting disks allow the fixing of soft tissue (joint capsule, ligaments) to bone without producing extensive pressure necrosis (see Fig. 230 11).

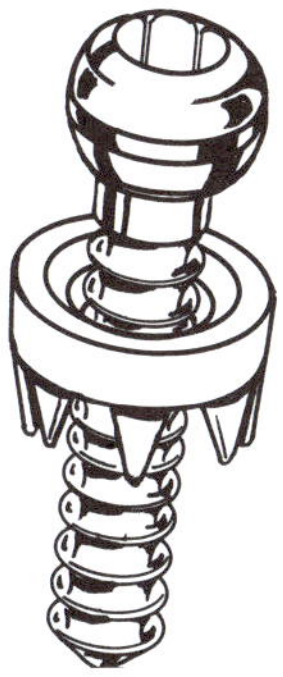

Cortical screw

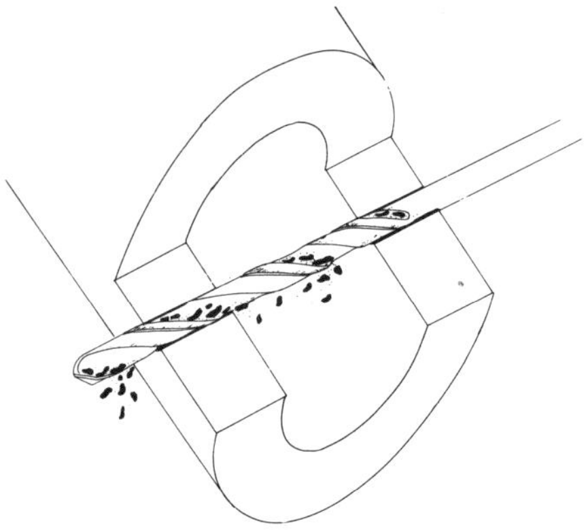

1

Preliminary drilling with a 3.2 mm drill. The cuttings are thrown from the drill holes.

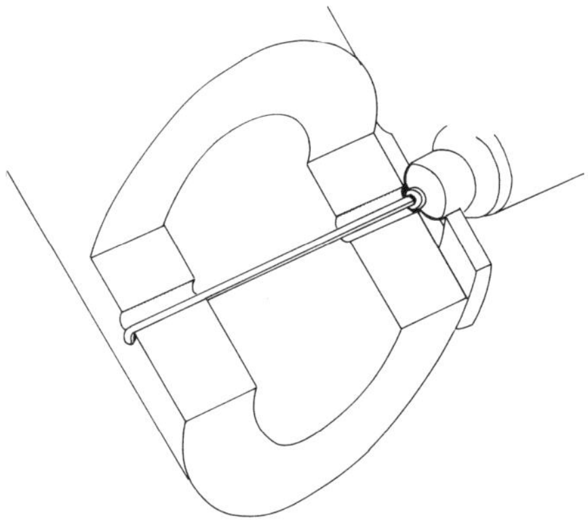

2

Determining the screw length with the screw measuring device.

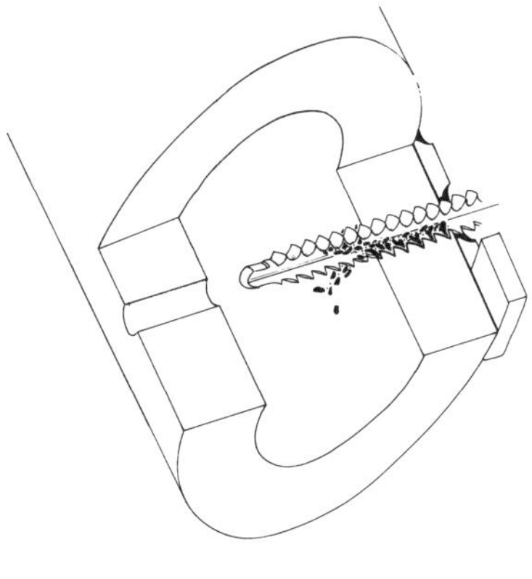

3

Tapping the thread: The cuttings milled from the turns of the thread fall into the longitudinal groove of the tap and then normally are thrown out of the hole. Increased difficulty in turning the tap can be caused by the cuttings getting stuck. This can lead to destruction of the bony thread. A reverse of the tool of 180° will remove the jammed material.

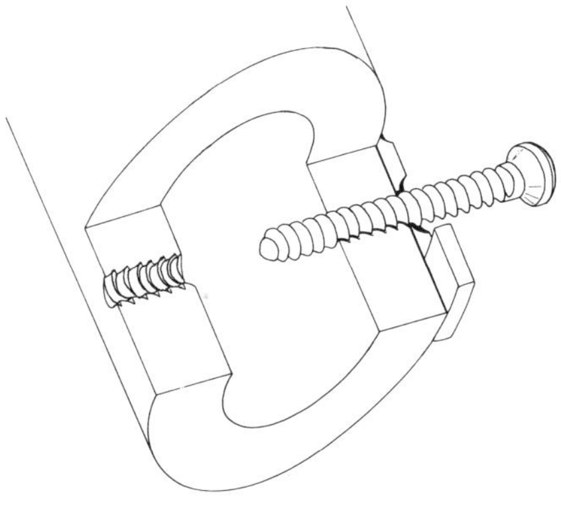

4

The screw can now be easily and accurately introduced into the prepared bony thread.

Cancellous Bone Screw

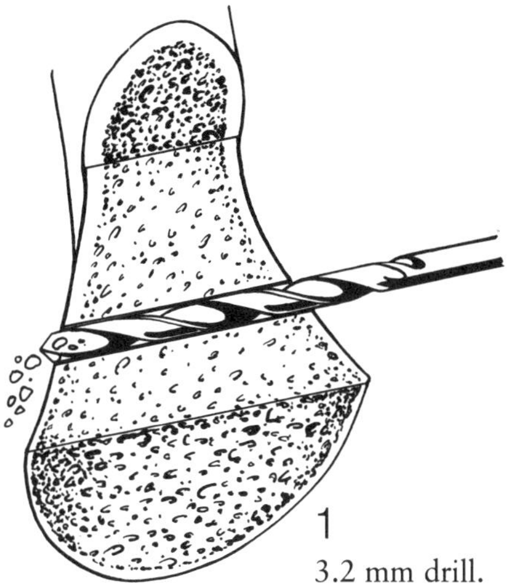

1
3.2 mm drill.

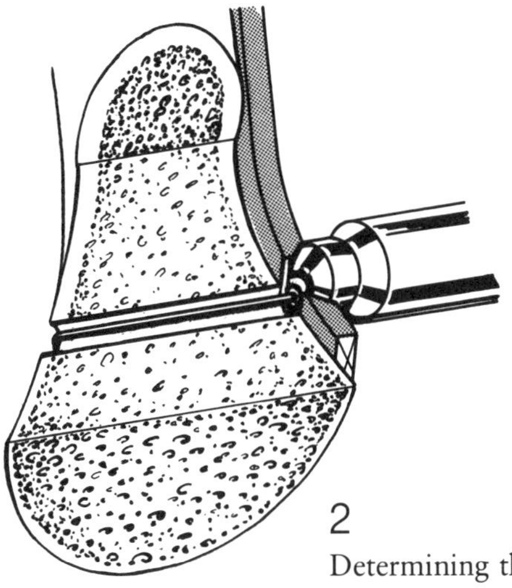

2
Determining the screw length.

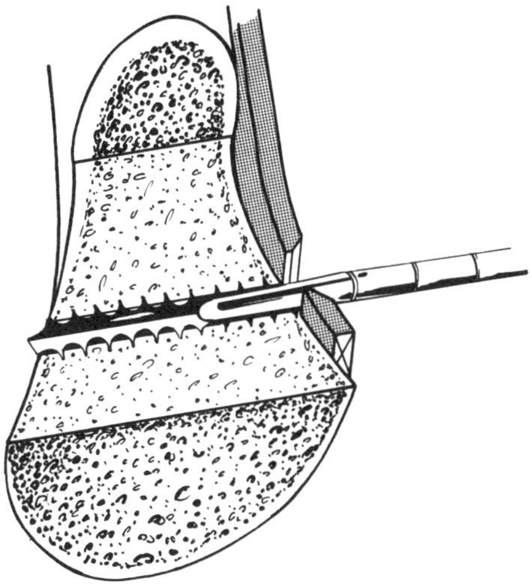

3
Tap for cancellous bone (with scale for checking the predetermined screw length).

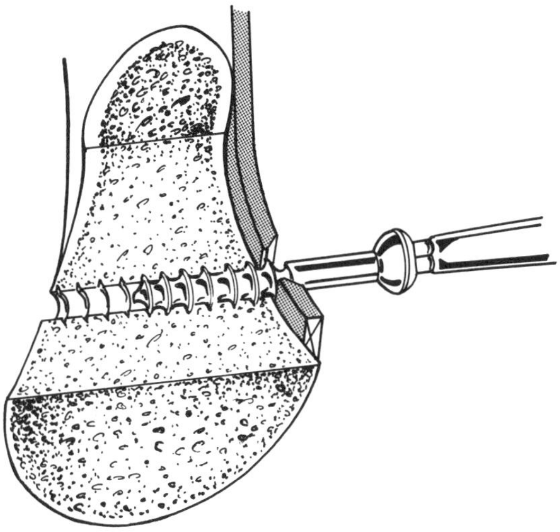

4
Screw (about ½ thread track) projects 1–2 mm, see Fig. 20–7.

Traction screws

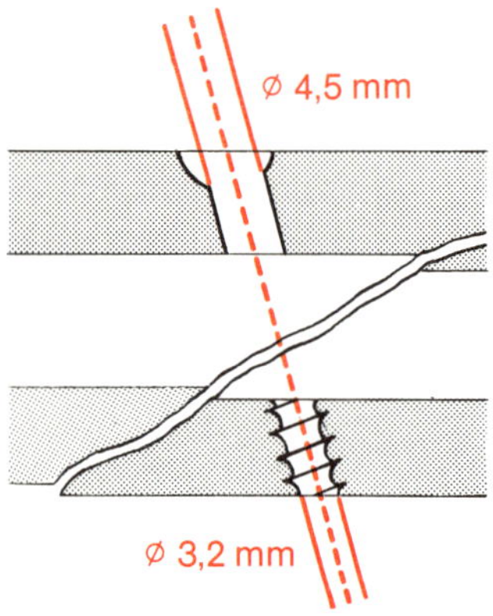

1
The corresponding application...

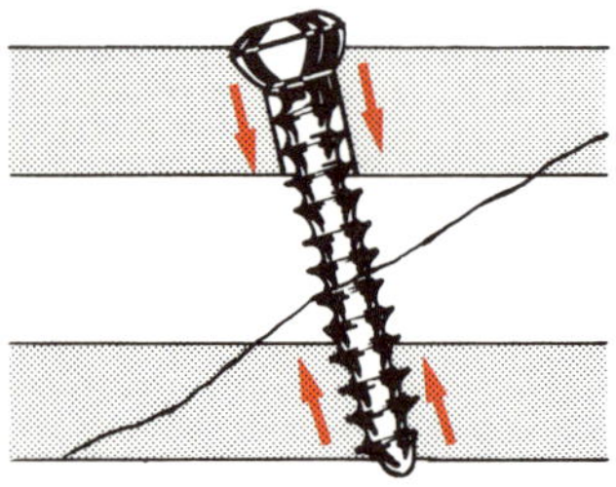

2
... turns the normal *cortical screw* into a *traction screw*.

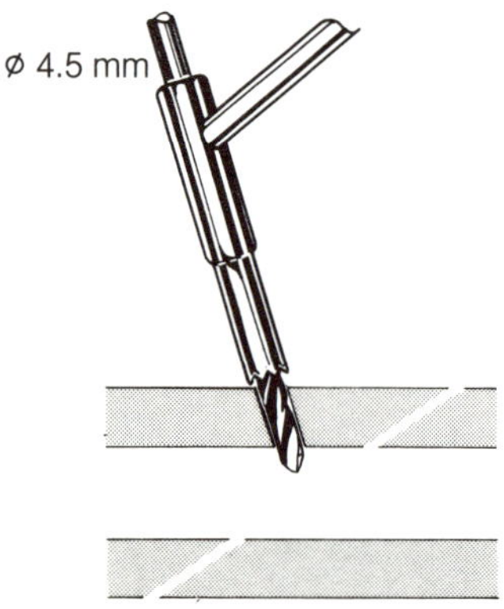

3
Start with the 4.5 mm drill.

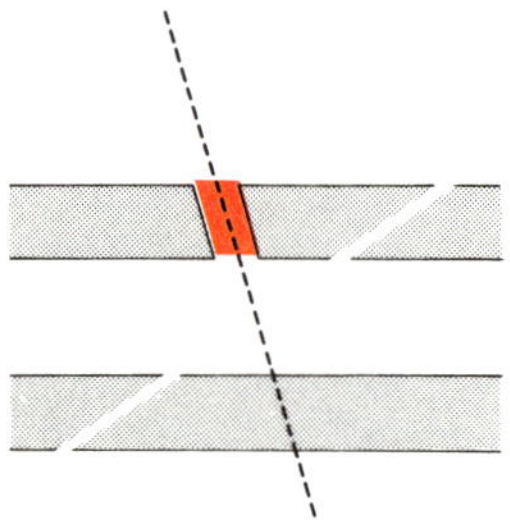

4
The drilling cylinder ensures the correct centering of the drill hole in the opposite cortex so that the screw cannot get stuck.

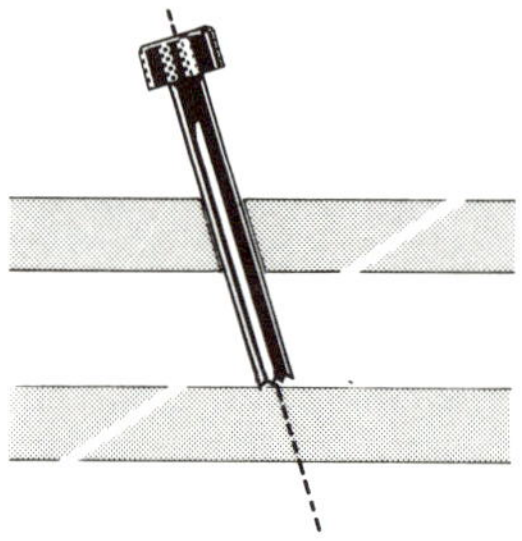

5
Only one cortical bone is perforated.

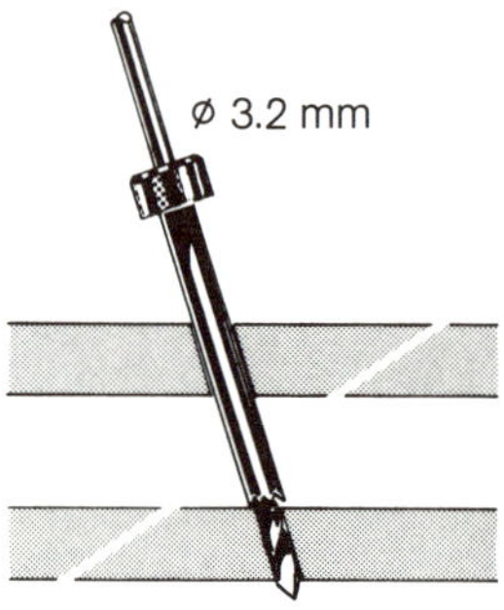

6
Use of the 3.2 mm drill.

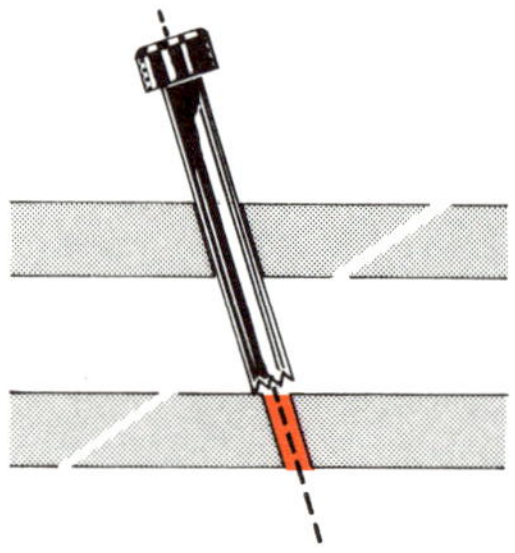

7
Drilling cylinder is removed.

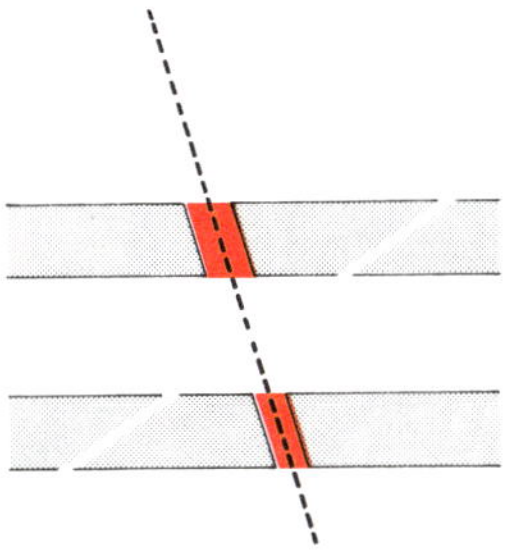

8
There are now two concentric drill holes in the two cortical bones. The diameter of the first is greater than that of the screw thread so that the screw slides through smoothly.

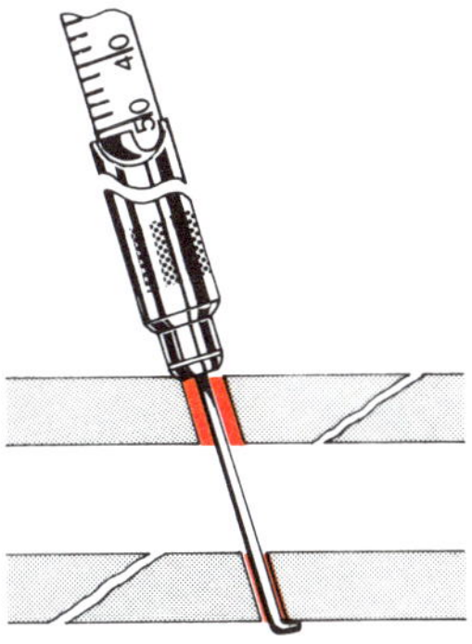

9
Measure the screw length prior to cutting the thread so as to prevent the tool from damaging a thread that may have already been cut in the bone.

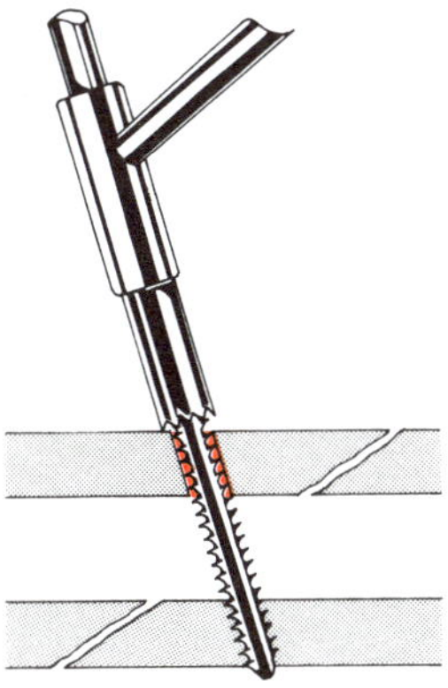

10
Cutting the thread.

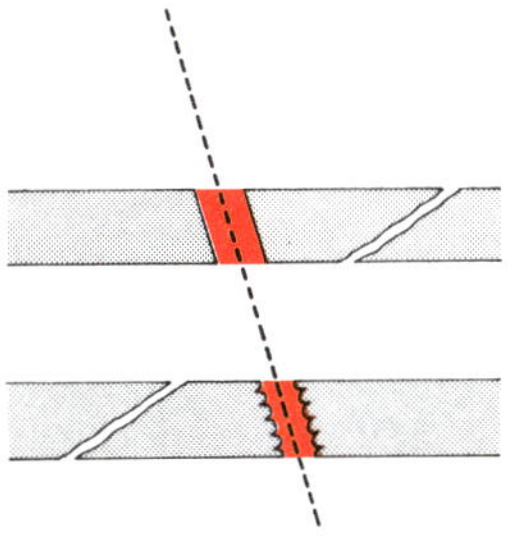

11
A thread has been made only in the second drill hole; only there can the screw get some purchase.

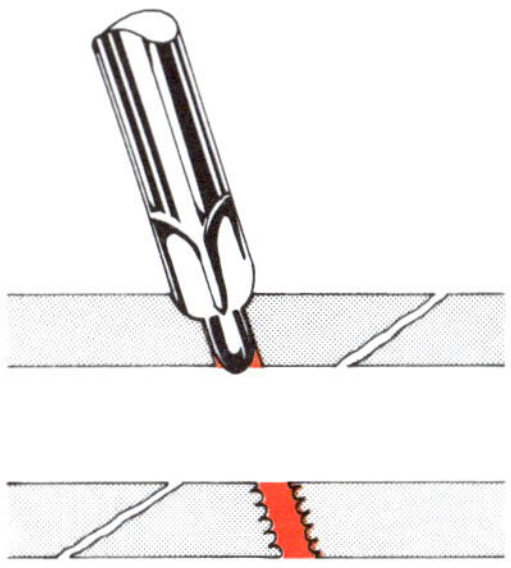

12
With the use of a cap cutter, a broader contact surface for the screw head in the bone is obtained.

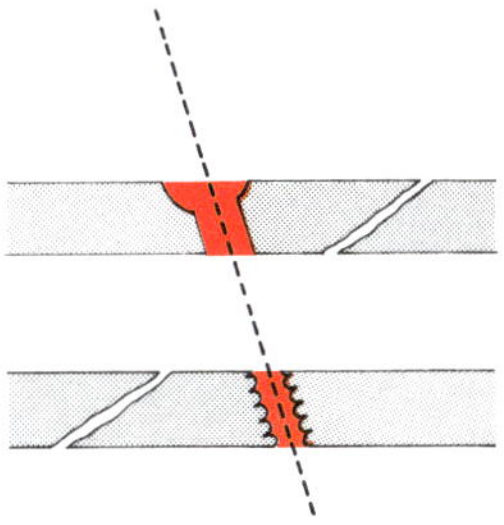

13
In this way, the screw does not get support only on the edge of the drill hole. Beware of cutting too deeply lest the cortex become too thin and break on tightening the screw.

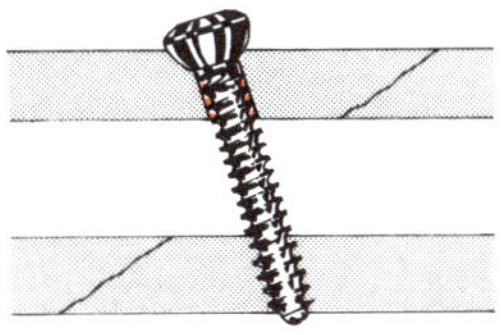

14
On tightening the screw, the two fragments are pressed together.

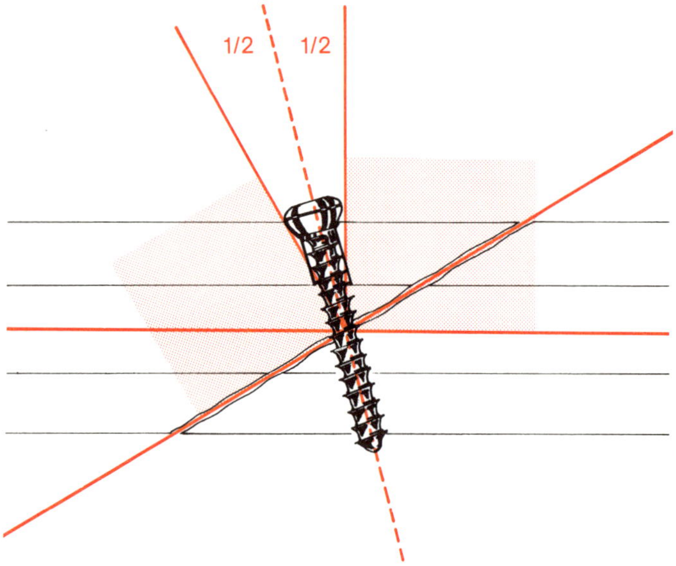

15

The direction of the traction screw is the bisector of the angle between the fracture and the perpendicular on the axis of the shaft.

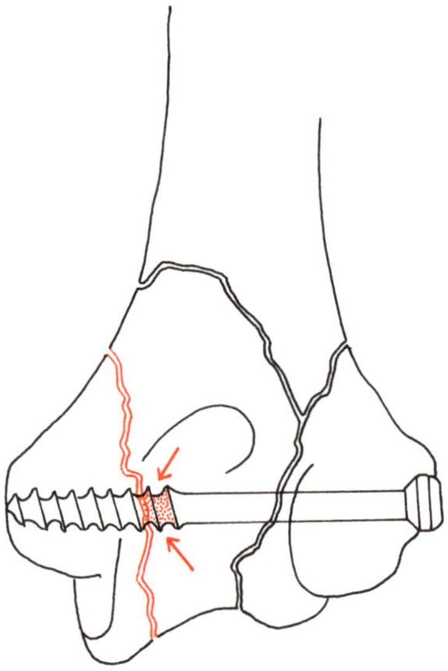

16

Cancellous screw used as traction screw:
When a traction screw with a long thread is used, the fracture site is not completely traversed by the thread and a blocking effect comes about (See Fig. 257–12).

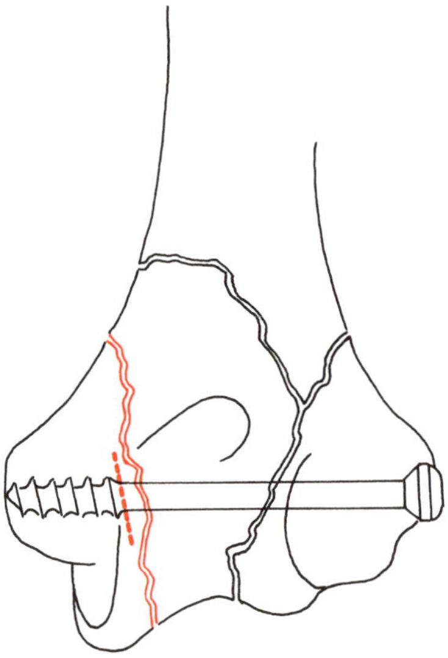

17

Cancellous screw used as traction screw:
When a cancellous screw with a short thread for the same fracture is used, the screw traverses the entire fracture site and produces pressure between the two fragments.

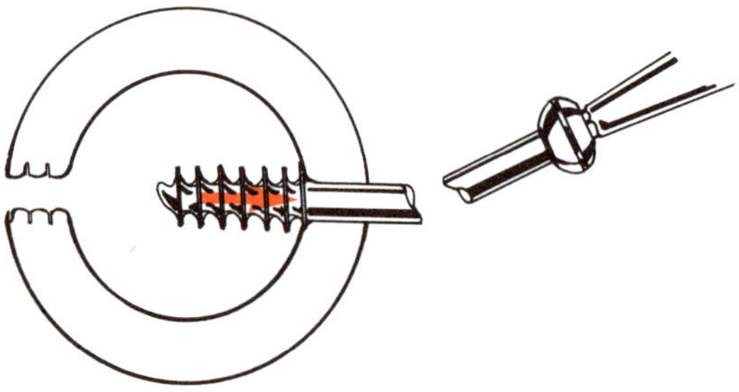

18

The use of malleolar, cancellous or navicular screws in areas with solid cortical bone is risky; the thread cut into the cortex for the screw closes up again around the smooth body of the screw. On removing the screw, the screw thread can no longer return through the cortex; it strips or breaks.

19

A cortical screw used as a traction screw can also be applied without difficulty through a plate, provided it is possible to place a neutralizing plate. Here, the traction screw creates the interfragmental pressure and the plate serves only as an internal splint. With a round-hole plate, however, the screw can be inserted only in the vertical direction through the plate hole. The bisector of the angle between the level of the fracture and the axis of the bone shaft (See Fig. 24–15) can therefore hardly be met.

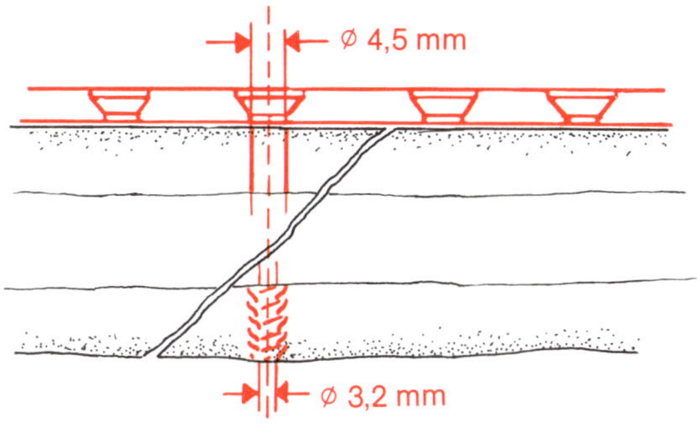

20

By contrast, in slotted plates, the screw can also be inserted at an angle.

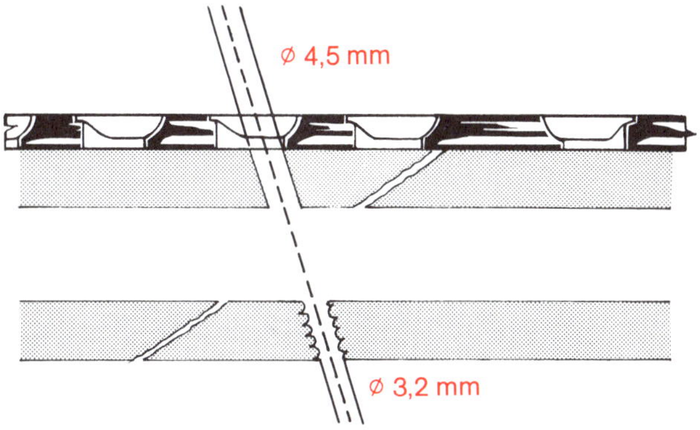

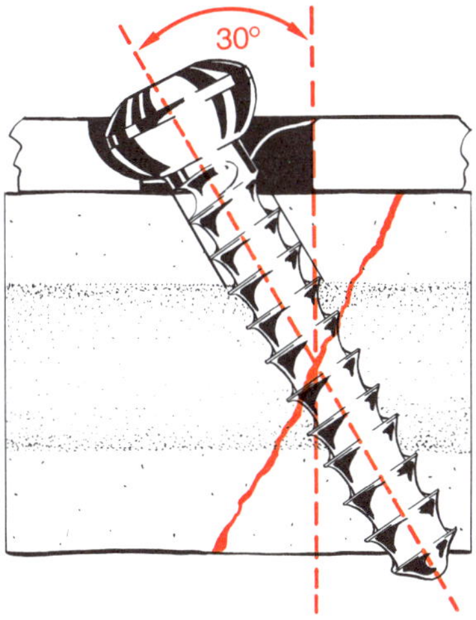

21

The angle of the oblique direction may amount to 30° longitudinally (not with round-hole plates!).

22

The rounded head of the screw, even in an oblique position, adapts itself smoothly and without pressure from the edges to the adequately shaped hole in the plate.

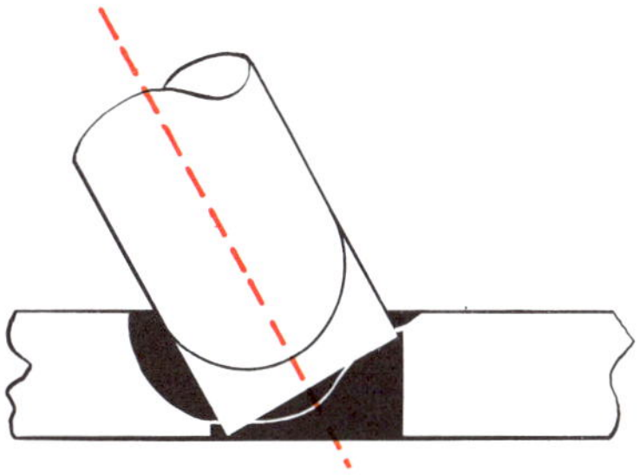

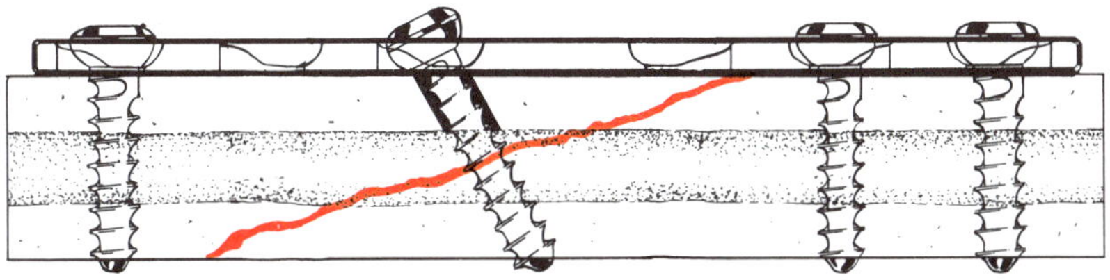

23

With a long-hole plate, the screw can also be inserted according to the rule stated in Fig. 24–15.

Broken screw

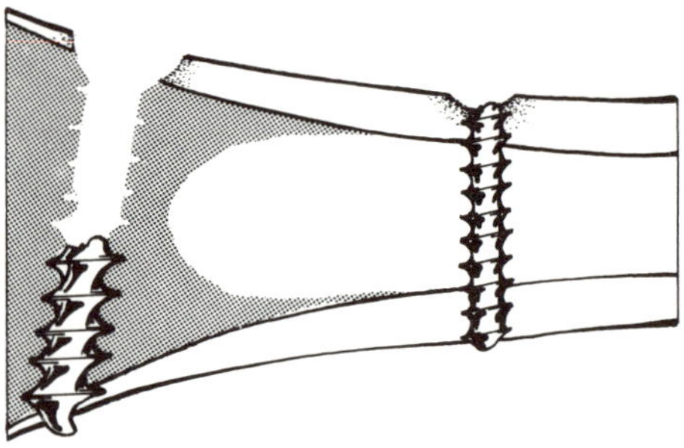

1
Broken screws inside and near the surface.

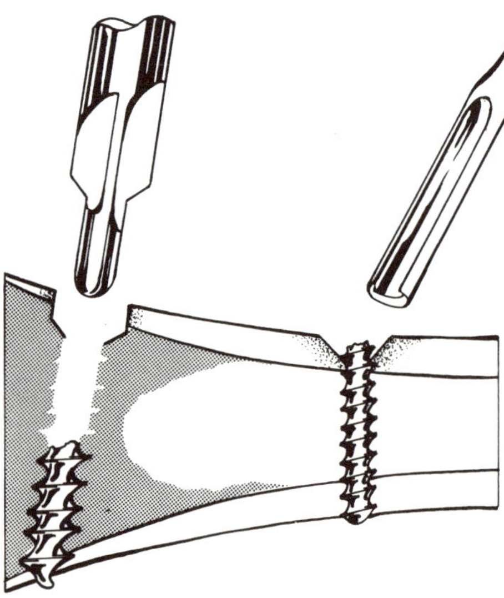

2
The tracks of the broken screws are exposed with use of a small gouge or a grooved cutter.

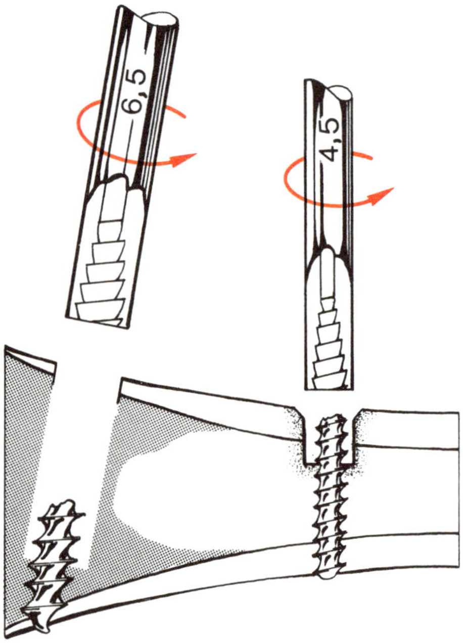

3
A centering bolt in the grooved cutter guides the instrument along the correct axis to the screw fragment.

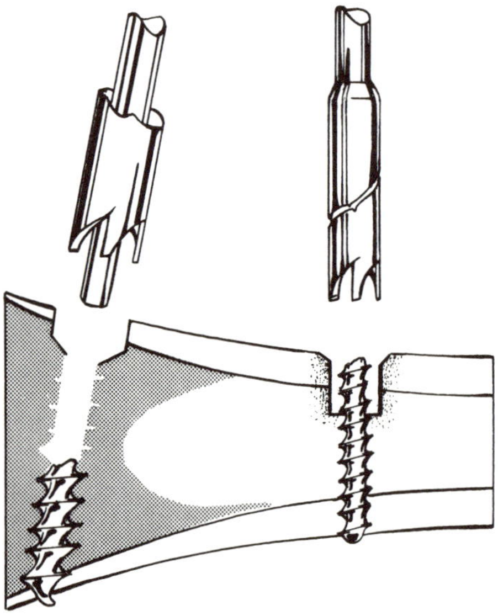

4
For the various screw diameters extractors are available measuring 3.5, 4.5 and 6.5 mm in diameter.

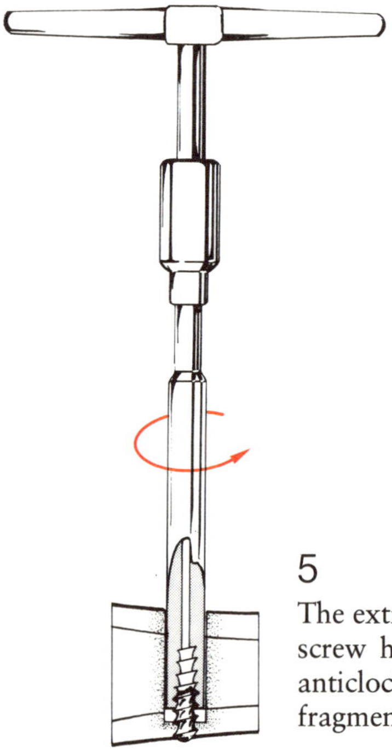

5
The extractor is pressed onto the screw head and a simultaneous anticlockwise rotation brings the fragment out.

Plates

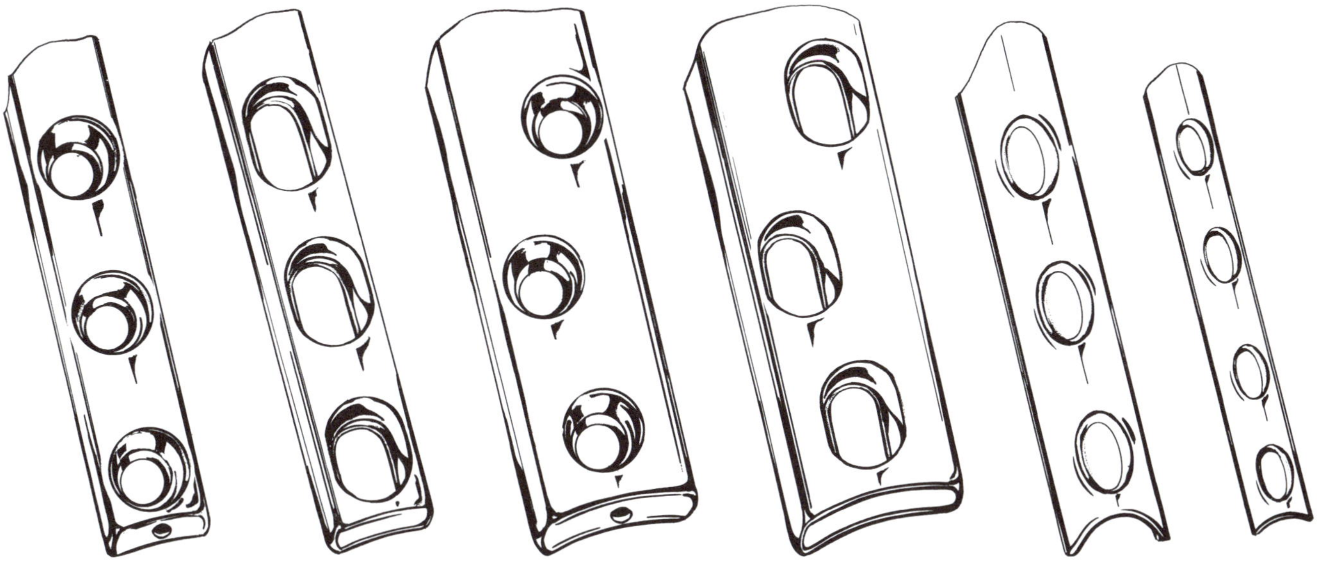

1

Narrow plates are used principally in the forearm and the lower leg. *Broad plates* are applied exclusively to the humerus, exceptionally also to the femur, although angular plates are preferable here when intramedullary nailing is not feasible.

Half-tubular plates are used in special instances for the forearm, as well as in all those situations where a narrow plate would occupy too much space. The half-tubular plate is weak; therefore, it should be used exclusively for the adaptive fixation of bone fragments and never as a neutralizing plate.

One-third tubular plates are applied principally to the external malleolus.

2

The first screw used to fasten the plate must be inserted *in the vicinity of the fracture.*

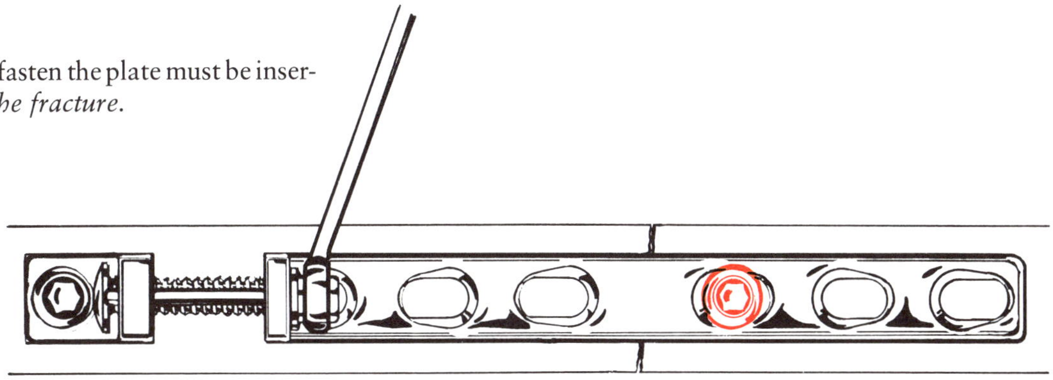

3

If this rule is disregarded, the fragments will deviate laterally on initial tightening of the plate (or as shown in Fig. 28–5), without producing substantial interfragmental pressure.

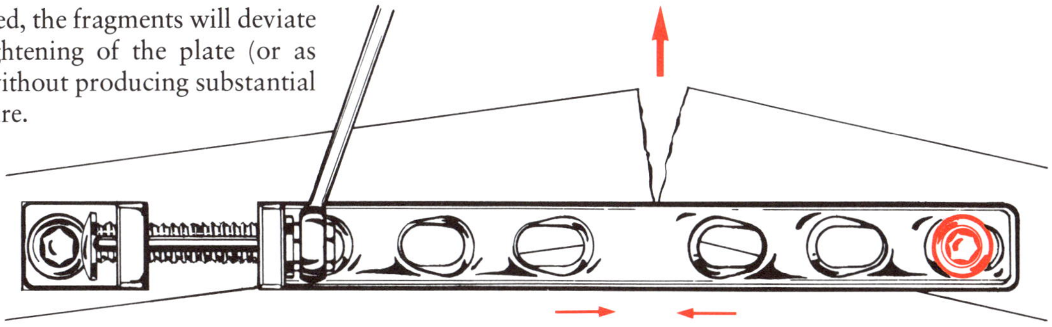

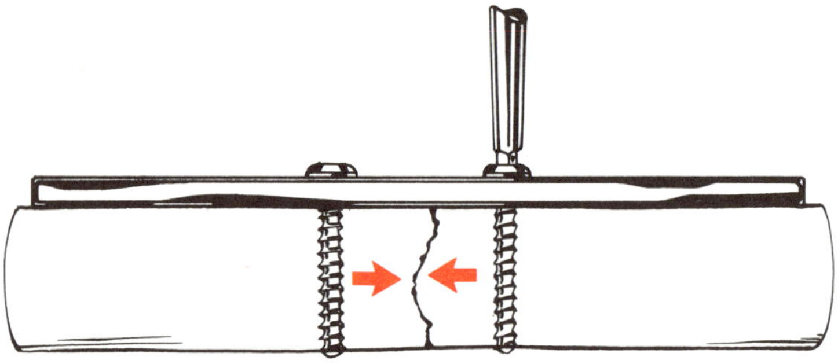

4

Also with use of a slotted plate, the tensing screws must be inserted first in the vicinity of the fracture.

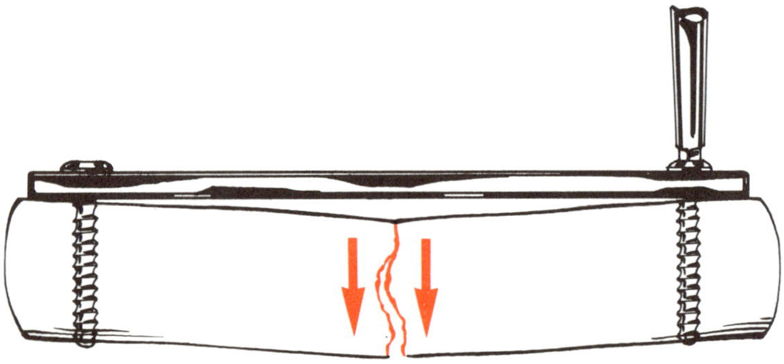

5

Tensing the plate with screws inserted *near its ends* tends to cause the fragments to deviate. This phenomenon can, however, also be utilized in a positive way, namely, to develop increasing interfragmental compression by proceeding as shown in Fig. 28–8 and 28–9.

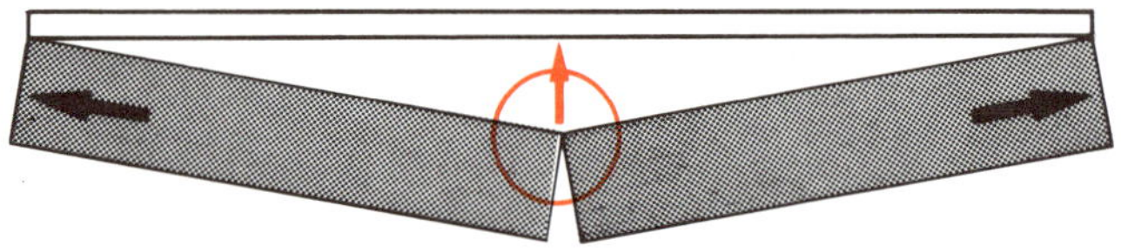

6

By placing a plate upon a broken, concavely-curved bony surface and, with a screw, drawing the most inferior point in the fractured area in the direction of the plate...

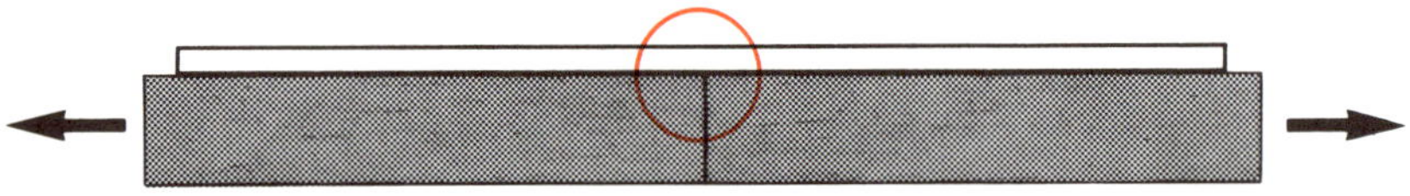

7

... the bone becomes displaced beyond the ends of the plate. The fragments are joined together at the fracture site without any pressure.

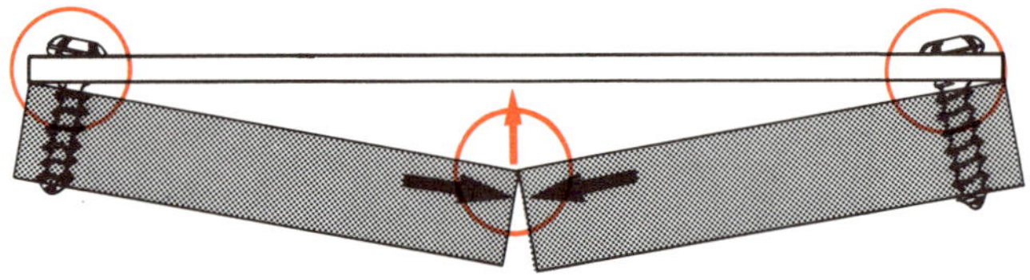

8

When, however, the bone is prevented from deviating by inserting screws into the ends of the plate, and...

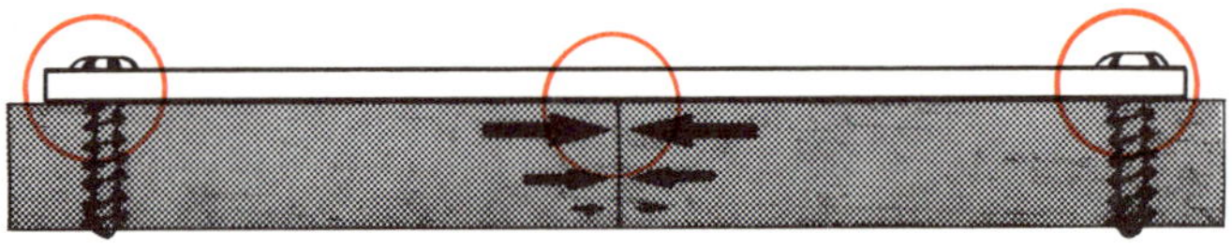

9

... the middle screw is tightened, pressure is bound to originate in the fractured area.

10

An important point in compression plate fixation is to bend the plate concavely before applying it.

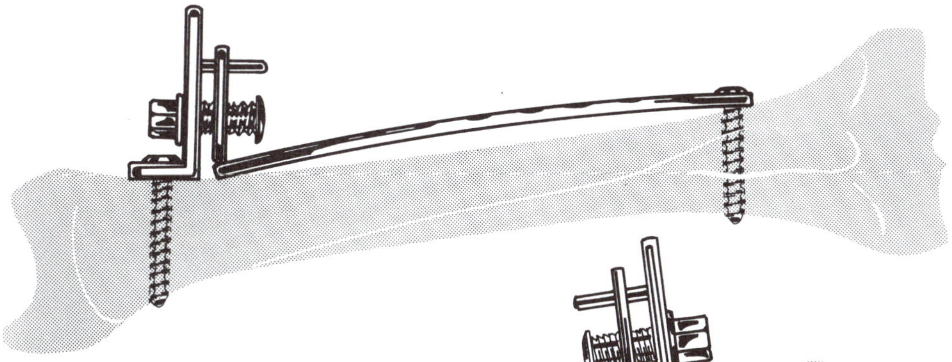

11

In applying, for example, a ten-hole plate to a straight long bone, the following rule of thumb holds good: keep the center of the plate in the fractured area at a distance of about 5 mm.

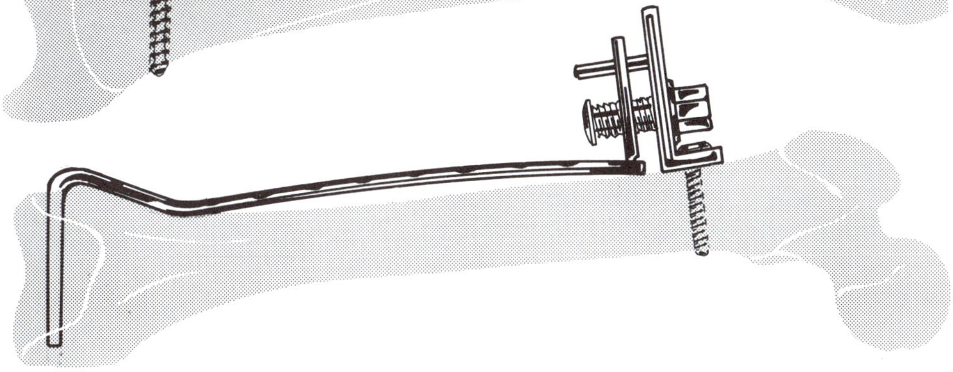

12

When a plate is tensed without first having been concavely bent, the fracture site underneath the plate closes up and great pressure is produced there. At the fracture site opposite the plate no pressure develops and there may even be a tendency for the cleft to gape open.

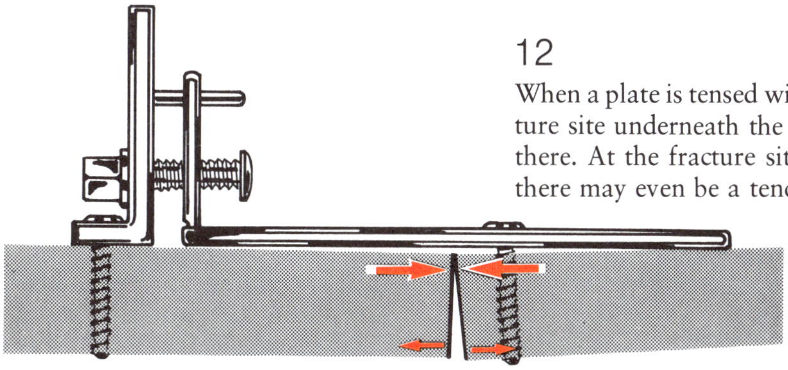

13

On tensing a concavely-bent plate, pressure first develops at the fracture site opposite the plate.

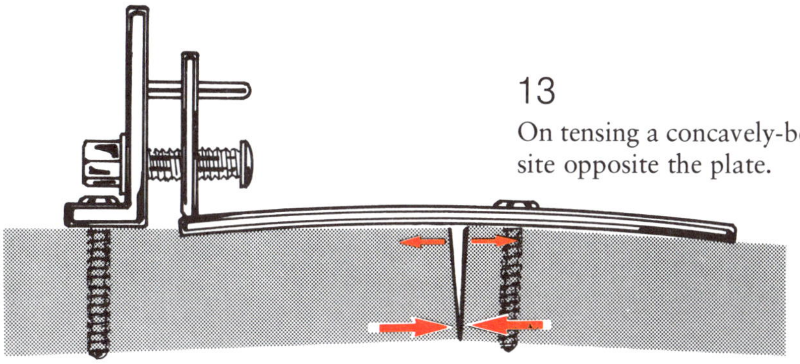

14

On tensing the plate further, pressure gradually develops which is equally divided over the entire surface of the fracture.

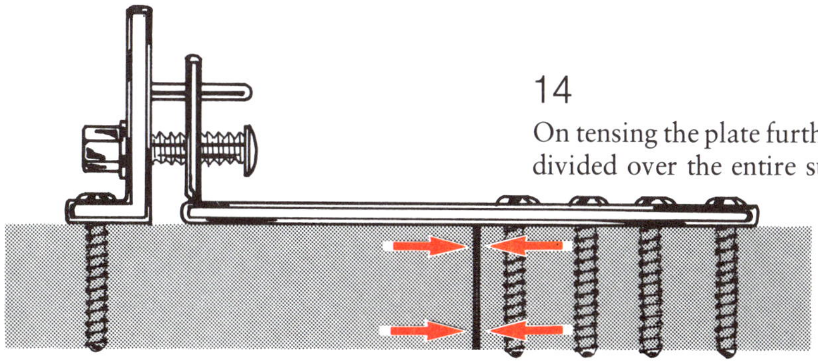

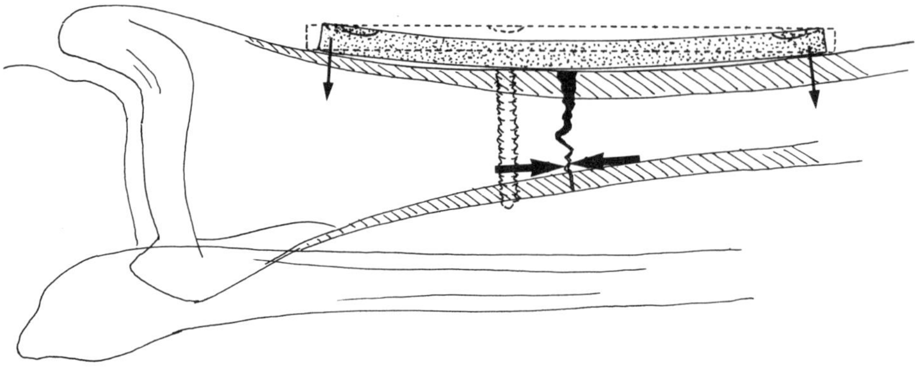

15

With concave bony surfaces, the intrinsic elasticity of the plate can be exploited for the production of an even pressure upon the *entire surface* of the fracture, without bending the plate concavely. On attempting to draw the center of a straight plate onto a concave surface it is shown that the ends of the plate exert pressure on the bone and that the cleft of the fracture closes up on the opposite side but gapes just under the plate.

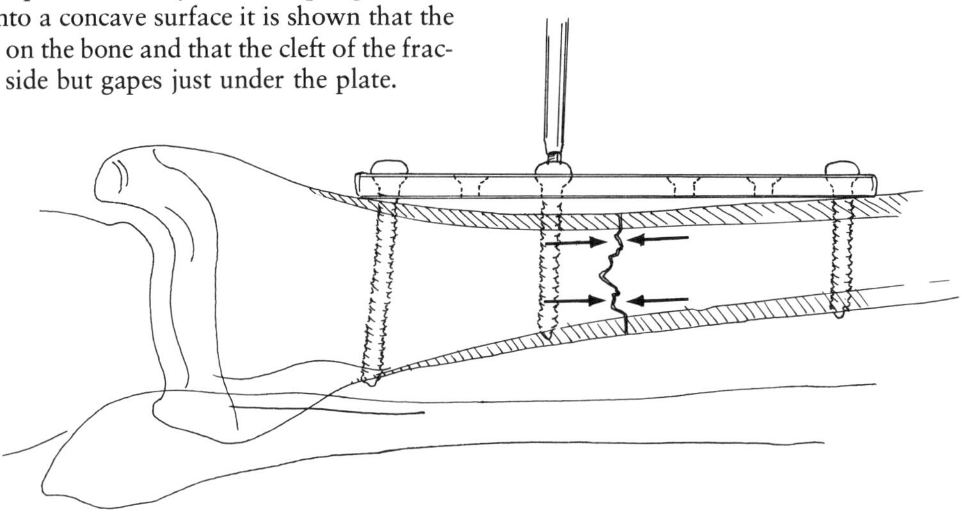

16

By combining these two processes, interfragmental pressure develops in the cleft of the fracture.

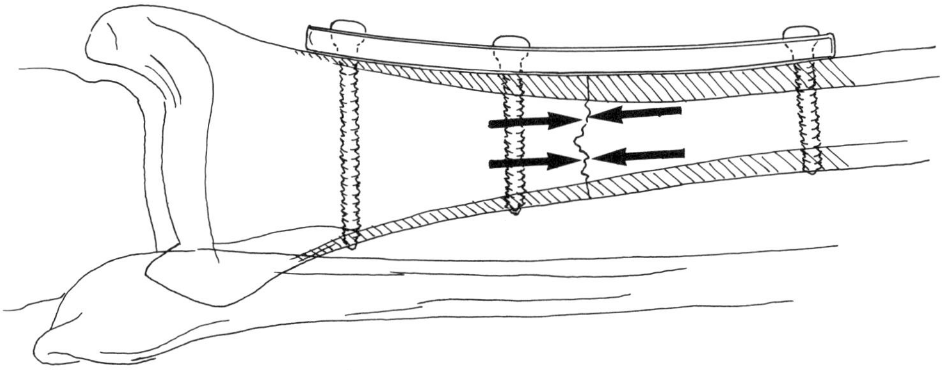

17

Interfragmental pressure develops *in the vicinity nearest the plate* through its apparent shortening. The same pressure develops *at a distance from the plate* through the intrinsic tension of the bending plate via leverage at its ends.

This principle can always be made use of, provided the plates are bent in such a way that their ends are closely applied to the bone while their centers are a few millimeters distant from it. By proceeding in this manner one causes the compression plate to produce pressure that is not confined only to the vicinity nearest the plate.

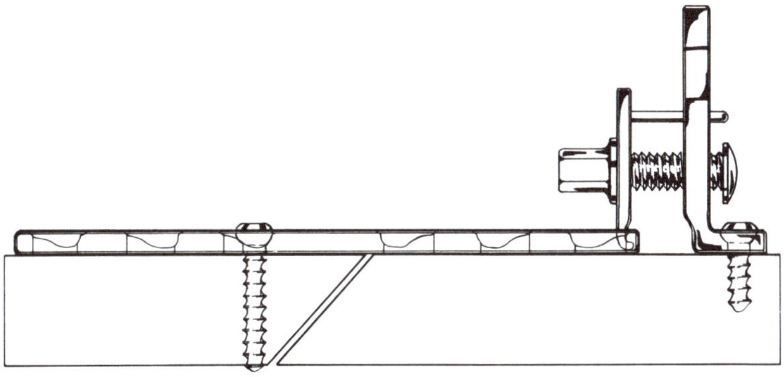

18
Oblique fractures can also be brought under pressure by compression plate fixation. The result, however, depends on which side the plate is applied to. When pressure is exerted by a plate fitted in the manner shown here, the fragments are bound to slip.

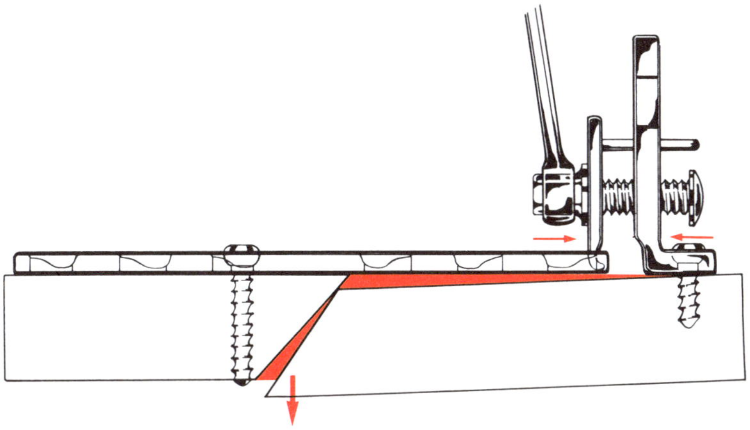

19
Slipping of the fragments with displacement; interfragmental pressure cannot possibly occur.

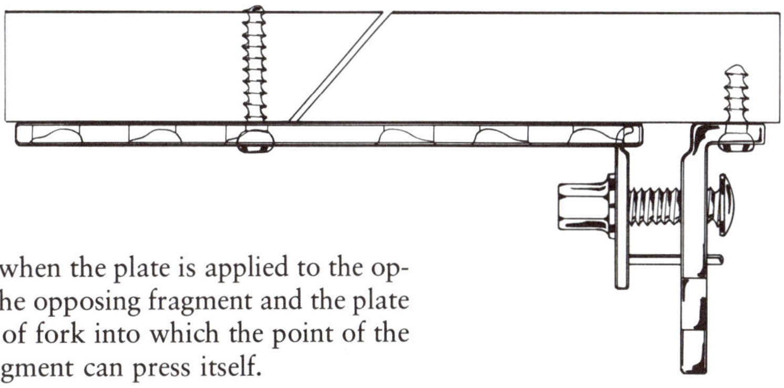

20
Conversely, when the plate is applied to the opposite side, the opposing fragment and the plate form a kind of fork into which the point of the stretched fragment can press itself.

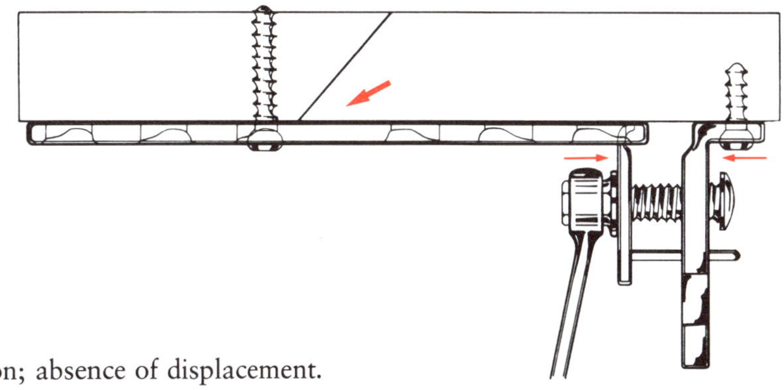

21
Compression; absence of displacement.

Errors in compression plate fixation

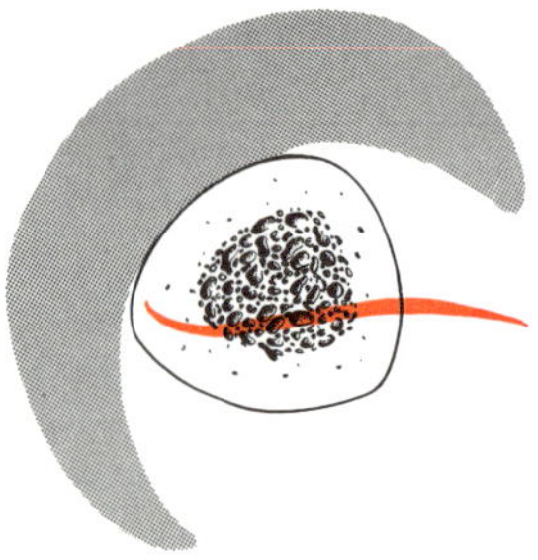

22

Detachment of *soft tissue* amounts to *more than one-half the circumference* of the bone.

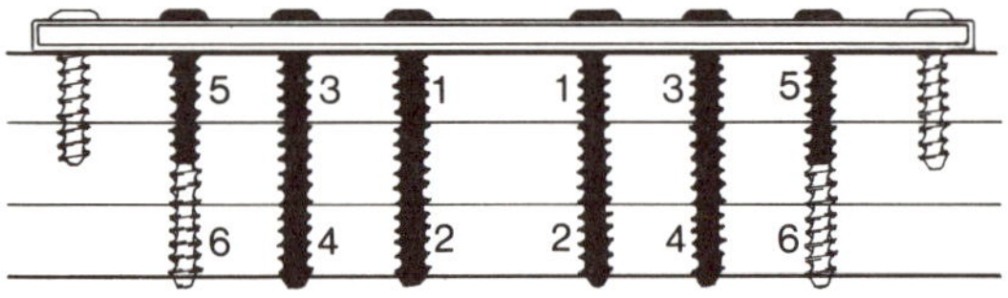

23

Plate is too short: At least 5 to 6 mm of cortex on each side of the fracture should be securely gripped by the screw threads. Since, in tubular bones, the screws at the ends of the plate should pass through one cortex only, this circumstance alone requires a greater length of plate than would be expected initially.

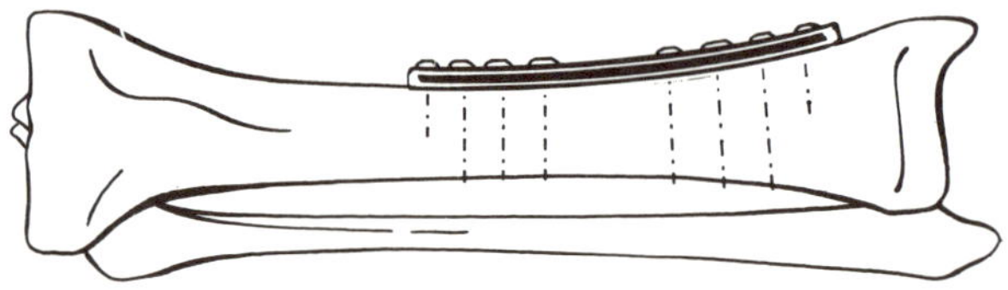

24

Plate is too massive and therefore occupies too much space (See Anterior Tibial Syndrome, Figs. 281–1 ff.); disorders of circulation result. Therefore, broad plates should not be applied to the tibia, for example.

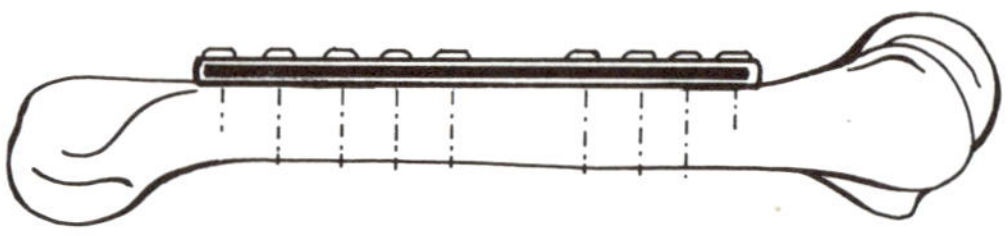

25

Plate is too weak. The humerus can, and should, be stabilized by a broad plate. Here, no disorders of circulation through lack of space are to be feared.

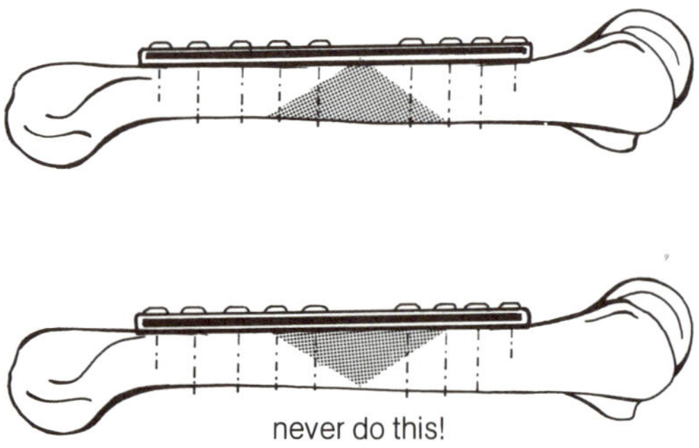

26

The plate destroys too much bone. It must never be placed over the base of a bending wedge, a point to consider when choosing the mode of approach. A possible consequence is undue prolongation of the healing process and danger of fracture of the plate by fatigue.

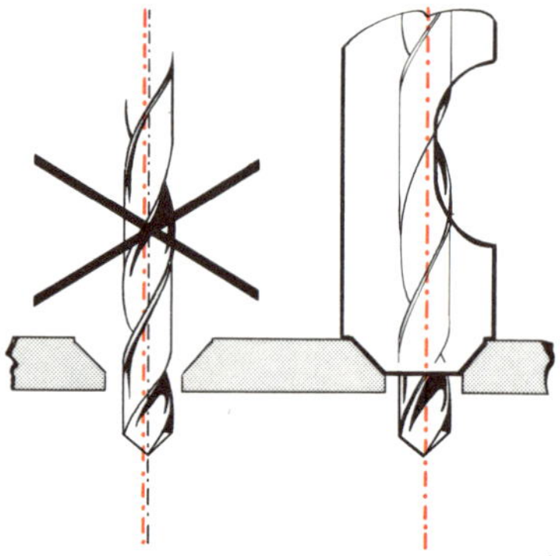

27

Compression plate fixation should never be undertaken by tensing the plate or by employing traction screws. The compression obtained initially can also be nullified by not using a correct, centering drill guide or by applying the plate to the concave side of the bone.

Half-tubular plate

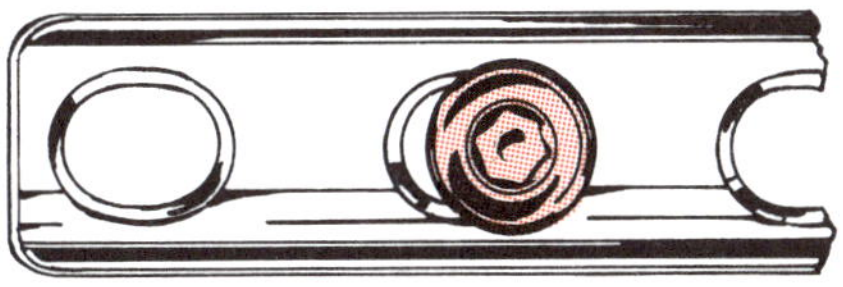

1

In the half-tubular plate, the holes are oval (not to be confused with slots). This kind of plate can, like the slotted plate, be tensed within certain limits solely by placing the screws eccentrically.

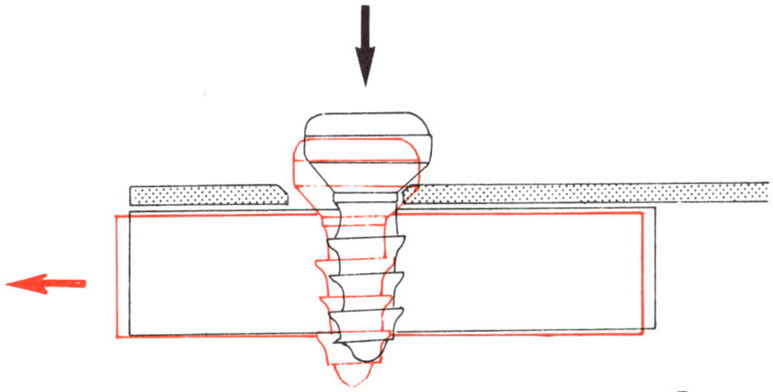

2

If one thinks of the plate as being fixed, the eccentrically-placed screw will, on sinking its head into the screw hole, be forced to migrate toward the center of the hole, taking with it the attached fragment.

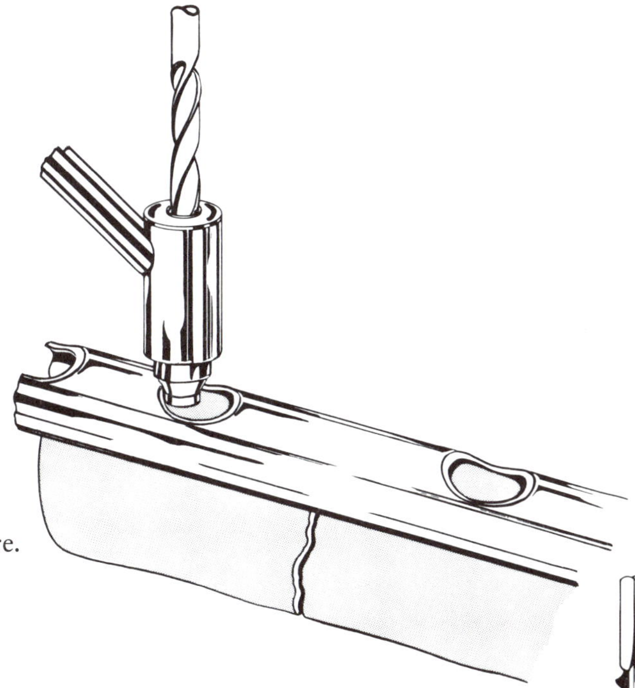

3

The first hole is drilled nearest the fracture.

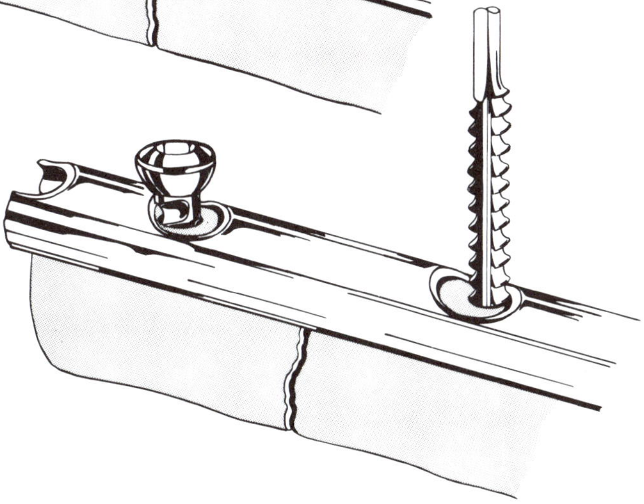

4

The head of the first screw should be sunk into the hole in the plate only *after* the second screw has been fitted. The second screw is also inserted into a hole near the fracture. *Within the plate holes, the screw holes are placed away from the fracture.* To do this, the cleft of the fracture must already have been narrowed as far as possible with the use of hooks or repositioning forceps.

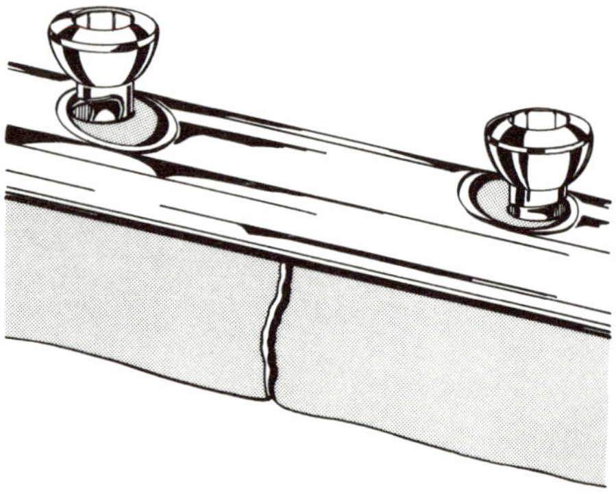

5

Both screws near the fracture have been fitted; their heads, however, have not yet been sunk into the plate hole. The cleft of the fracture still gapes slightly.

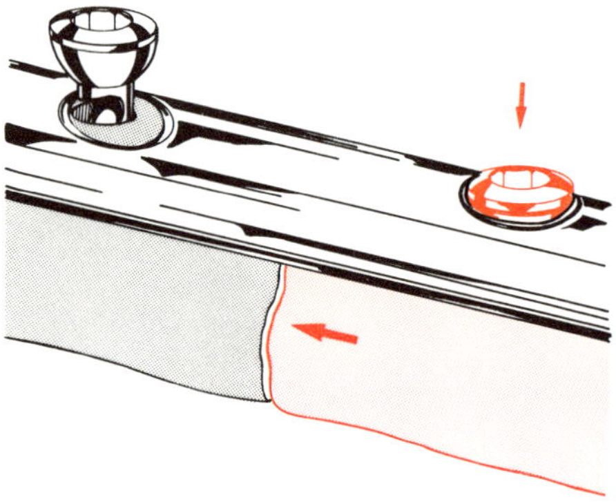

6

As the first screw head is sunk, it is pushed through the edge of the plate hole in the direction of the fracture cleft, taking the fragment with it. The other screw prevents the fragment from moving aside, and the fracture cleft thus closes up.

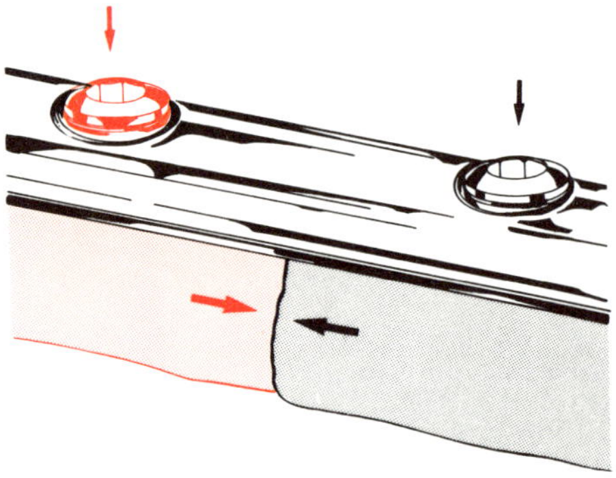

7

When the other screw head is sunk, the process is reversed and pressure develops in the fracture cleft.
The half-tubular plate can be readily tensed with the plate tightener.

Round-hole plate

1

The first screw is inserted near the fracture. This can be done prior to the definitive reduction.

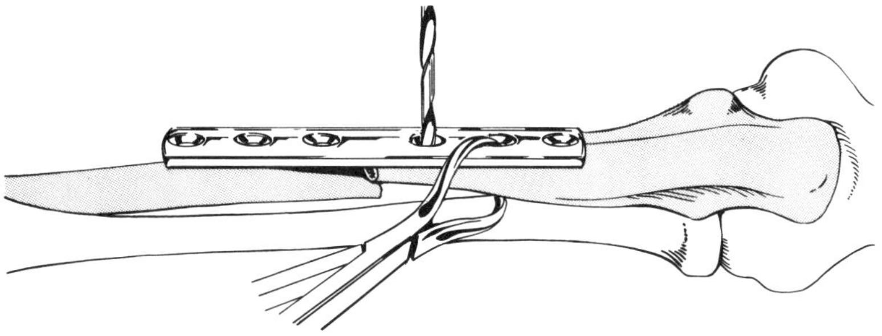

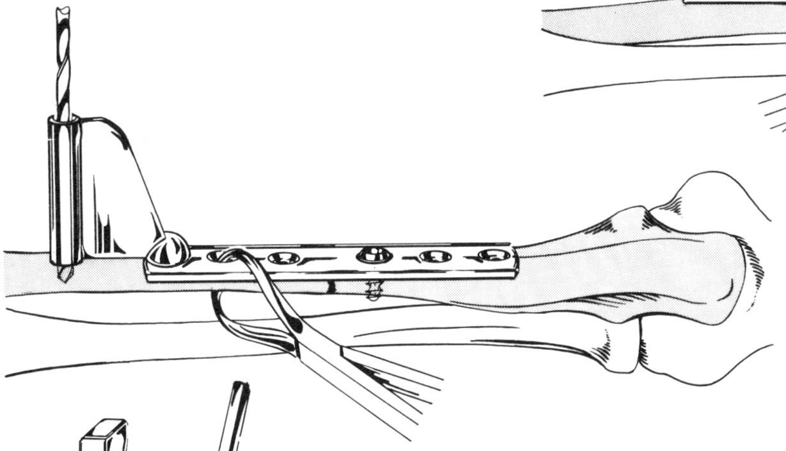

2

After reduction, the drill hole for the plate tightener is made at an appropriate distance, using the correct drill guide.

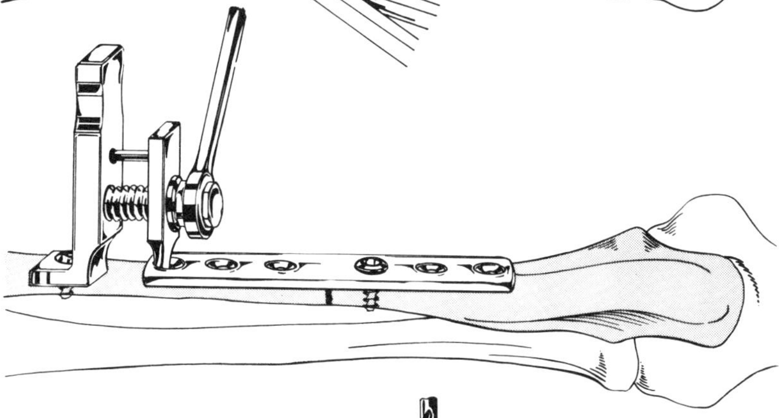

3

Initial slight compression allows proper alignment of the fragments (See also Fig. 27–2).

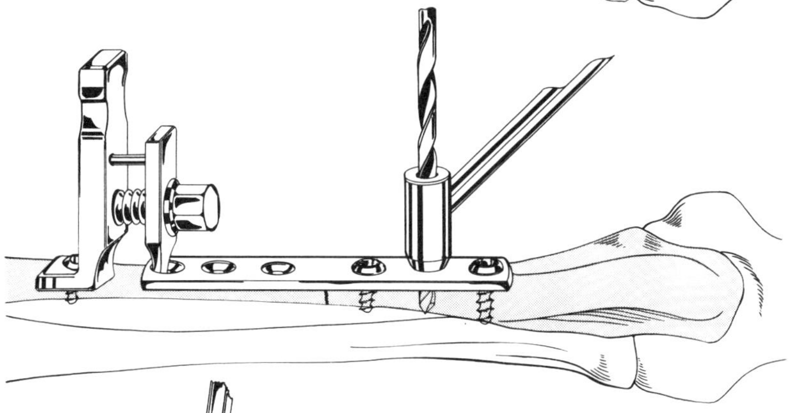

4

The remaining screws are fitted into the fragment opposite the plate tightener.

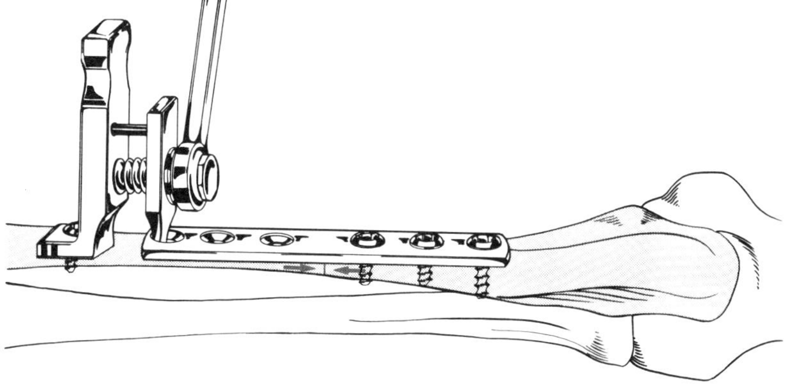

5

Definitive compression. Whenever possible, a ring spanner should be used to spare the hexagonal nuts of the instruments.

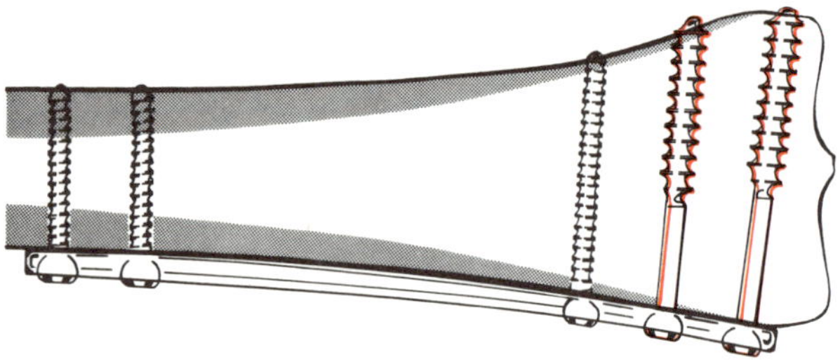

6

Since one end of the plate frequently rests on an area where the cortex is extremely thin and cancellous bone is prevalent, the two holes *near the ends* of each plate permit the insertion of cancellous screws.

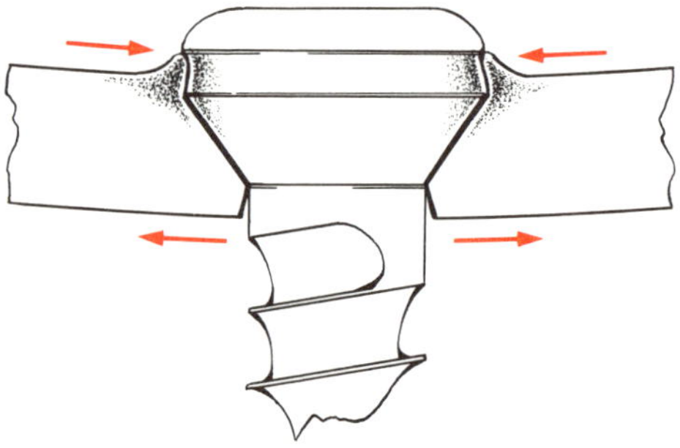

7

Even *minor* bending of the plate in the region of the screw holes makes it impossible for cancellous screws to pass through. Plates should always be bent *between* the screws.

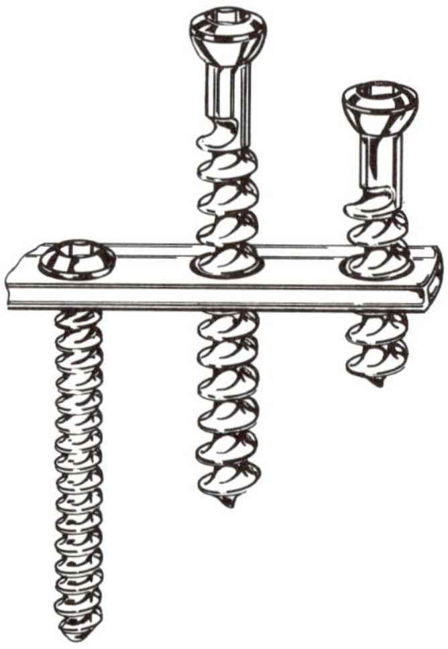

8

Cancellous screws cannot, like cortical screws, be put through the hole in the plate, but have to be screwed in.

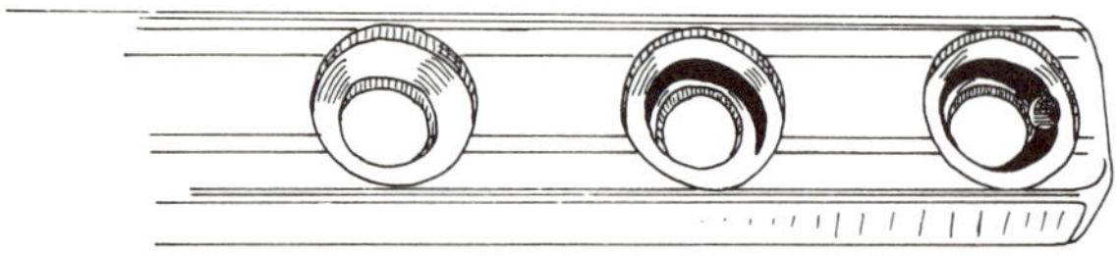

9

The screws are guided through the corresponding holes by a cut-out thread. At each end of the plate there is a hole or notch to which the plate tightener can be attached.

Slotted plate

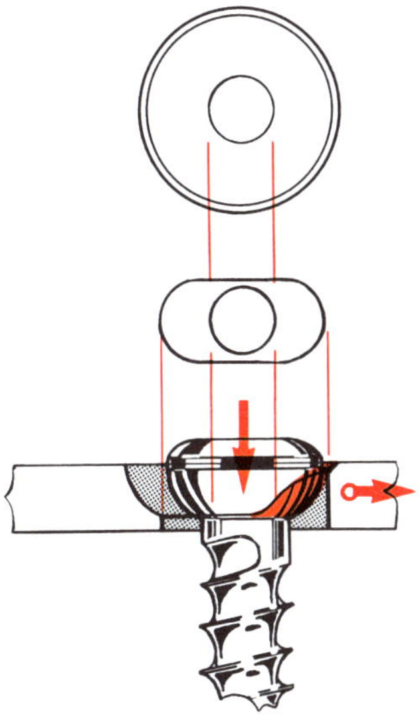

1

Sinking of the screw head forces the plate to become displaced longitudinally. Lateral displacement is impossible.

Moreover, manifestations of bone resorption at the fracture site do not impede further longitudinal displacement: the fragments can move closer together and no blocking effect ensues.

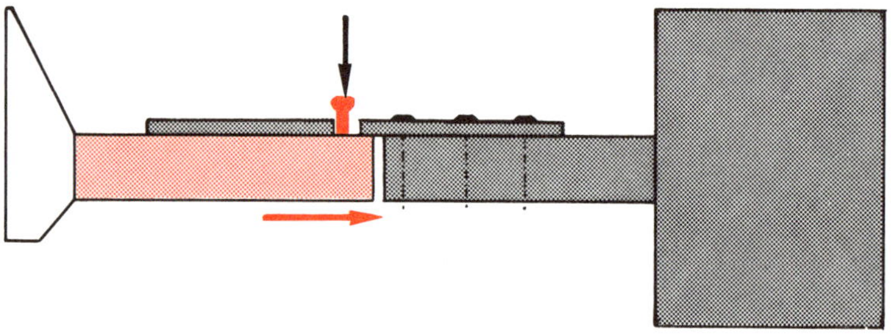

2
The plate is fixed to the "immovable" fragment and the screws to the "movable" one.

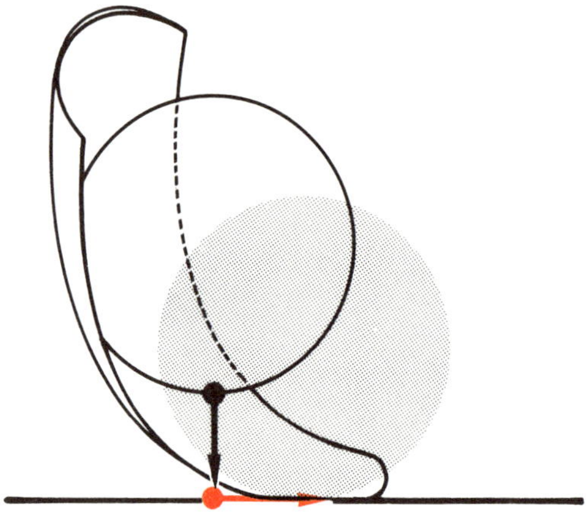

3
The slide way is fixed and the ball, in sliding down, is forced to change its course.

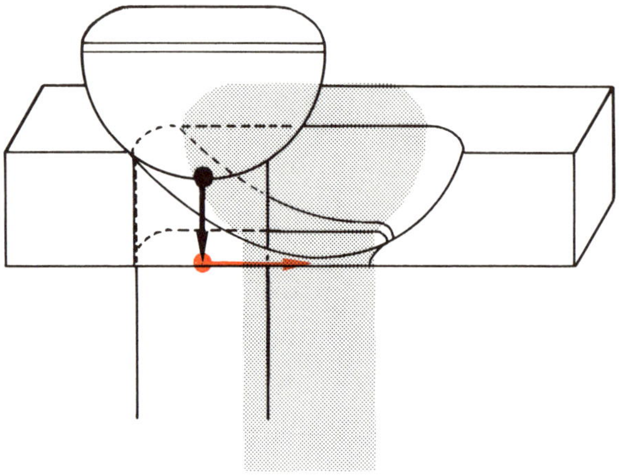

4
The plate is "fixed" and the screw, on being inserted into the hole in the plate, moves along the slide way in the direction of the arrow, taking "its" fragment with it.

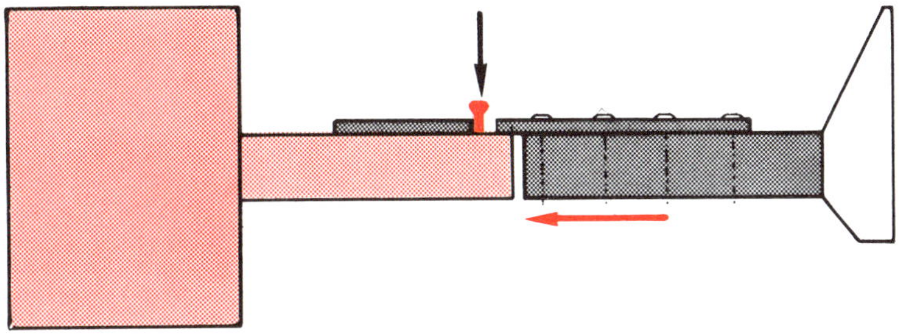

5
The plate is fixed to the "movable" fragment, and the screw to the "immovable" one.

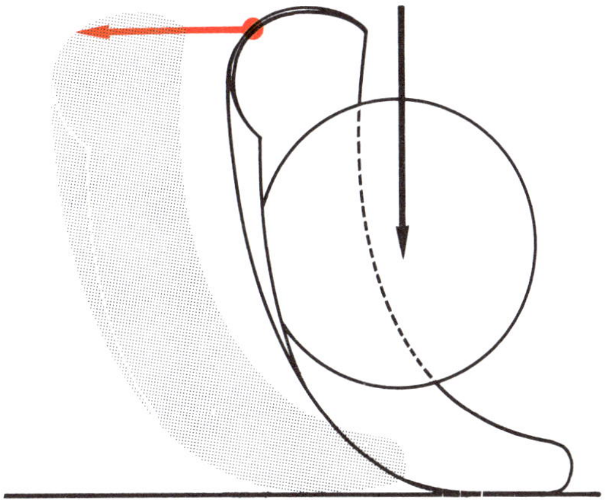

6
The ball, in sliding down, keeps to its direction and the slide way is thereby forced to deviate.

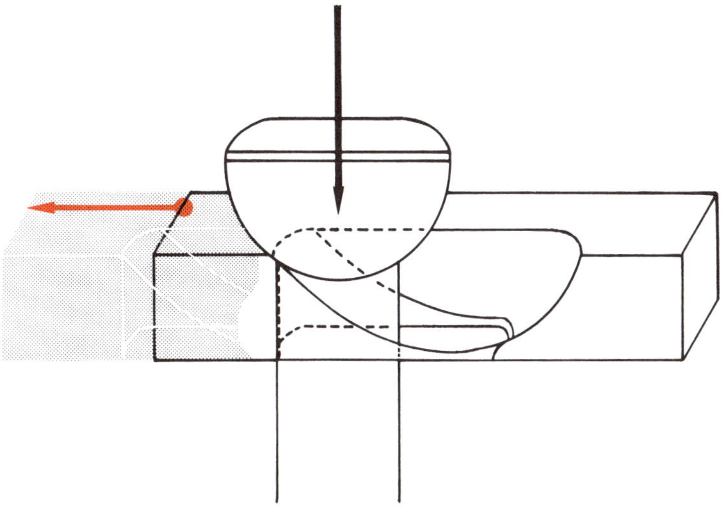

7
The plate is free to move with "its" fragment, whereas the screw is "fixed".

For drill guides marked with an arrow, one should remember:
the arrow points toward the fracture.

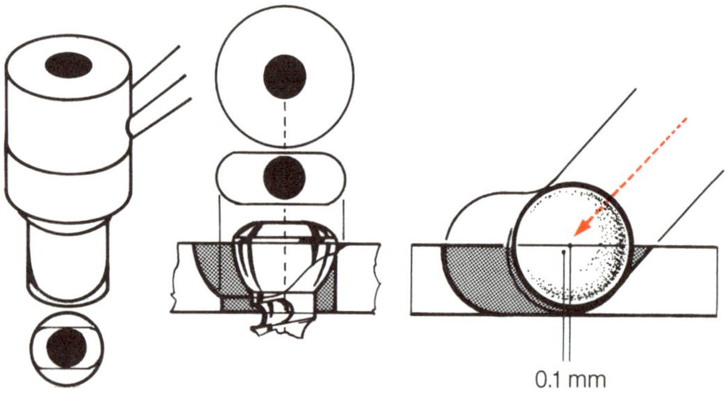

8
With use of a central drill guide, the shape of the holes in the plate inevitably leads to a thrust of 0.1 mm. Thus (contrary to the round-hole plate), no blocking effect can develop.

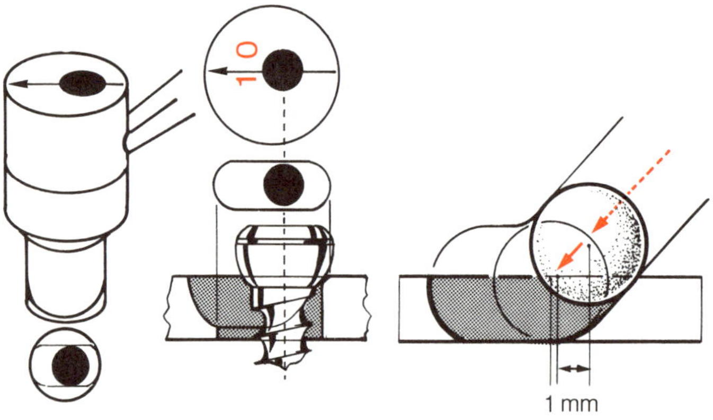

9
In a confined space, the tension range of 1 mm allows one to dispense with the plate tightener. However, it is advisable to employ the tightener routinely, also when using a slotted plate. The tension range of 1 mm is very small and often does not suffice to approximate the fragments to such an extent that interfragmental compression can be developed.

10
The slotted plate used as a *supporting plate* by adequate employment of the drill guide.

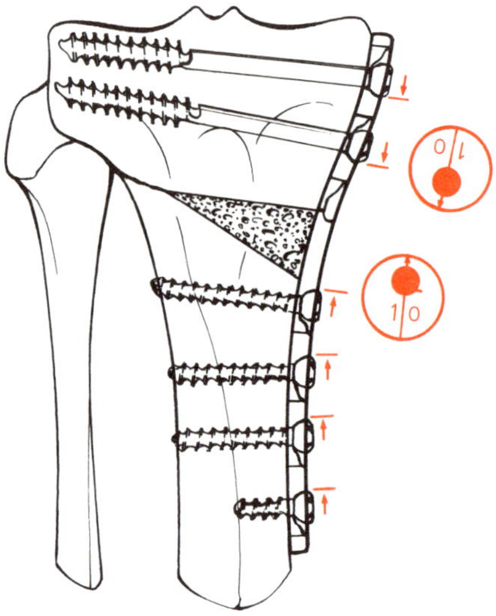

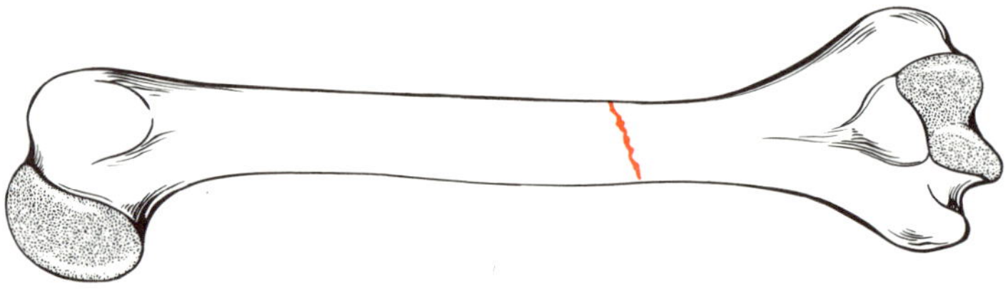

11
Fracture of the shaft. Here, the use of a plate tightener presents some difficulty.

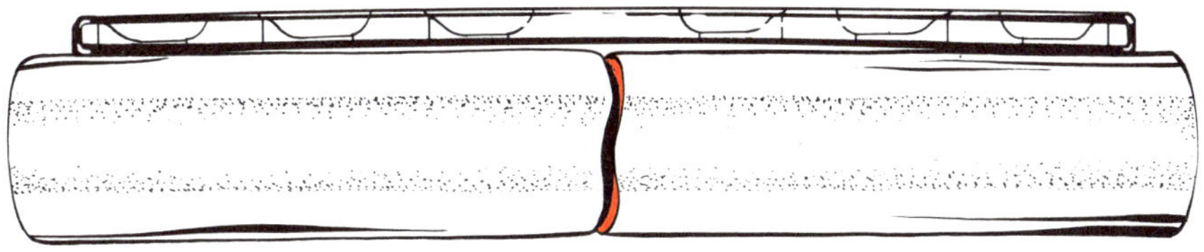

12

The slide ways in the plate holes are so arranged that they always push the screw heads toward the center of the plate.

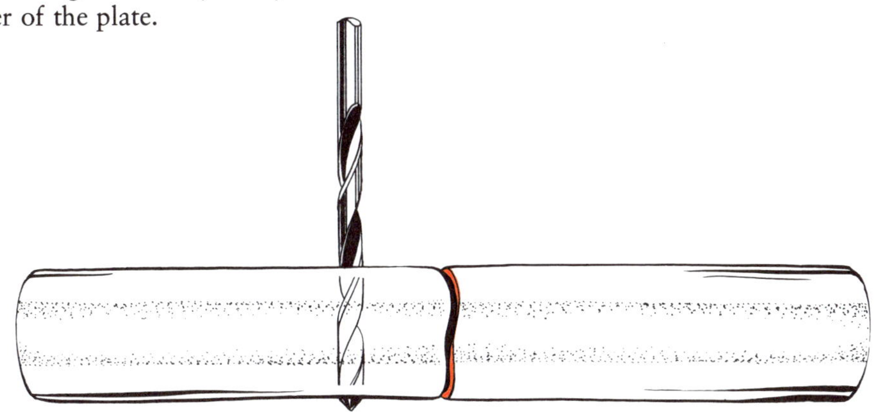

13

The first drill hole is made *near the fracture,* without a plate and as a rule without a centering drill guide. The distance "d" from the fracture should be at least 5 mm, preferably 8 mm. This often means that one hole in the fracture area is not occupied by a screw.

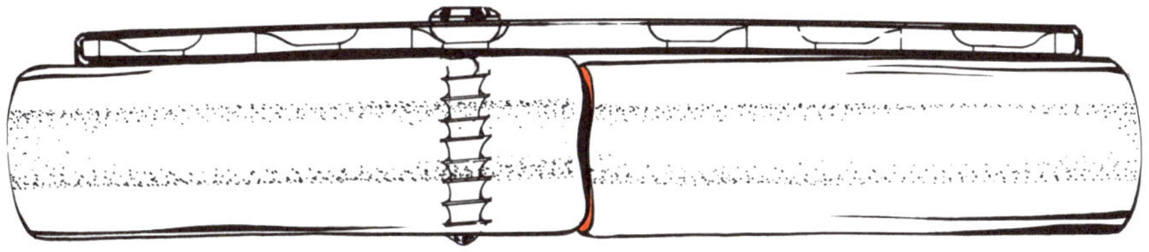

14

When the screw is sunk into the slot, its head becomes centered in such a fashion that, should bone resorption take place at the fracture site, some space will remain for the fragments to move closer together.

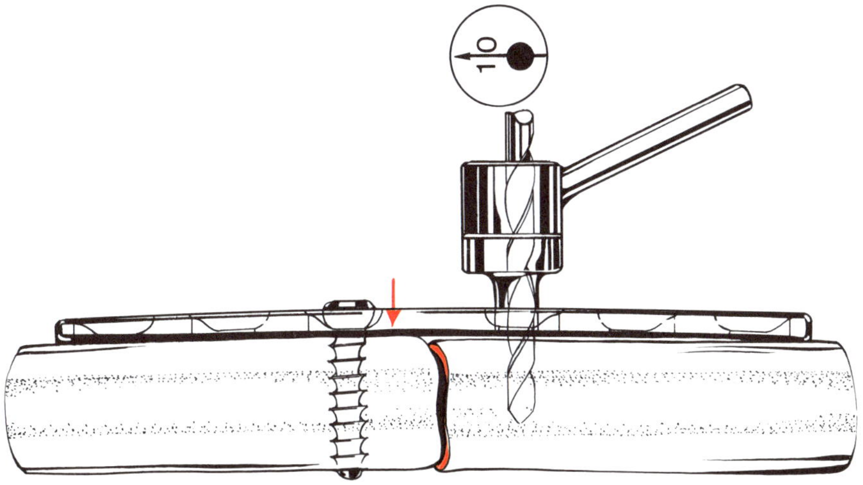

15

The second screw is *similarly inserted near the fracture,* always by means of a centering drill guide.

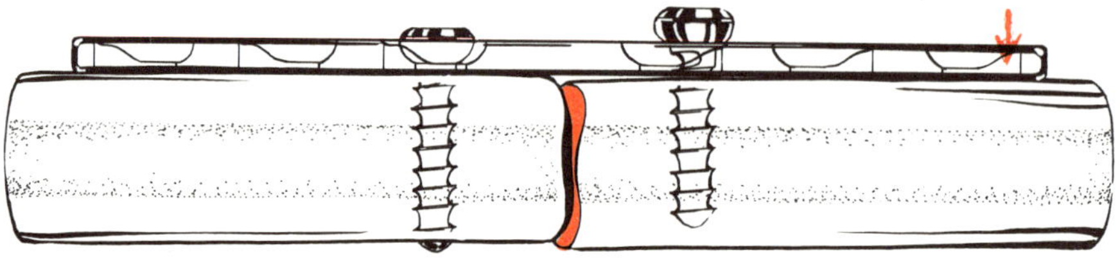

16

As the screw head is sunk, it slips along the slide way of the hole toward the center of the plate, taking its fragment with it.

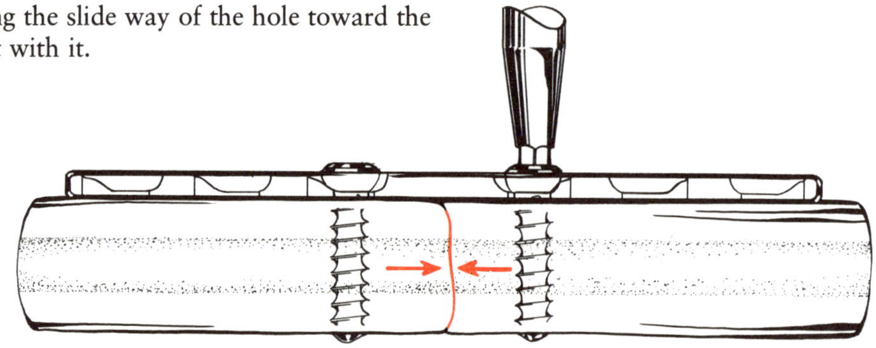

17

Interfragmental compression has developed. Despite this, enough residual space in both slots (as well as in all the others) remains, which allows the fragments to move somewhat closer together later on.

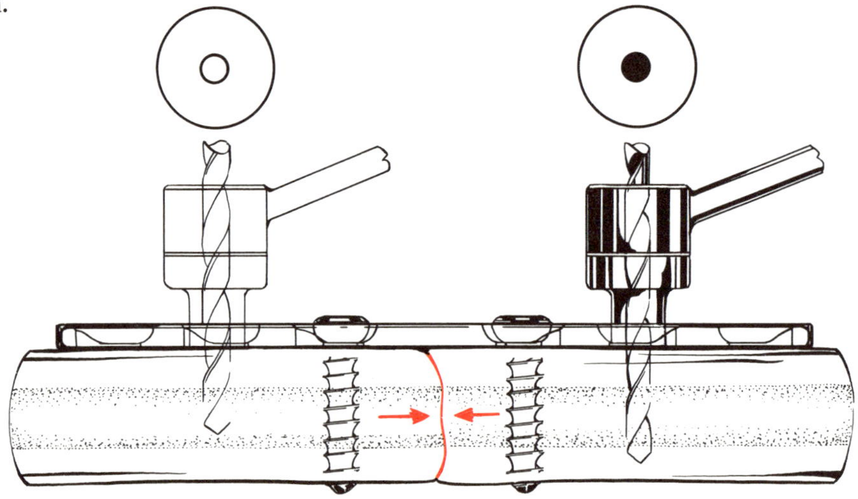

18

All the remaining screws are emplaced, not using the 1.0 mm eccentric drill guide, but...

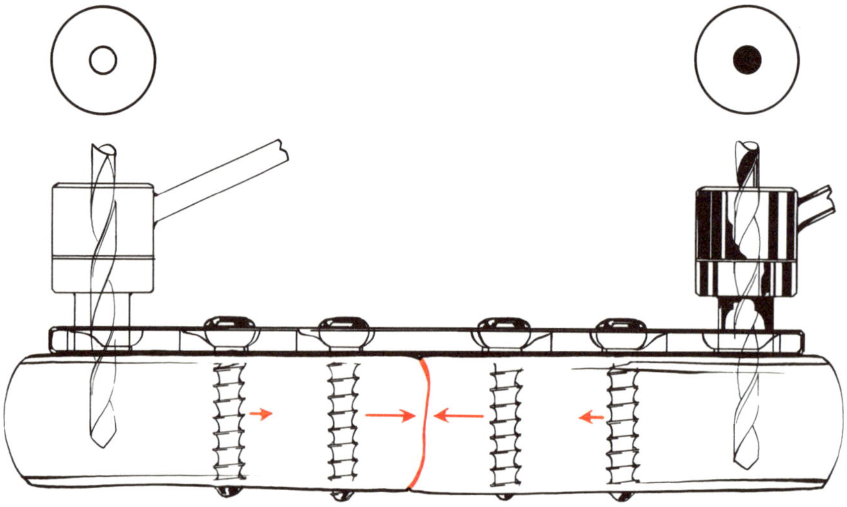

19

... using exclusively the neutral drill guide with a central hole.

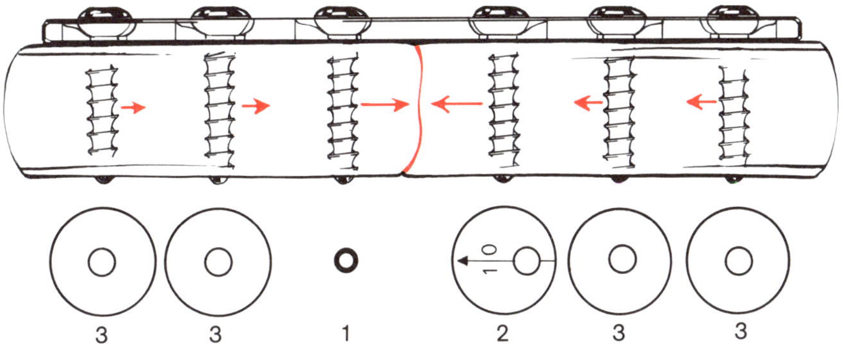

20

In the lower row of the figure, the drill guides are again assigned to their corresponding screws. Only by proceeding consistently can a dependable osteosynthesis be achieved. Any change in the order or omission of individual steps is sure to invite complications.

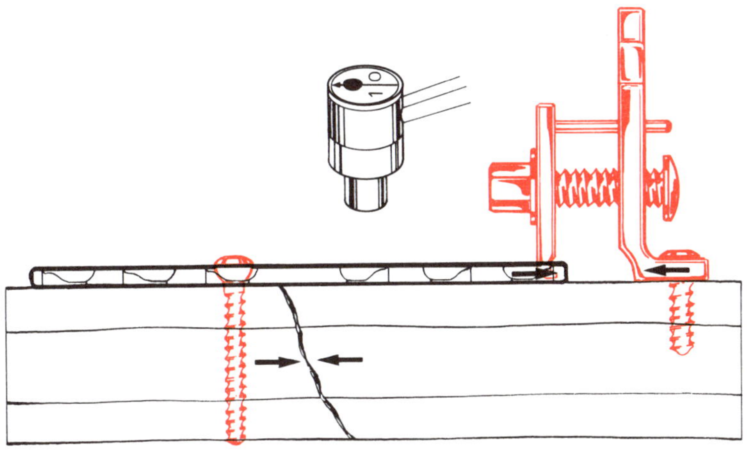

21

Routine use of the slotted plate with *plate tightener* and *neutral drill guide.*

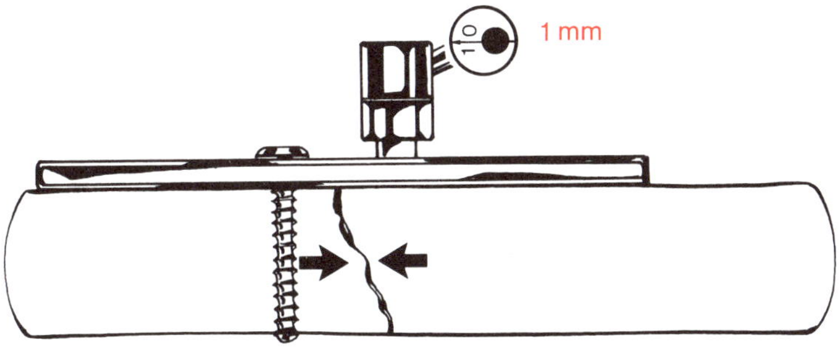

22

Exceptional use of the slotted plate solely with 1.0 mm tightening drill guide.

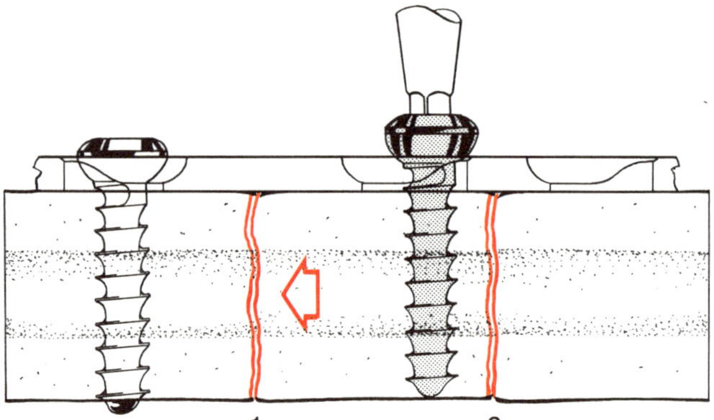

23

In *comminuted fractures* that cannot be brought under pressure with the plate tightener, the slots allow interfragmental pressure to develop succesively at both levels of the fracture.

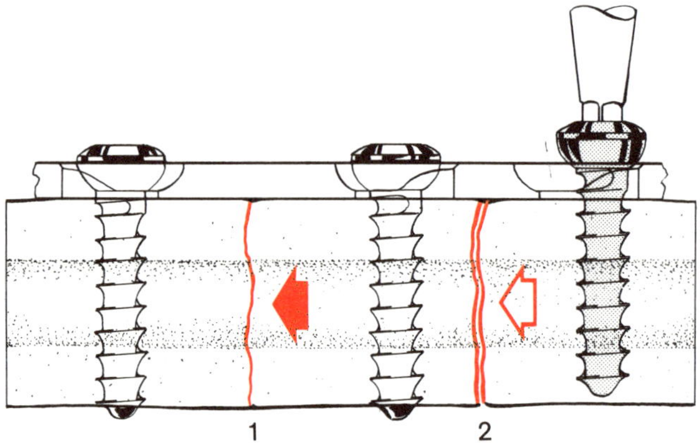

24

The first screw is inserted with the 1.0 mm drill guide near the center of the plate and produces compression within fracture cleft 1. The *second screw is also* inserted with the 1.0 mm drill guide and...

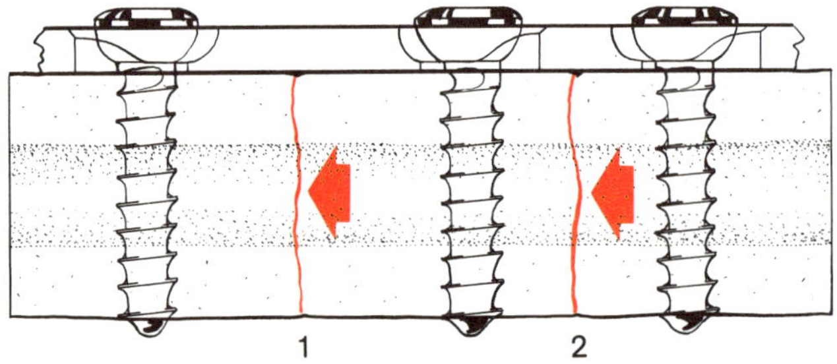

25

... produces compression in fracture cleft 2.

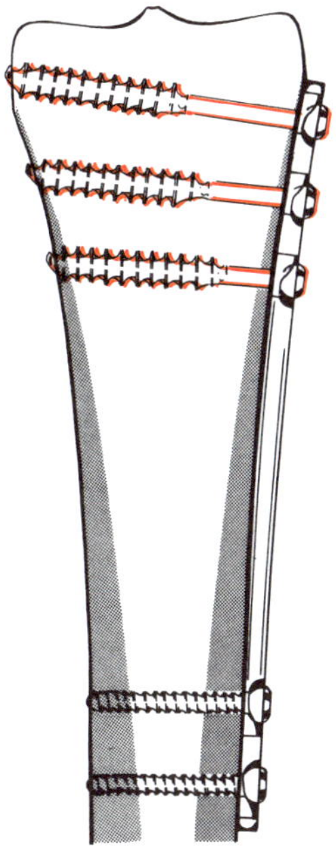

26

A cancellous screw can also pass through each hole in the plate.

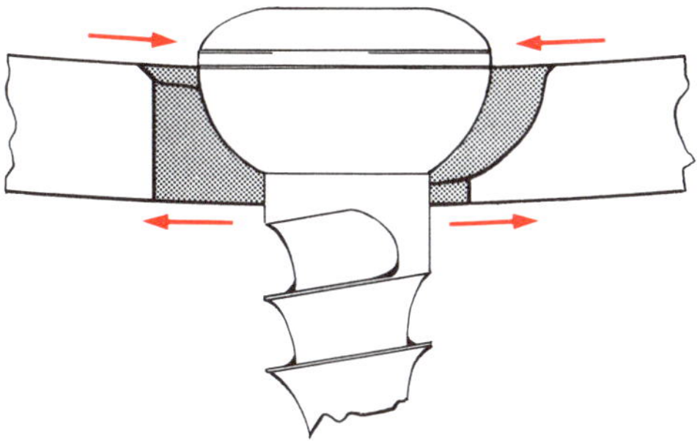

27

Slight bending in the region of the hole in the plate does not cause the head or thread of the screw to get stuck.

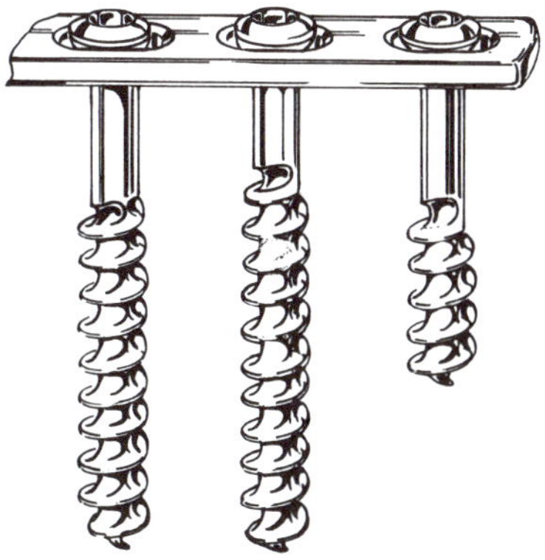

28

The cancellous screws can be inserted through all holes with the same ease as the cortical screws.

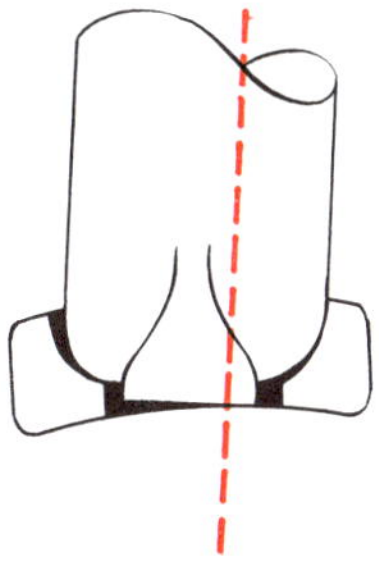

29

With use of the slotted plate, the screw can also be inserted obliquely without risk of the screw head becoming wedged.

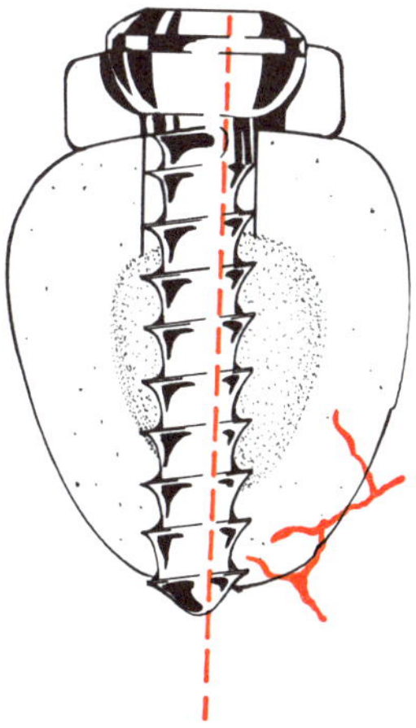

30

Thus it is easier to keep out of the way of clefts and debris in the cortex opposite the plate.

Device for external skeletal fixation

Preferential indications

1. First-degree and second-degree open fractures.
2. Infected pseudarthroses.
3. Arthrodeses and metaphyseal osteotomies.

Principles of application

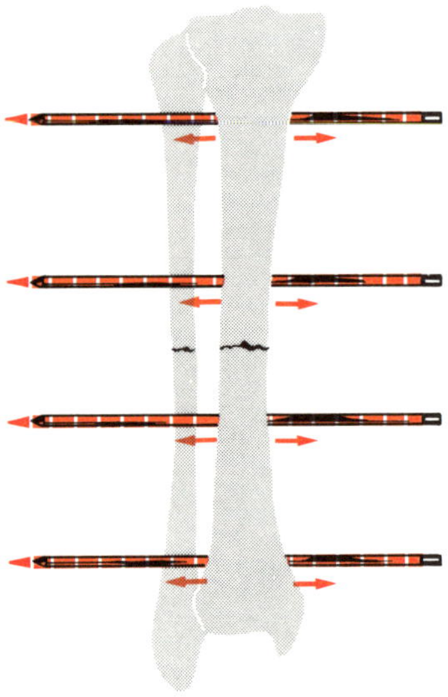

1
Nail-induced infections can only be obviated by preventing the nail from becoming displaced while it remains in the bone.

2
Such lateral movement can be prevented either by fastening the nails to each other…

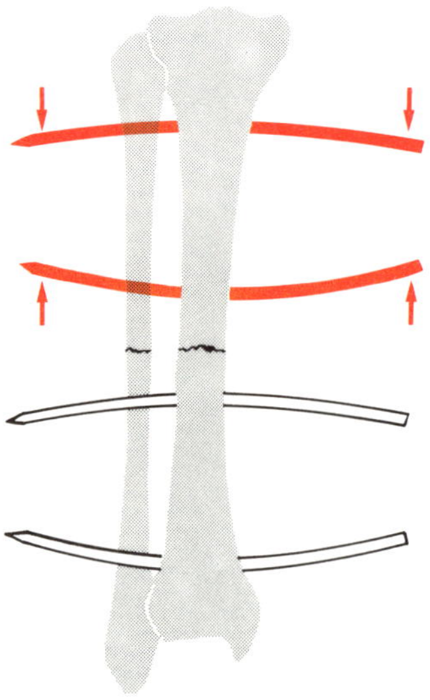

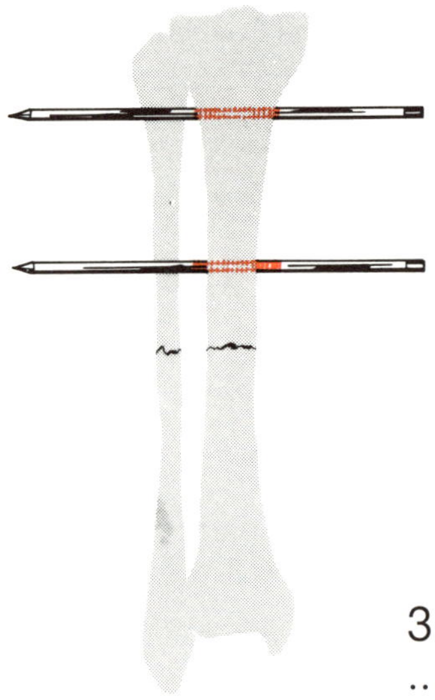

3
… or by employing nails with a partial thread at their middle.

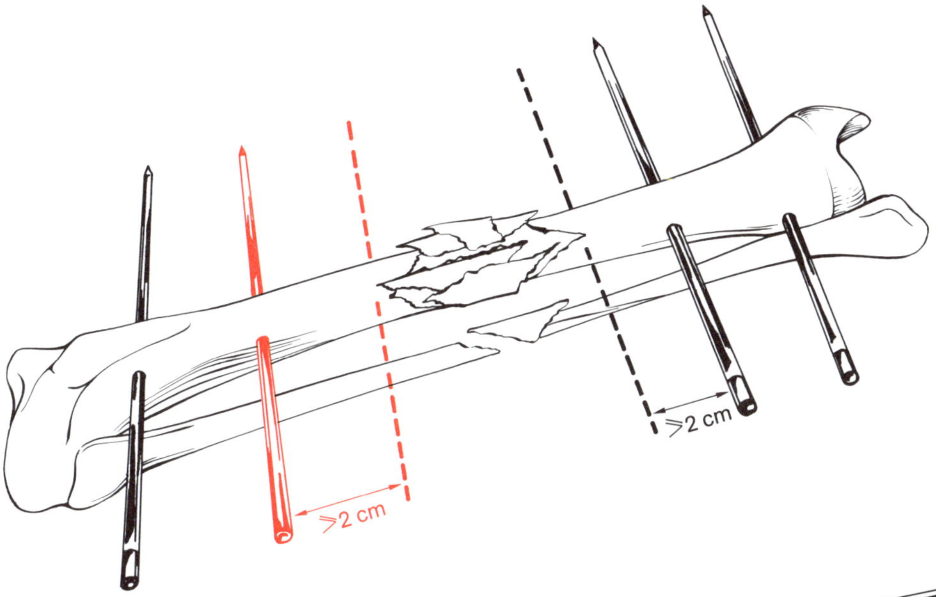

4

Nails are inserted as far as possible from the site of fracture.

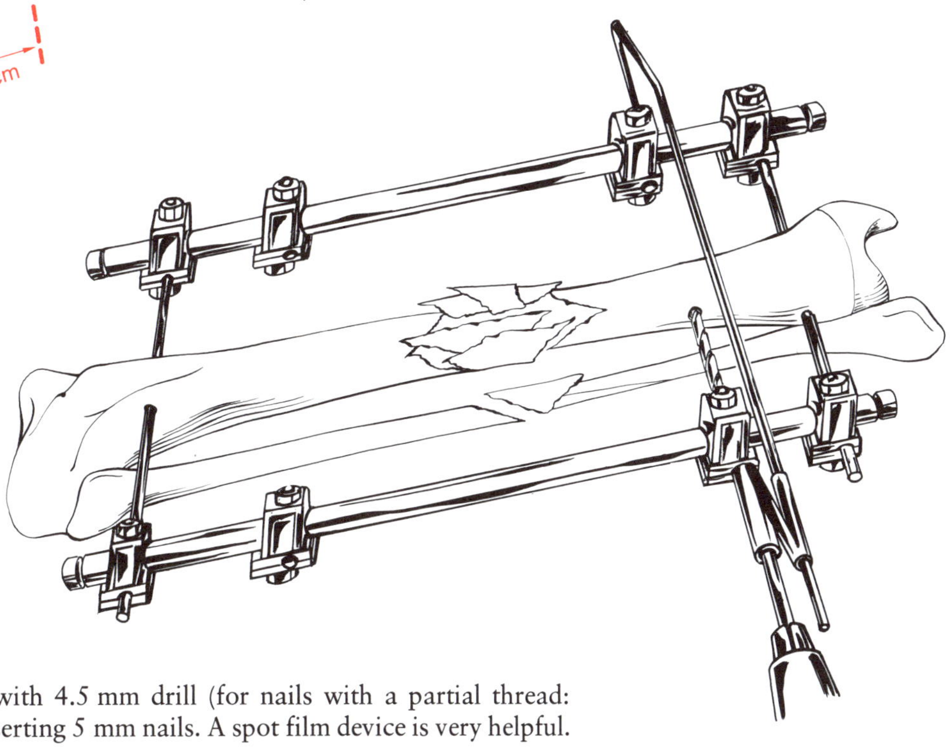

5

Previous drilling of nail holes with 4.5 mm drill (for nails with a partial thread: 3.2 mm; and thread cutting). Inserting 5 mm nails. A spot film device is very helpful.

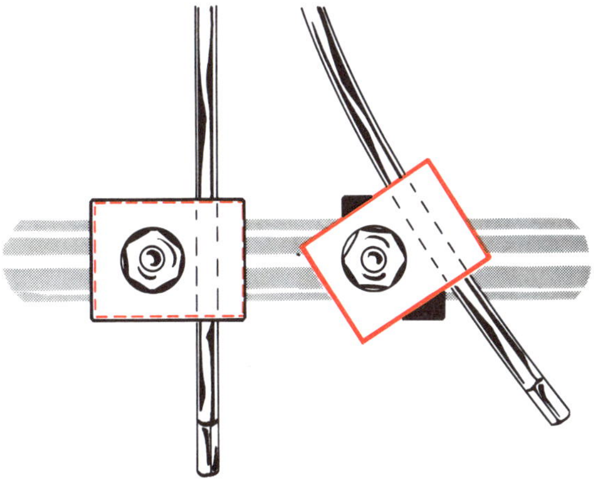

6

Use of individual rotating jaws.

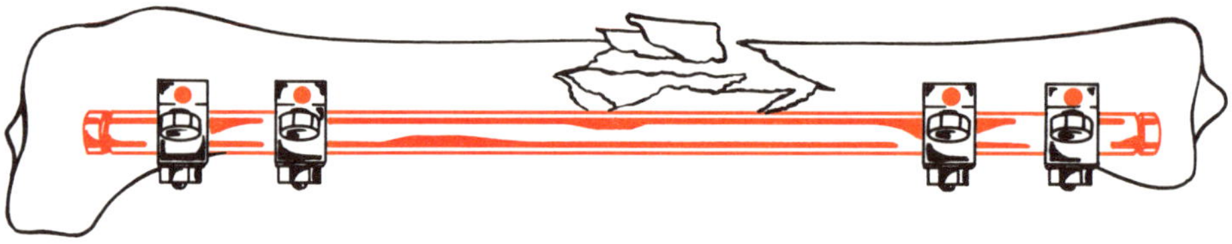

Tube dorsal to nails.

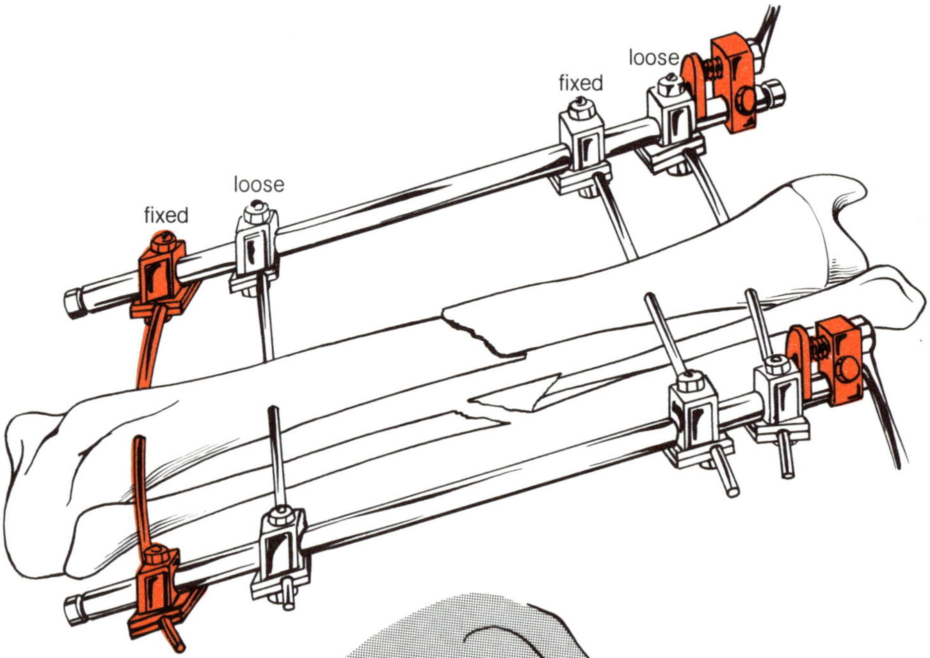

8
Interfragmental compression (if possible) and subsequent...

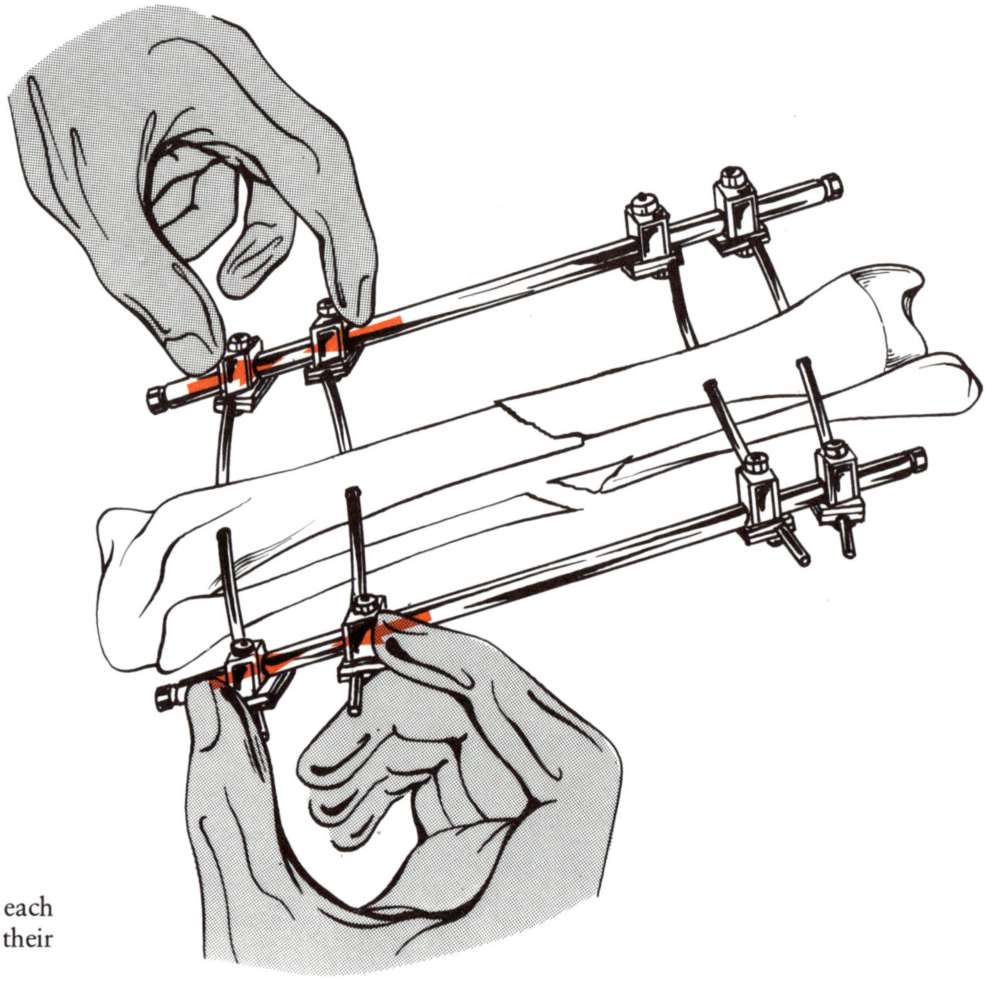

9
... fastening of the nails to each other (or using a thread at their middle).

Short fragments

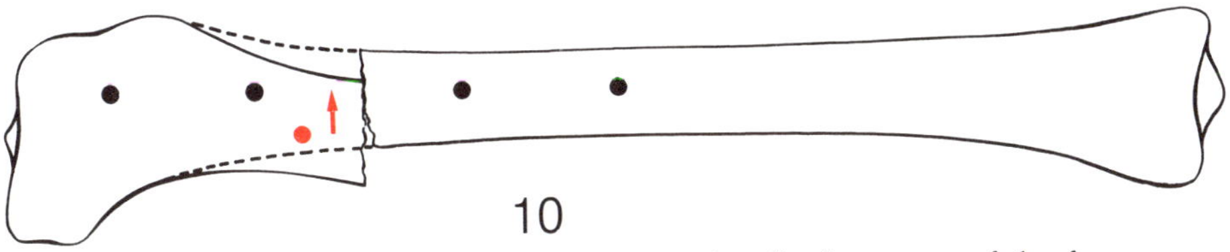

10
Anteroposterior displacement of the fragments can be prevented by use of a second nail (For other possibilities see Fig. 49–12).

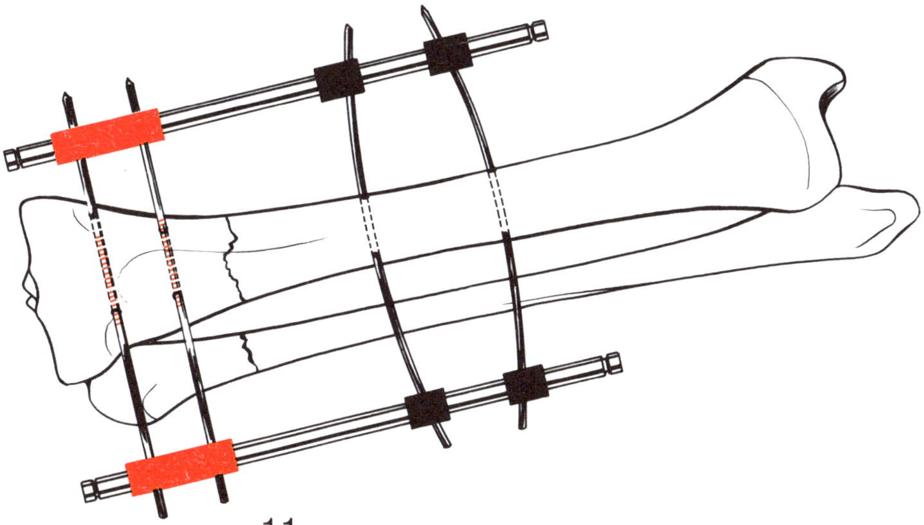

11
If this procedure is chosen for a very short fragment, a double jaw is available. Since, in the latter technique, the nails cannot be fastened to each other, nails with a partial thread at their middle are a must.

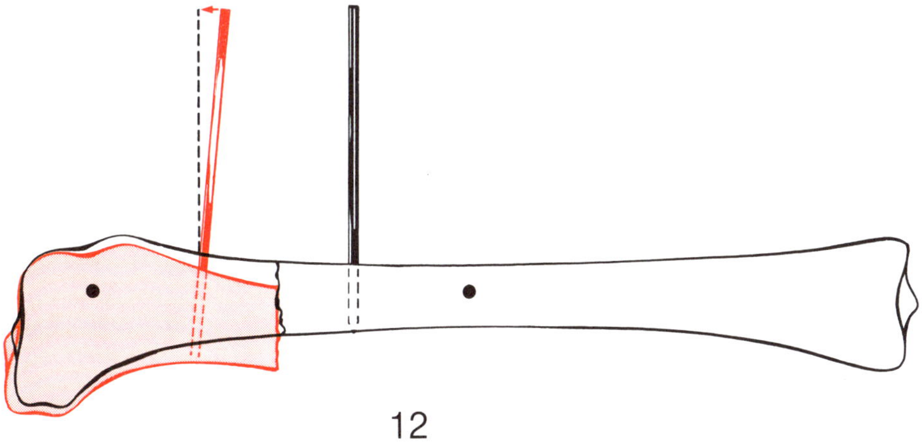

12
Fixation of the fragments in the anteroposterior direction is feasible using a second nail (Schanz screw) perpendicular to the first one. The rigidity provided by this technique corresponds approximately to that of the procedure depicted in Fig. 49–10.

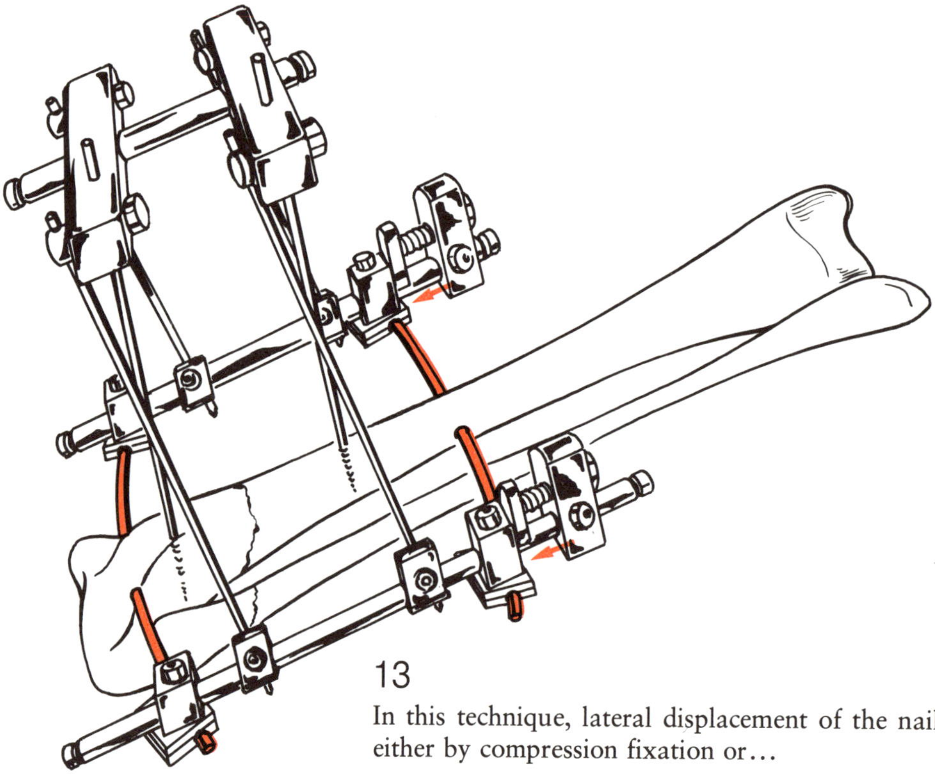

13

In this technique, lateral displacement of the nails must be prevented either by compression fixation or...

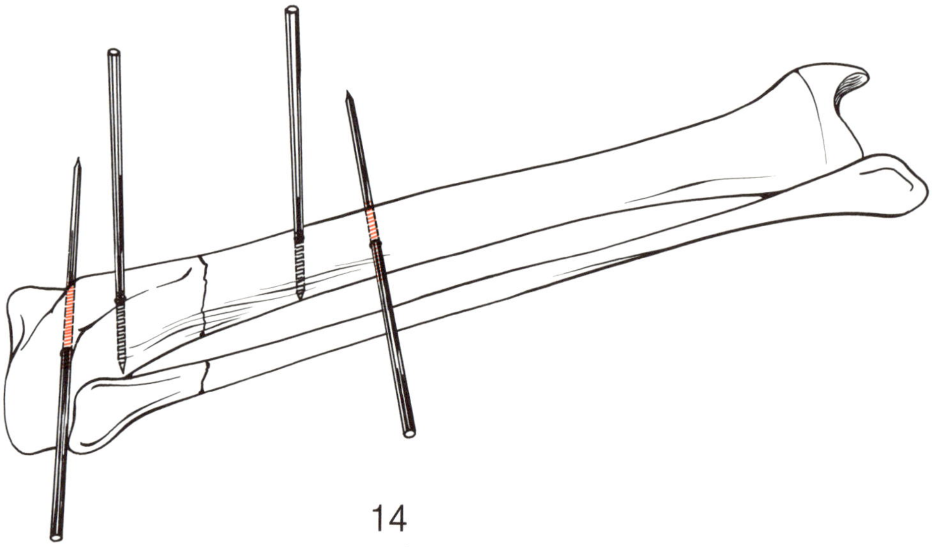

14

... by using nails with a partial thread.

Particular features

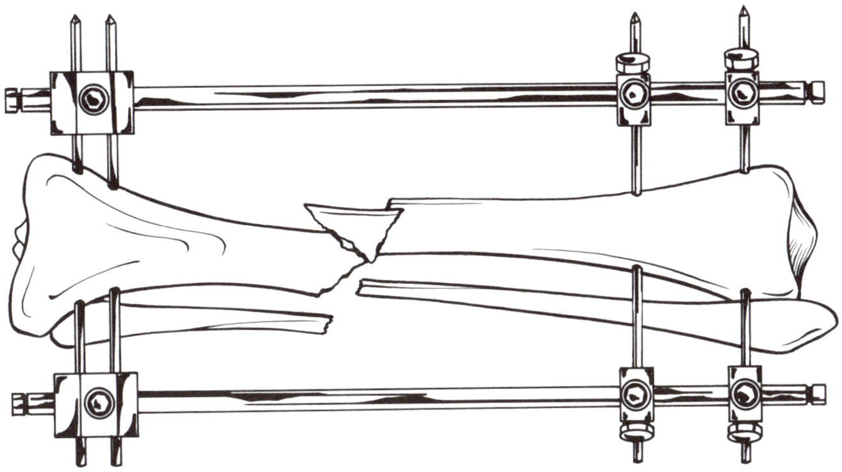

15

Lateral displacement of fragments is corrected by…

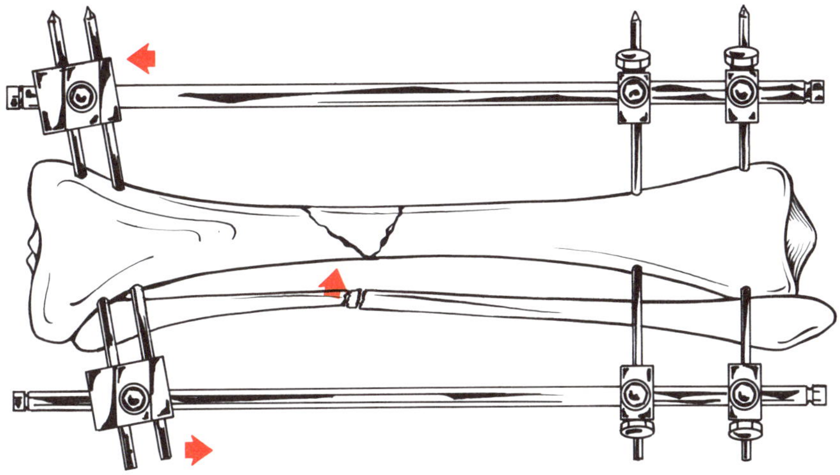

16

… corresponding displacement of the rotating jaws along the tube. The same effect can be obtained with use of special individual swiveling jaws.

17

Displacement *in the frontal plane* can be corrected by…

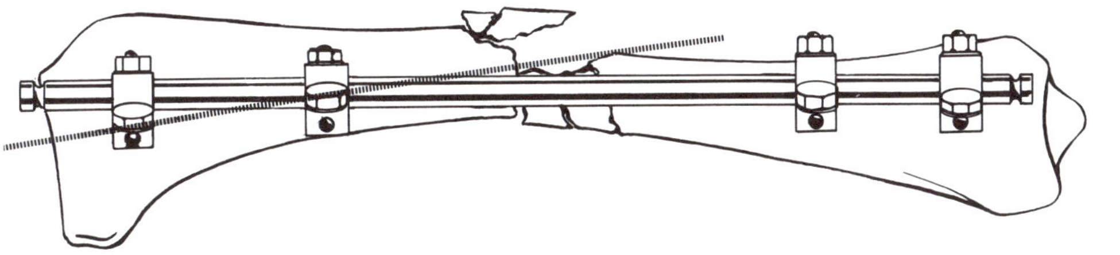

18

… interposing a link and…

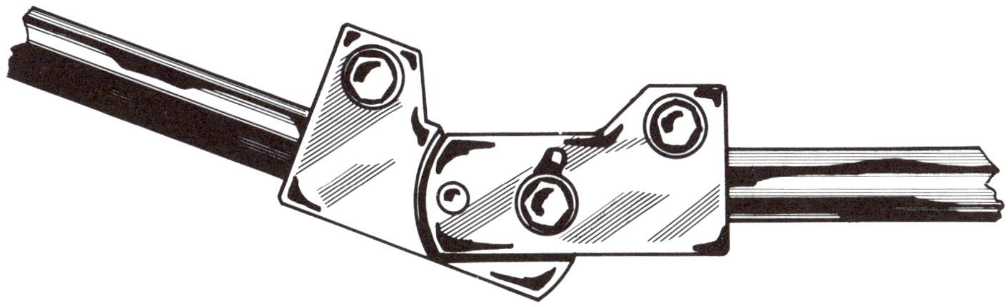

19

… replacing the long tubes by two correspondingly shorter ones.

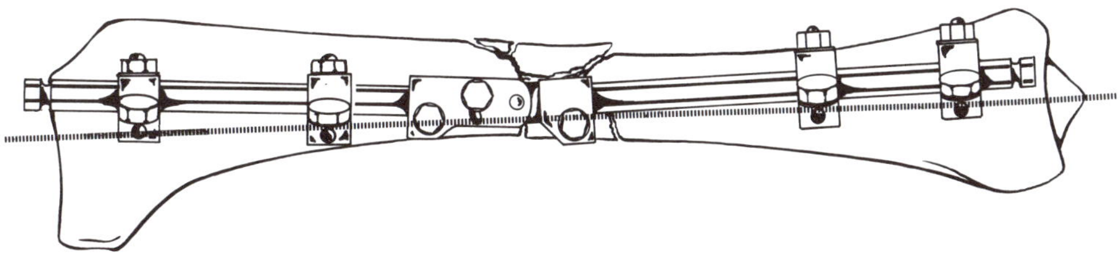

Fixation with a wire suture

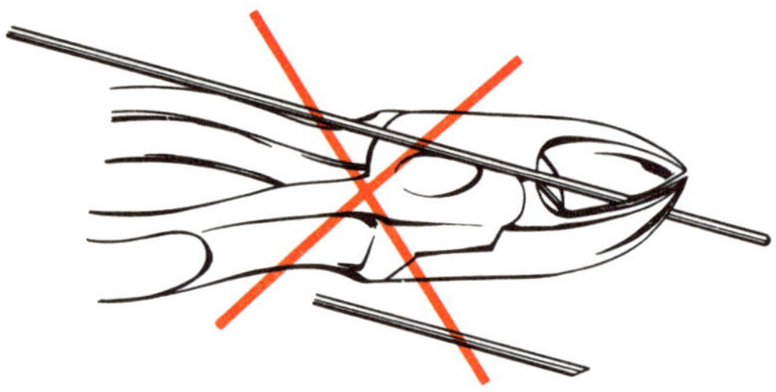

1

In applying a wire suture, for example, when the free end of the wire must be pushed through the soft tissues, the ends of the wire are sharpened. A long cutting point is obtained by applying the wire cutter – contrary to one's first impulse – not from the long end...

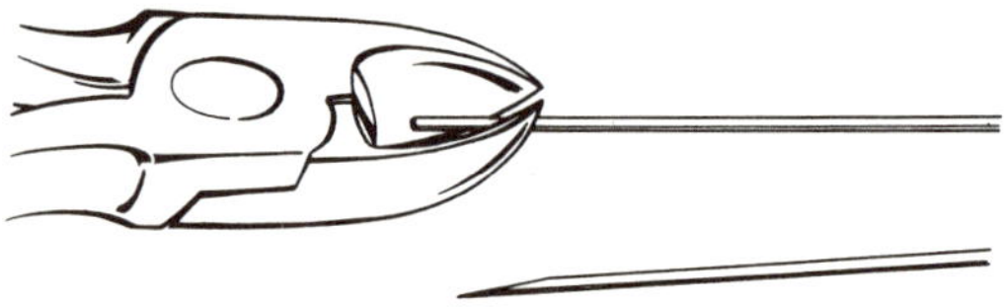

2

... but from the short end of the wire.

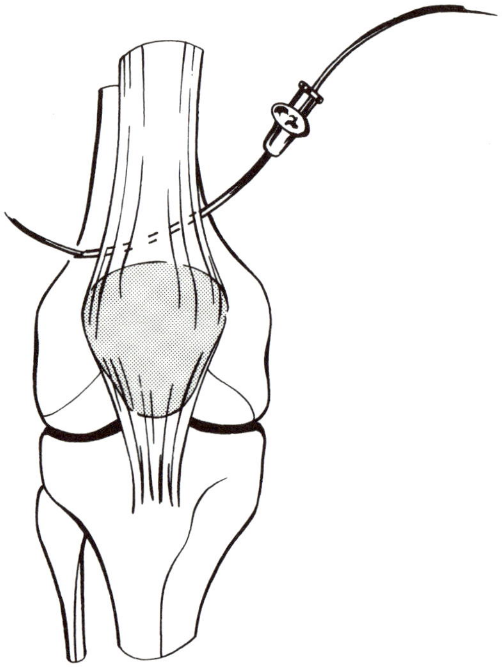

3

To be able to guide the soft wire accurately, a suitably bent, long cannula is very helpful since it possesses the necessary rigidity.

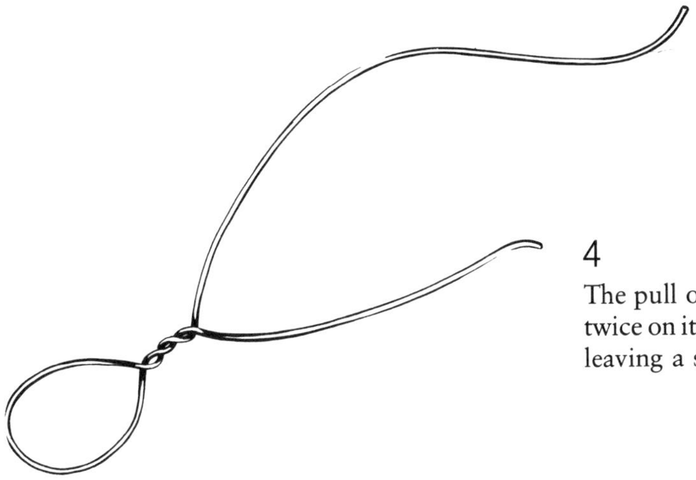

4
The pull of the wire suture can be reinforced by twisting the wire twice on itself. Prior to applying the suture, the wire is twisted once, leaving a small loop.

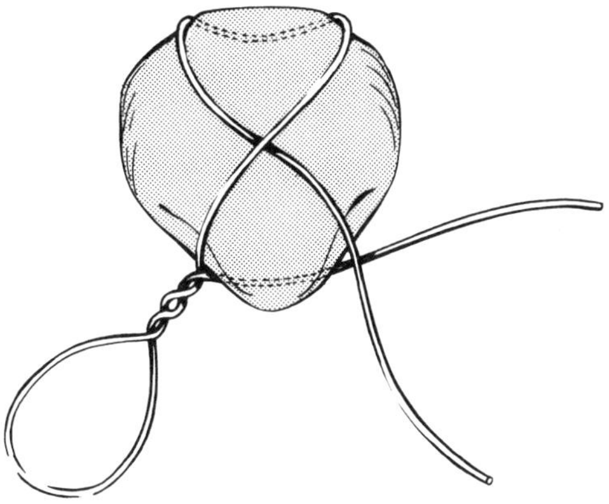

5
The wiring is in place; the second twist of the wire is formed with use of its free ends.

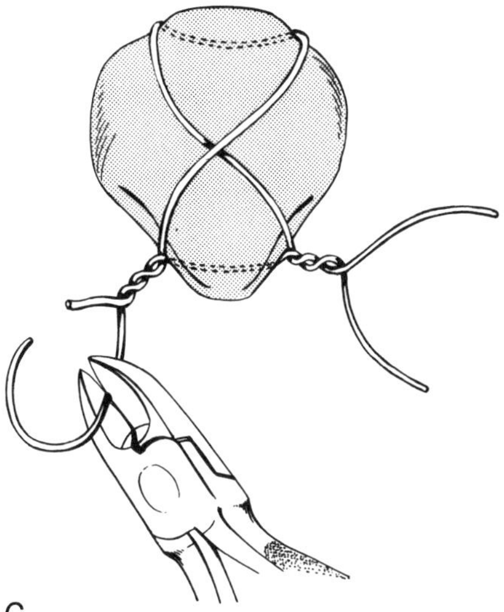

6
The small wire loop is cut off. Additional twisting will considerably reinforce the pull.

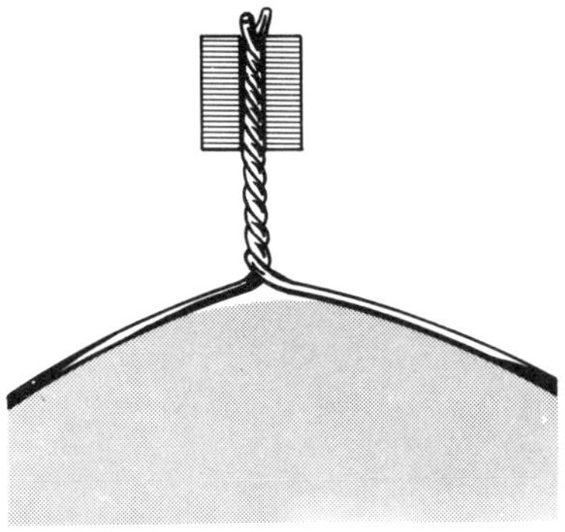

7
The twisted end of the wire should not be cut off too sparingly, so that it can be better embedded in the soft tissue. To this end, first the base (not the end) of the twisted wire is grasped with flat pliers ...

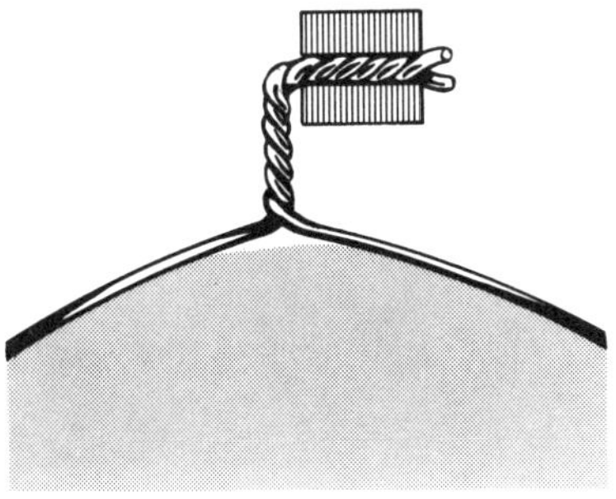

8
... and bent inward.

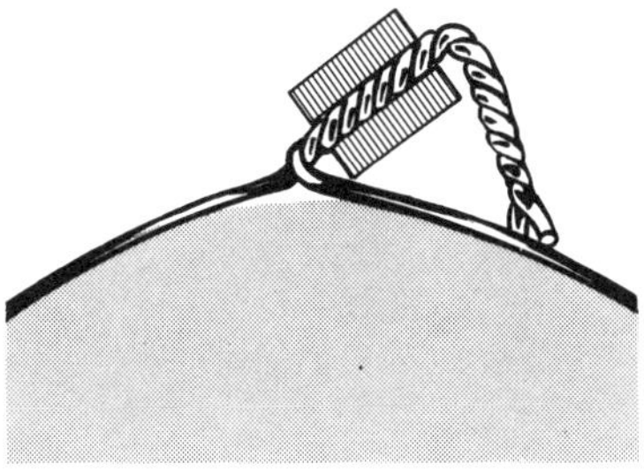

9
Only then is the twisted wire grasped at its base. Now the end of the twisted wire can be suitably adapted to the bone, so as to prevent it from perforating the soft tissues and from being bent open by movement.

Drilling wires should check only lateral displacement and must not be used to prevent fragments from becoming approximated.

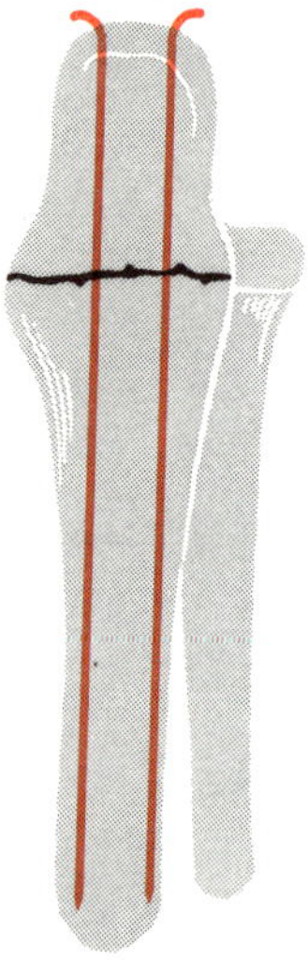

10

Parallel drilling wires *act as splints.*

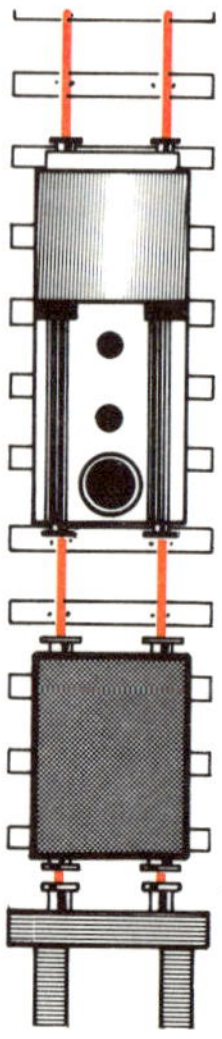

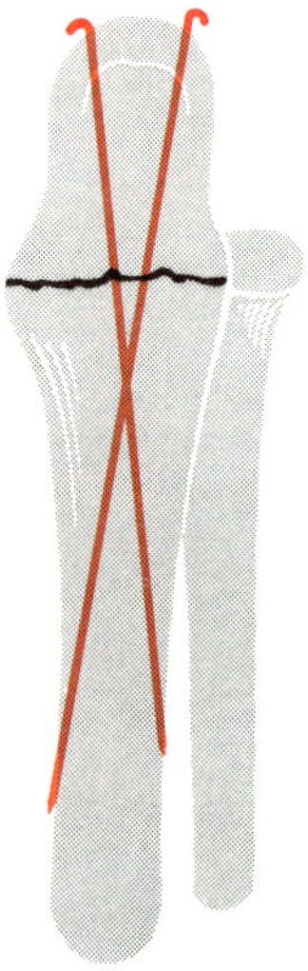

11

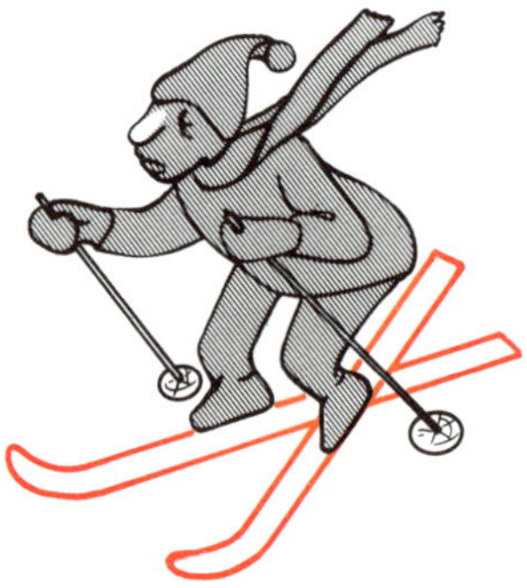

Crossed drilling wires primarily check the approximation of the fragments when bone resorption takes place in the cleft of the fracture.

Intramedullary nail

Stable nailing is feasible only after the marrow cavity has been trephined.

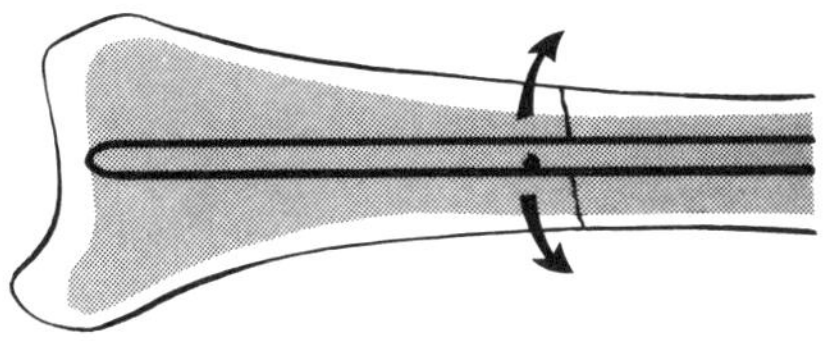

1

The nail must be strong enough to impede any movement in the cleft of the fracture.

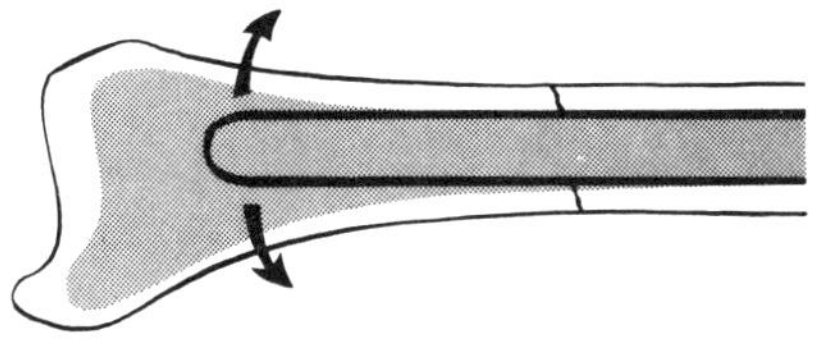

2

For the same reason ist must be long enough.

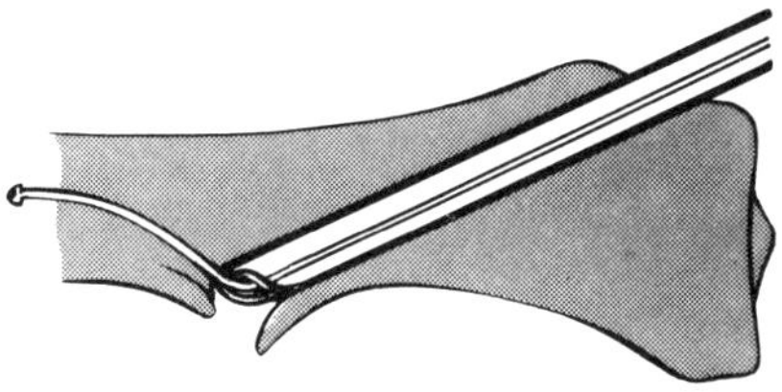

3

In view of the inherent elasticity of the AO nail, and with use of the 4 mm guide rod, such a perforation is not possible. It is, however, advisable to insert the nail slowly until its tip has passed this critical spot.

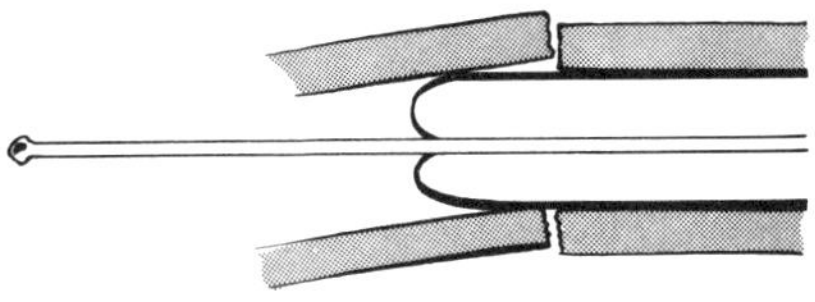

4

The distal end of the nail should be adequately bent so as to prevent the cortex...

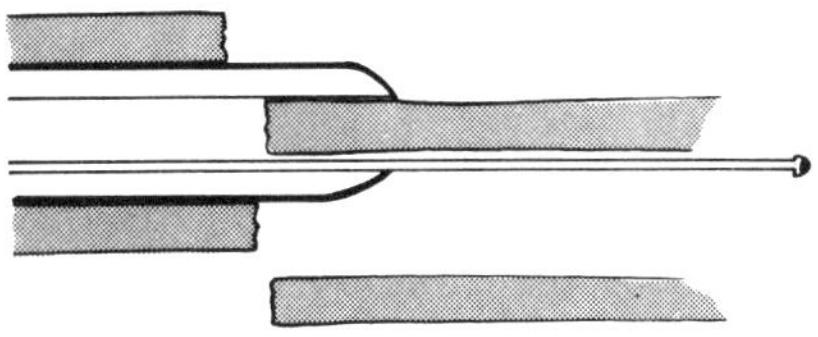

5

... from being interposed between the 4 mm guide rod and the wall of the nail when a minor displacement persists after reduction.

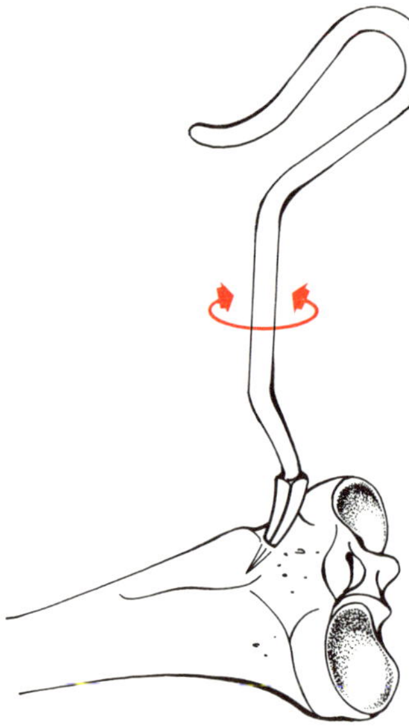

6

The marrow cavity is opened by continuous turning of the reamer.

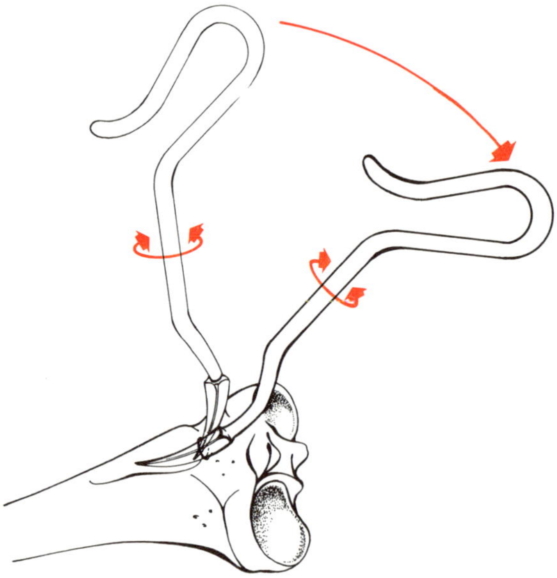

7

While turning, the reamer is simultaneously driven into the marrow cavity, and its handle slowly lowered to prevent the point from perforating the cortex at the posterior aspect of the tibia. Clasping the tibial tubercle with one's thumb and index finger will be of assistance in keeping within the longitudinal axis of the shaft.

8

Drill pin (3 mm) with button at the end.

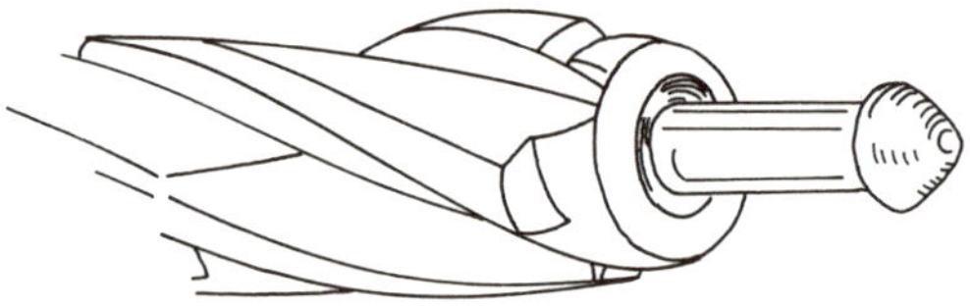

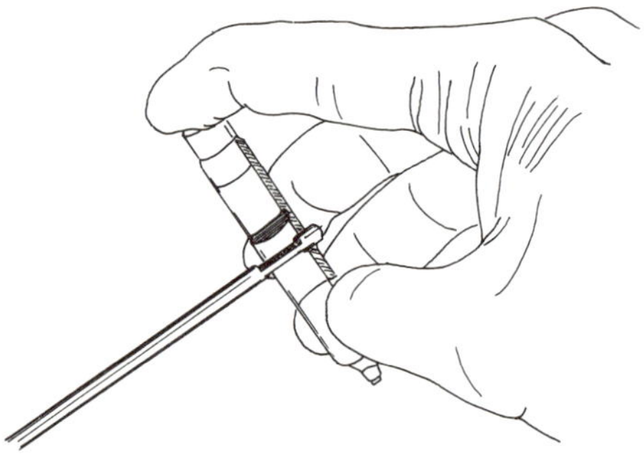

9

The handle fits the drill pin and the guide rod equally well. It is used for directing the drill (rotating the broken end of its pin) in driving the pin in, for holding the pin tight in trephining the marrow cavity, and for clasping the guide rod while knocking the nail home. By pressing a button, one push up the handle laterally.

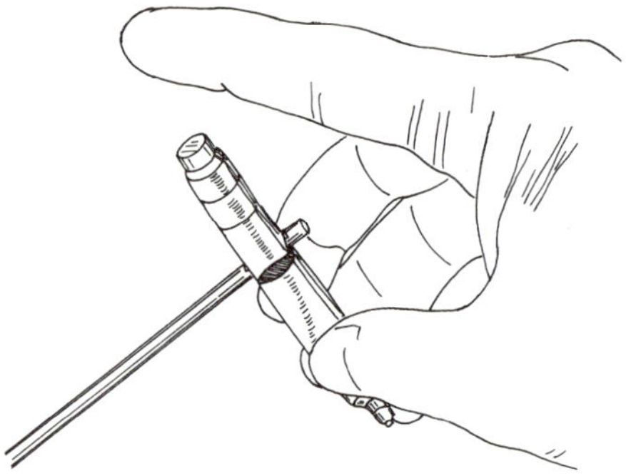

10

After release of the button, the handle becomes locked on the pin or the rod and can no longer fall down. One should be able to apply the handle, and take it off, with one hand.

11

The drill pin should be slightly bent at its anterior end. It is useful to have such an adequately bent pin on hand in one's set of instruments.

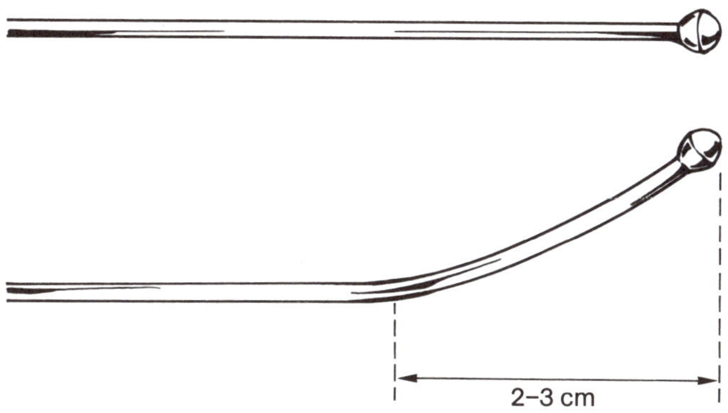

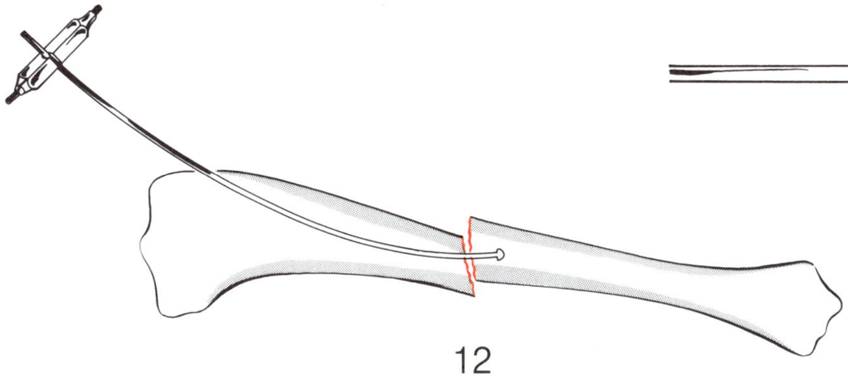

12

By adequate turning of the pin it is easier to pass its end over a fracture site that has not been accurately reduced and, above all – distally – to keep it exactly in the center of the bone.

13

Beware of vigorous hammer blows! An assistant holds the guard plate to protect the tissues with one hand while, with the other, he prevents the pin from springing back and forth as it is being hammered.

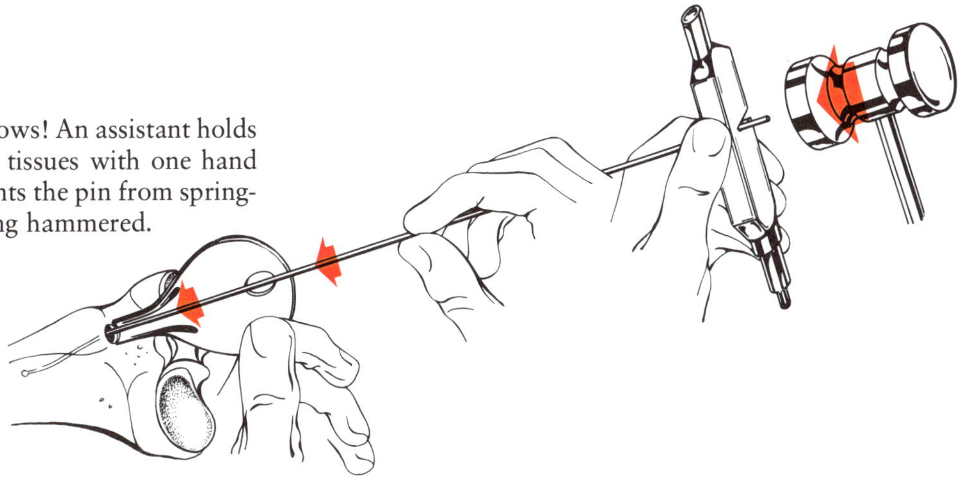

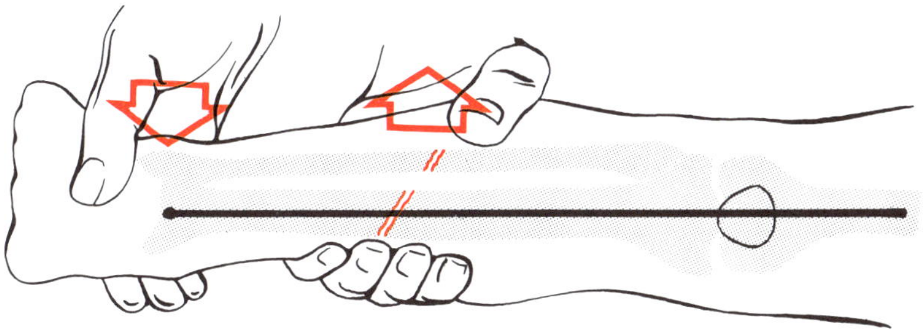

14

Even during the first turn of the drill, it is important that the valgus position be corrected by holding the limb appropriately. In closed nailing, release of the longitudinal traction facilitates such a maneuver. While it is true that the tendency for recurvation is thus reinforced, this can, however, be counterbalanced by holding the limb in a suitable position. In this way a straight canal is drilled for correct guidance of the nail.

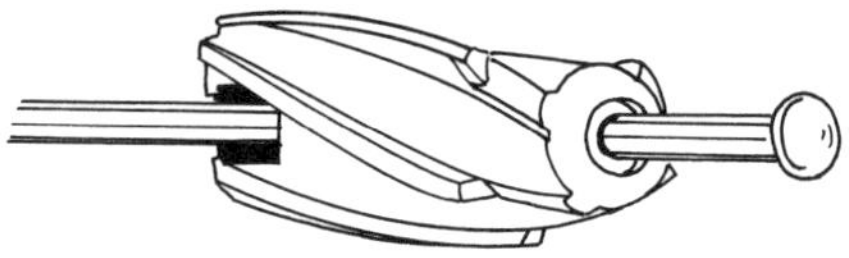

15

Blunt drill. Available diameters: (increasing by 0.5 mm) from 9.5 mm upward.

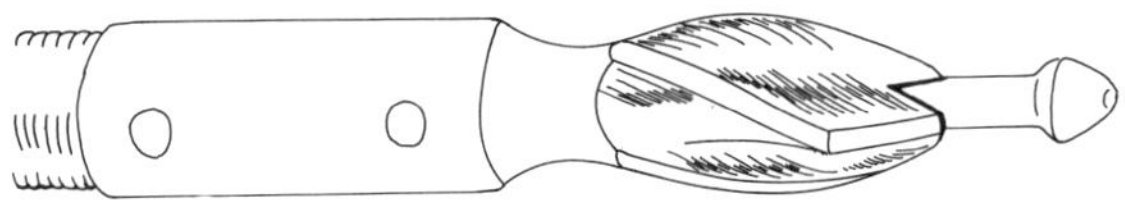

16

Sharp drill head. Diameters: 9 mm (used for the first turn of the drill in the tibia and sometimes the femur) and 12 mm (for the first turn of the drill in a femur with a wide marrow cavity).

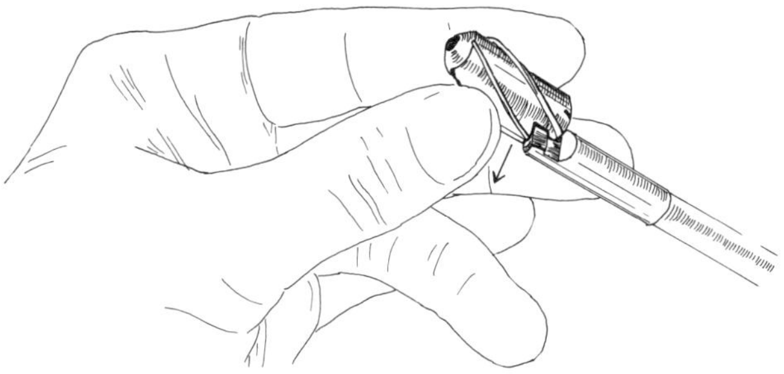

17

The removable drill heads are pushed, laterally, onto the flexible shaft of the drill. They fall off again if not fastened to the drill pin together with the shaft.

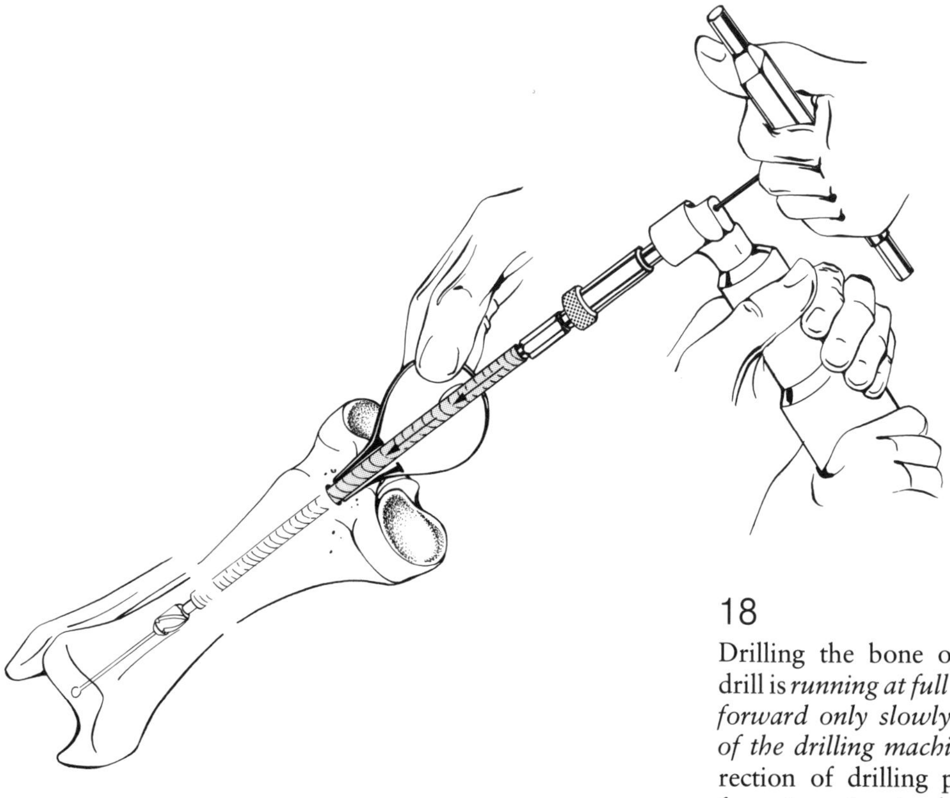

18

Drilling the bone open: Though the drill is *running at full speed*, it is *pushed forward only slowly*. *Correct holding of the drilling machine* against the direction of drilling prevents the head from jamming in the marrow cavity. The handle presses the drill pin steadily into the marrow cavity.

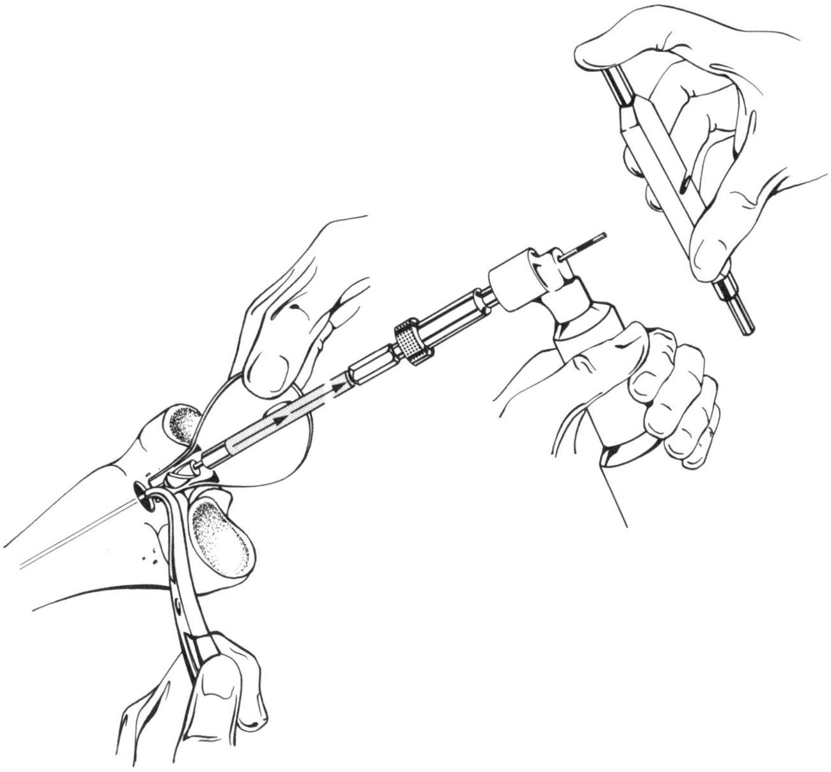

19

On withdrawal of the drill prior to removing the handle, the drill pin is held firmly with a pair of pincers so that it cannot be pulled out inadvertently.

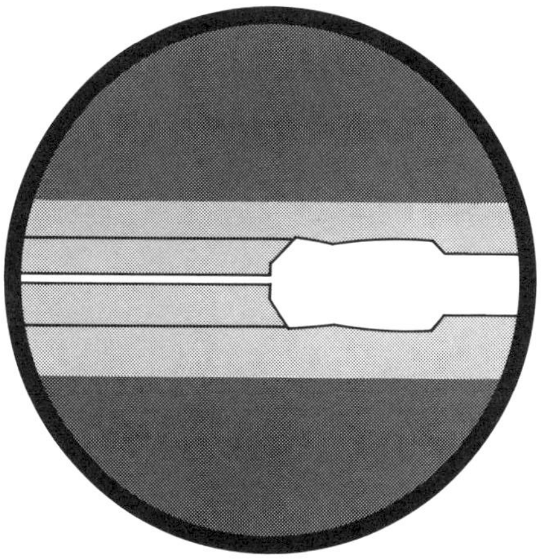

20

Drilling is continued until distinct contact with cortical bone is established. At this moment the roentgenogram should show that the small clear border between the drill head and the inner aspect of the cortex at the narrowest site is just about to vanish.

The following points apply in **measuring the diameter of the nail:**

1. In solid bone, the effective size of the nail should correspond to that of the drill head; in "soft" bone (i.e., osteoporotic) 3 weeks following a fracture, it should be 1/2 mm larger.
2. New AO nails are actually 0.2 to 0.5 mm thinner than the engraved number indicates.
3. Old AO nails are actually 0.2 to 0.5 mm thicker than the engraved number indicates.
4. The diameter of the drill head corresponds to the millimeters indicated.
5. AO nails are only available in gradations of full millimeters. As a consequence, when the hole drilled in solid bone measures, say, 12.5 mm, a new "number 13" nail or an old "number 12" should be chosen.

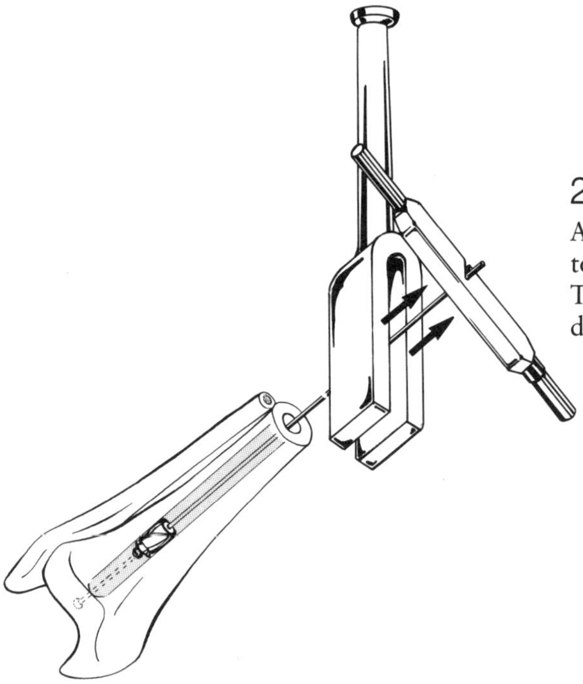

21

A broken or jammed drill head can be removed with aid of the button at the end of the drill pin, using an arbor and a slit hammer. Traction on the flexible shaft of the drill remains ineffective and destroys the shaft.

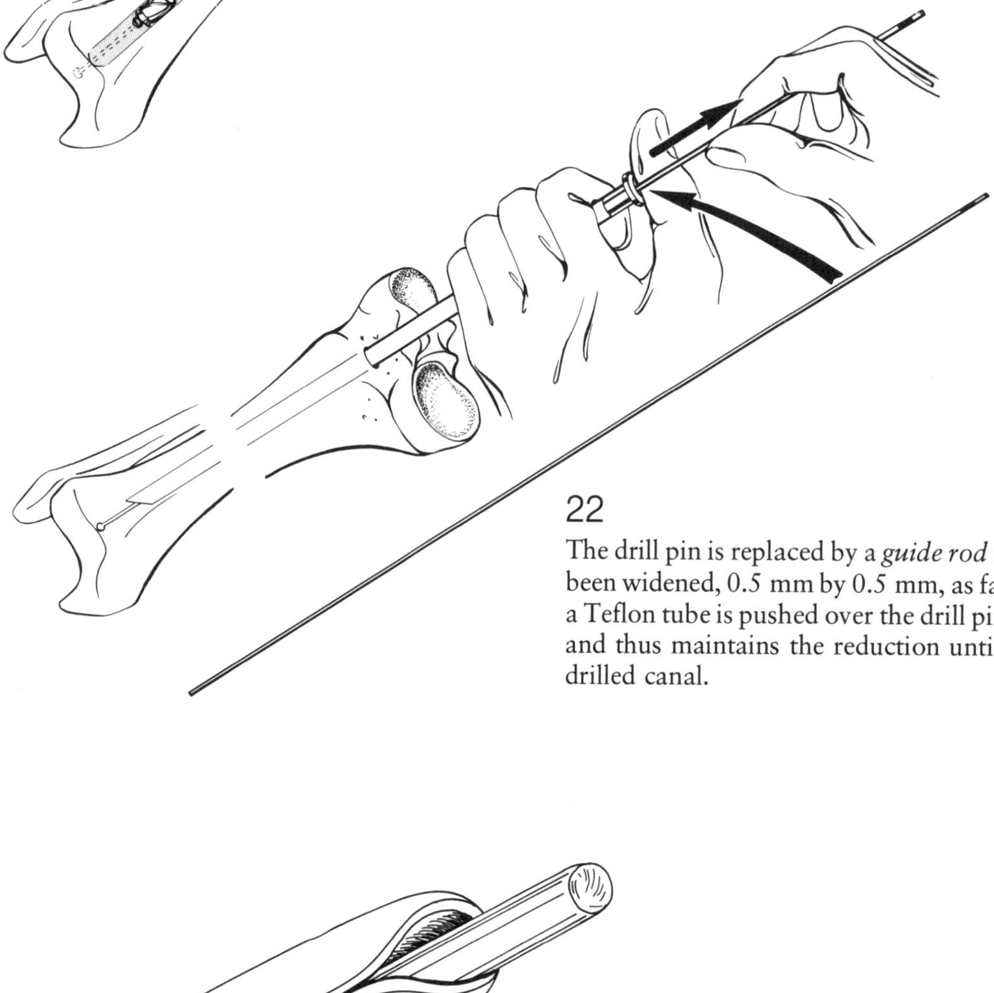

22

The drill pin is replaced by a *guide rod* after the marrow cavity has been widened, 0.5 mm by 0.5 mm, as far as the cortex. To this end, a Teflon tube is pushed over the drill pin; it crosses the fracture site and thus maintains the reduction until the rod is placed into the drilled canal.

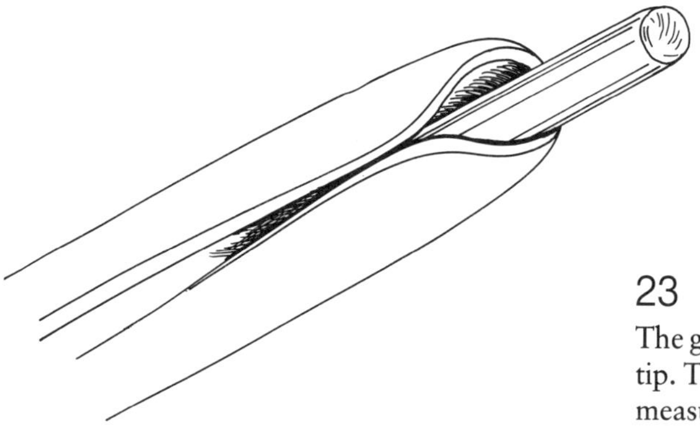

23

The guide rod measures 4 mm in diameter and has no button at the tip. The nail must not be driven in over the drill pin since the latter, measuring no more than 3 mm, is too weak and complications – such as the one depicted in Fig. 55–3 – are liable to supervene.

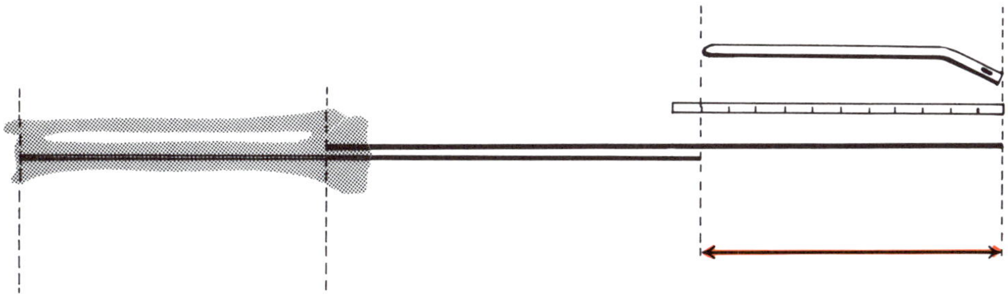

24

Measuring the nail length with a second guide rod of equal length.

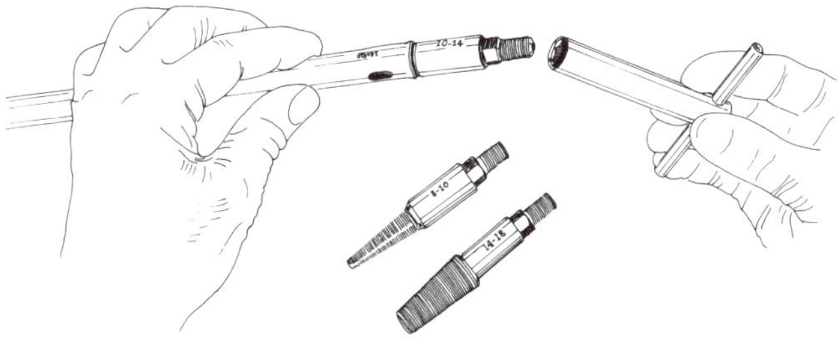

25

The parts to be driven in are fitted to the nail. Depending on the thickness of the latter, various conical pieces are available. The appropriate cone is firmly screwed to the end of the nail.

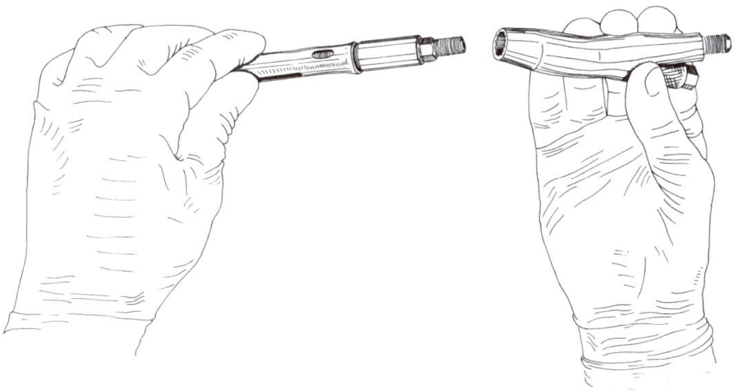

26

Attaching the device for driving the nail home. The device neutralizes the curvature of the nail so that the blows can be struck parallel to axis.

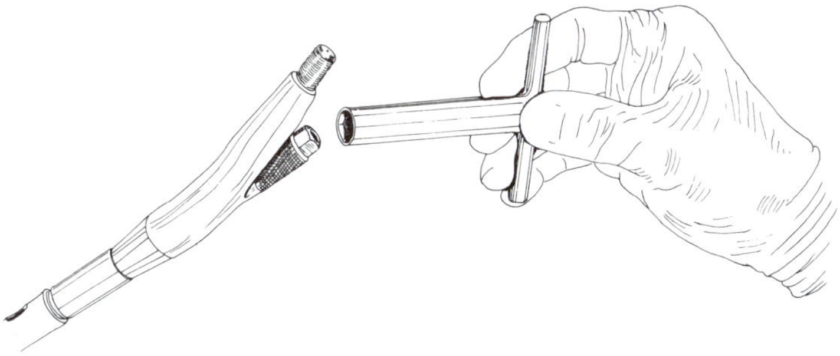

27

The nut is only slightly tightened. The instrument is fitted with a clamping thread which, when tightened too firmly, is difficult to unscrew.

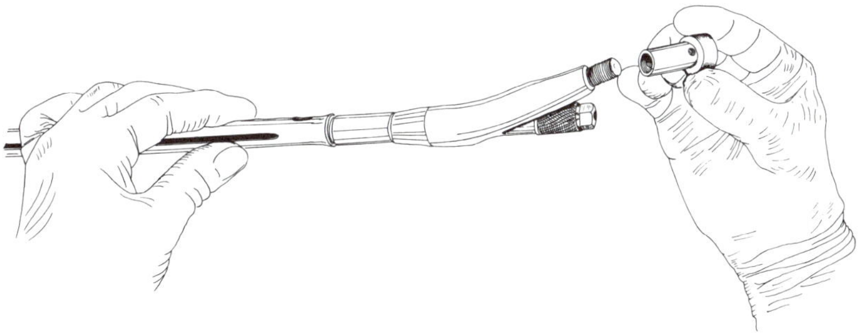

28

Screwing on the drive head. In its place one can also screw on the device for driving the nail out (and in).

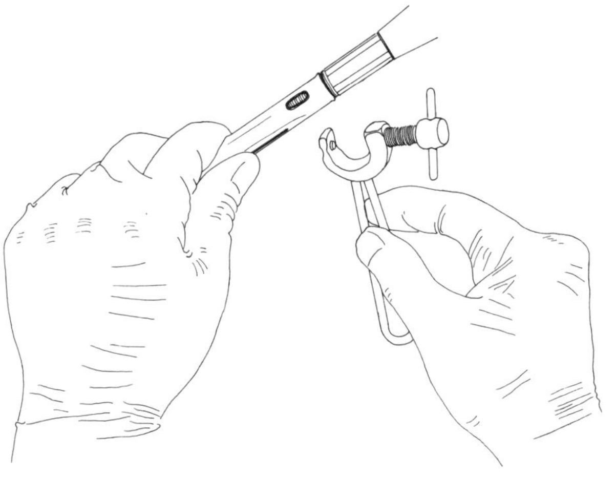

29

The holding device is mounted and screwed into the anterior or posterior nail hole only after the unit has been pushed over the guide rod. Otherwise, the end of the rod is apt to get jammed in the device.

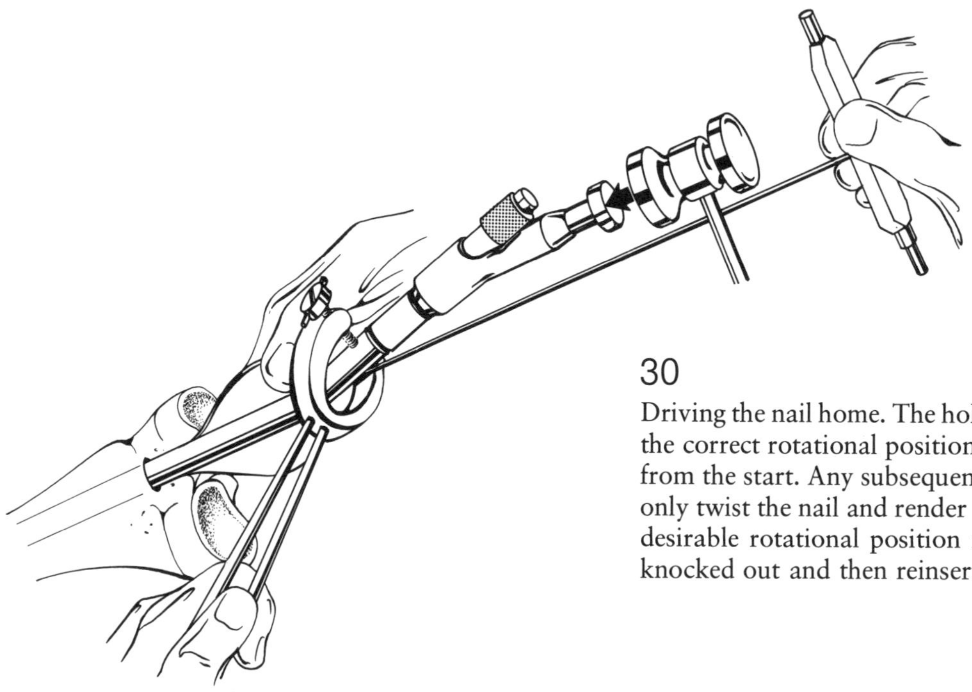

30

Driving the nail home. The holding device serves to maintain the correct rotational position of the nail – a factor to heed from the start. Any subsequent attempt at correction would only twist the nail and render it unserviceable. When an undesirable rotational position results, the nail must first be knocked out and then reinserted in the correct position.

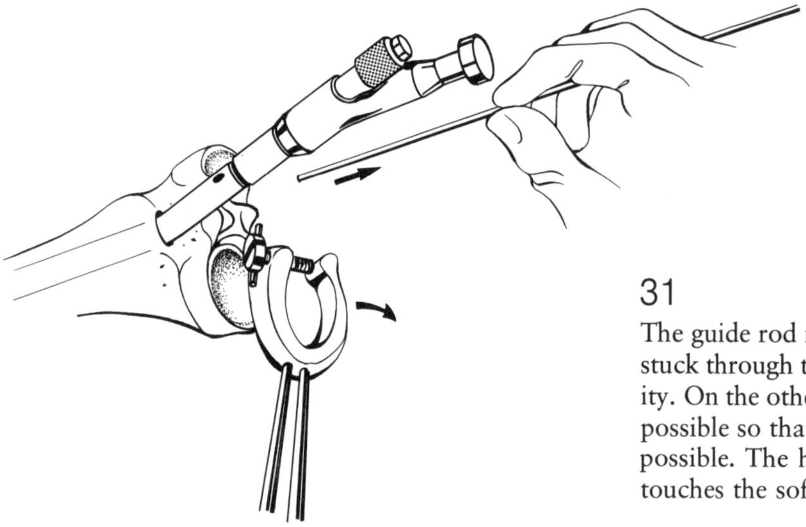

31

The guide rod must be removed in good time, before it gets stuck through the curve of the nail entering the marrow cavity. On the other hand, the rod should be removed as late as possible so that it can guide the point of the nail as long as possible. The holding device is also removed as soon as it touches the soft tissue.

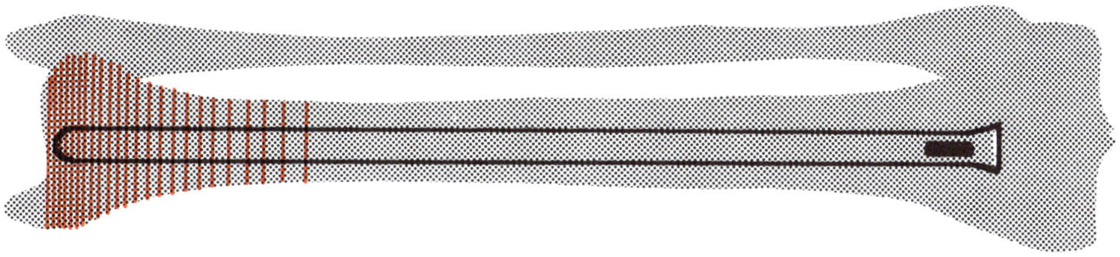

32

The point of the nail should lie close to the joint line. Thereby it becomes seated in firm subchondral cancellous bone and the nail is guided a long distance in the distal fragment. Its position is checked on the lateral roentgenogram; in so doing, the central ray must be directed vertically onto the joint line.

Up to 360 mm, the nail lengths are graduated at intervals of 15 mm; from 360 mm upward, at intervals of 20 mm.

When intermediate lengths have been measured, these can be taken into account by driving the nail into different depths of the marrow cavity, so that at any event the nail comes to lie as far distally as possible. On no account must the end of the nail project beyond the anterior aspect of the tibia. This would give rise to persistent discomfort as long as the nail remains in place.

3. Clavicle

Anatomy

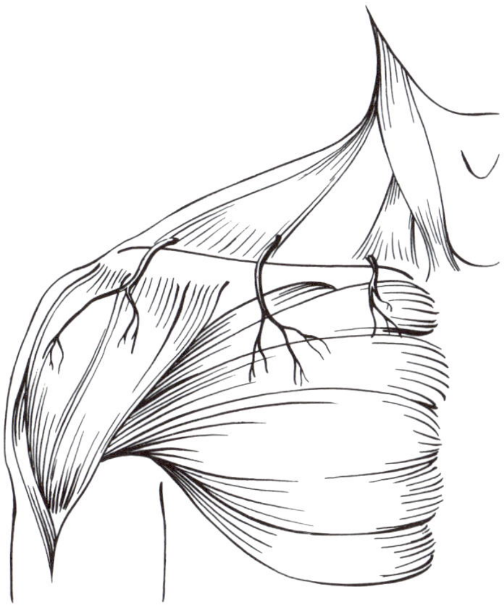

1
The sensory nerves of the skin (supraclavicular nerves) cross the clavicle from rostral to caudal. Therefore it is preferable to make a vertical skin incision.

Approach

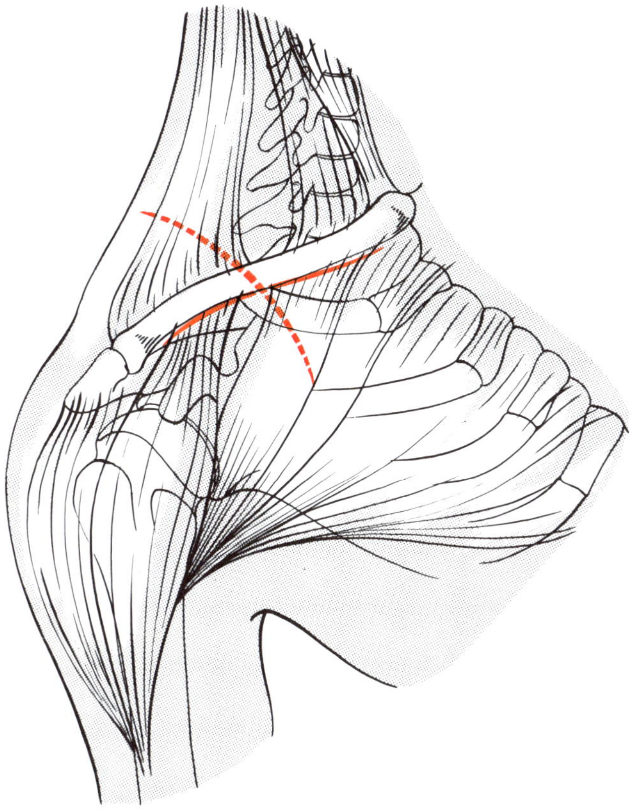

2
The sagittal incision is more favorable than one running parallel to the inferior border of the clavicle.

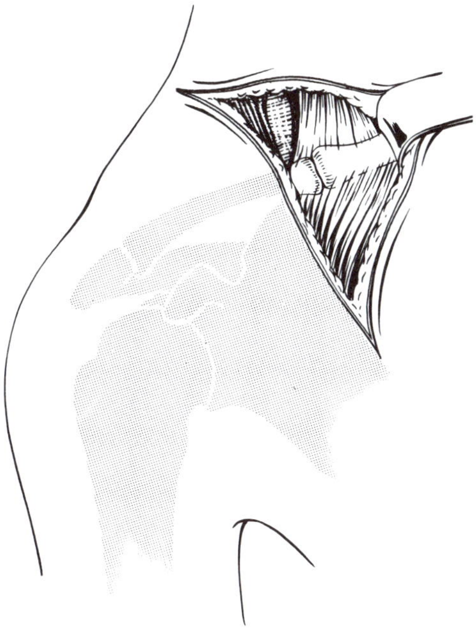

3
The soft structures overlying the fascia are mobilized *medialward*...

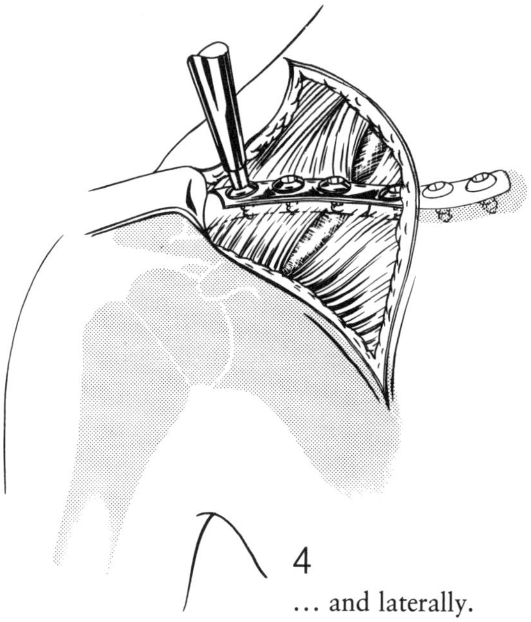

4
... and laterally.

Tactics

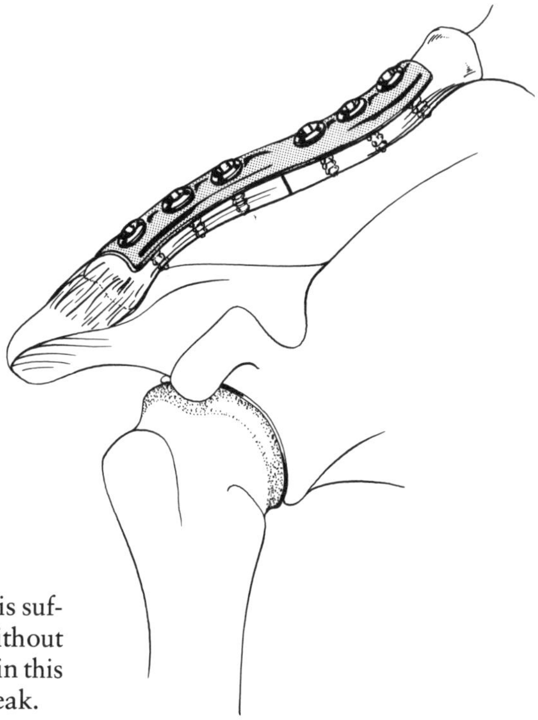

5
The plate of choice is the half-tubular plate. This is sufficiently flexible and possesses enough stability without unduly filling up the soft tissues which are sparse in this location. A third-tubular plate would be too weak.

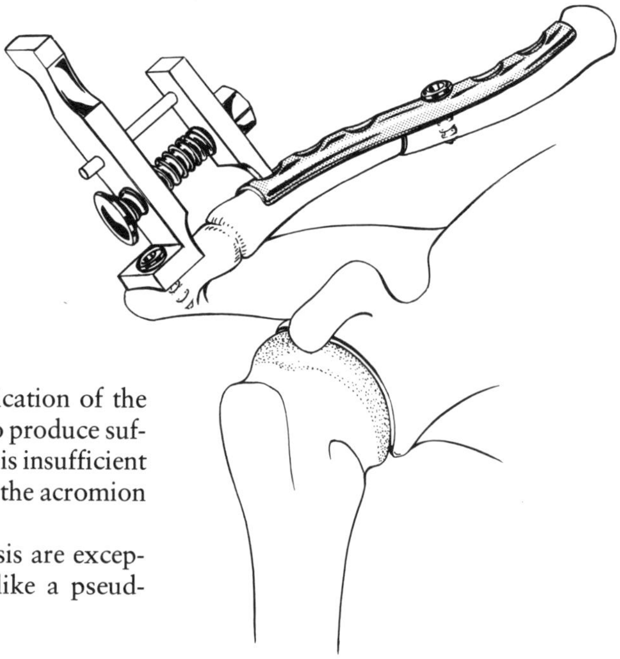

6
With use of the half-tubular plate, application of the plate tightener is indispensable in order to produce sufficiently strong compression. When there is insufficient space, the instrument can be mounted on the acromion without adverse consequences.
Fresh fractures requiring an osteosynthesis are exceptional. Such a case is then dealt with like a pseudarthrosis.

4. Acromioclavicular Joint

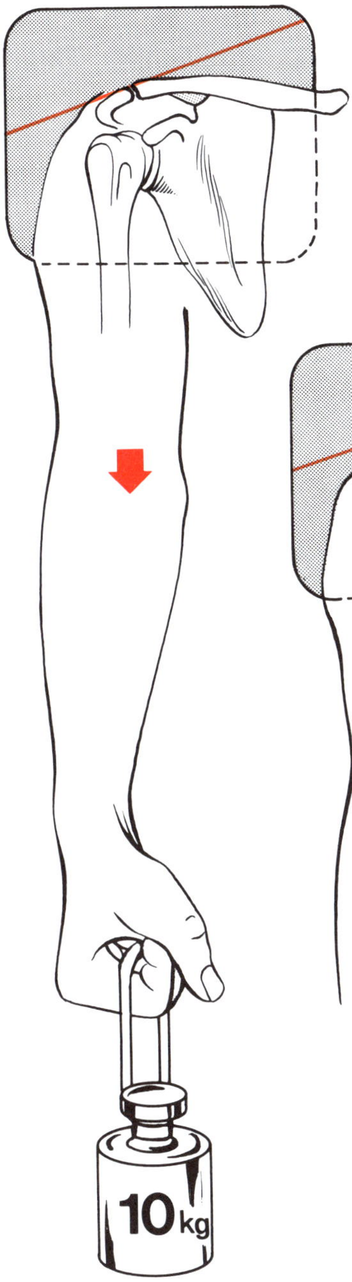

Diagnosis

1

In the absence of injury the tip of the acromion aligns with the lateral end of the clavicle, even under weight bearing.

Indication

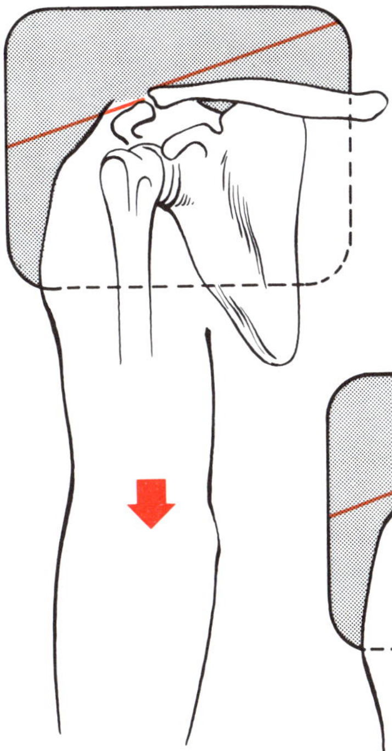

2

Displacement amounting to less than the breadth of the clavicular shaft constitutes no indication for surgical intervention.

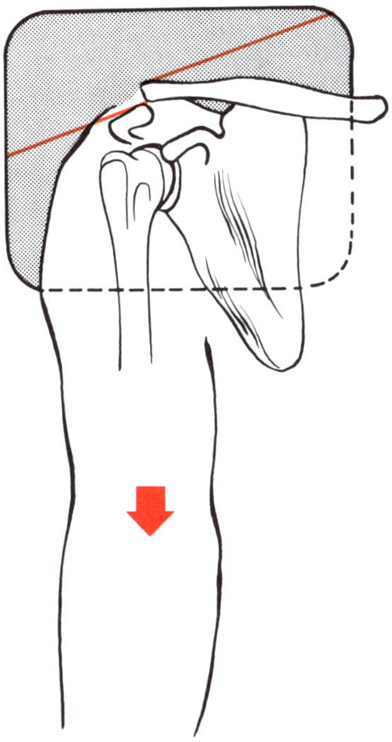

3

Displacement amounting to the breadth of the clavicular shaft or more is an absolute indication for surgery.

Principle

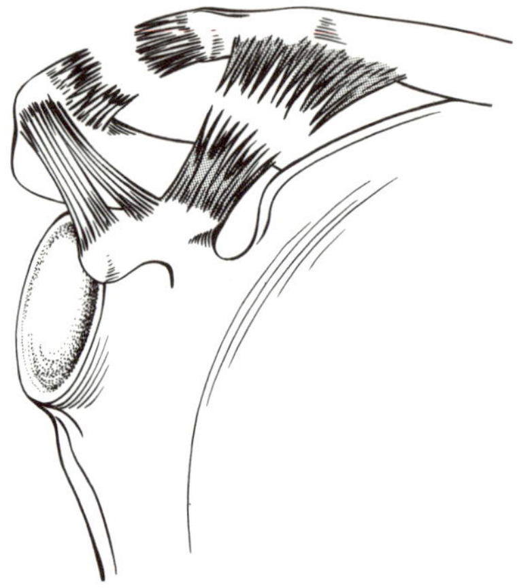

4
In complete dislocation – which in itself requires operative management – the coracoclavicular ligament also is always torn and must be sutured. Wiring serves only to protect the suture.

Anatomy

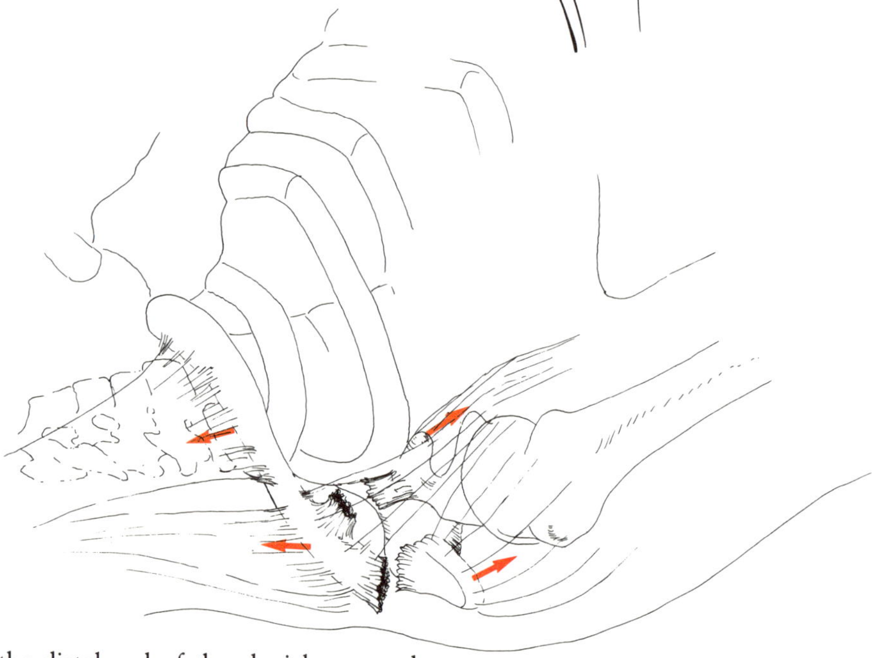

5
The sternocleidomastoid muscle pulls the distal end of the clavicle upward, while gravity pulls the shoulder girdle downward.

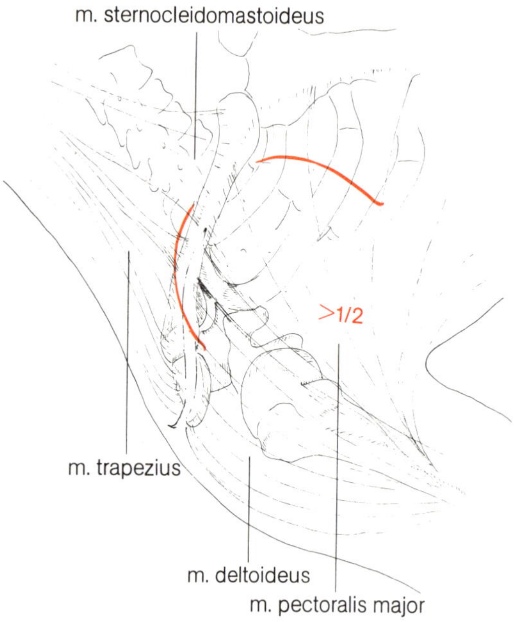

Approach

6
Sagittal or S-shaped skin incision, encircling the acromion and carried a short distance beneath the clavicle.

Tactics

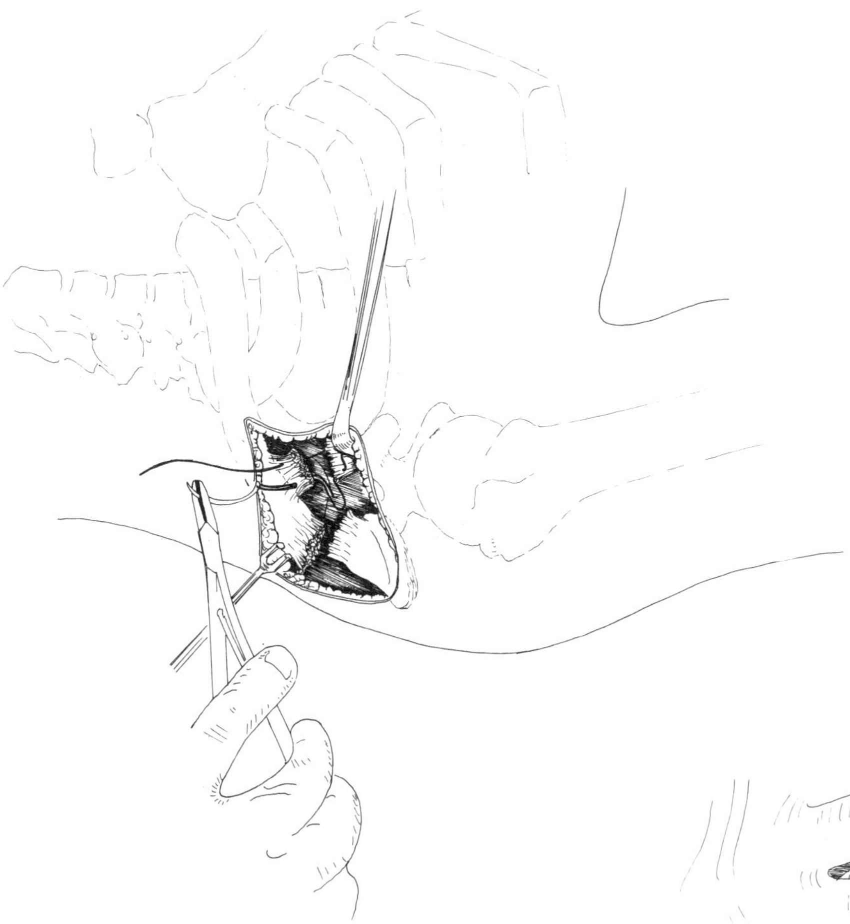

7

Prior to applying the wire, the suture (consisting on a strong nonabsorbable thread) is placed through the stumps of the coracoclavicular ligament, but it is not yet tied.

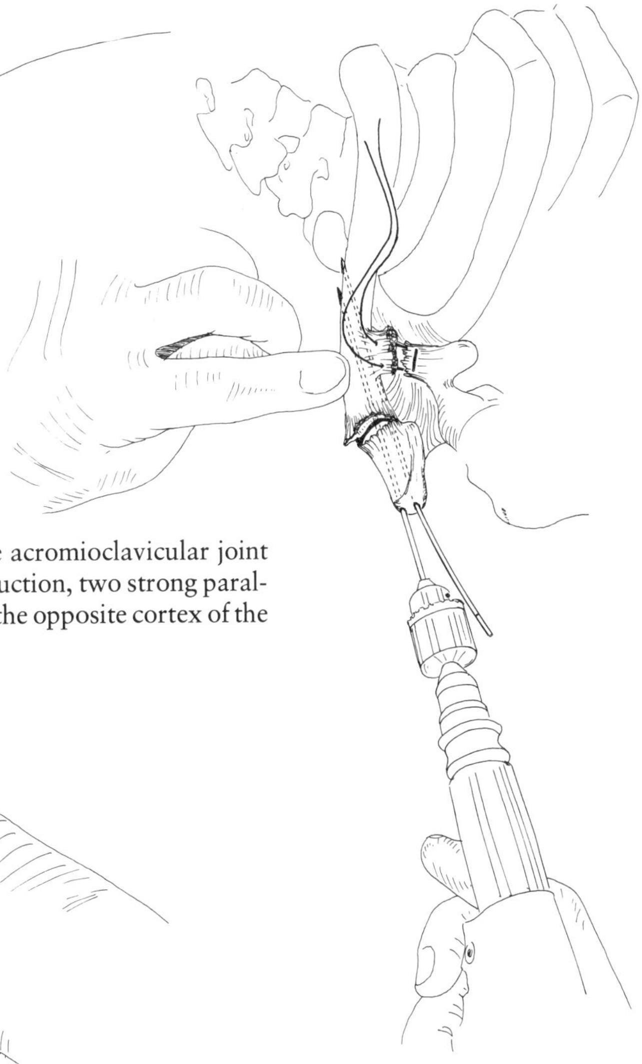

8

Inverted remains of the joint capsule are removed from the acromioclavicular joint and sutured after the wiring has been applied. Following reduction, two strong parallel wires are bored in; the points of the wires are anchored in the opposite cortex of the clavicle.

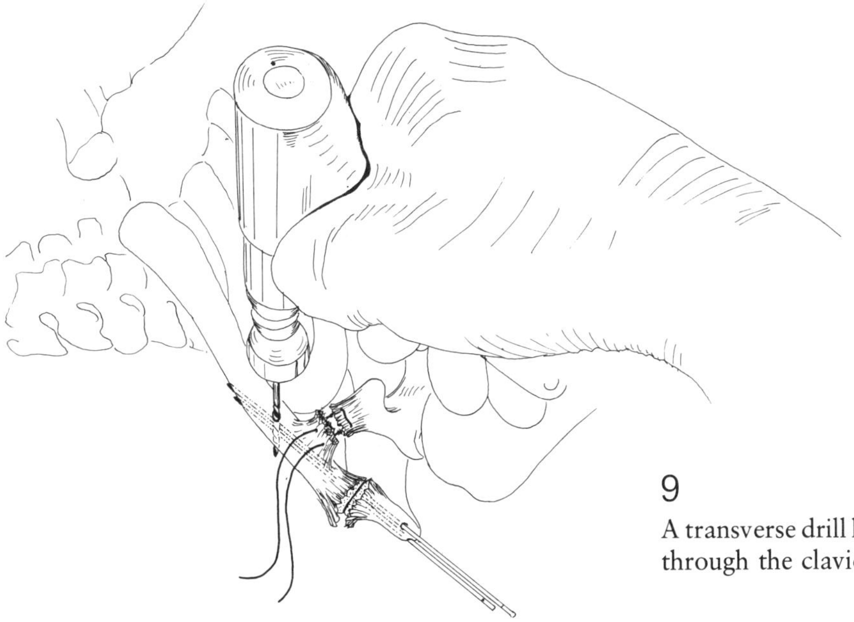

9

A transverse drill hole (made by using a 2 mm drill) is created through the clavicle.

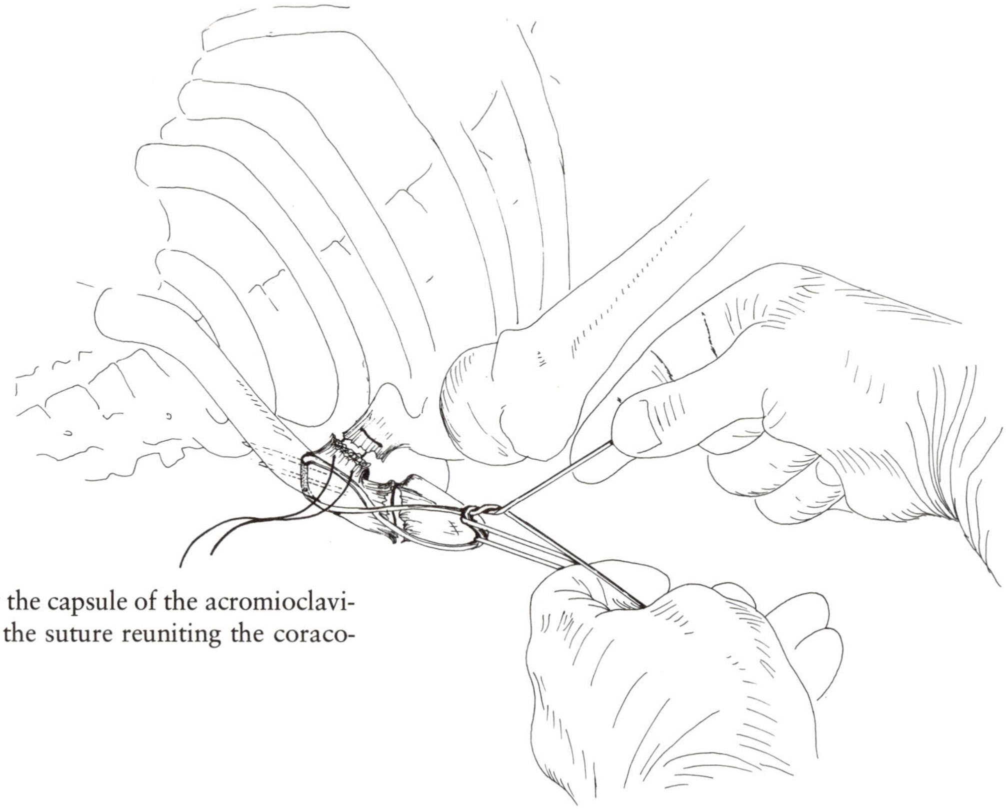

10
The wiring is applied. Now the capsule of the acromioclavicular joint is sewn up and the suture reuniting the coraco-acromial ligament is tied.

Techniques of reconstruction

11
For old axiocervical breaks, cuneiform osteotomy is recommended.

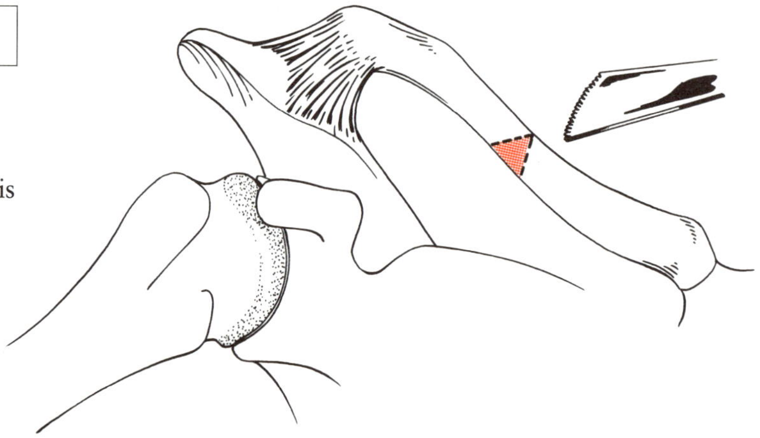

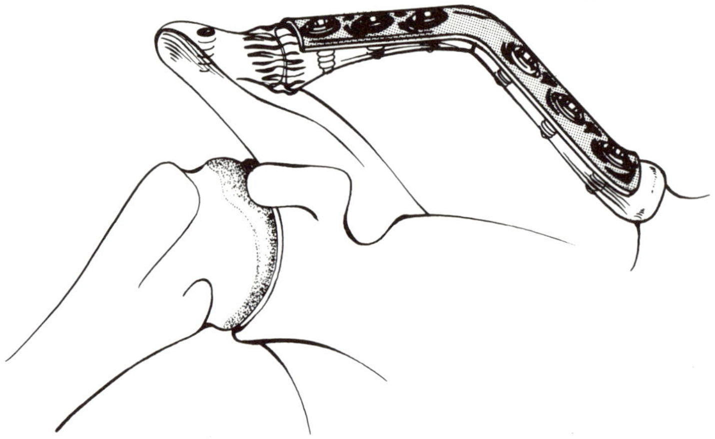

12
In most cases, the joint itself can be left untouched; only occasionally is it necessary to free it from cicatricial tissue so that the peripheral end of the clavicle can properly adjust itself. Fixation with a half-tubular plate.

5. Humerus

Humerus – proximal part

Anatomy

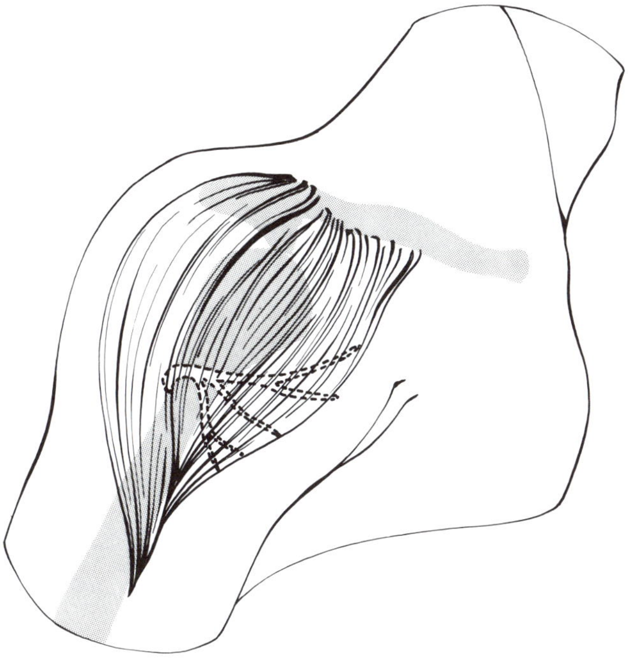

1
The transmuscular approach to the humerus through the deltoid muscle should be avoided by all possible means. Otherwise, the nervous supply of the ventral portions of the deltoid muscle is destroyed.

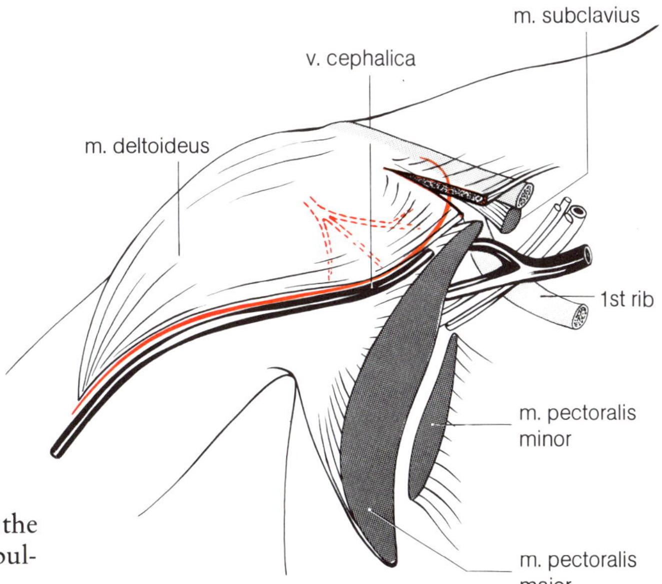

2
Therefore, if necessary, only the clavicular insertion of the deltoid muscle should be notched or partly detached and pulled laterally.

Indication

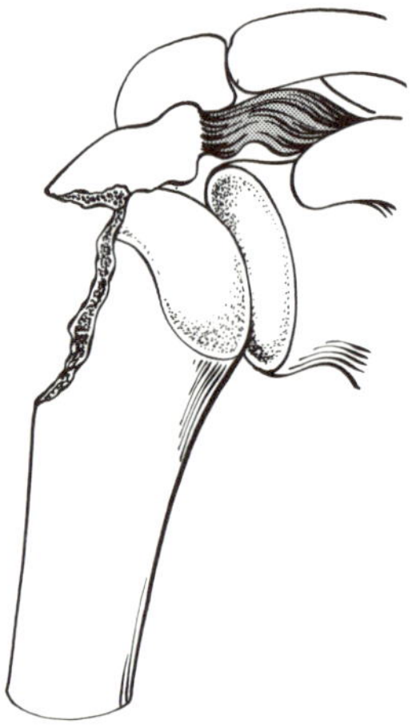

3

Displaced avulsions of the great tuberosity or in its neighborhood: operative management.

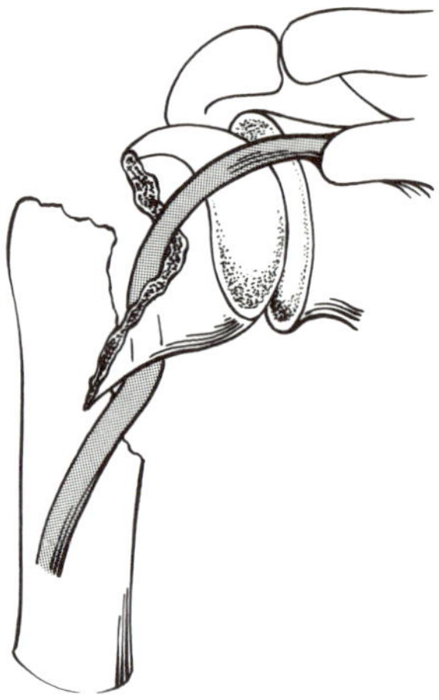

4

Fracture-dislocations with interposition of the long biceps tendon: operative management, no immobilization for patients older than 30.

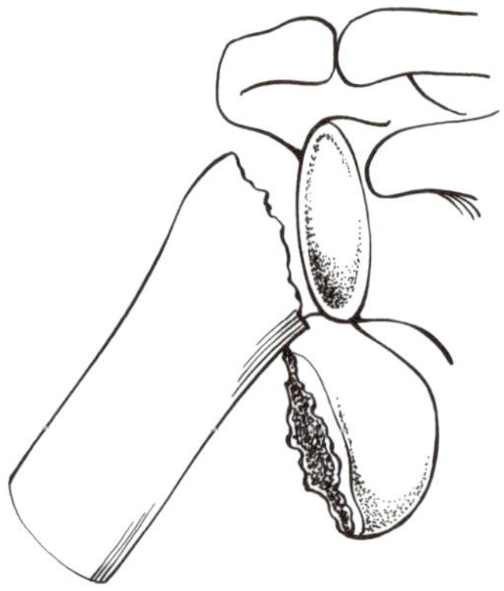

5

Subcapital fractures: as a rule, conservative management. Osteosynthesis may be considered for fracture-dislocations that cannot be reduced under general anesthesia. With conservative management, an immobilizing dressing is to be avoided in patients older than 30.

Operative means ... Principle

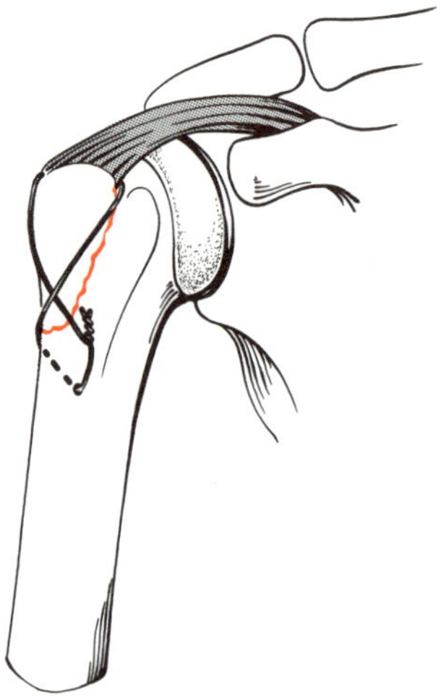

6

Great tuberosity: wire suture, or...

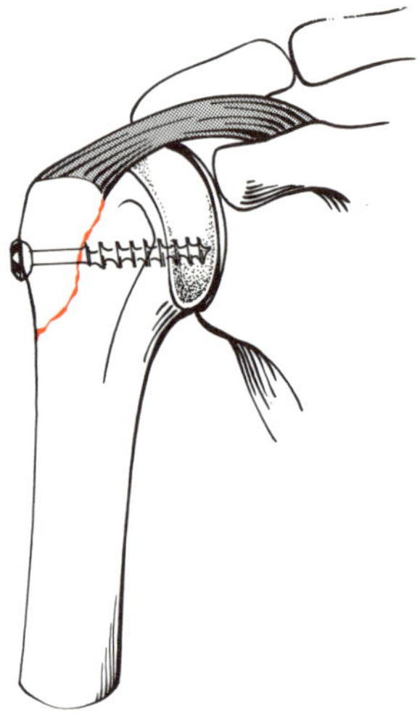

7

... cancellous or cortical screw.

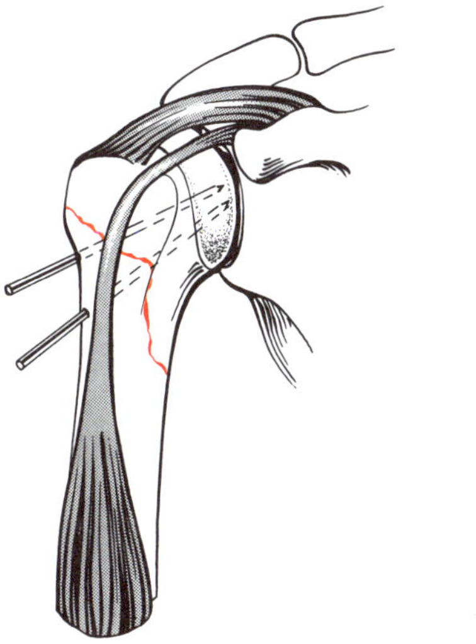

8
Subcapital fracture-dislocation: osteosynthesis with drilling wires, or...

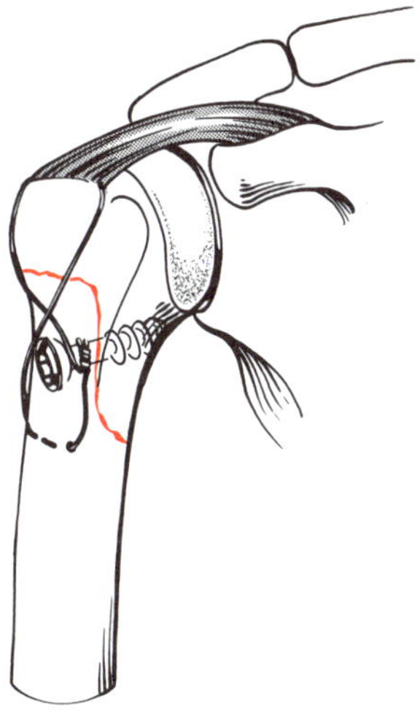

9
... a combination of wiring and screw, or...

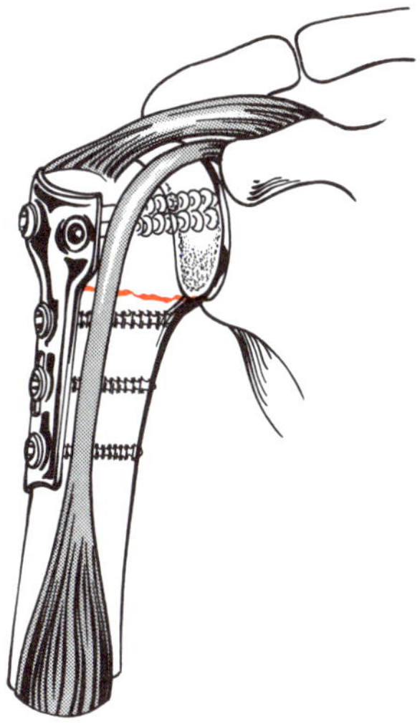

10
... osteosynthesis with use of a T-plate or an L-plate.

Positioning

Supine position. A narrow pillow or roll is placed between the scapulas so that the shoulders can "fall away" to either side.

Approach

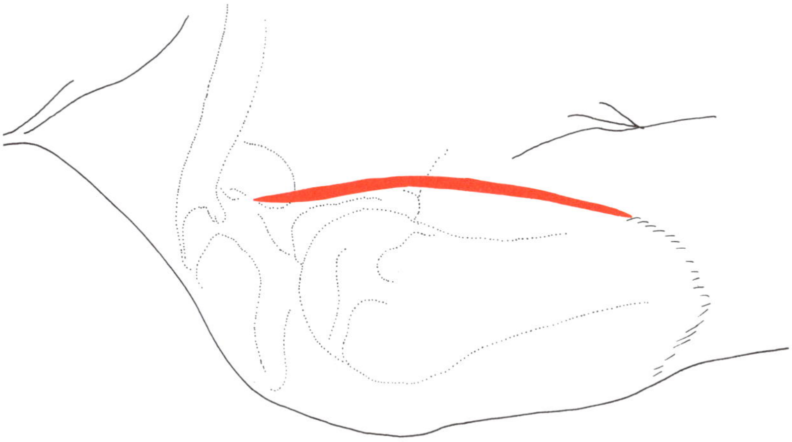

11
Skin incision in the deltoid sulcus (See also Fig. 71–2).

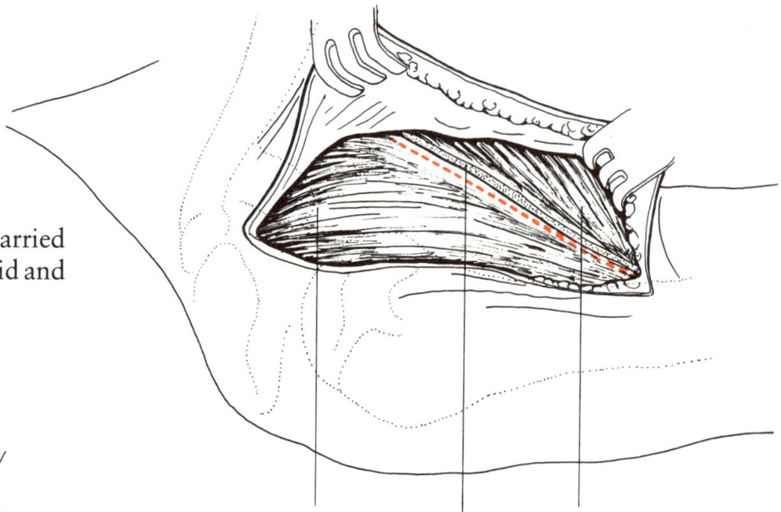

12

The cephalic vein is identified. The incision is carried lateral to the vein in the groove between the deltoid and the pectoralis major muscle.

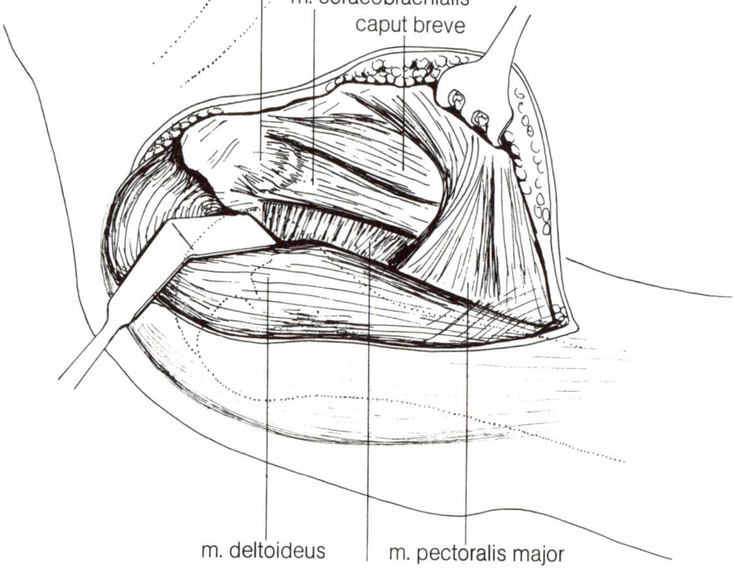

13

One then gets to the insertion of the subscapular muscle, the joint capsule and the tendon of the long head of the biceps muscle.

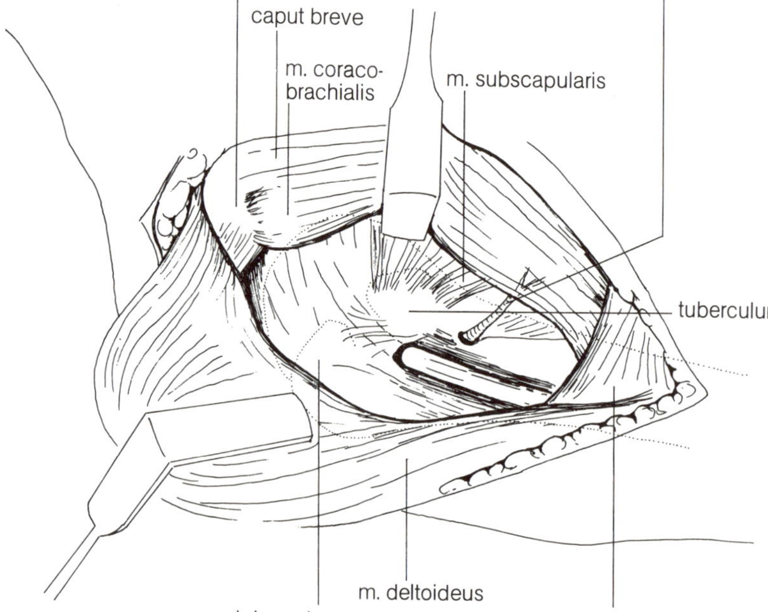

14

By rotating the arm internally, the tendon of the long head of the biceps becomes accessible. The incision can be extended distally, as shown in Figs. 83–22 ff.

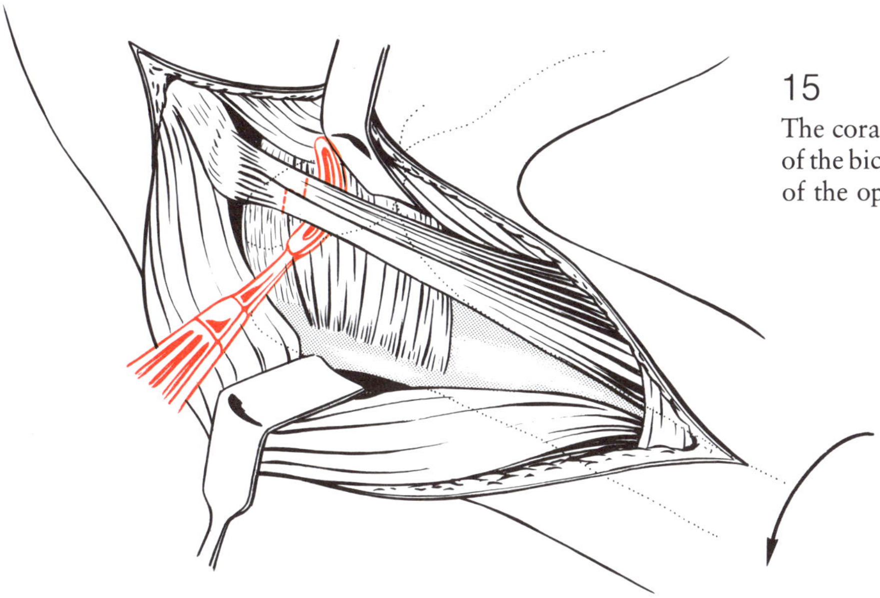

15

The coracobrachialis muscle and the short head of the biceps can be detached to gain a fuller view of the operative field.

16

It is often necessary to detach the subscapularis muscle to gain sufficient access to the joint and, above all, to the inferior margin of the glenoid. The muscle then is marked with retention sutures medial to the proposed line of separation. To this end the arm is externally rotated.

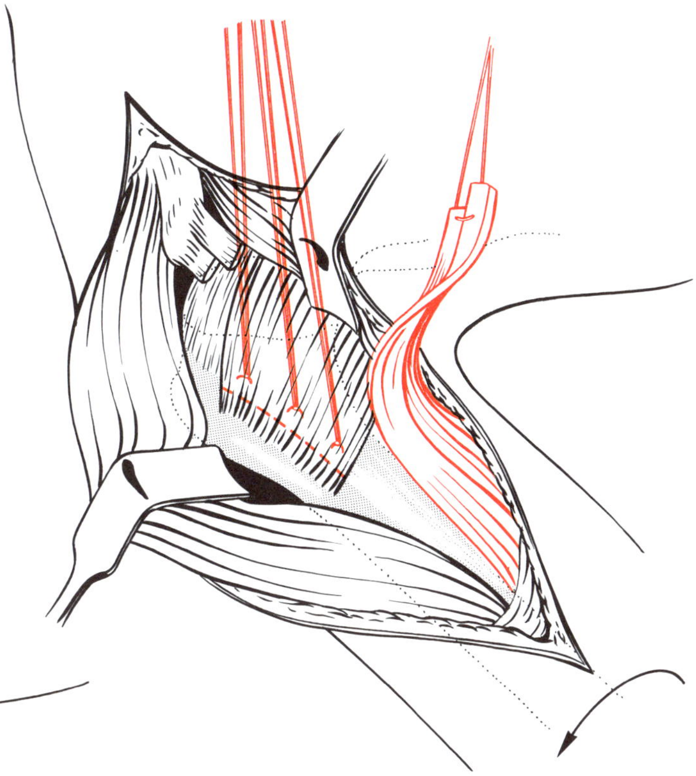

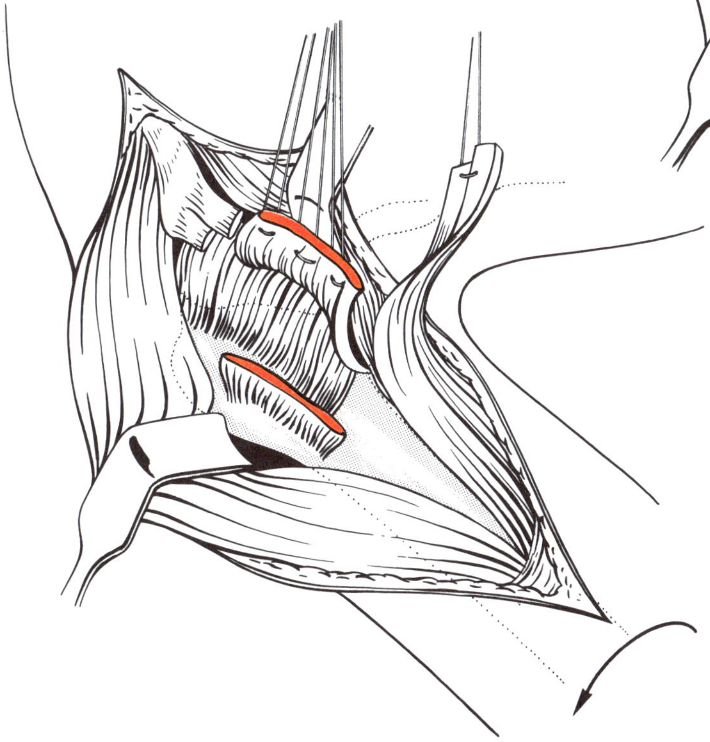

17

When the subscapularis muscle is turned back, the joint capsule appears. Now the glenoid margin can be readily palpated through the capsule and the operator is enabled to get a proper orientation on the anatomical relationships.

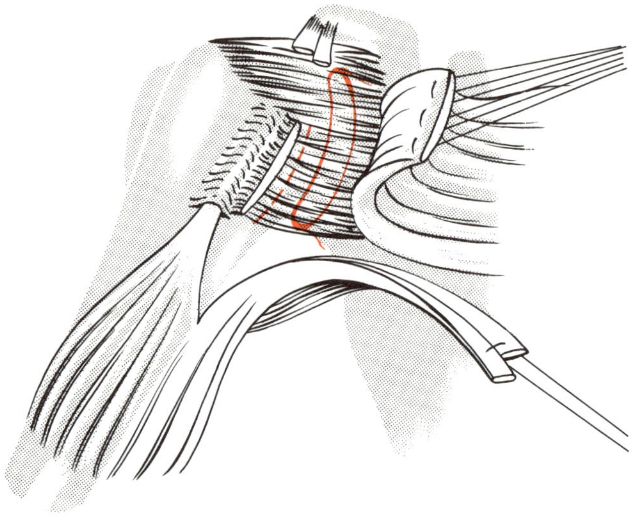

18

The capsule is opened parallel to the glenoid margin, leaving a narrow border for resuturing. The later suture of the capsule is best undertaken in overlapping fashion with concomitant plication.

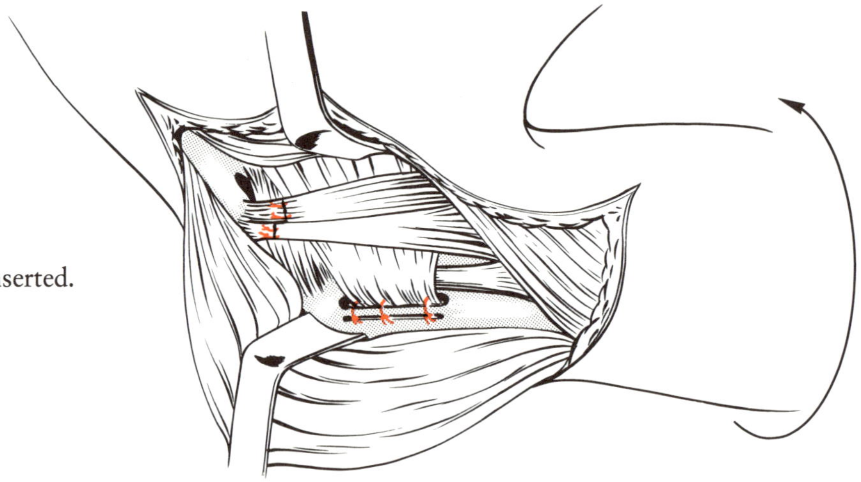

19

The severed muscle attachments are reinserted.

Tactics

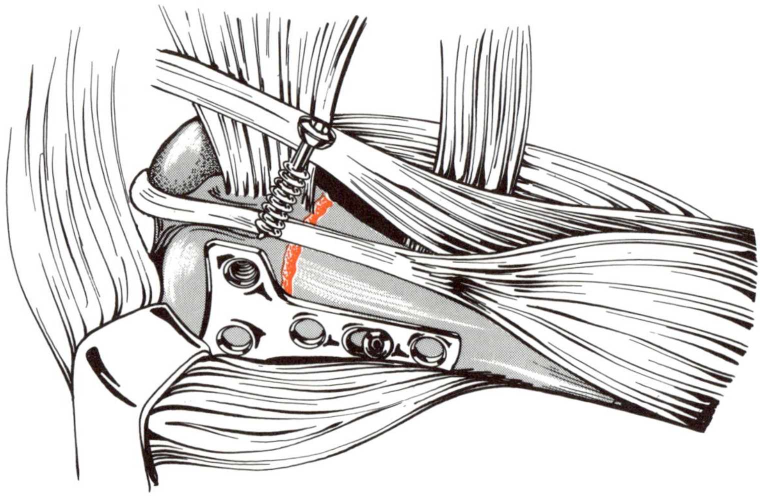

20

The T-plate should be applied lateral to the intertubercular groove. If this is not feasible, the long biceps tendon can be detached from its origin; subsequently, however, it must be reinserted in the region of the coracoid process.
Following reduction of the fracture, the plate is fastened with a screw in the oval screw hole, the screw being placed in the distal part of the hole. Only then are drill holes made in the head of the humerus and the cancellous screws fitted.

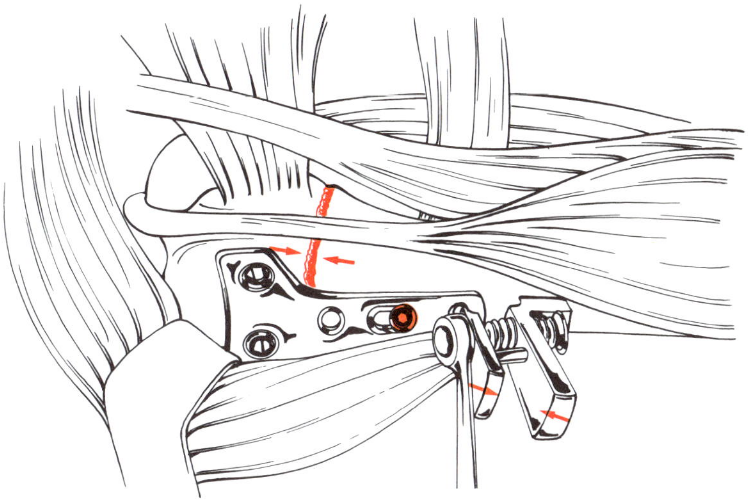

21

The plate tightener is mounted and the plate is tightened. Owing to the oval shape of the hole, the plate – together with the humeral head – can be pressed on the distal fragment without the previously-inserted screw needing to be removed.

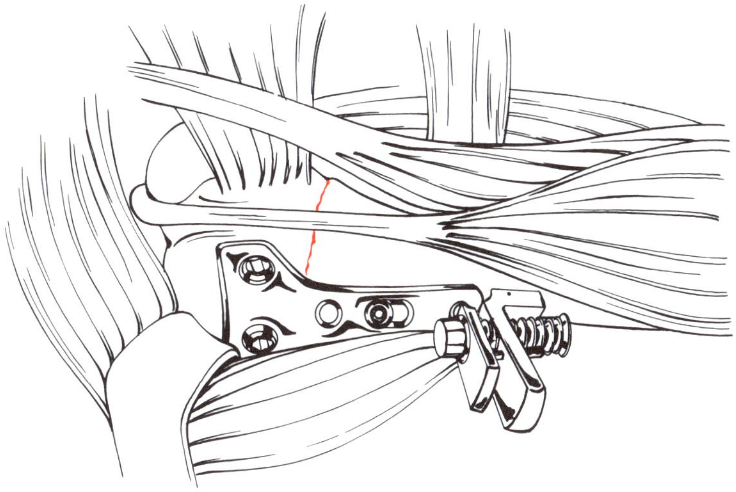

22

When the plate is tightened the previously-inserted screw lies in the proximal part of the oval hole in the plate.

Humerus – middle part

Types of injuries

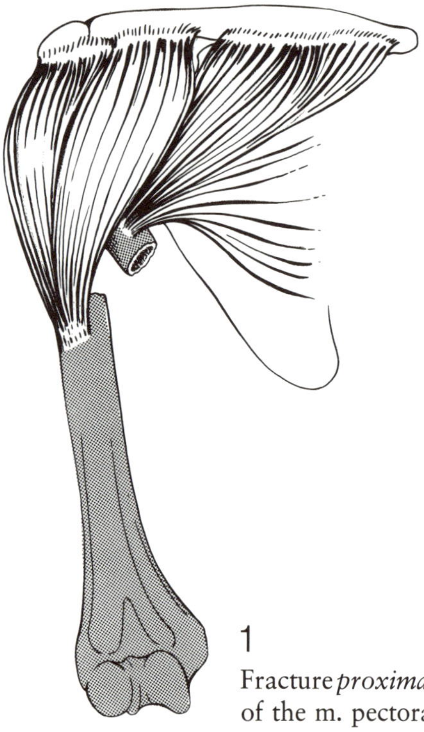

1
Fracture *proximal* to the attachment of the m. pectoralis.

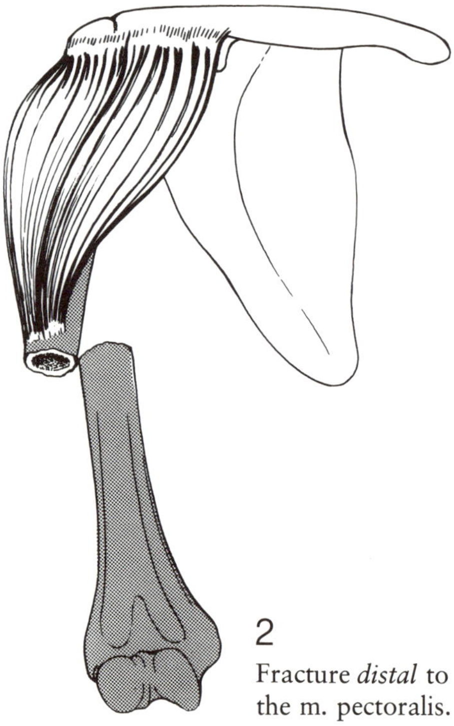

2
Fracture *distal* to the attachment of the m. pectoralis.

Indication

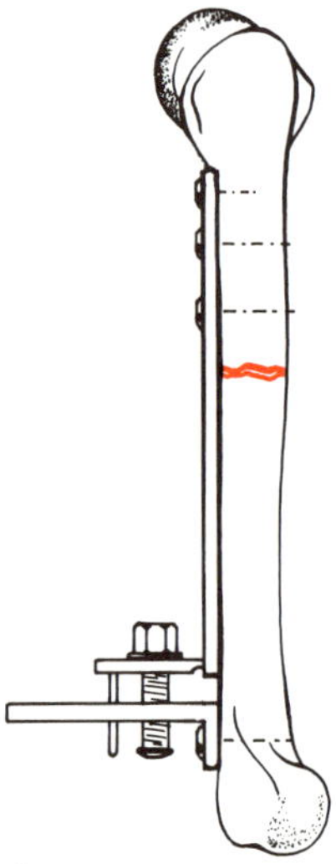

3
Operative: Transverse fractures.

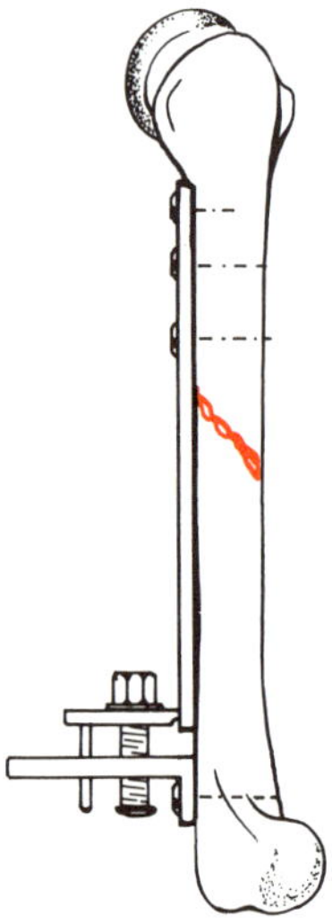

4
Operative: Short oblique fractures.

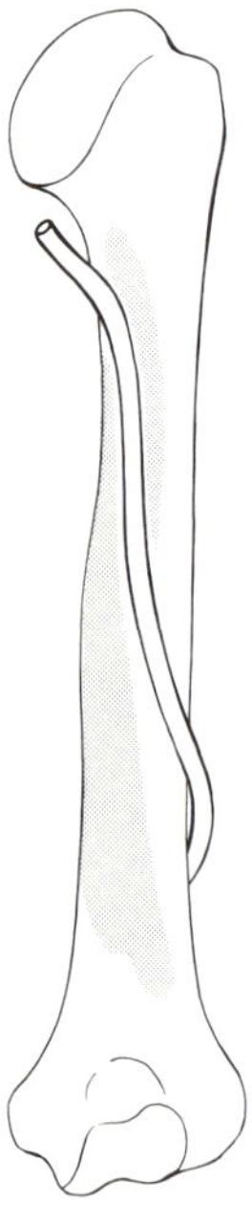

5
Operative: Involvement of nerves or disorders of circulation.

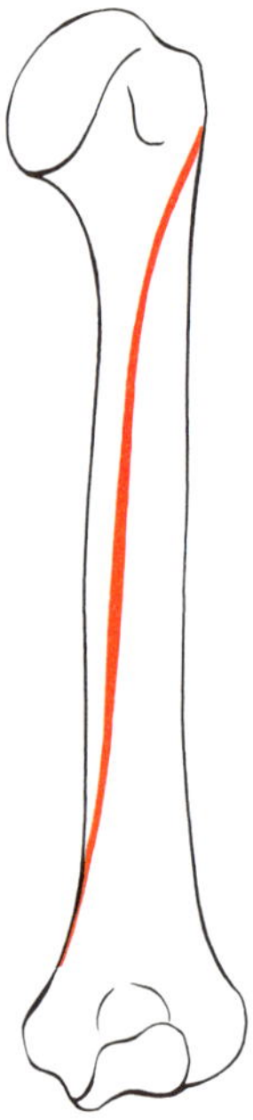

6
Conservative (e.g., hanging cast): Long oblique fractures, fractures with multiple fragments and comminuted fractures.

Positioning

Supine position:

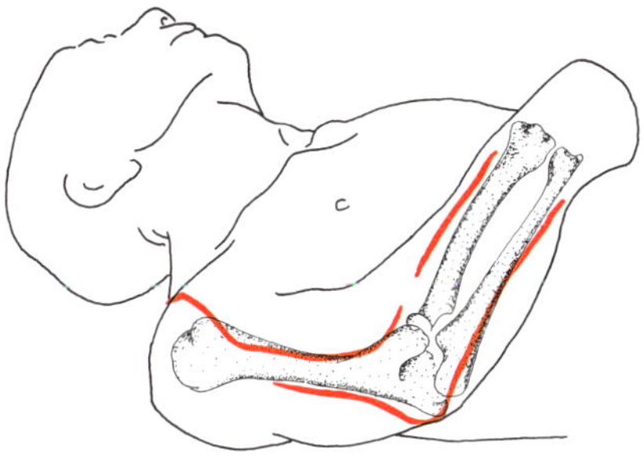

7

Advantages:
- Anesthesia not problematic
- Sterility not problematic
- Reduction maneuvers easy
- All modes of approach possible

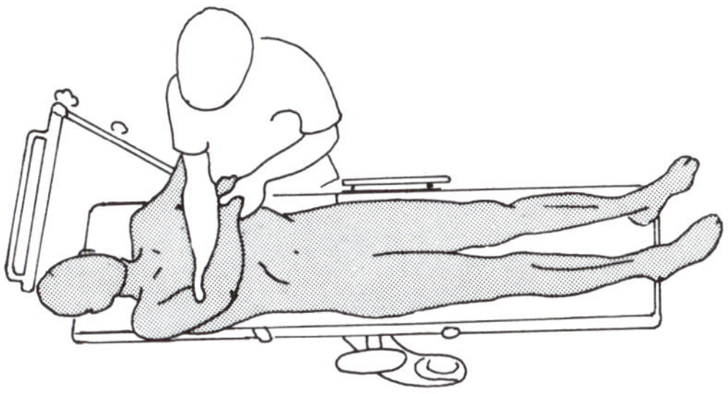

8

Disadvantage:
- Assistance exacting

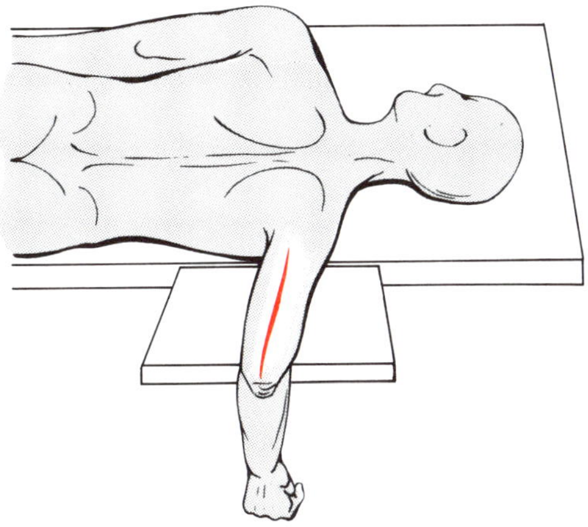

Prone position:

9

Advantage:
- Little dependence on assistants. Consequently, operative field commonly unimpaired.

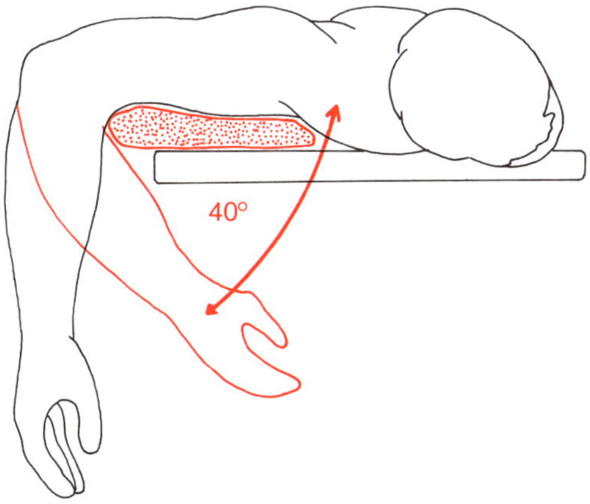

10

Disadvantages:
- Problems in anesthesia
- Problems of sterility, owing to the deeply dependent position of the hand
- Only dorsal approach possible

Dorsal approach

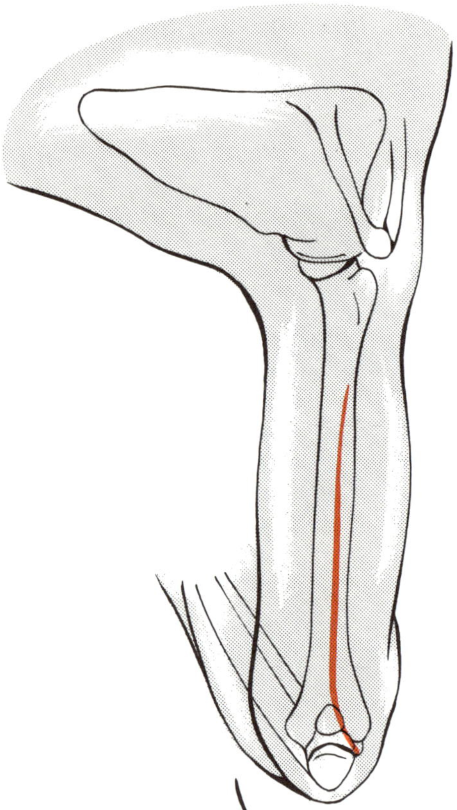

11

Skin incision of adequate length, i.e., sufficient for broad 8-hole plate plus plate tightener.

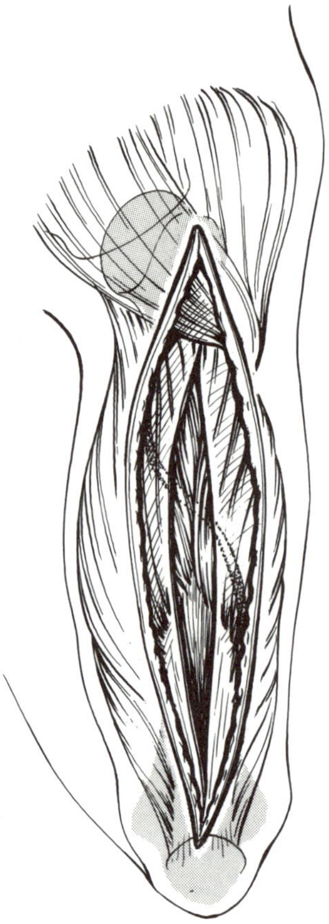

12

First, careful hemostasis, then splitting of the fascia and the triceps tendon.

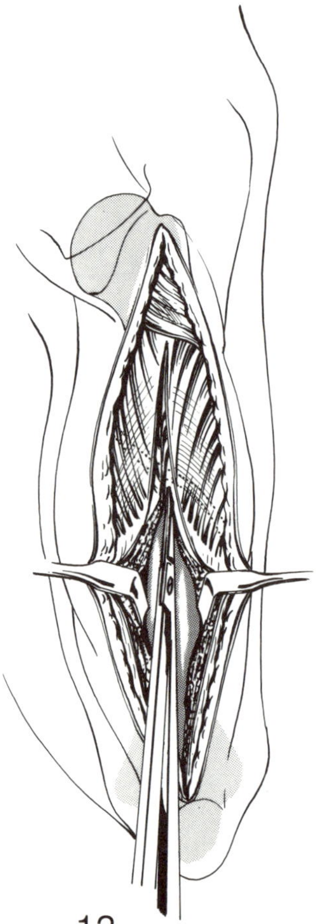

13

Proximally, the muscle fibers are then separated (not severed), layer after layer, with the slightly opened scissors and under direct vision, beginning from the surface. Any bleeding must be controlled.

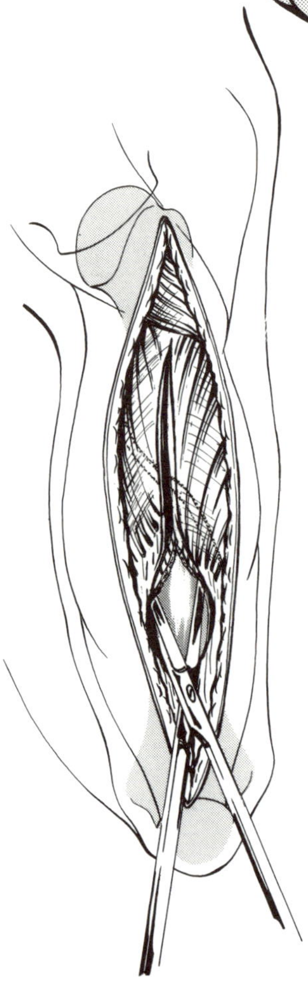

14

In the distal half of the wound the scissors penetrate between the muscle fibers toward the bone. On the bone, the scissors are opened transversely to the direction of the muscle fibers and retractors are inserted step by step.

15

In between, one feels repeatedly for the pencil-thick cord of the radial nerve.

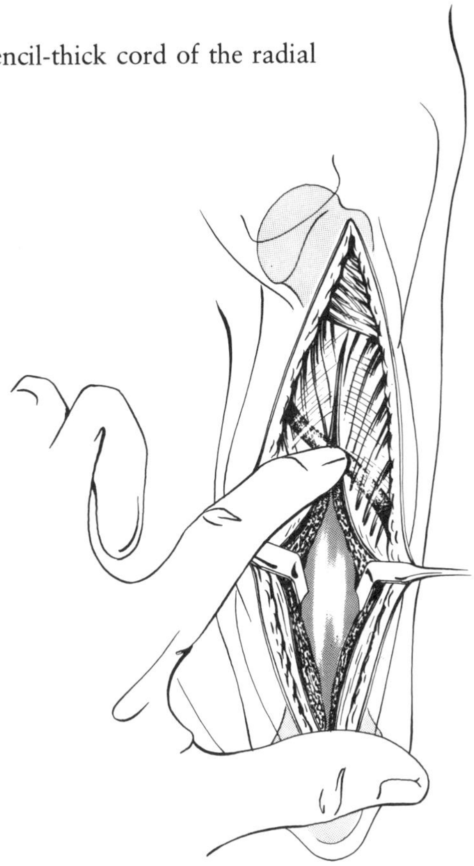

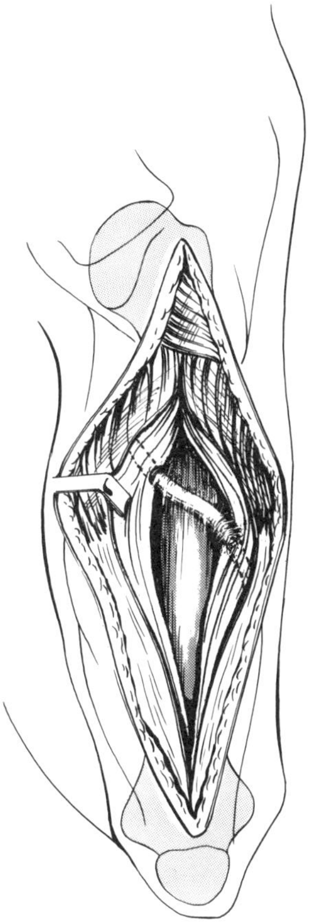

16

Finally, the whitish cord of the radial nerve becomes palpable and visible between the muscle fibers, often heralded by injury of one of its small companion vessels.

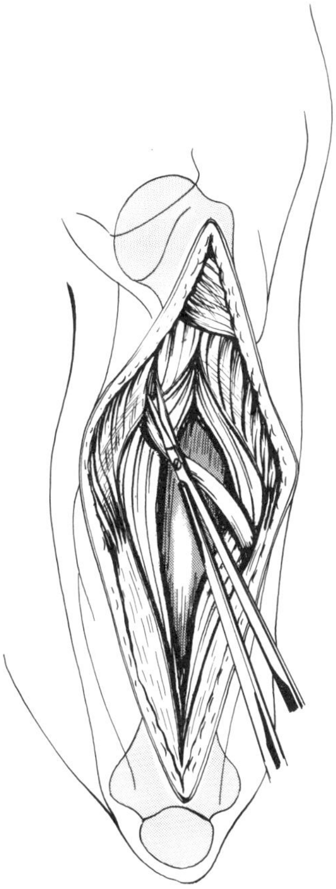

17

The nerve is not isolated over its entire length but only confidently identified in one location. The entire cord (consisting of nerve, companion vessels and enveloping connective tissue) is undermined and sufficiently isolated medially and proximally, as well as laterally and distally, so that it can be adequately mobilized and transposed.

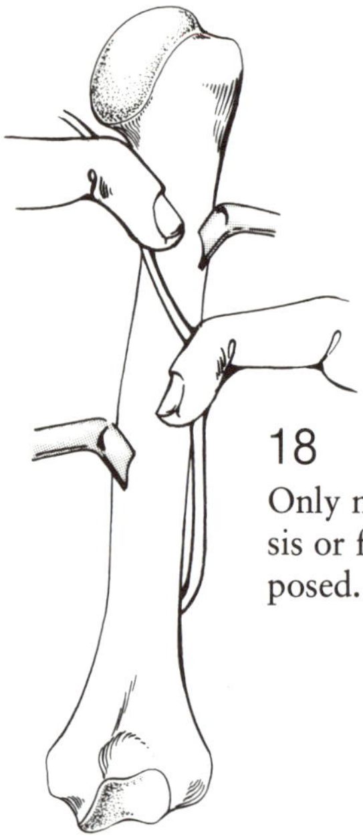

18
Only now is the pseudarthrosis or fracture located and exposed.

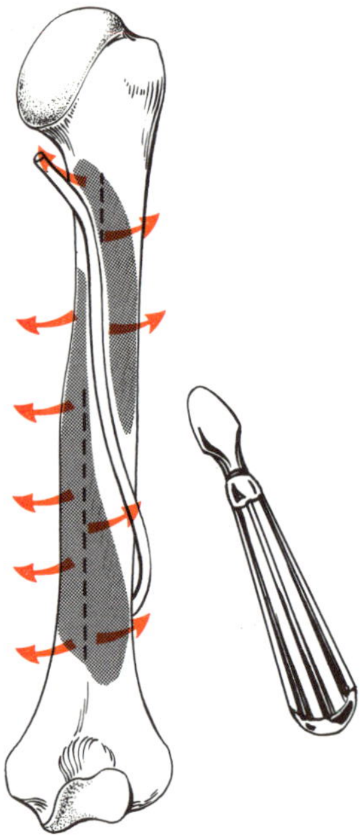

19
The medial head of the muscle is split and pushed away to expose the distal and the middle part of the posterior surface of the humerus. The same procedure is applied to the lateral head to expose the proximal part of the posterior surface of the humerus.

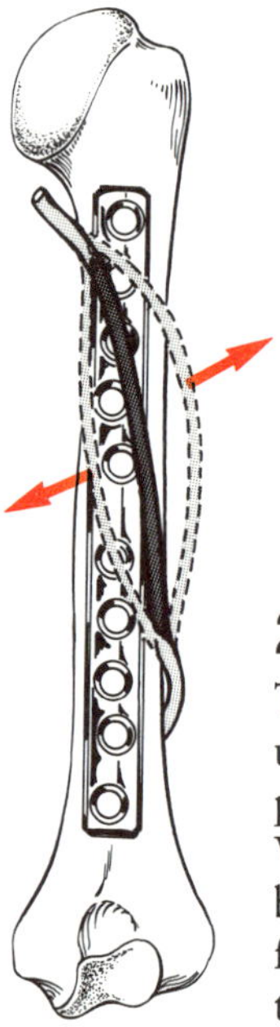

20
The radial nerve can be lifted up without difficulty and a plate fitted underneath it. When the nerve is tense it can be transposed between the fragments to the volar side of the humerus.

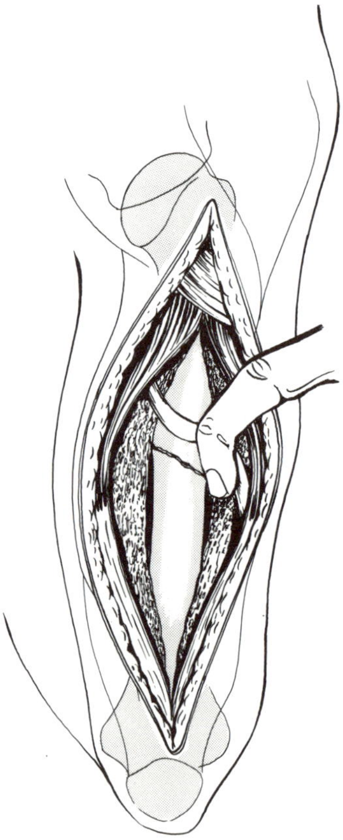

21
No retractors, let alone elevators, should be used on the side of the nerve, much as one may be tempted to do so. The fingers are much gentler and thus safer.

Lateral approach

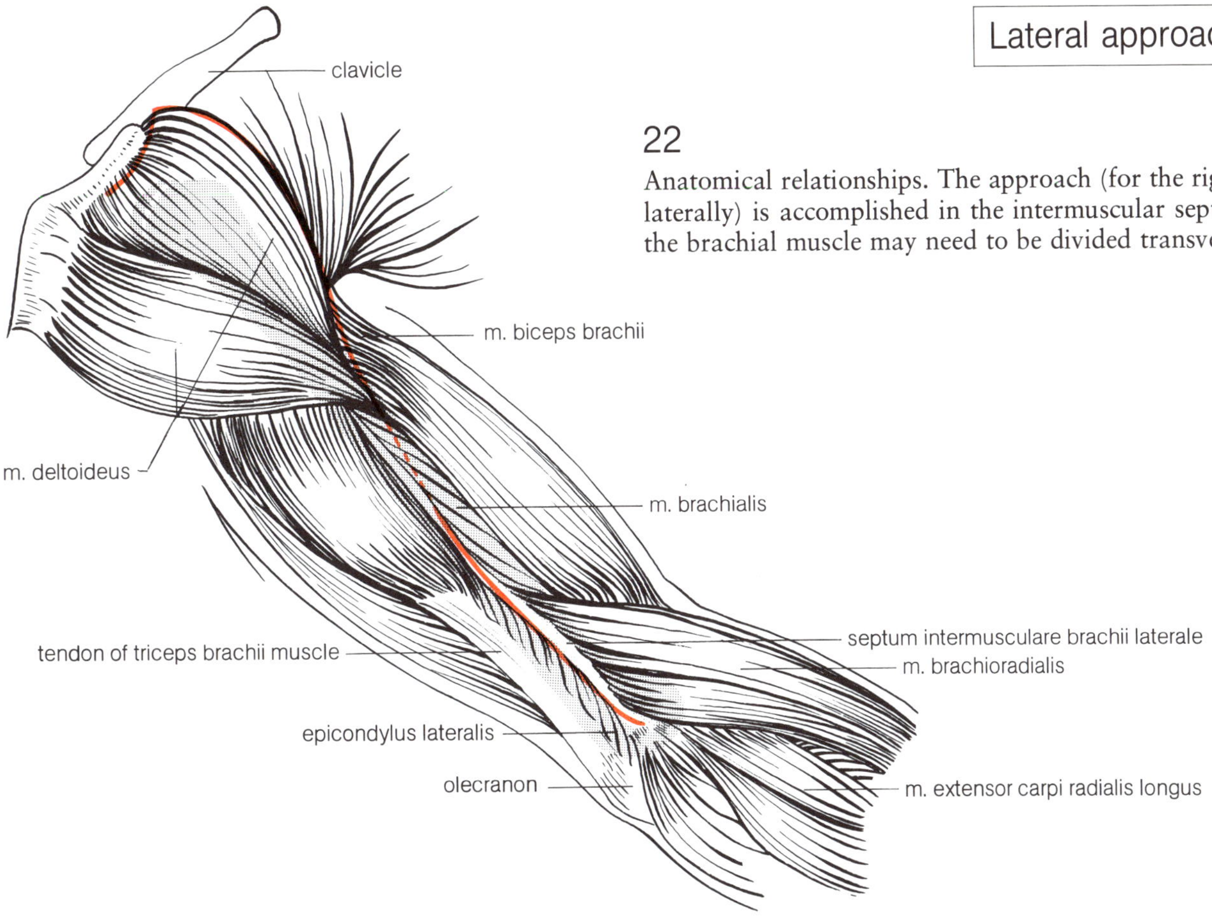

22

Anatomical relationships. The approach (for the right arm, laterally) is accomplished in the intermuscular septa. Only the brachial muscle may need to be divided transversely.

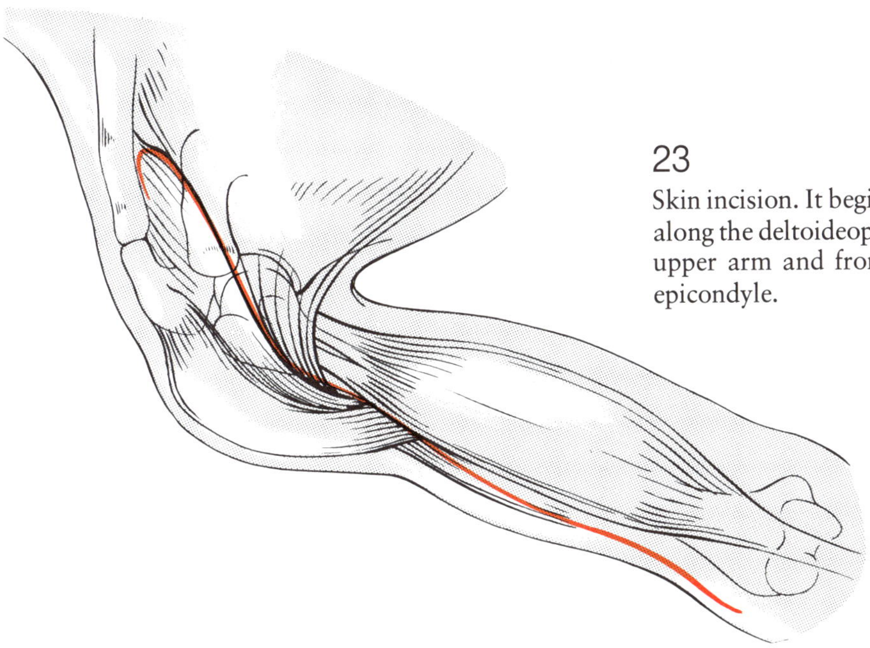

23

Skin incision. It begins at the clavicle, and is carried in an arc along the deltoideopectoral groove to the lateral aspect of the upper arm and from there in a straight line to the lateral epicondyle.

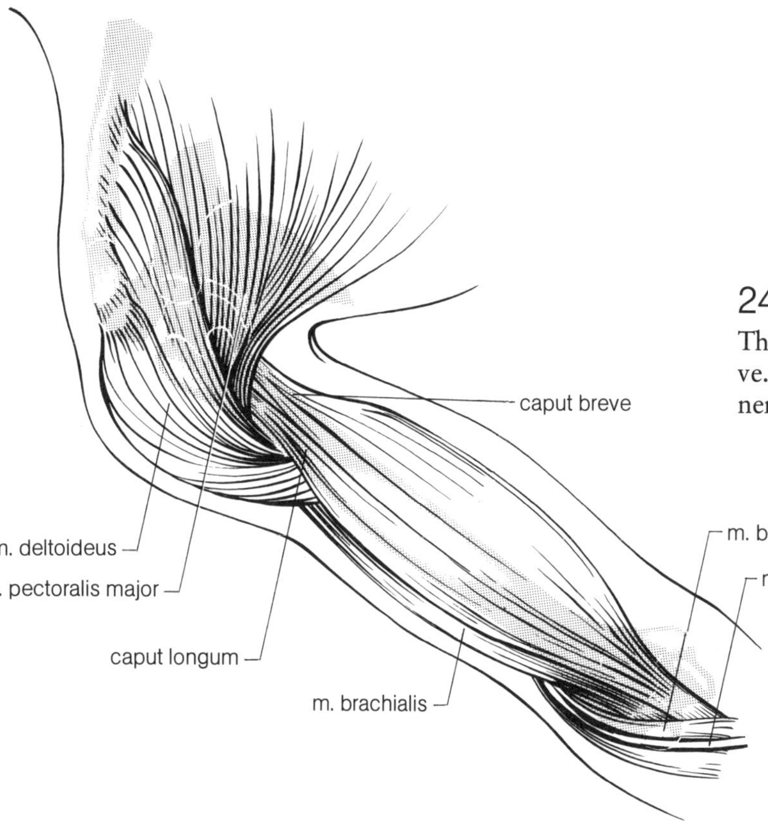

24

The brachioradial muscle protects the radial nerve. Until the brachial muscle is divided, the radial nerve is only endangered by pull on the retractor.

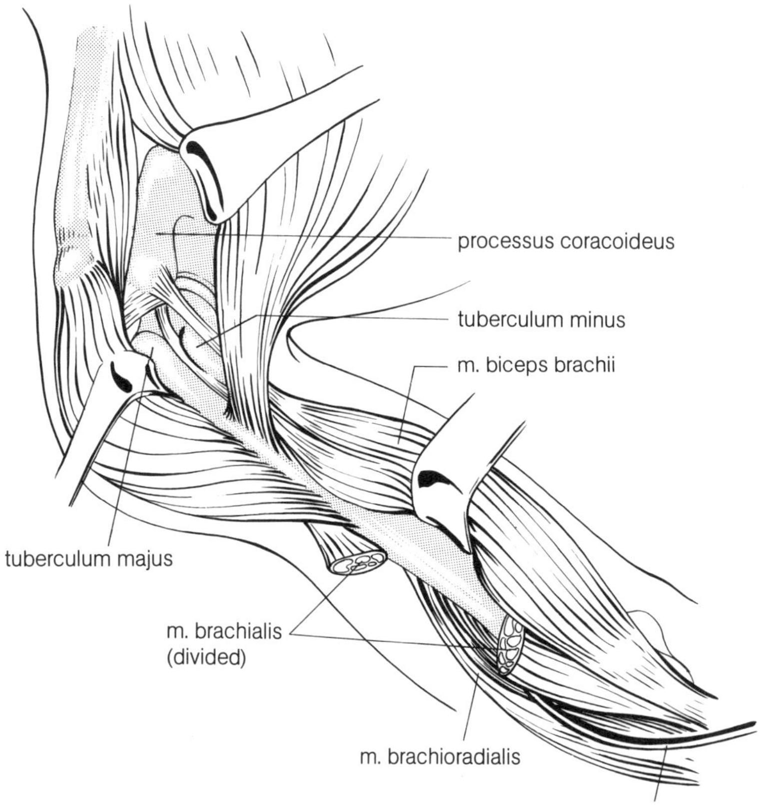

25

After the brachial muscle has been divided, the radial nerve is identified. The lateral surface of the humerus is exposed.

Humerus – distal part

Types of injuries

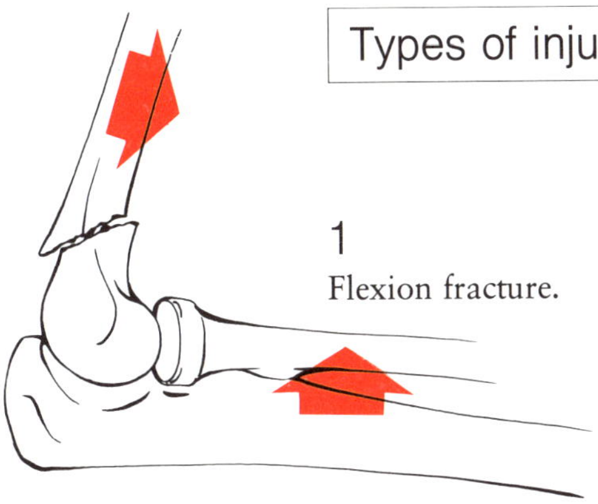

1
Flexion fracture.

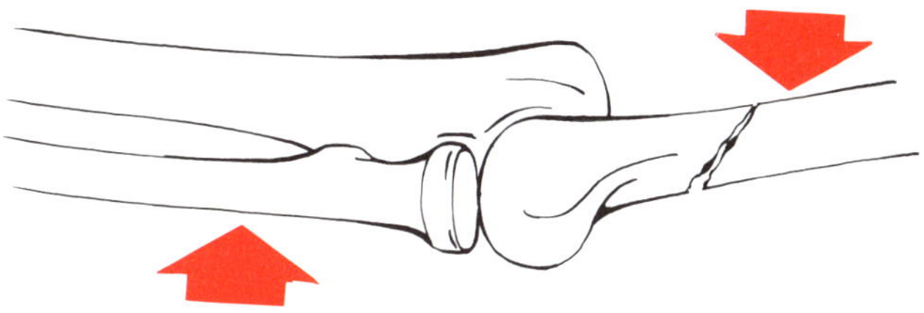

2
Hyperextension fracture.

Indication

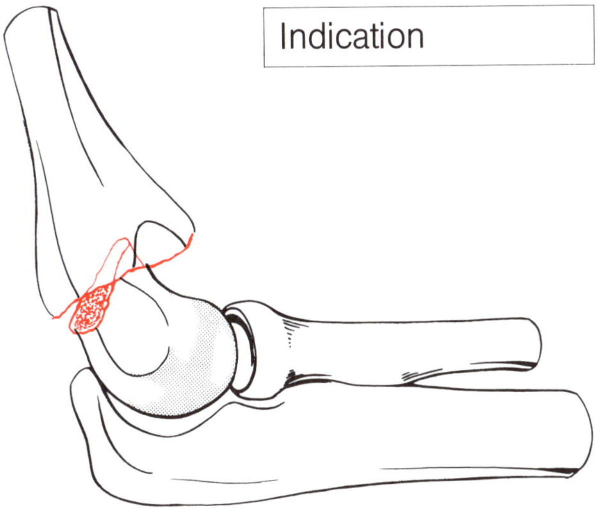

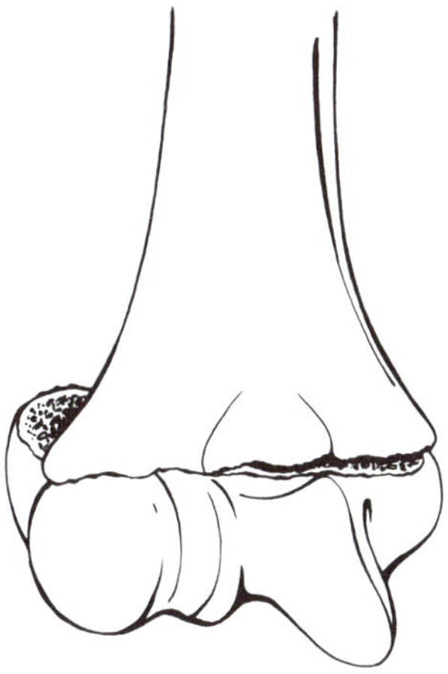

3 and 4

- Rotary deformity. This type of injury is the most difficult to correct. In the lateral roentgenogram it is manifested as a thorn-like projection of the proximal end of the fragment on the flexor side. When the deformity exceeds 10° (which can hardly be ascertained without operative exposure) open reduction should be performed.
- Disorders of arterial circulation and neural disturbances.
- Combination with intra-articular fractures (p. 101 ff.).

Timing of the operation

The most favorable moment is within the first 12 to 24 hours.

Operative possibilities

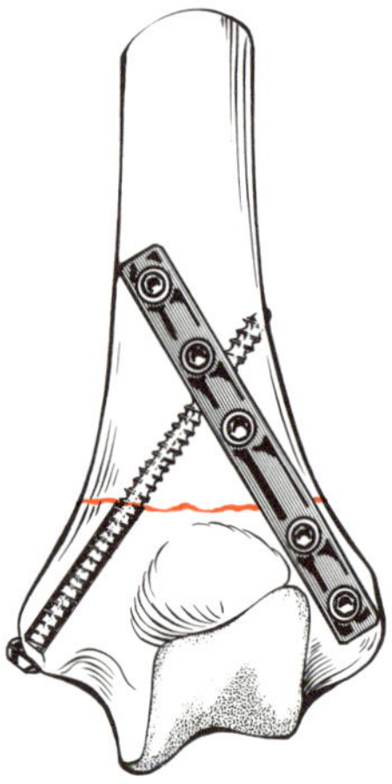

5
Osteosynthesis of the radial pillar with a plate, and with a screw in the ulnar pillar, if necessary with additional transposition of the ulnar nerve (See Fig. 87–9 f.).

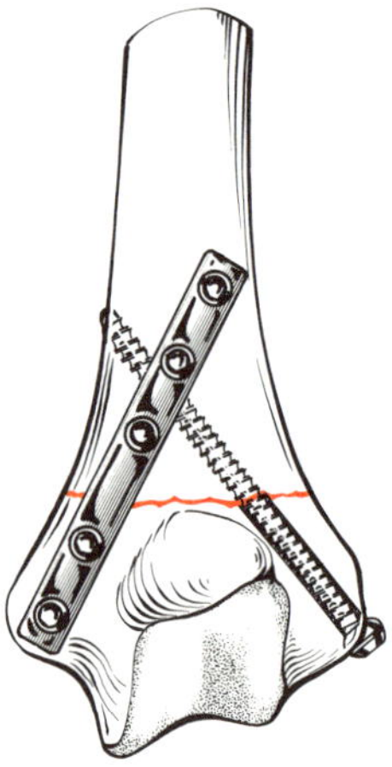

6
Osteosynthesis of the ulnar pillar with a plate, and with a screw in the radial pillar, if necessary combined with transposition of the ulnar nerve (Figs. 87–9 f.).

Principle

See also Figs. 102–6 ff.

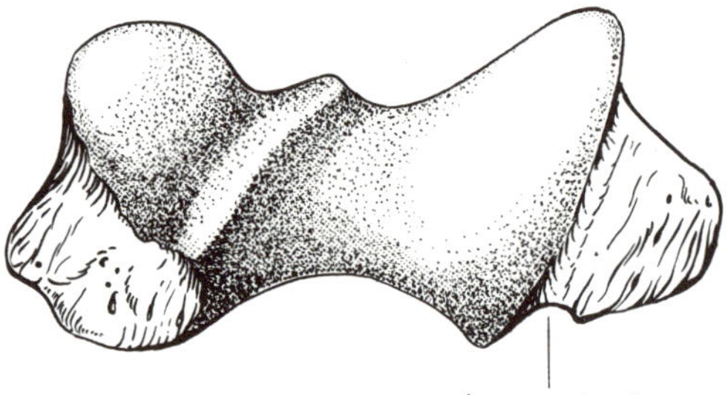

7
The ulnar nerve lies in a groove on the dorsal side of the ulnar epicondyle, close to the edge of the trochlea.

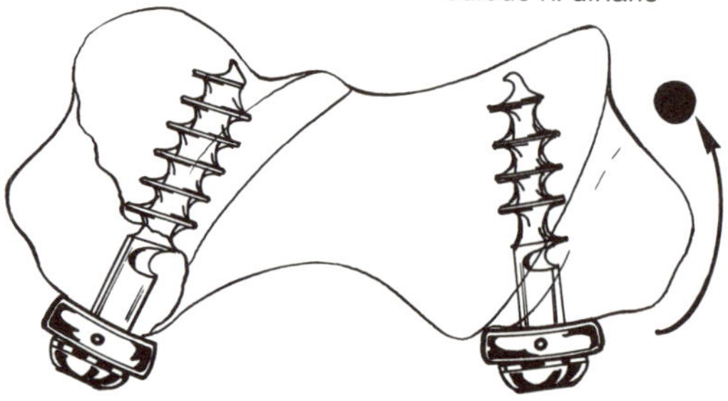

8
Transposition of ulnar nerve to the flexor side, thus enabling the ulnar plate to be placed as far distally as wanted.

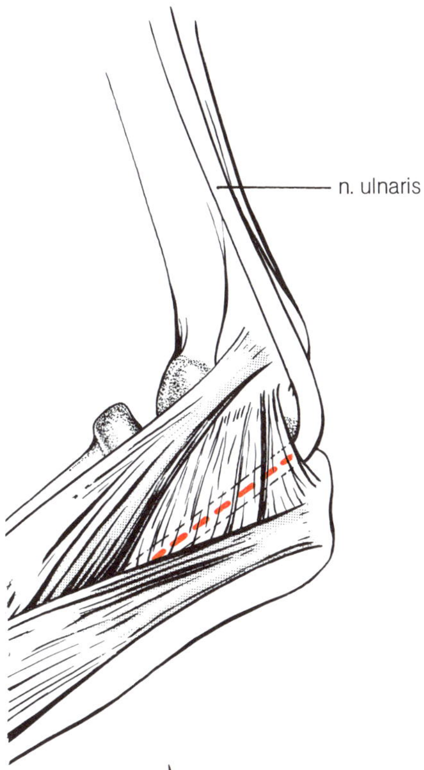

9

After locating and exposing the ulnar nerve dorsally (most securely by repeatedly feeling for the almost pencil-thick cord during continuing dissection), the ulnar collateral ligament is divided.

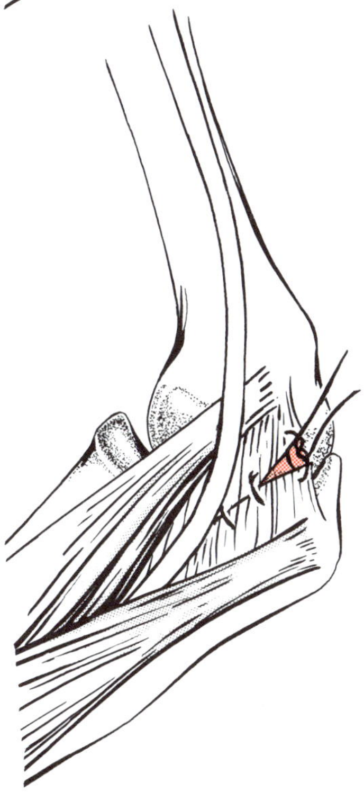

10

Adequate transposition is feasible only by carrying the incision far enough distally into the musculature. Subsequently, the ligament is reunited.

Approach

Dorsal (89–2 f.) or radial (95–1 ff.).

Tactics

As shown in Figs. 102–6 ff.

6. Elbow Joint

General features

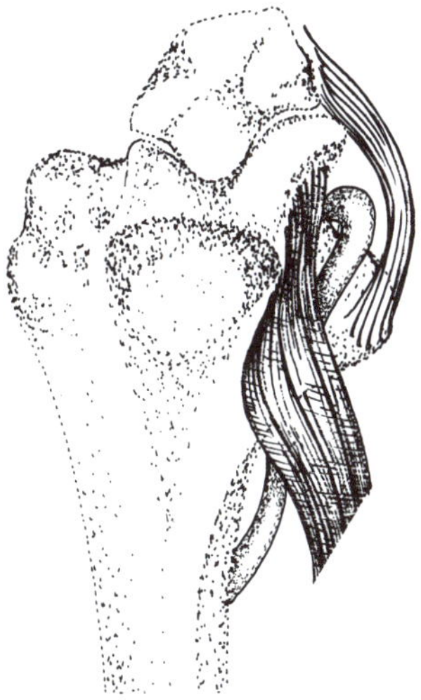

Anatomy

1
Position of the ulnar nerve with the joint flexed, dorsal view.

Dorsal approach, with turned-down triceps tendon

This approach allows only partial inspection of the articular surface. It is therefore only suitable for simple joint fractures.

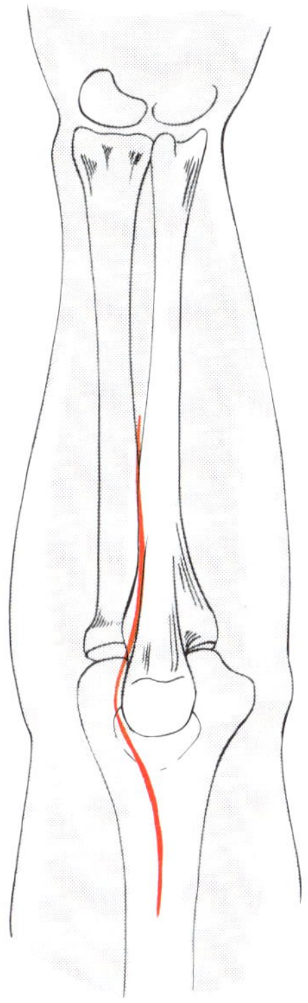

2
The skin incision is carried around the tip of the olecranon.

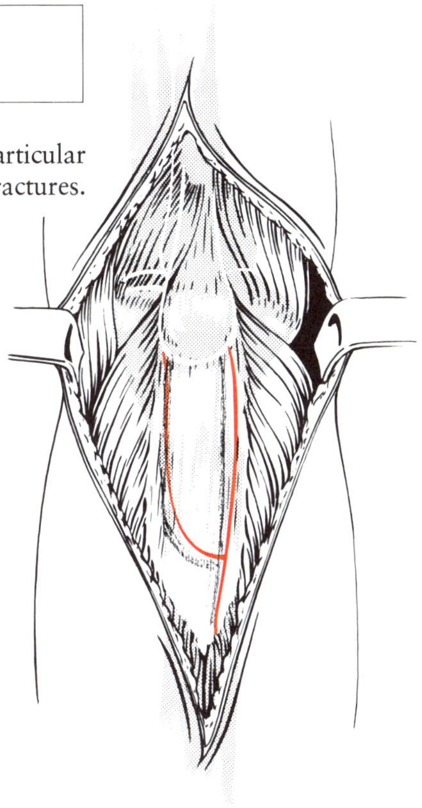

3
Simple longitudinal incision of the triceps tendon does not fully expose the operative field. The mode of incision shown in the figure encircles the triceps tendon in tongue-like fashion and, when necessary, can be extended proximally between the muscle bundles. In this way a free operative field is obtained. Following the operation, the strong edges of the tendon facilitate stable reinsertion of the tendon to the muscle.

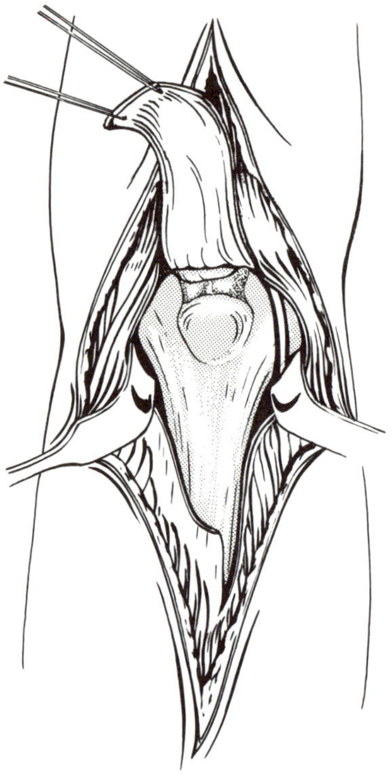

4

The attachment of the tendon is kept aside with a retention suture. The ulnar nerve is located prior to inspection of the fracture. It is absolutely essential to identify the nerve.

Dorsal approach by osteotomy of the olecranon

In joint fractures.

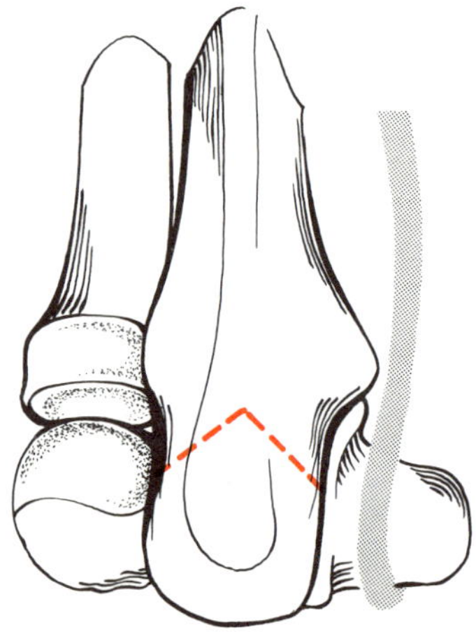

1

Following the skin incision shown in Fig. 89–2, the ulnar nerve is exposed. It is expedient to perform not a straight but a V-shaped incision.

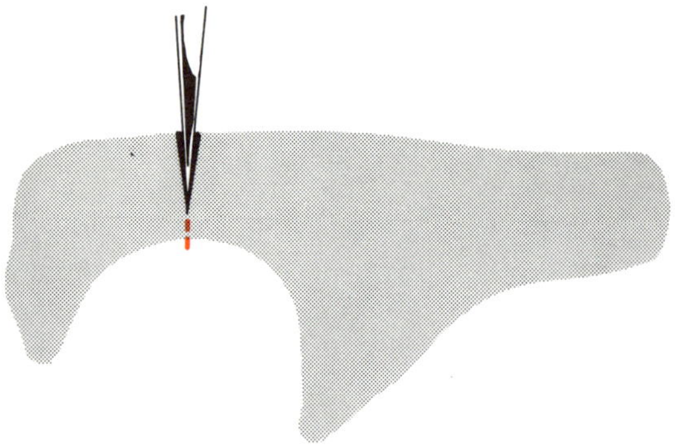

2

The saw should not enter the joint; the osteotomy is preferably completed with the chisel.

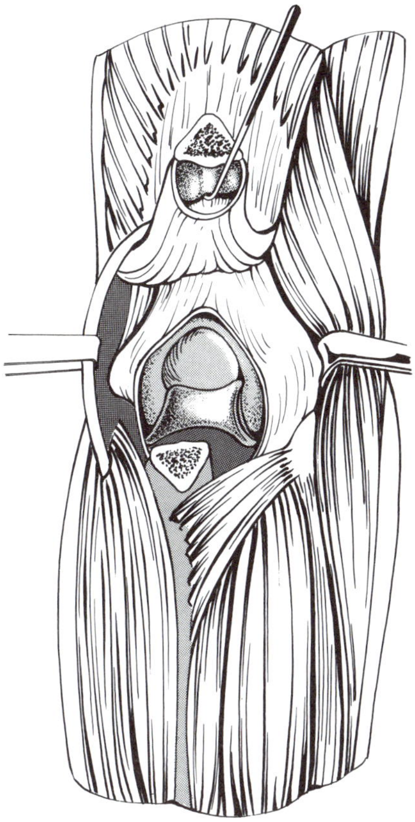

3
Incision is made on either side of the triceps tendon and the olecranon is lifted up cranially. It is important to identify the ulnar nerve with certainty at this point.

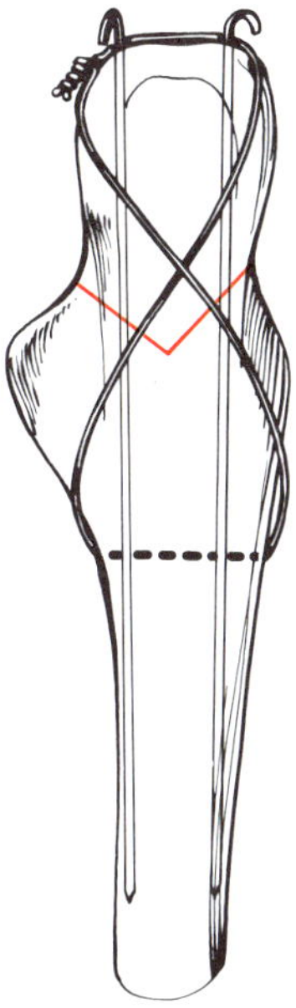

4
The V-shaped osteotomy is of value in reinsertion through wiring. Subsequent osteosynthesis with use of a screw (even if the thread is cut prior to the osteotomy) can easily lead to displacement and is not efficient enough.

Ulnar approach

only to the anterior compartment of the joint; useful for ligament injuries and fractures of a single condyle or the coronoid process.

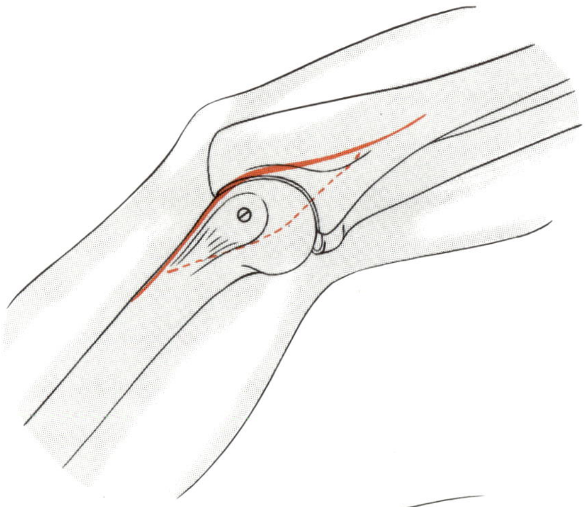

1

Skin incision encircling the ulnar epicondyle on the flexor surface.
Variant: skin incision encircling the epicondyle dorsally (e.g., for the management of a condylar fracture) with identification and, possibly, transposition of the ulnar nerve.
On penetrating too far ventrally (for fear of the ulnar nerve), one is very apt to make the approach unclear.

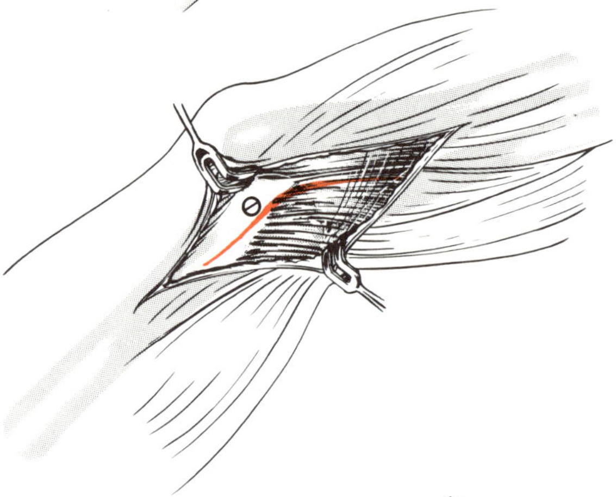

2

The lateral condyle and the lacertus fibrosus are identified with certainty; the ulnar muscular septum is visible. The ulnar nerve should always be safely exposed so that it can be constantly observed.

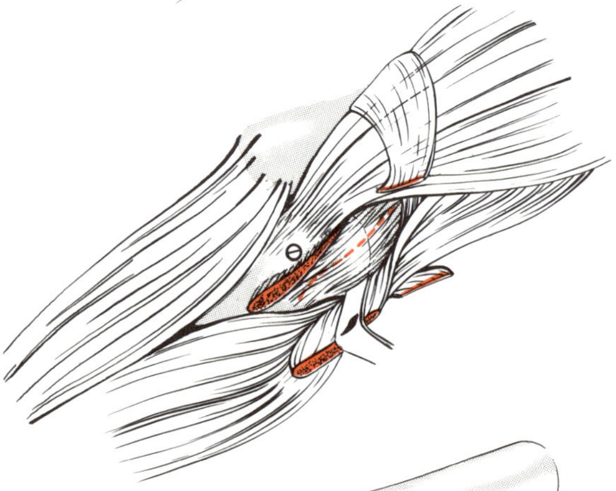

3

The pronator teres muscle is detached from its proximal origin. Underneath it, the ventral capsule comes into view. The joint capsule is opened at its humeral attachment.

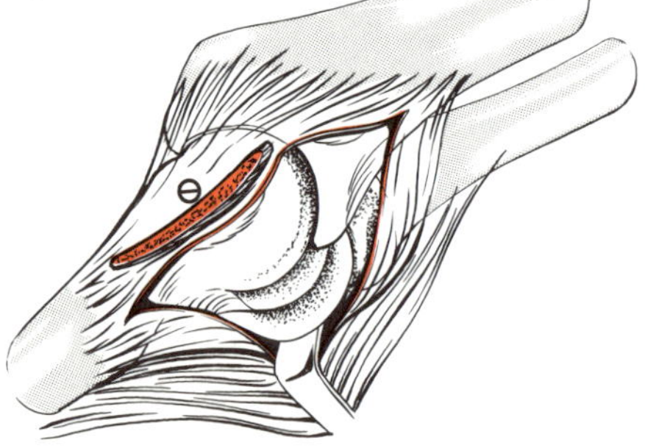

4

View of the anterior ulnar compartment of the joint as far as the head of the radius.

Approach through the dorsal side

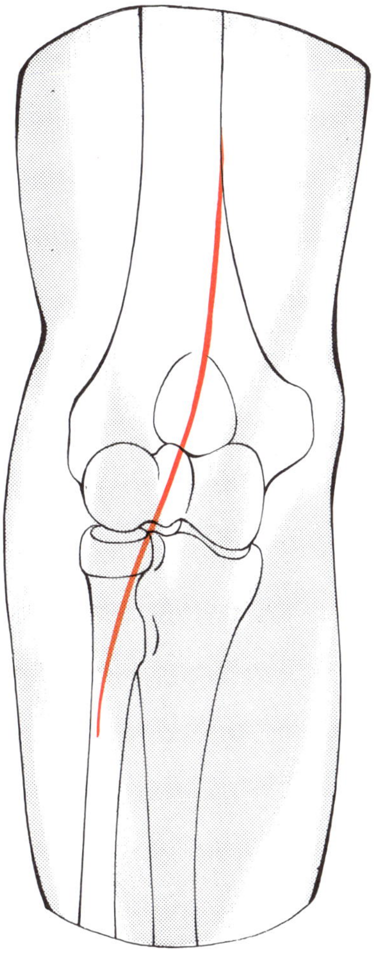

1
S-shaped skin incision in the antecubital fossa.

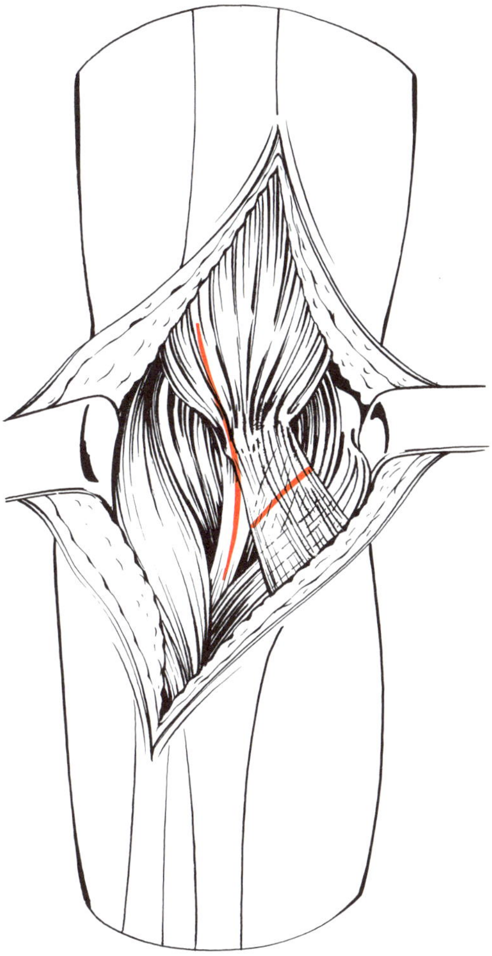

2
The biceps tendon, the lacertus fibrosus and the radial cutaneous nerve of the forearm are exposed. The lacertus fibrosus, which interferes with a sufficient opening of the wound, is divided.

Advantages of the approach: little danger of iatrogenic damage to nerves and vessels.

Disadvantage: relatively less view of the joint and restricted approach. The approach is adequate for the removal of small fragments of the coronoid process which cannot be fastened with a screw.

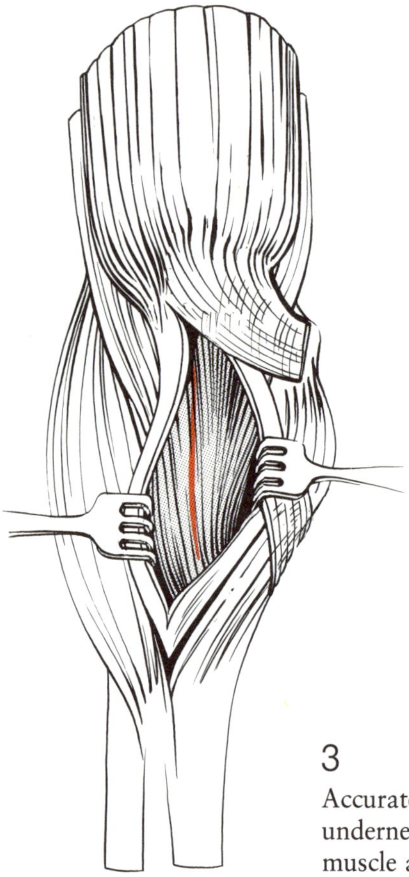

3
Accurate longitudinal splitting of the biceps tendon; underneath it, the longitudinal fibers of the brachial muscle are visible.

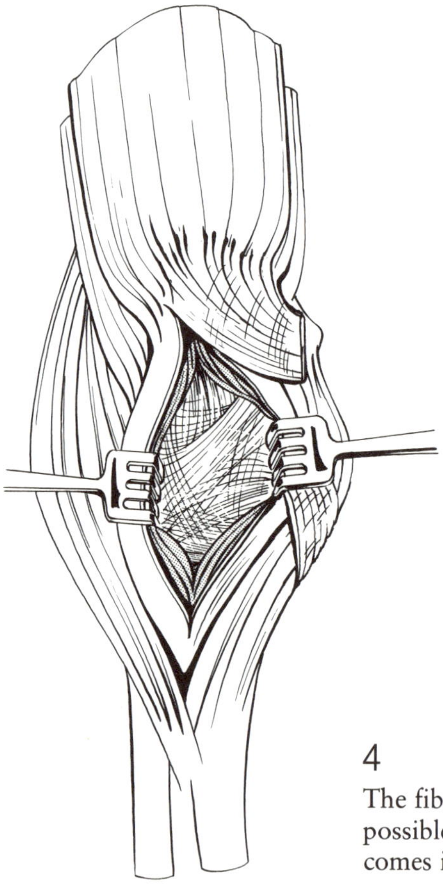

4
The fibers of the brachial muscle are forced apart, as far as possible by blunt dissection; underneath them, the capsule comes into view.

Radial approach

(ligament injuries, fractures of one condyle, loose bodies)

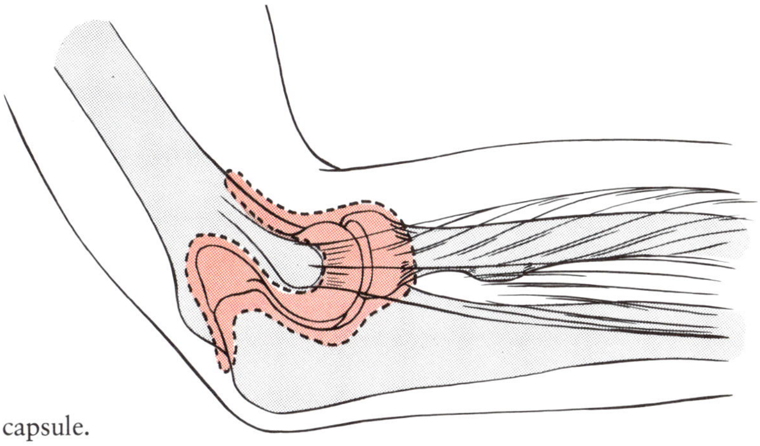

1
Outline of the joint capsule.

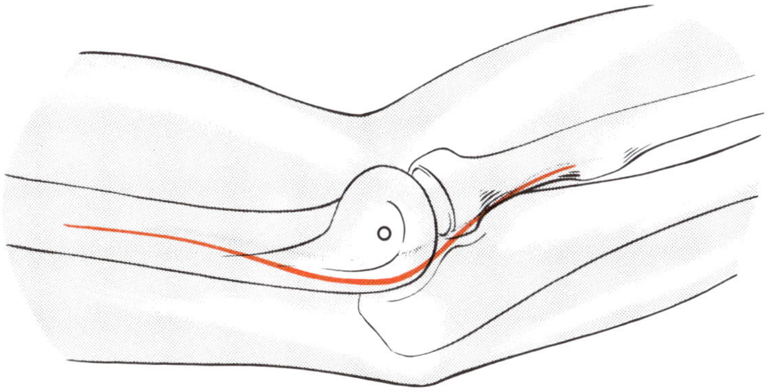

2
Skin incision. Most frequent mistake made: the incision is placed too far to the volar side so that the situation tends to become unclear. One should be meticulous in placing the skin incision a little dorsal to the radial condyle and in keeping it there until the fascial and ligamentous layers are exposed.

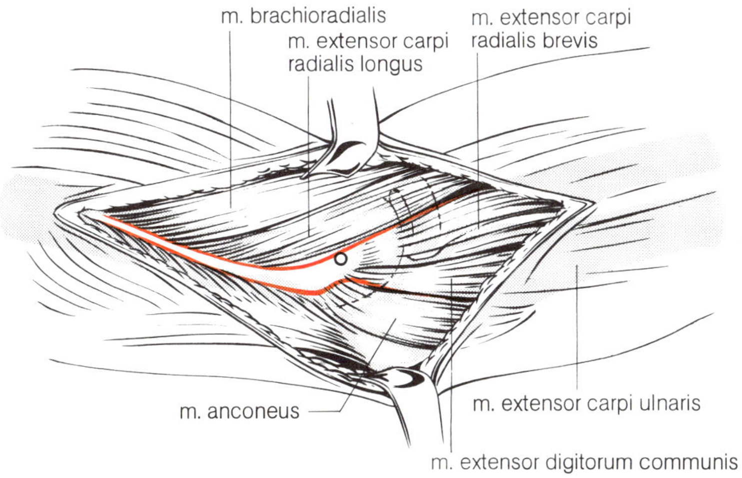

3
Approaches to the ventral and the dorsal compartment of the joint. With this approach, important nerves or vessels are neither visible in the wound nor liable to be injured. The radial nerve courses under the brachial muscle along the anterior and lateral portions of the joint capsule of the elbow. Only in this area, therefore, must caution be exercised in applying traction to the retractors.

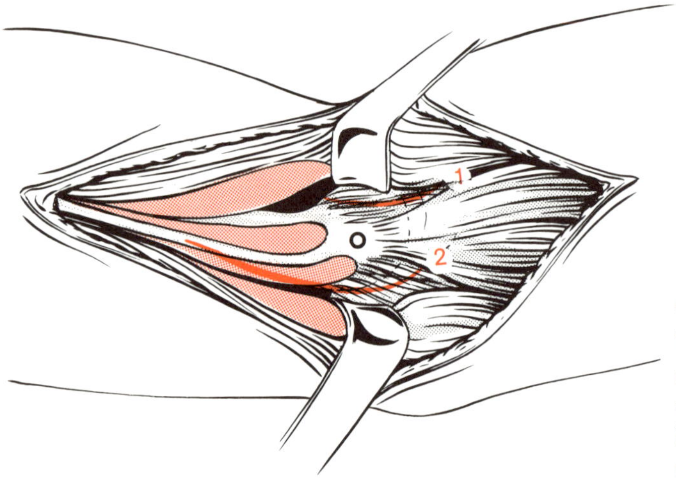

4

The brachial and the extensor carpi radialis longus muscles are detached at their origins. Underneath them, the ventral capsule (1) comes into view; it is opened near its humeral insertion. The anconeus muscle is detached and the dorsal compartment of the joint is opened at site (2).

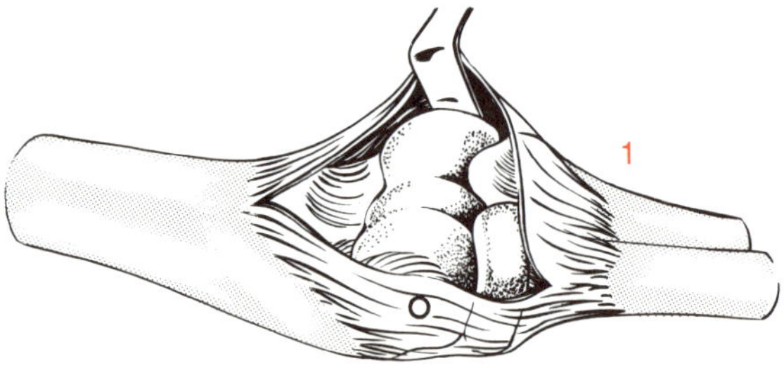

5

The anterior joint cavity...

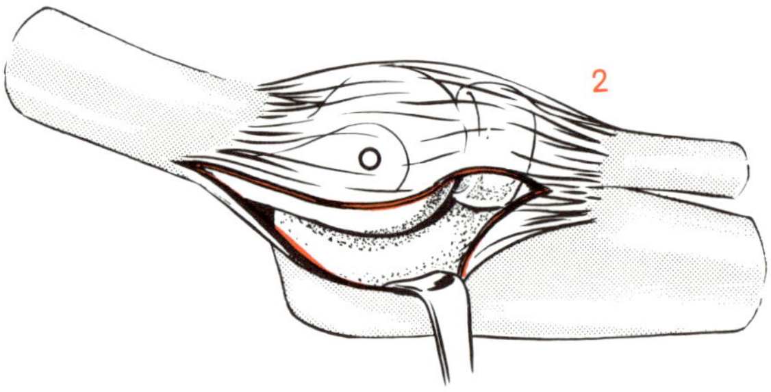

6

... and the dorsal joint cavity can be inspected as far as the ulnar border of the capsule.

The subperiosteal dissection is then continued ventral and dorsal to the humerus so as to obtain an adequate view of the inferior end of the humerus, the interior of the joint, the coronoid process and the head of the radius.

Distal portion of the biceps tendon

Anatomy

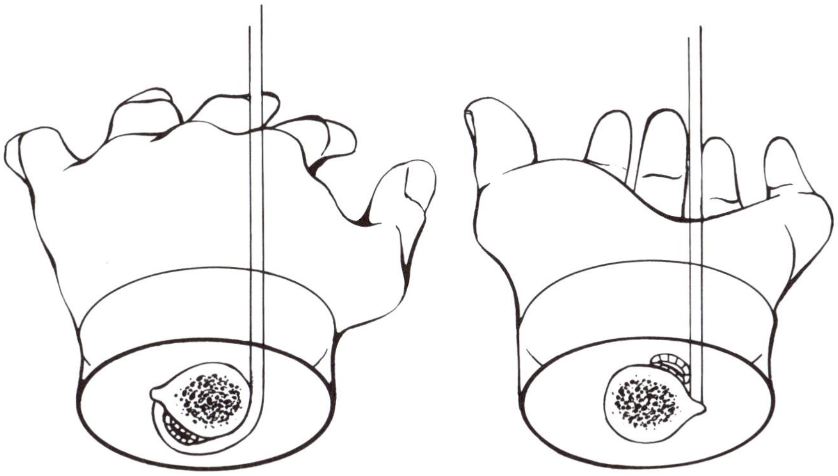

1
The biceps muscle is not only the strongest flexor but also the strongest supinator of the forearm. Both functions can only be restored by reinserting the tendon to the tuberosity of the radius.

Types of injuries

The tendon is almost always avulsed from the tuberosity of the radius, only exceptionally from a point higher up. Therefore, reinsertion of the tendon is practically always required and simple suturing is not feasible.

Diagnosis

The diagnosis can be made by physical examination: with flexion of the elbow joint at a right angle and *maximal supination*, the antecubital fossa is "empty". A movable swelling is palpable in the distal and, sometimes the middle, third of the flexor side of the humerus. Vigorous flexion and supination are restricted.
Differential diagnosis: isolated function deficit of the musculocutaneous nerve.

Indication

Without exception operative.

Operative possibilities

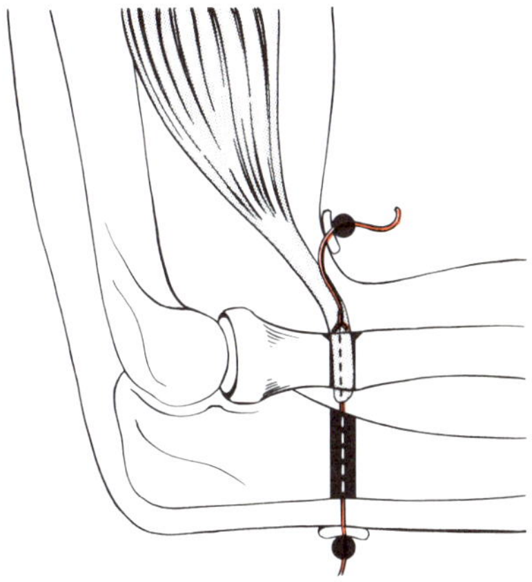

2
Bunnel technique: drill hole through radius and ulna, anchoring with use of a pull-out wire.

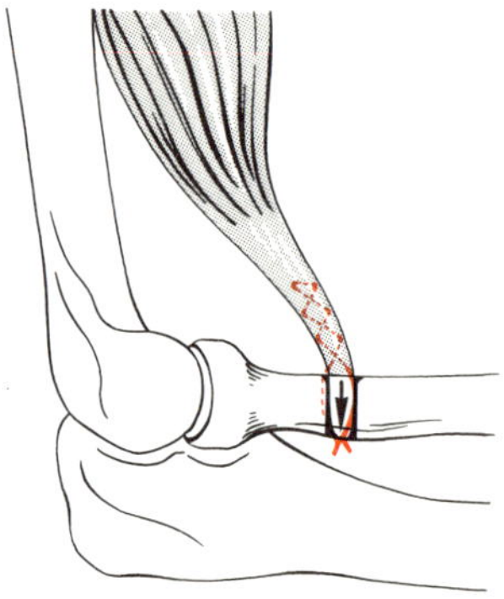

3

Drill hole only in radius. The wire is knotted around the radius.

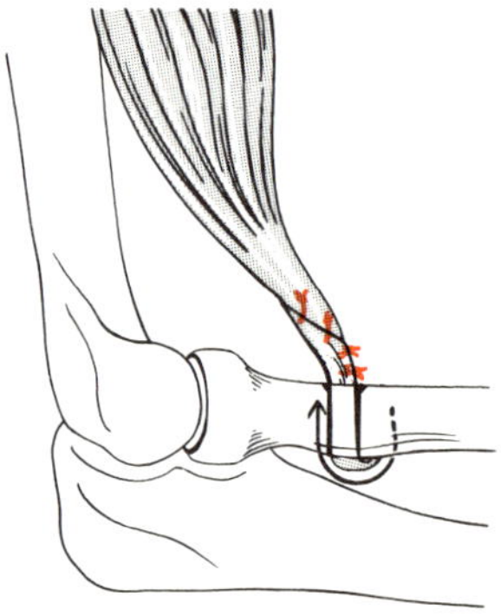

4

If it is feasible to pull the tendon down to that extent: pass the tendon (or part of it) through a drill hole in the radius and suture it to itself.

Positioning

Supine position, arm on a table, pneumatic tourniquet (or elastic bandage).

Approach

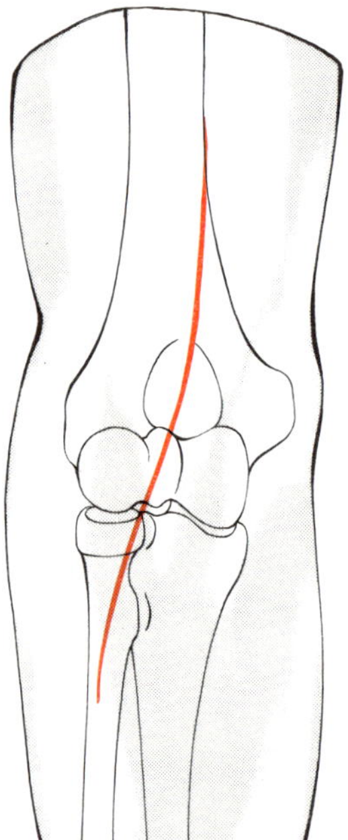

5

Skin incision and approach as shown in Figs. 93–1 ff.

Tactics

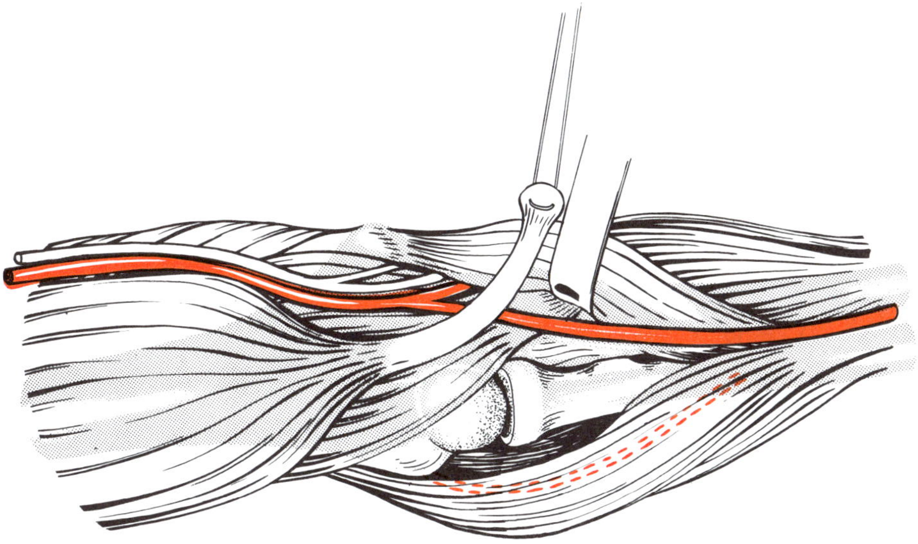

6
After dividing the subcutaneous adipose tissue, one sees the end of the tendon, which mostly shows a bulbous enlargement.
Full supination greatly facilitates penetrating to the tuberosity of the radius. If possible, retractors should not be inserted on the radial side, to spare the radial nerve.

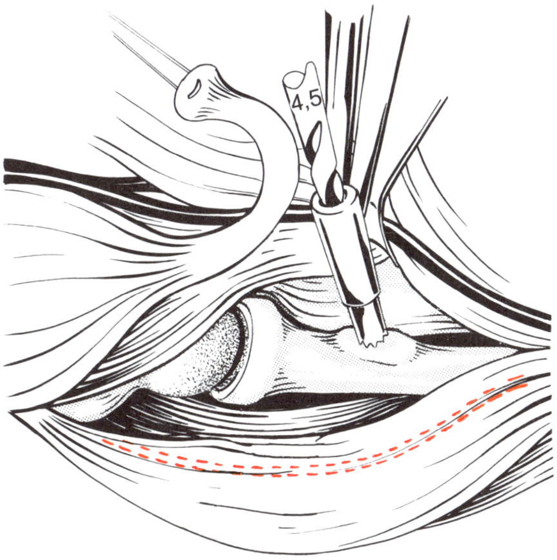

7
The tuberosity of the radius is perforated in the anteroposterior direction, using a 4.5 mm drill.

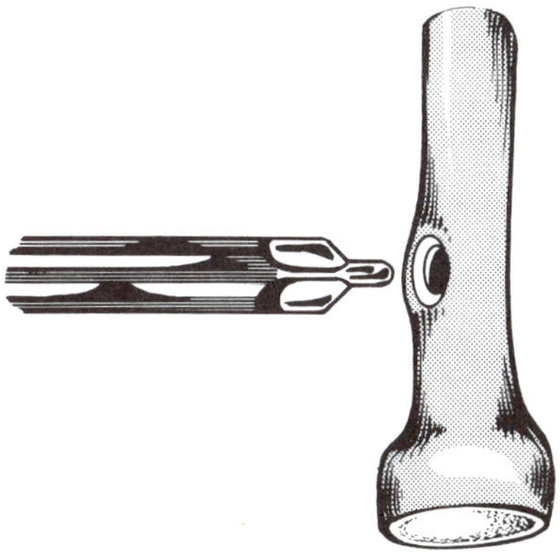

8
The use of a grooved bur facilitates the insertion of the tendon (See also Fig. 5–1 f.). Supporting disks and small lead balls are threaded on.

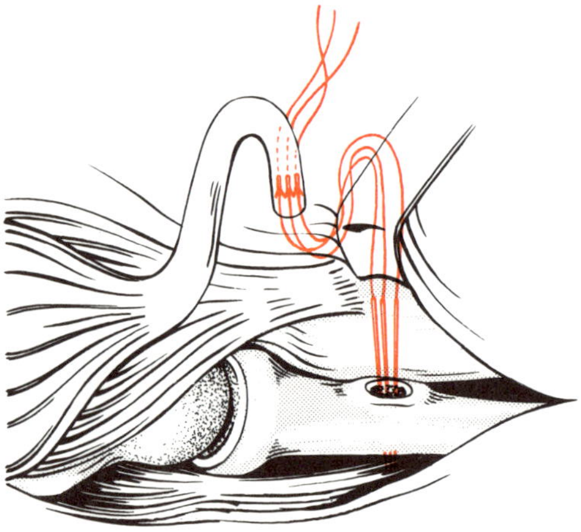

9

Insertion of 2 to 3 Lengemann wire threads form the proximal into the distal stump of the tendon. The wires are passed together through the drill hole and are run dorsally through the skin. The lead seals are fastened.

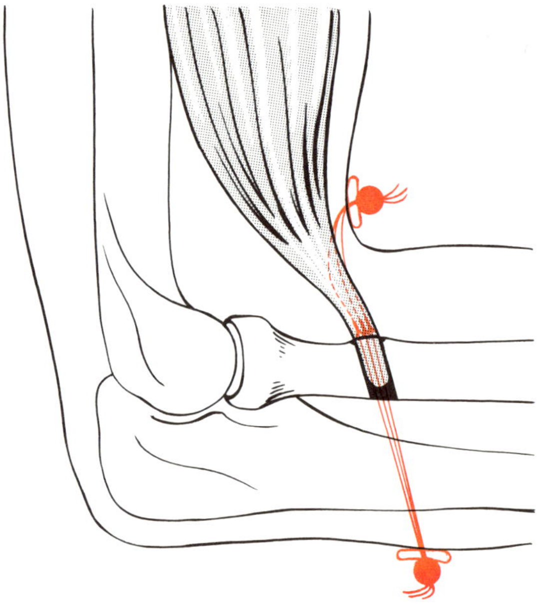

10

The elbow joint is flexed at a right angle and the tendon is inserted into the drill hole.

Postoperative management

Cast applied to upper arm for 5 to 6 weeks with flexed position of the elbow joint and slight supination of the forearm. Then, removal of wire and active exercises.

Distal part of humerus

Types of injuries

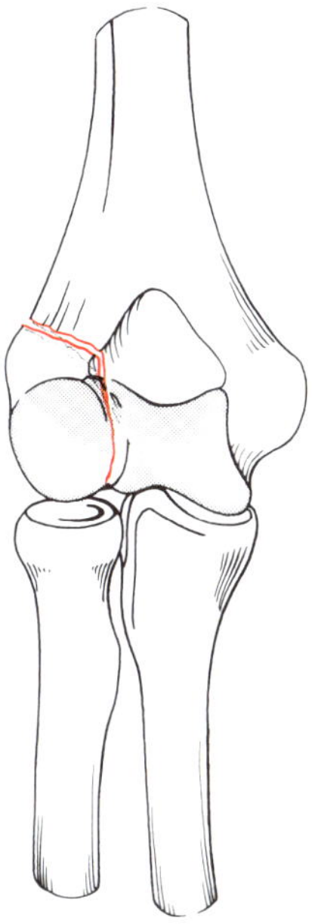

1
Fracture of radial condyle and epicondyle.

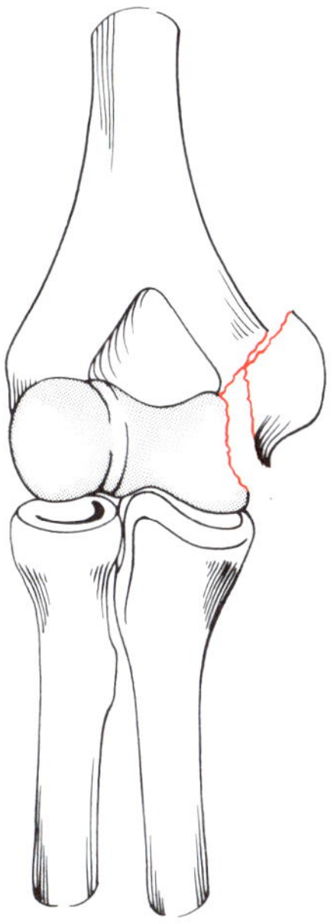

2
Fracture of ulnar epicondyle and condyle.

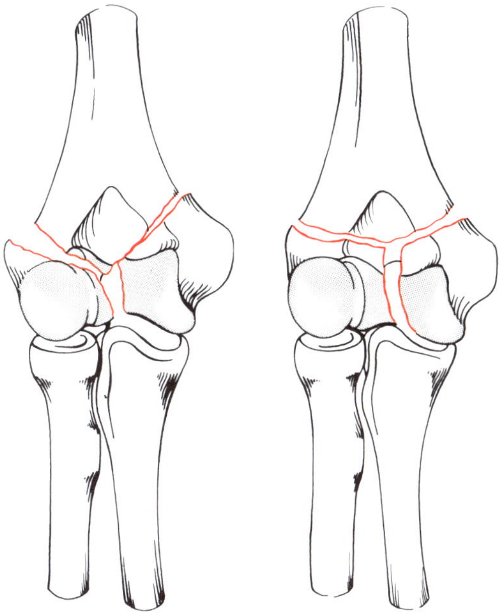

3
Transcondylar and intercondylar fracture (Y and T fractures).

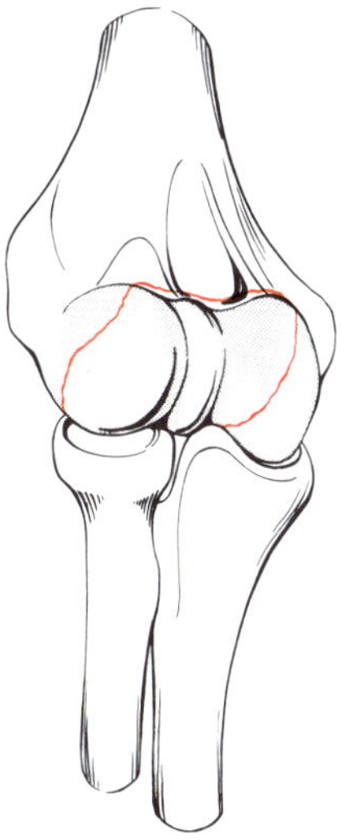

4
Intra-articular transverse fractures.

Approach See Figs. 90–1 ff.

Principle

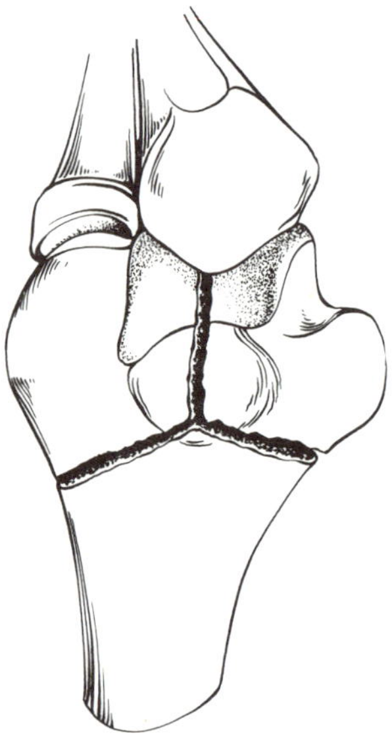

4
As with any intra-articular fracture, a satisfactory result can only be obtained if…

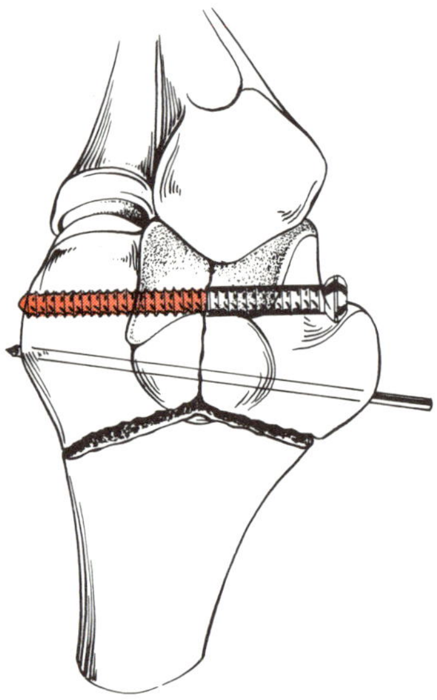

5
… one first succeeds in restoring the articular surface without a residual step. Particularly in fractures of the elbow joint there may be a great temptation first to fasten an articular fragment to the proximal chief fragment. For selection of the screw, Figs. 24–16 and 24–18 should be borne in mind.

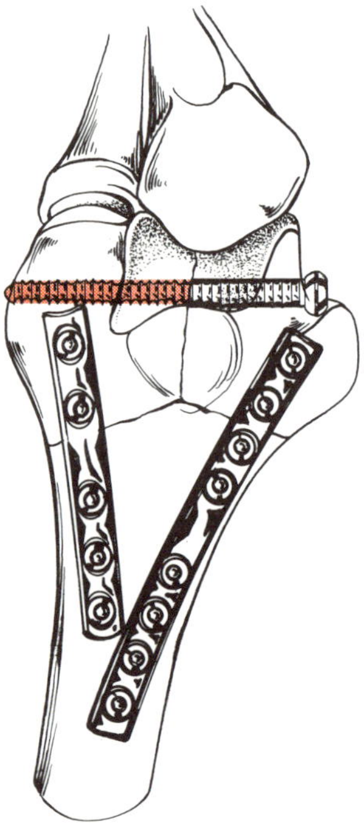

6
Most stable mode of fixation. If possible a narrow, so-called standard plate should be used on the side of the radial condyle. DC plates are particularly helpful there.

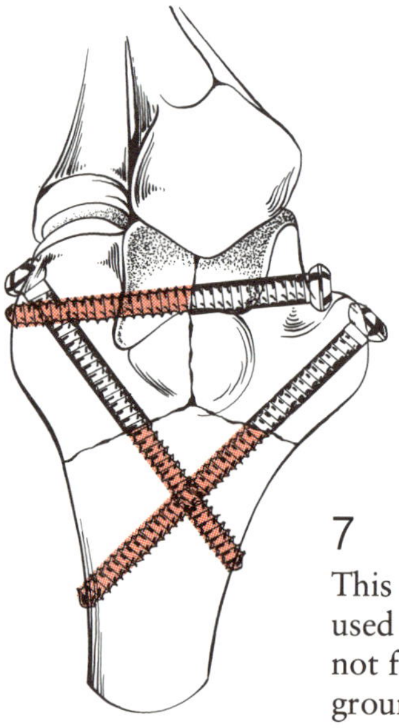

7
This kind of fixation should be used only when plate fixation is not feasible (rare) on anatomical grounds.

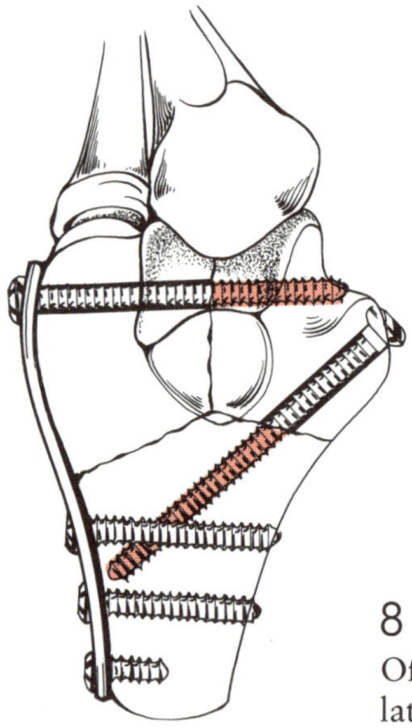

8
Often, plate fixation can still be performed if the plate is applied laterally.

Tactics with large fragments

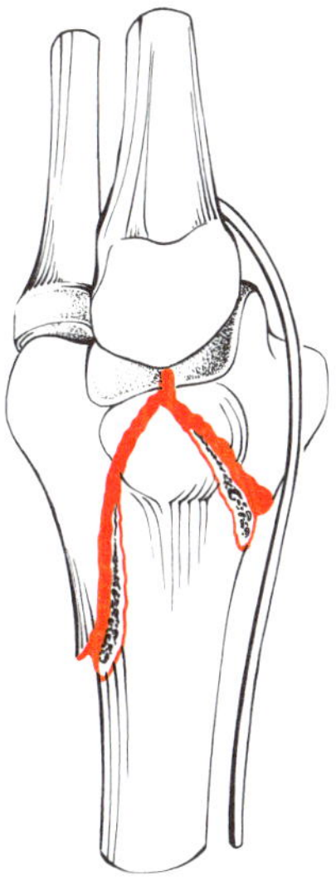

9

The approach shown in Fig. 89–2 is often adequate. It is important to expose the ulnar nerve from the very beginning to such an extent that it can be closely watched during the operation.

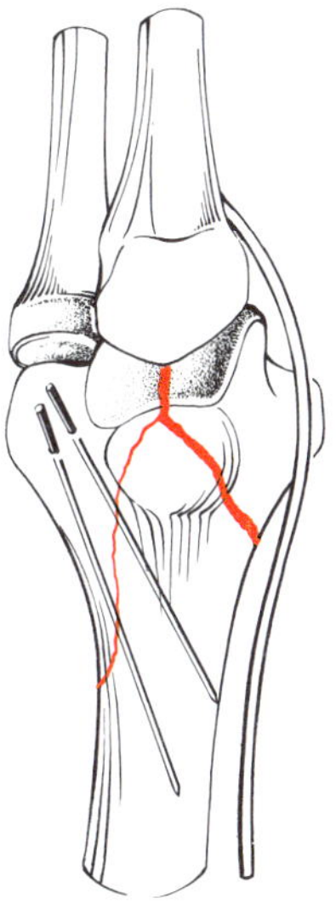

10

Here, the fragments are relatively large. In such a case it may be easier first to fasten the larger fragment and only secondarily to restore the articular surface without a residual step.

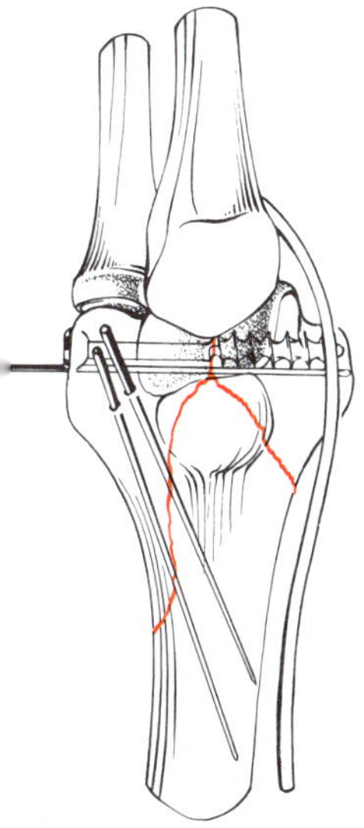

11

In every case, however, definitive fixation is first done in the joint-forming fragments. Most important, the screw thread must completely, traverse the fracture cleft. Still better, employ a cortical screw for traction.

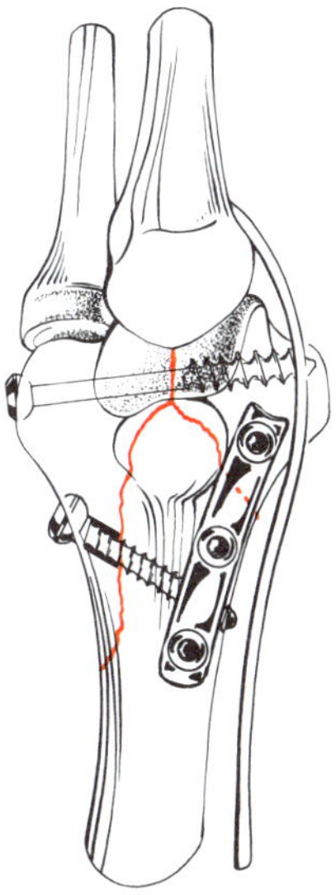

12

Additional fixation with screws passed through the distal fragments into the proximal chief fragment.

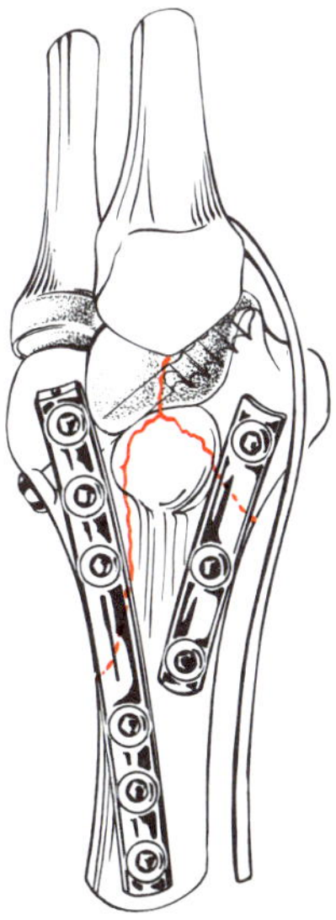

13

It is preferable to accomplish additional fixation with use of one or more narrow plates.

Tactics with small and multiple fragments

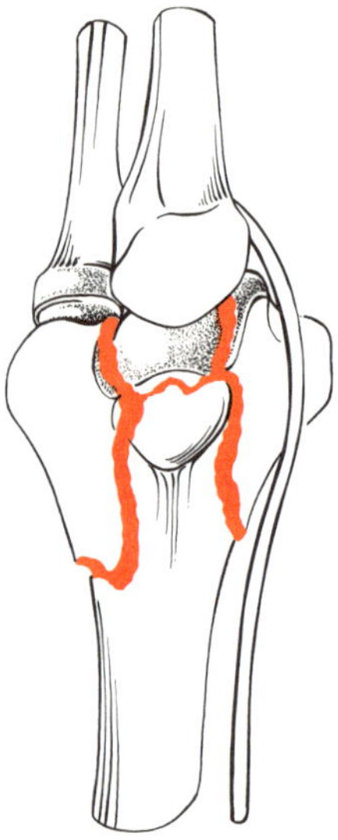

14
Approach as shown in Figs. 90–1 ff. In the presence of greater comminution it is advisable in every case first to reconstruct the articular surface. Prior to the first attempts at reduction, coagula must be thoroughly removed and the fragments identified, leaving them untouched. Removing the fragments first renders orientation very difficult.

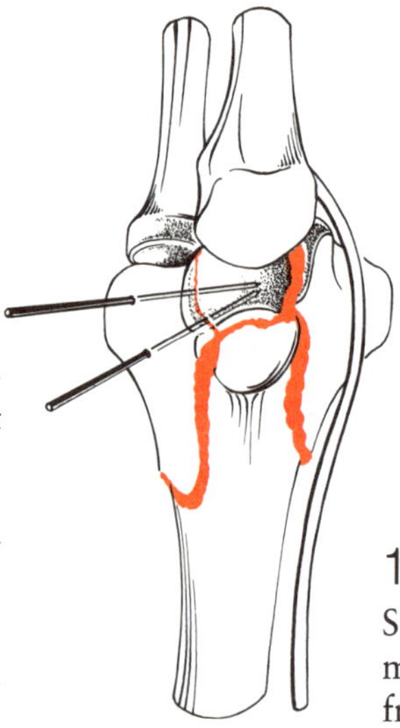

15
Stepwise reconstruction and preliminary fixation of the joint-forming fragments.

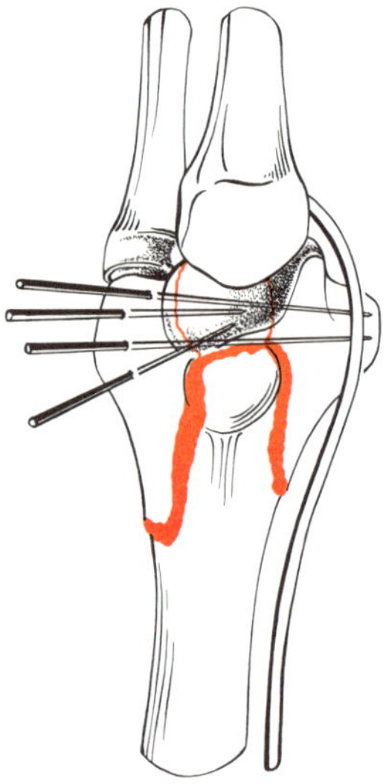

16
The first wires can now be removed to make room for the screw.

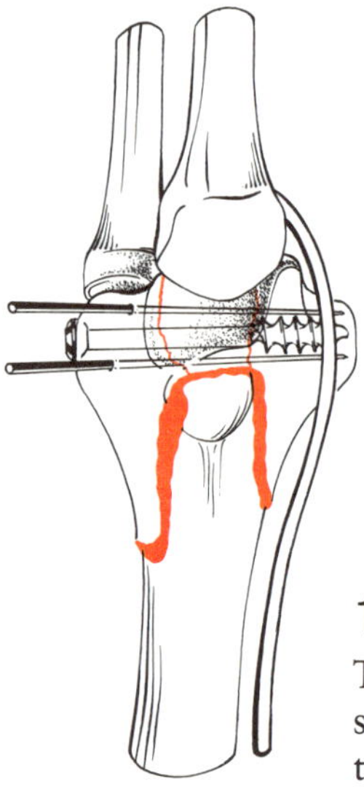

17
The joint-forming parts have been stabilized. Now they can be repositioned to the chief fragment.

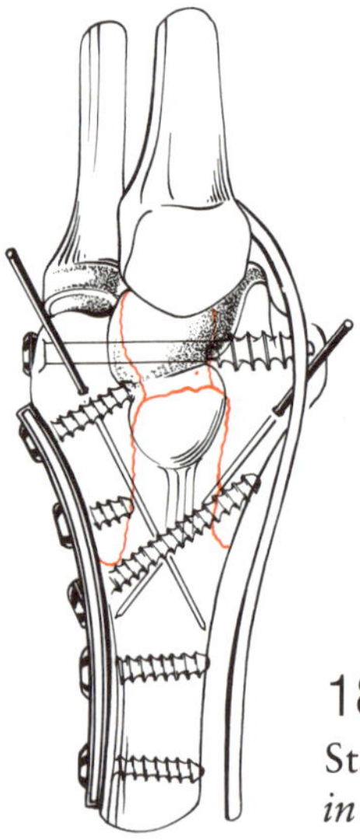

18
Stabilization by plate and screws. No wires should be left *in situ*.

Olecranon

Types of injuries

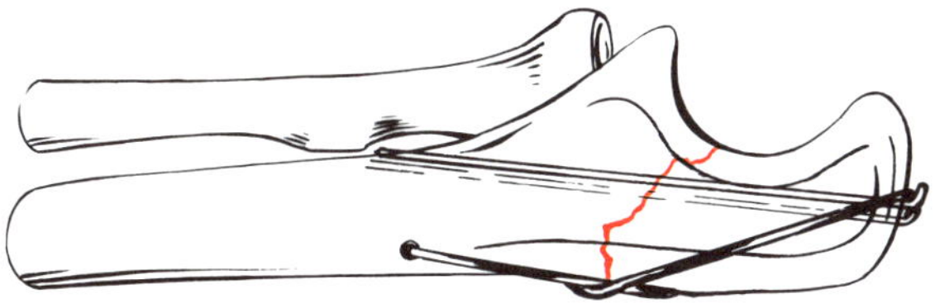

1
Simple (transverse) fracture. Management: wire suture (drilling wire 1.6 mm; fixing wire 2.0 mm, soft).

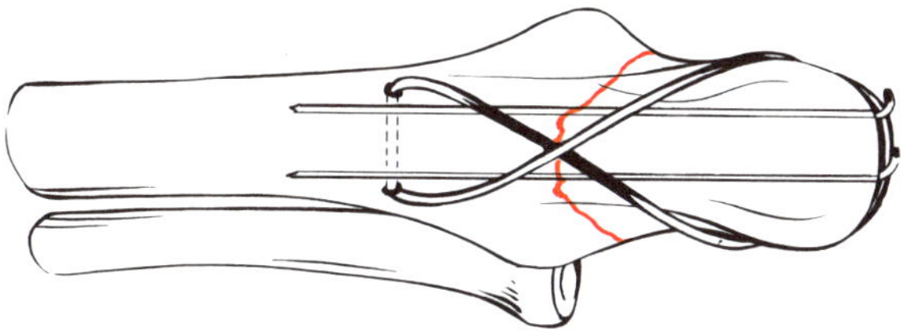

2
Drilling wires placed parallel to each other (See Figs. 54–10 ff.).

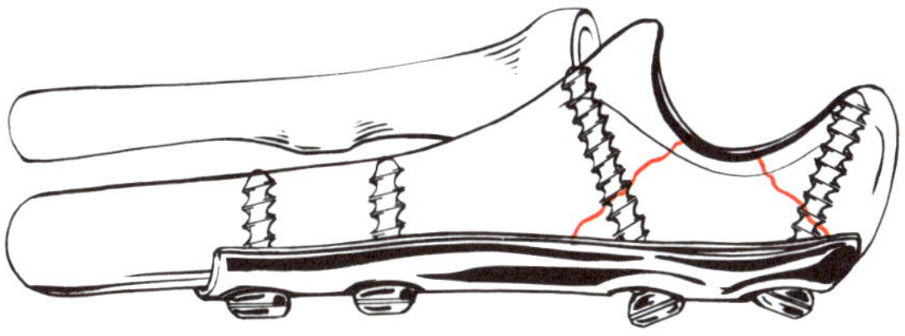

3
Comminuted multifragment fracture of the dorsal type. Management: half-tubular plate (possibly, one-third tubular plate).

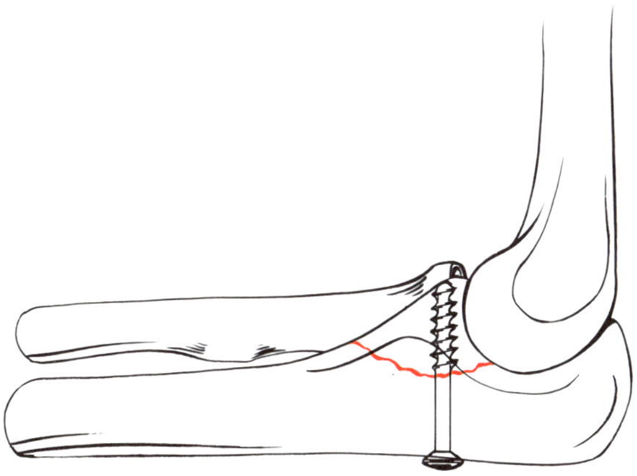

4
Comminuted multifragment fracture of the *ventral* type (unsuitable for wire fixation). In this category also belong fractures of the coronoid process. Ulnar approach as shown in Figs. 92–1 ff.

Principle

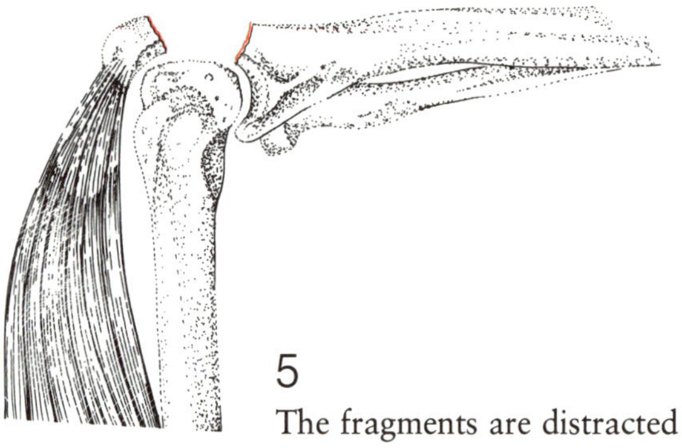

5

The fragments are distracted by flexion.

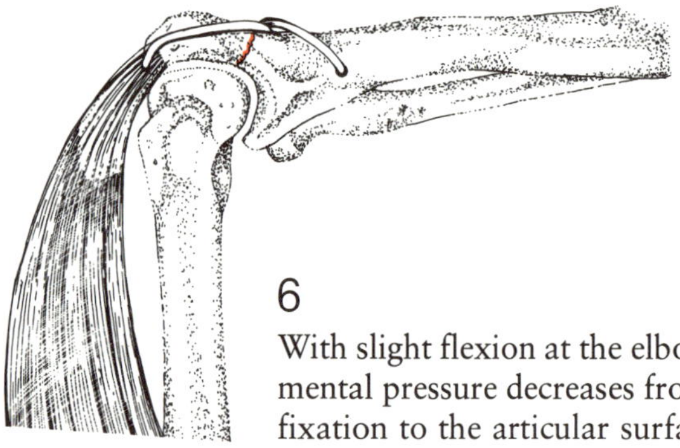

6

With slight flexion at the elbow joint, the interfragmental pressure decreases from the side of the wire fixation to the articular surface.

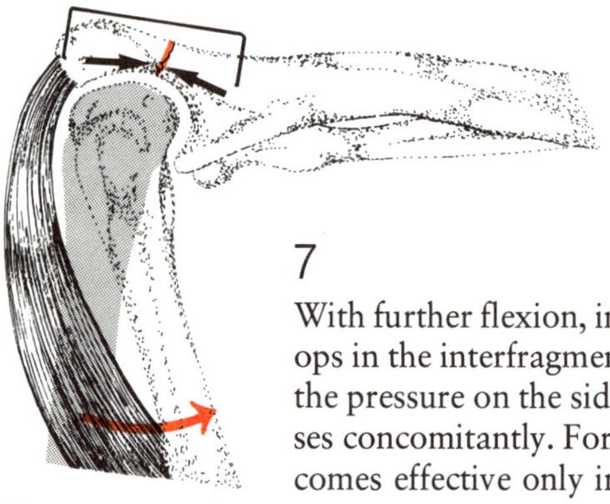

7

With further flexion, increasing pressure also develops in the interfragmental area near the joint, while the pressure on the side of the wire fixation decreases concomitantly. For this reason wire fixation becomes effective only in functional treatment.

Positioning See p. 79.

Approach

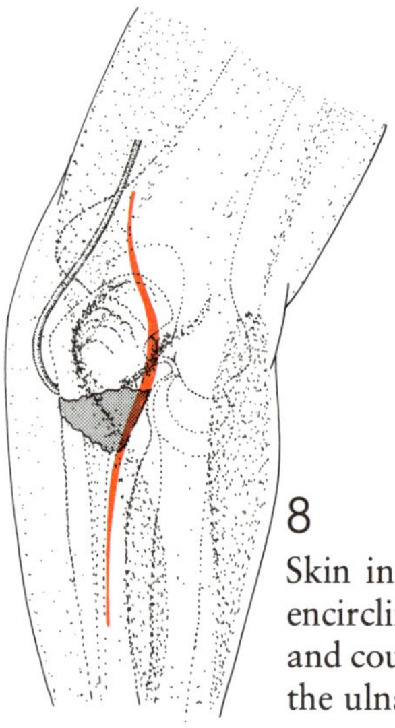

8

Skin incision on the radial side, encircling the tip of the olecranon and coursing radial to the edge of the ulna.

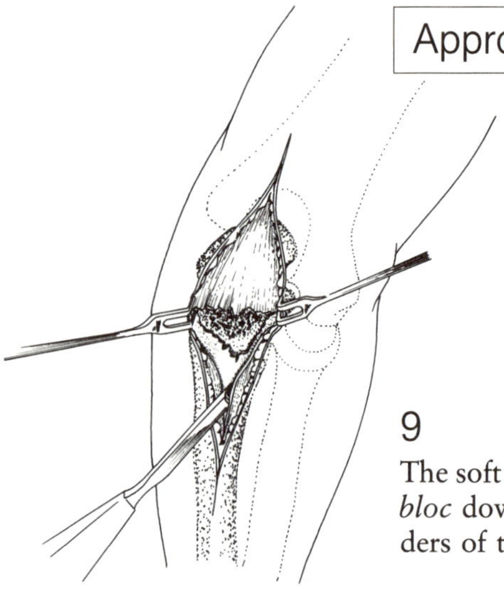

9

The soft structures are divided *en bloc* down to the bone. The borders of the fracture are exposed.

Tactics

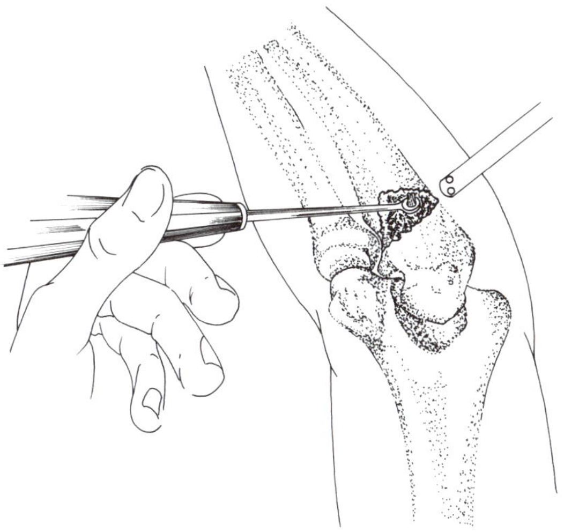

10

Coagula and enfolded tissue particles are removed. The borders of the fracture are neatly exposed.

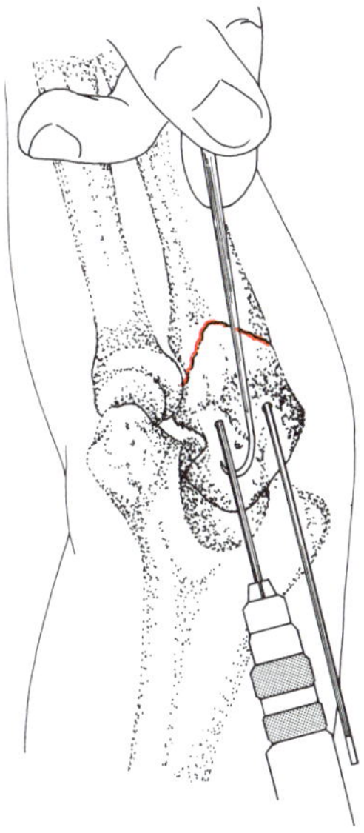

11

Reduction with a hook. Strong Kirschner wires are driven into place strictly parallel to each other.

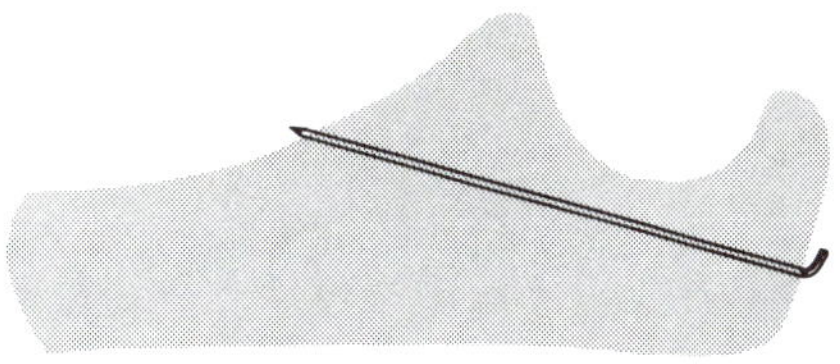

12

In most cases the drilling wires, which should always be anchored in cortical bone, can be driven into the cortex of the flexor side.

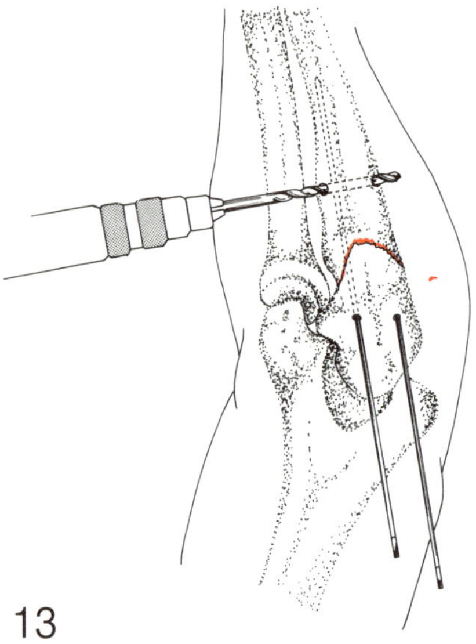

13
A transverse drill hole is made, also at sufficient distance from the tip of the olecranon, using a 2 mm drill.

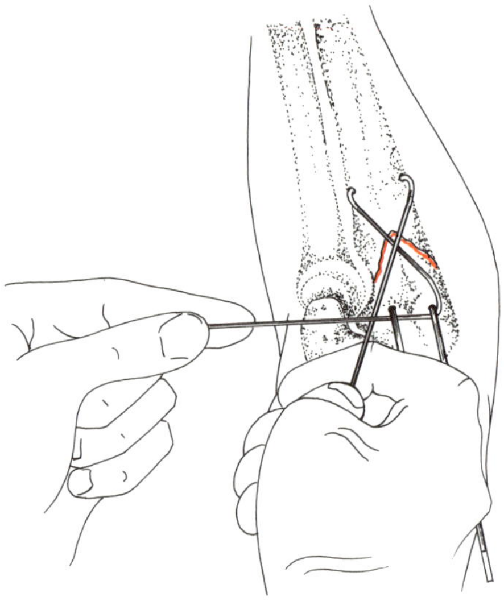

14
Applying the wiring for fixation.

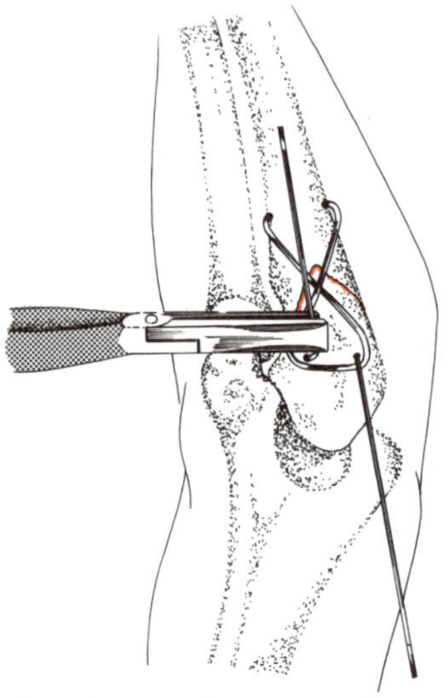

15
Next the wires are bent one after another in the direction of the fracture.

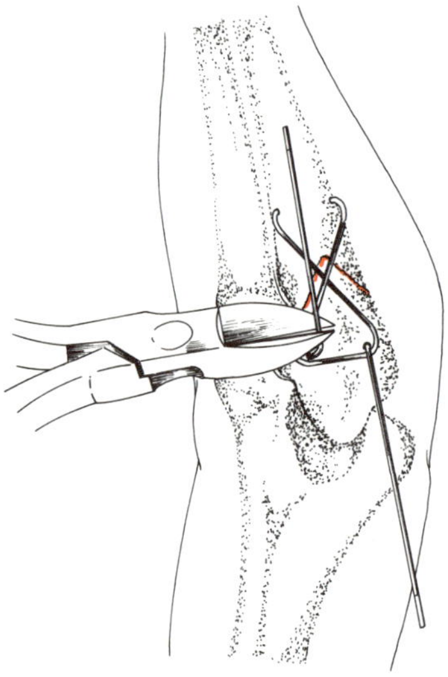

16
The wires are shortened to an excess length of 8 to 10 mm.

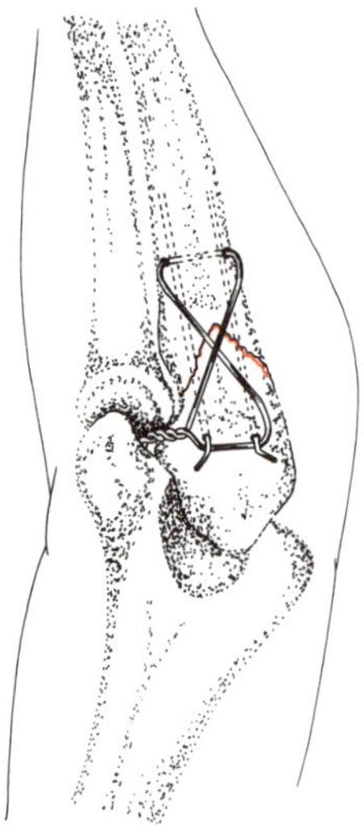

17
The wires are then turned back again so that they carry the loop of the wiring with them underneath the hook. In that way the hooks are concomitantly displaced into the soft tissues. The twisted part of the wire is also bent into the soft tissue.

Head of the radius

Types of injury

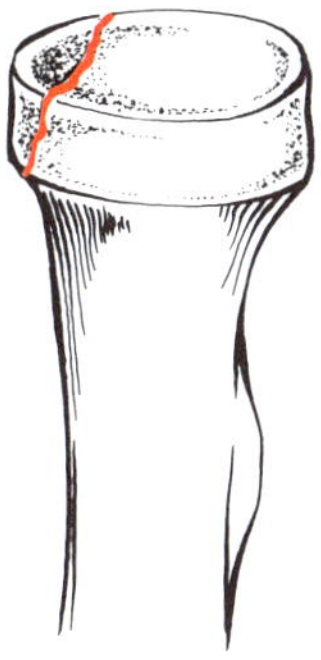

1

Marginal fractures. Small fractures are managed by resection, larger ones by osteosynthesis, and fractures without displacement by conservative means (three week's immobilization).

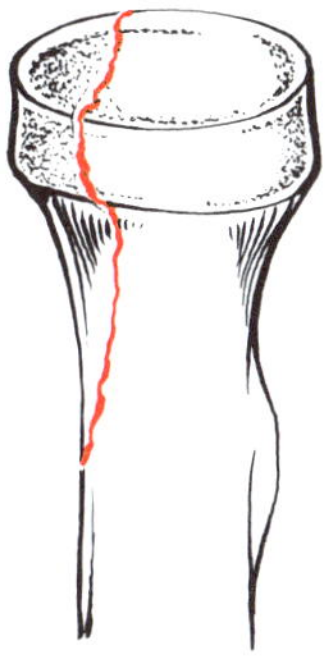

2

Chisel fractures are treated as shown in Fig. 109–1.

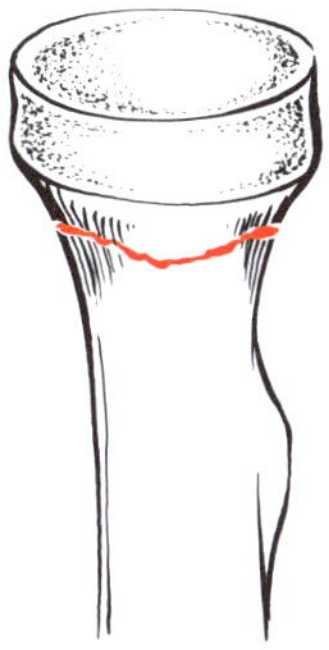

3

Fractures of the neck (in children, most often as Aitken-I fractures). Management by conservative means. Manifest displacement requires open reduction and transarticular fixation for 3 weeks.

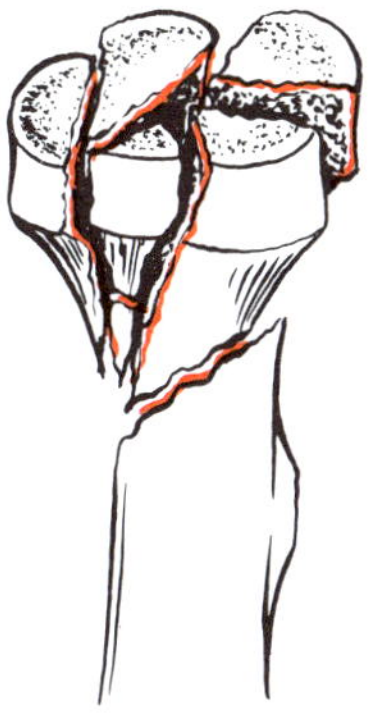

4

Comminuted fractures. Management: early resection, in exceptional cases, endoprosthesis.

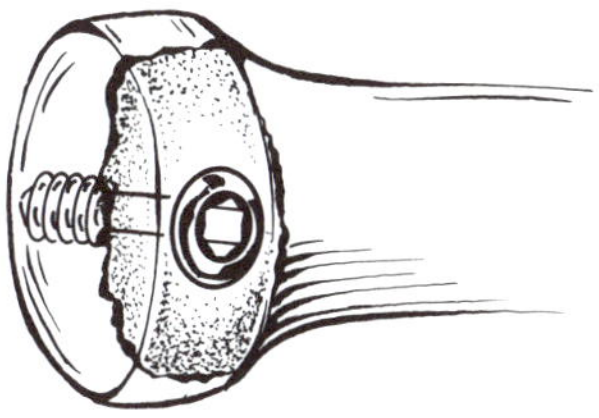

5

Transfixion by screw only in the presence of large solitary fragments (amounting in size to a quarter of the surface or more). Fixation with drill wire or the smallest fragment screw available. The earlier and the more atraumatic the operation, the less the danger of periarticular calcification. Transfixion from the opposite side is also feasible. Use of a fibrin glue may be contemplated.

Indication

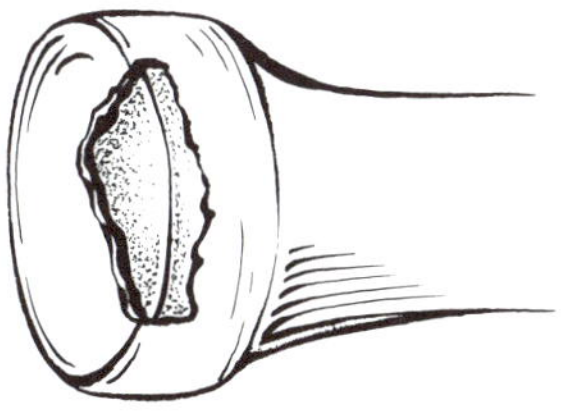

6

Small fragments are best removed. Comminuted fractures are treated either by conservative means or by resection of the radial head with or without replacement arthroplasty.

Principle

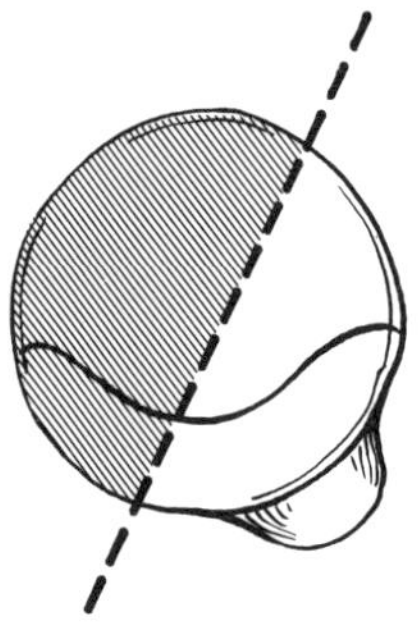

7

Applying wire or screw with the forearm pronated to prevent the heads from entering the articulating area between radius and ulna.

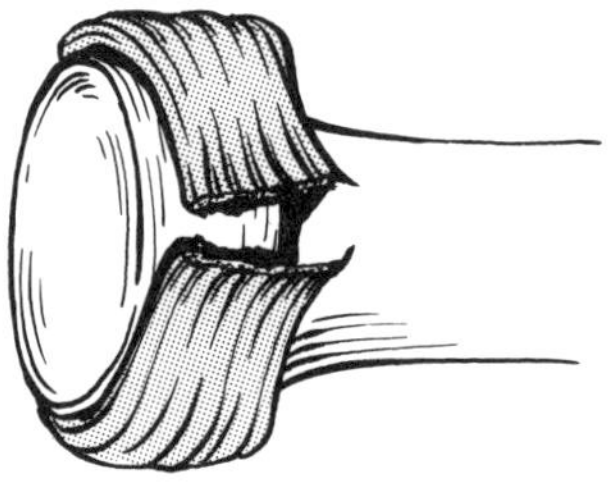

8

The anular ligament of the radius does not require suturing.

Approach See Figs. 95–1 ff.

Postoperative care

Excepting stabilized fractures, immobilization is required for 3 weeks. It should be noted however that, starting as early as the first postoperative day, the arm must be taken out of the plaster shell once or twice a day and small movements be performed to improve the nutrition of the articular cartilage. All the movements must be performed *below the pain threshold*. Considerable benefit from the exercises is very often experienced as late as 10 to 14 weeks after beginning them. Any irritation – for instance through forced therapeutic exercises – impairs the result the same as complete lack of regular exercises.

7. Forearm

General features

Anatomy

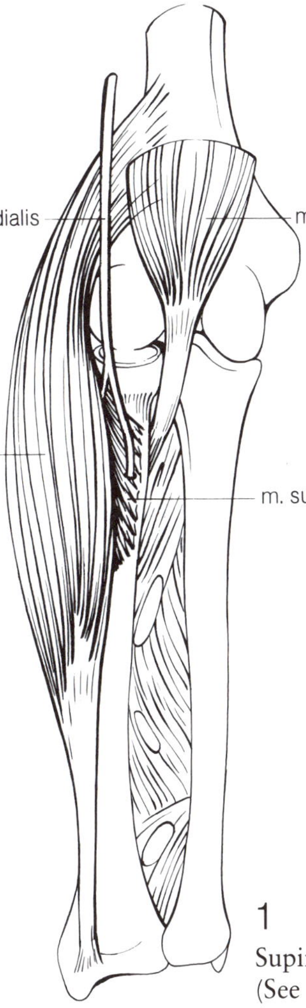

1
Supinator muscles
(See also Fig. 112–3).

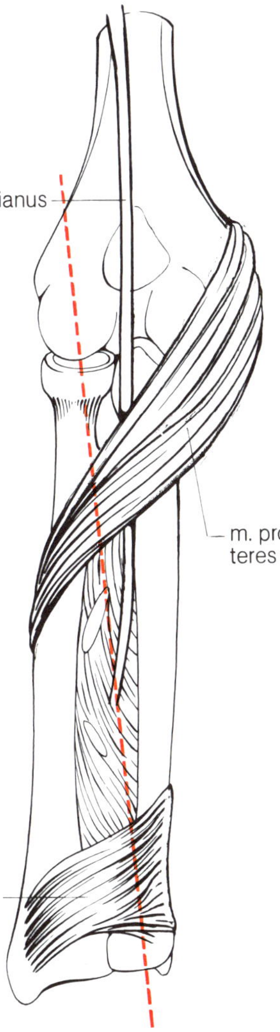

2
Pronator muscles.

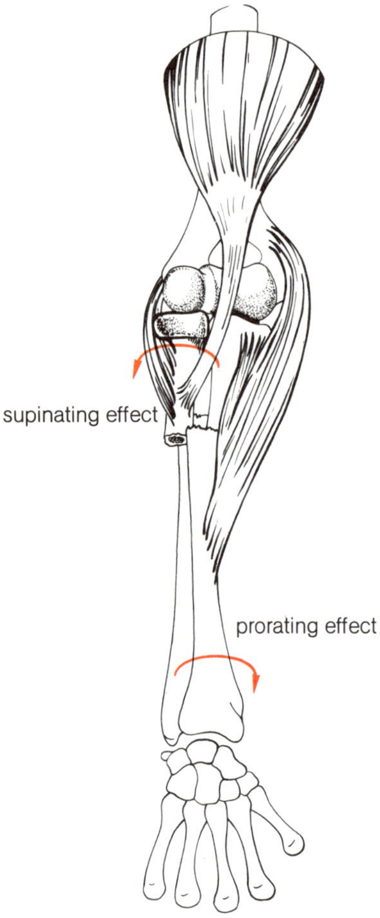

3

Displacement of the fragments with a *proximal* fracture. Reduction is facilitated by giving the hand a marked supinated position.

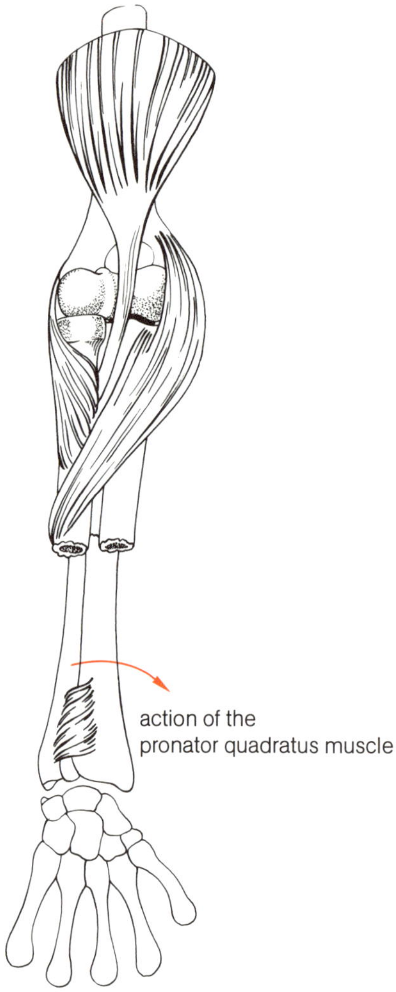

4

Pronating and supinating effects neutralize each other. With a fracture *in the middle of the shaft,* the intermediate supinated position facilitates reduction.

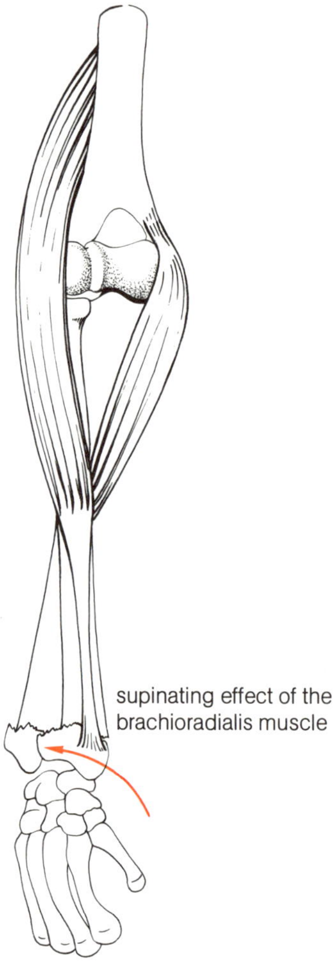

5

With a *distal* fracture, reduction is facilitated by marked pronated position of the hand.

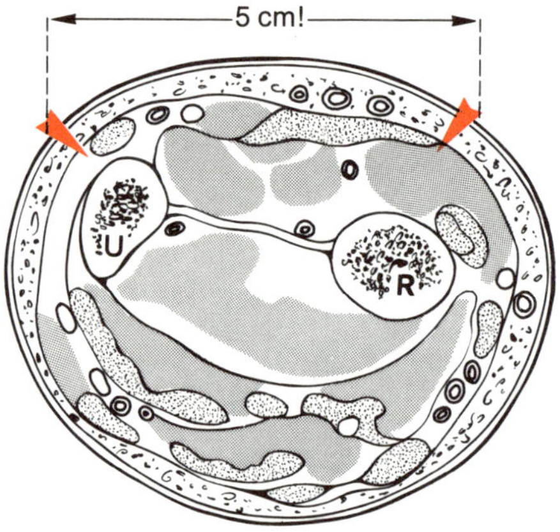

Principle

6

With forearm fractures, the dorsal bridge of skin and soft tissues must not become narrower than 5 cm, owing to the hazard of disturbed wound healing.

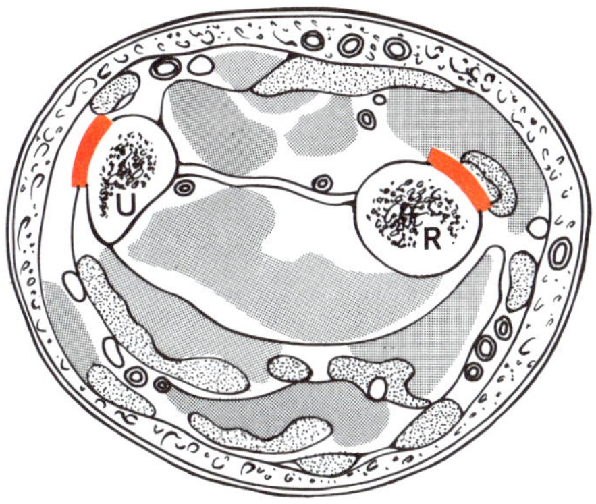

7

If possible a small standard plate (with use of the plate tightener) should be applied to the ulna as well as the radius. For a delicate skeleton, however, small DC plates in conjunction with correspondingly smaller screws are often adequate.

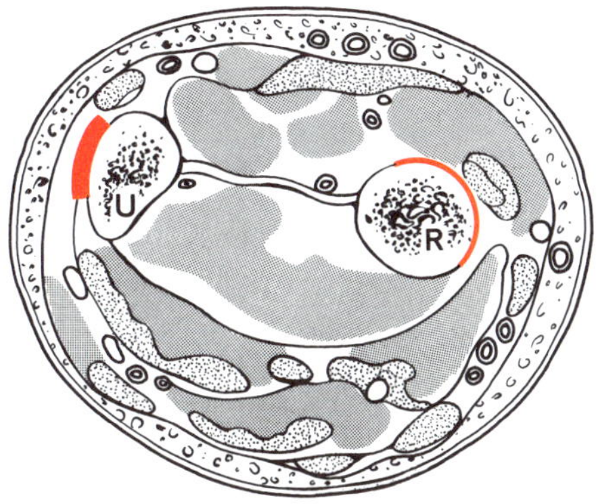

8

Excessive tension of the soft tissues frequently requires addition of a half-tubular plate. The latter, being the weaker plate, is applied to the radius which, as the pronating bone, must, above all, remain stable on rotation.

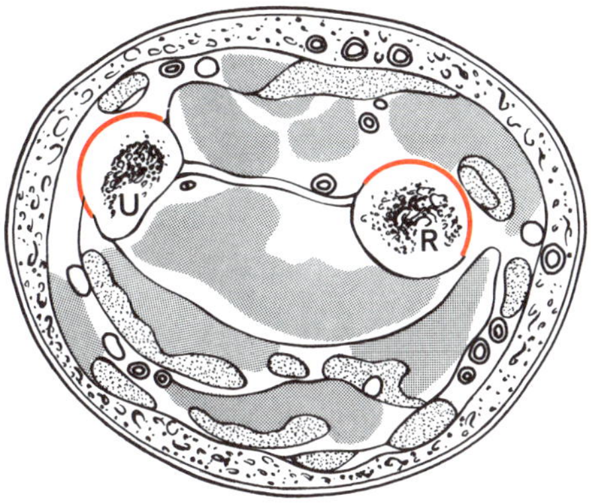

9

Only in exceptional cases do the soft tissues impede the application of two half-tubular plates.

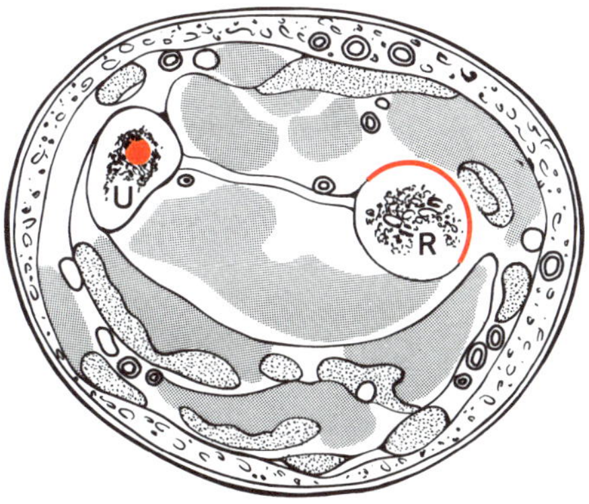

10

In such instances one can resort to the Rush pin, since this instrument is inserted into the ulna which, as the "carrier bone", is not subject to rotation. The pseudarthrosis, which frequently ensues, can be easily rectified by compression plate fixation.

Radius and ulna

Anatomy

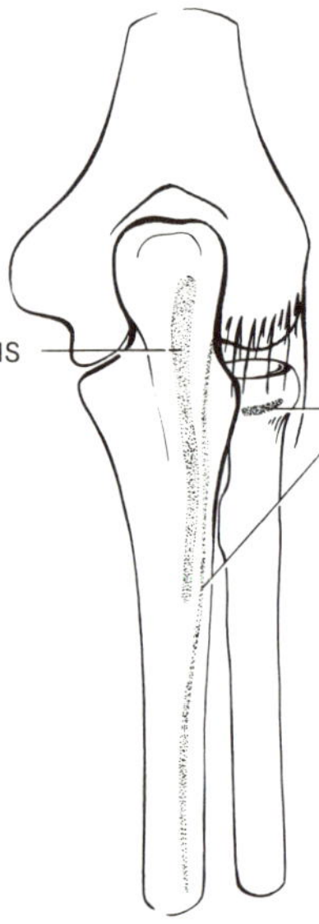

1
Origin of the anconeus muscle.

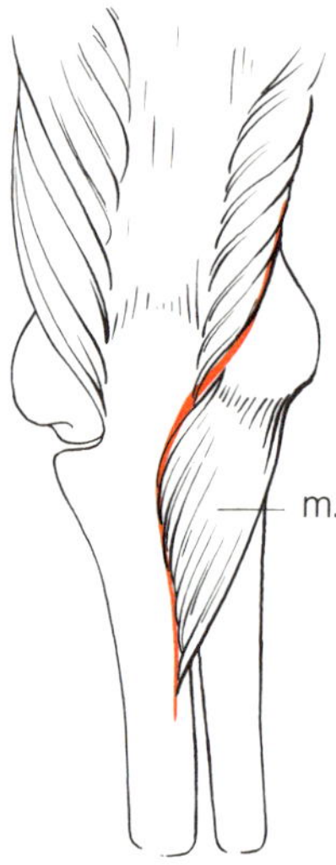

2
Shape and course of the isolated anconeus muscle.

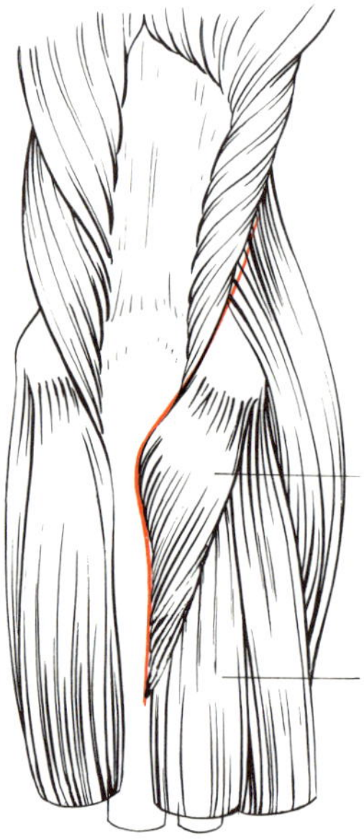

3
Anconeus muscle in the surrounding musculature.

Positioning See Fig. 79–8

Dorsal approach, after Boyd

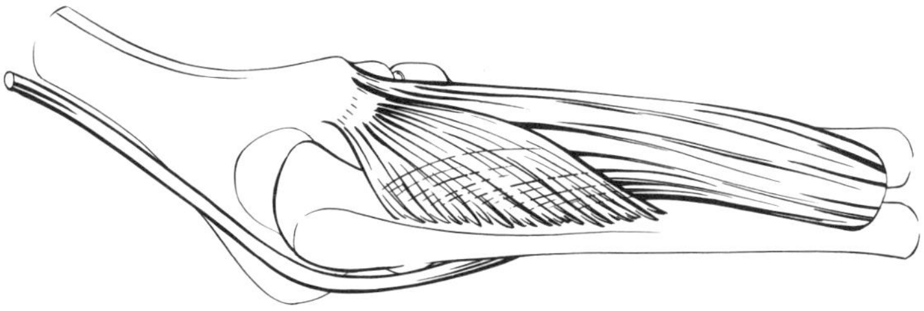

4
Skin incision one fingerbreadth radial to the posterior edge of the ulna.

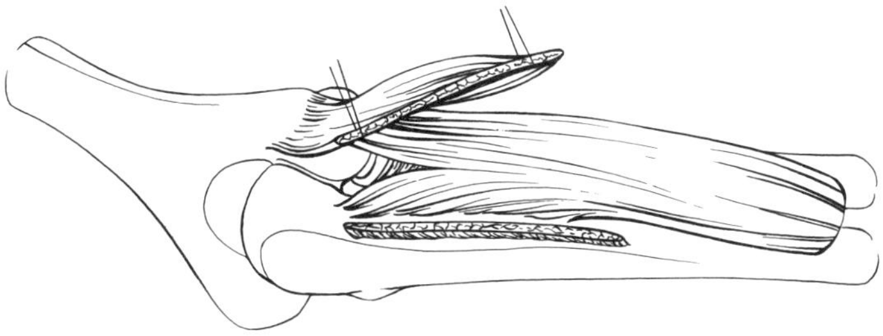

5
Detaching the origin of the anconeus muscle and...

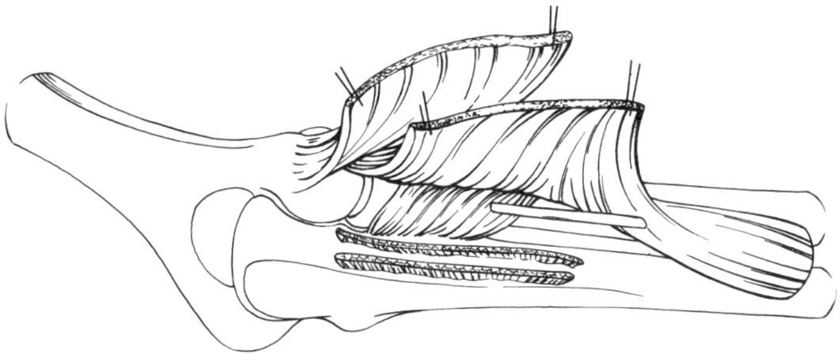

6
... the subjacent extensor carpi ulnaris muscle. The deep branch of the radial nerve, which penetrates the supinator muscle, is identified. (See also Figs. 111–1 and 117–3 ff.)

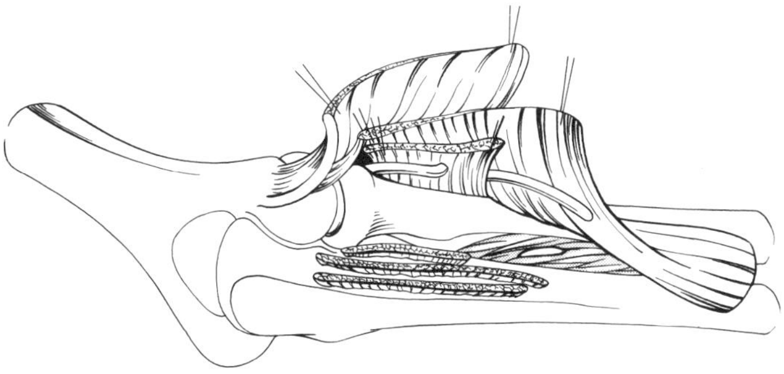

7
The radial insertion of the supinator muscle is detached. If the deep branch of the radial nerve is overstretched or injured, the thumb can no longer be abducted. Because the patient is postoperatively provided with a plaster cast, this anomaly may be overlooked for a long time, particularly since the other functions of the radial nerve have remained intact.

Ulna

Positioning See Fig. 79–8

Approach

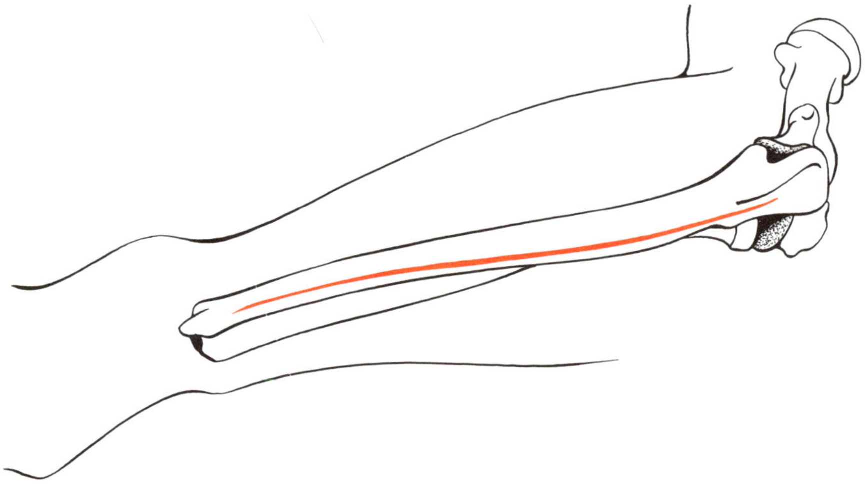

1

The skin incision is made on the extensor surface. It runs over a length of 0.5–1 cm, parallel to the palpable edge of the ulna.

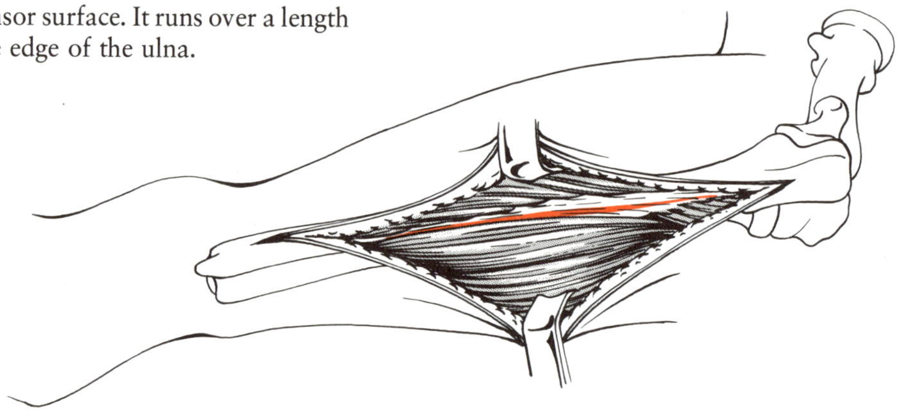

2

Without detaching the soft tissues layer by layer, the incision is carried down straight to the bone.

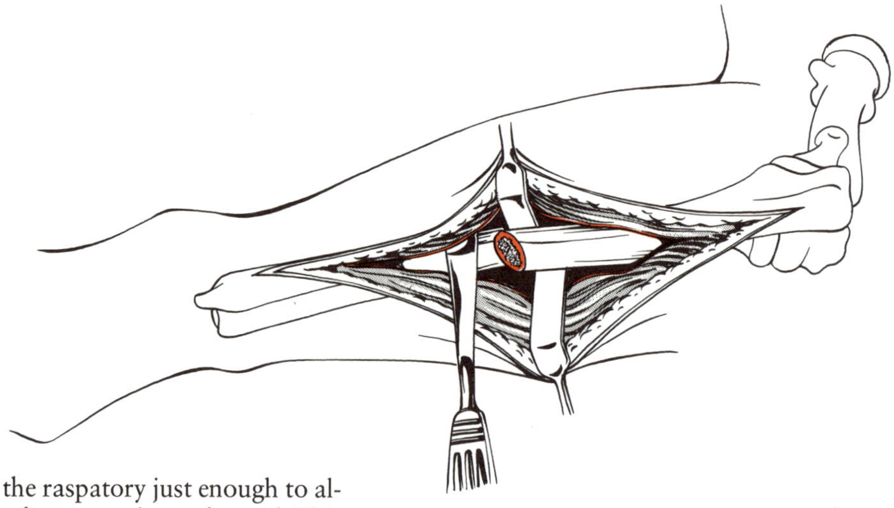

3

The soft tissues are pushed aside with the raspatory just enough to allow the fracture to be reduced and plate fixation to be performed. This means that in the fracture area complete detachment of the soft tissues, often as much as 1 cm proximal and distal to the fracture cleft, is usually unavoidable. Sometimes it suffices to make just sufficient room for the plate to be applied.

Radius – proximal part

Anatomy

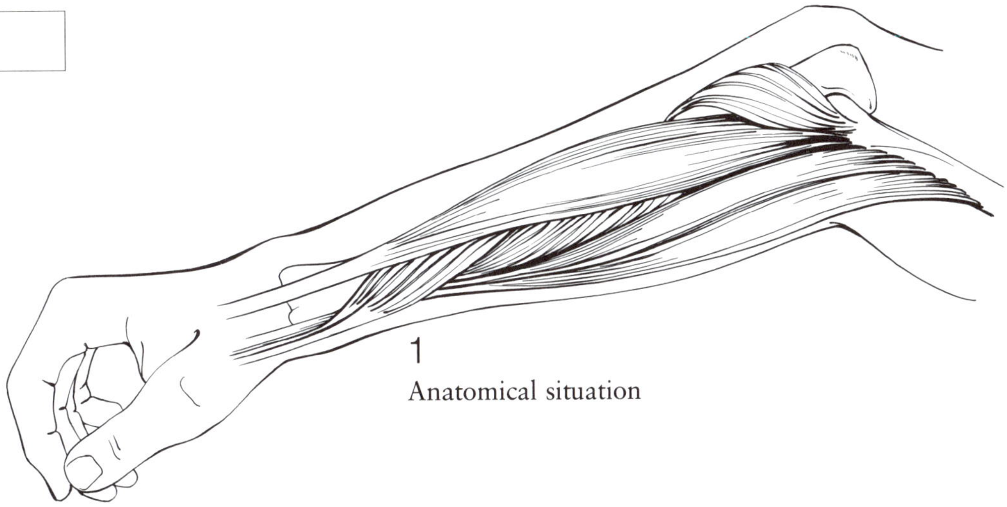

1
Anatomical situation

Positioning

See Fig. 79–8.

Approach

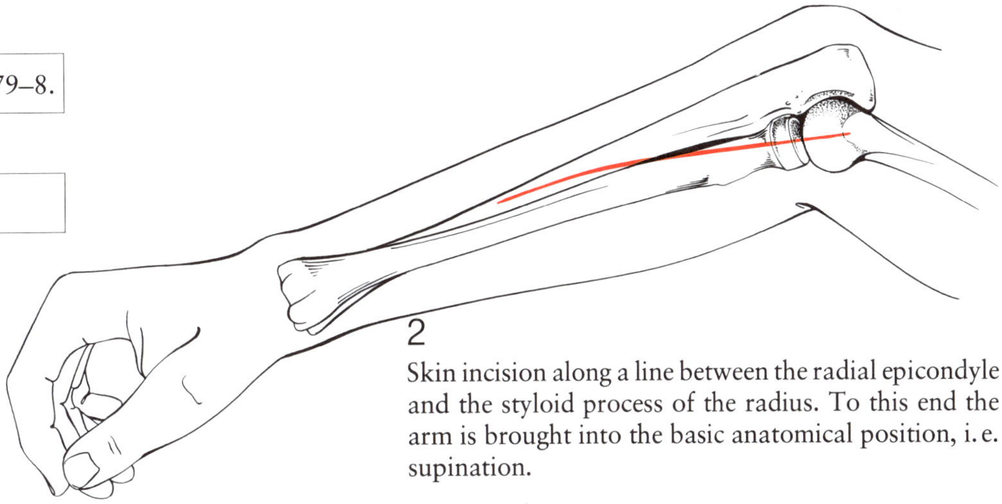

2
Skin incision along a line between the radial epicondyle and the styloid process of the radius. To this end the arm is brought into the basic anatomical position, i.e. supination.

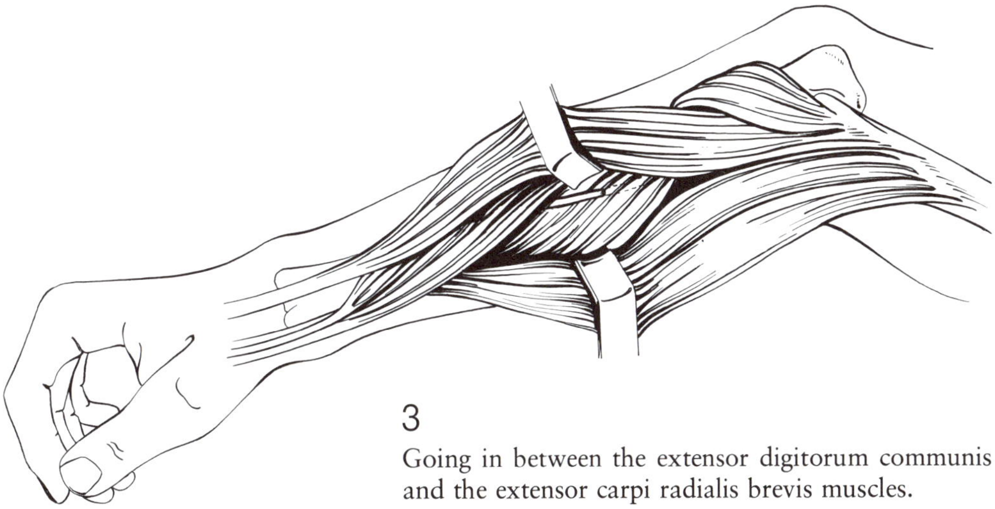

3
Going in between the extensor digitorum communis and the extensor carpi radialis brevis muscles.

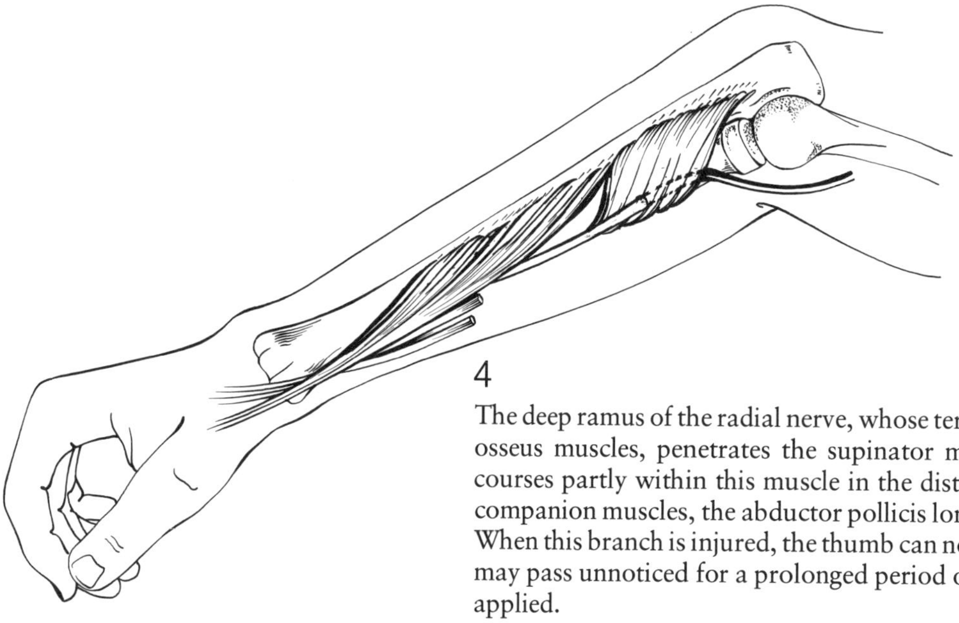

4

The deep ramus of the radial nerve, whose terminal branch supplies the interosseus muscles, penetrates the supinator muscle from the volar side and courses partly within this muscle in the distal direction to reach its further companion muscles, the abductor pollicis longus and the extensores pollicis. When this branch is injured, the thumb can no longer be abducted; this lesion may pass unnoticed for a prolonged period of time if a plaster cast has been applied.

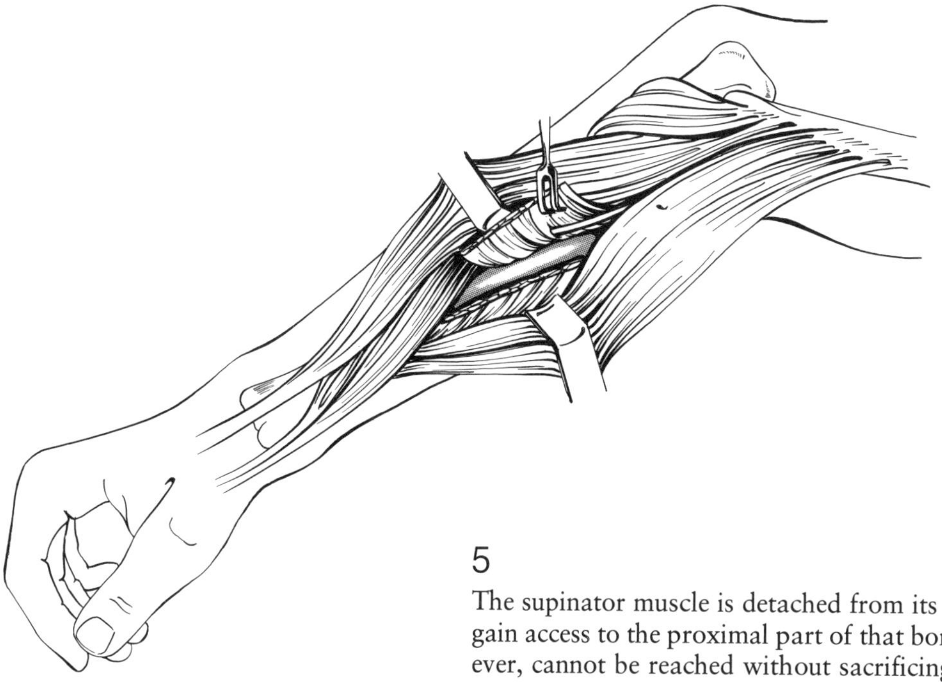

5

The supinator muscle is detached from its lateral insertion in the radius to gain access to the proximal part of that bone. The head of the radius, however, cannot be reached without sacrificing the nerve.

Middle part of radius

Positioning and approach

See Fig. 79–8.

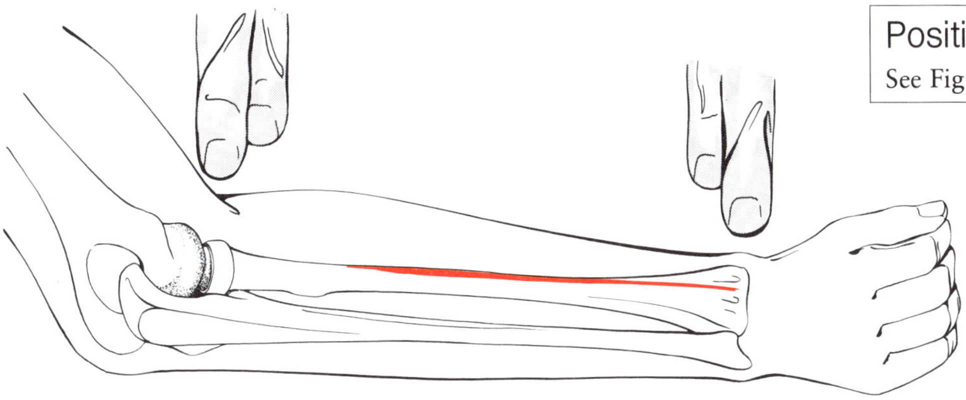

1

Skin incision a short distance dorsal to the palpable radius along a line connecting the styloid process of the radius and the lateral epicondyle. To this end the arm is flexed at the elbow joint and the forearm is supinated. When a medial incision has previously been made to gain access to the ulna, great care should be taken to assure that the bridge of soft tissues between the two incisions does not become too narrow.

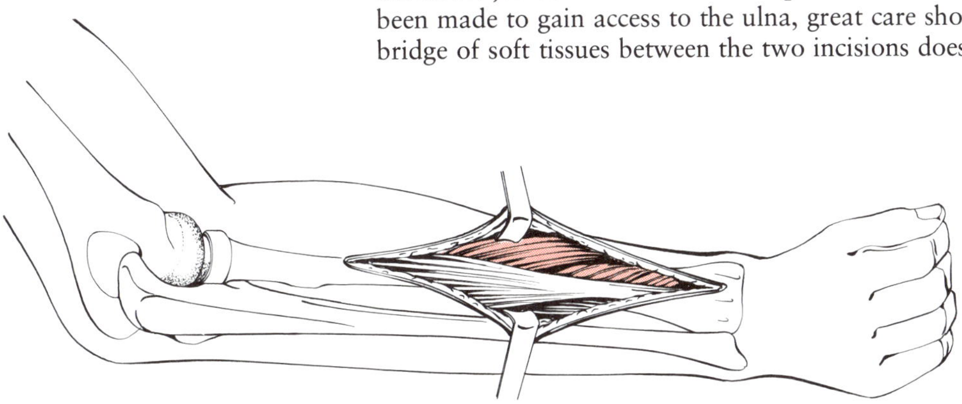

2

Going in between the extensor carpi radialis brevis and the extensor digitorum muscles in the middle third and in the distal part of the incision down to the bone.

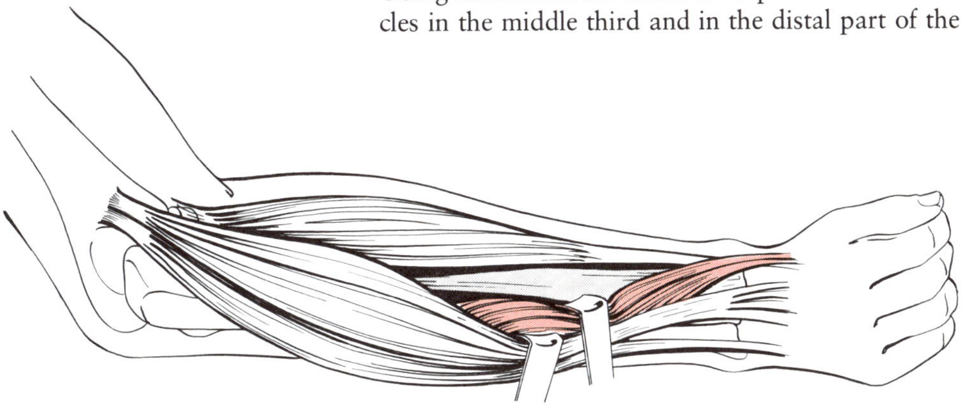

3

The abductor pollicis longus and the extensor pollicis brevis muscles course parallel to each other obliquely through the operative field. These muscles are detached from the gliding tissues, proximally on the radial side and distally on the ulnar side, and are undermined upon the radius.

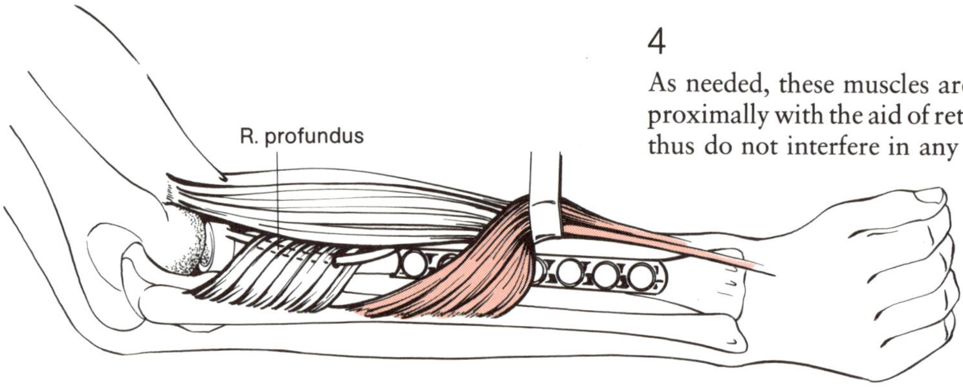

4

As needed, these muscles are pulled distally (Fig. 120–5) or proximally with the aid of retractors or retention sutures, and thus do not interfere in any way with the operation.

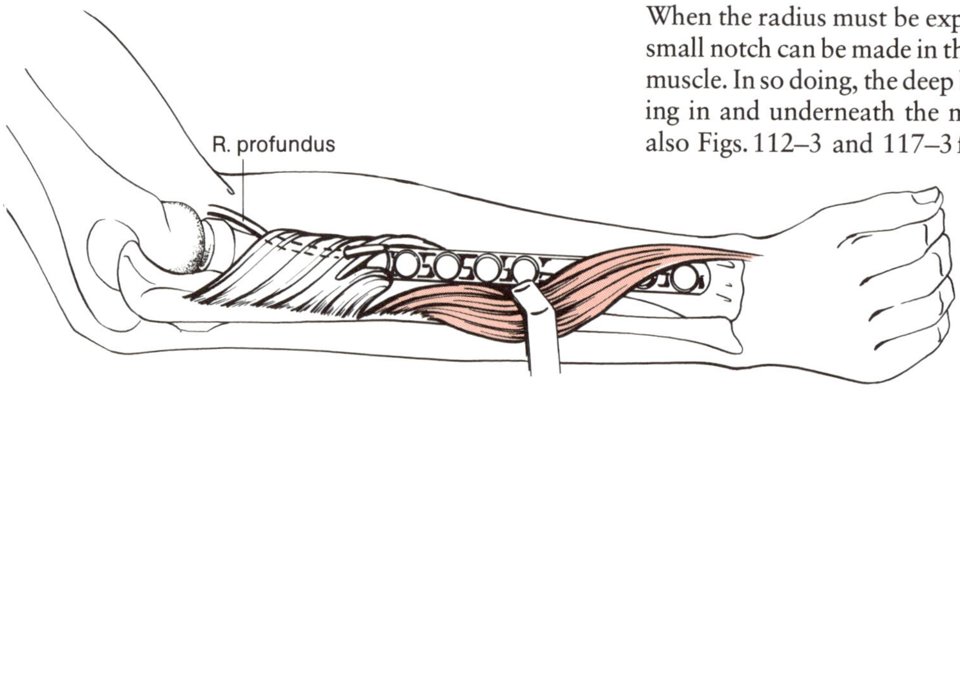

5

When the radius must be exposed a little more proximally, a small notch can be made in the distal portion of the supinator muscle. In so doing, the deep branch of the radial nerve coursing in and underneath the muscle must not be injured. See also Figs. 112–3 and 117–3 ff.

Radius – distal part

Anatomy

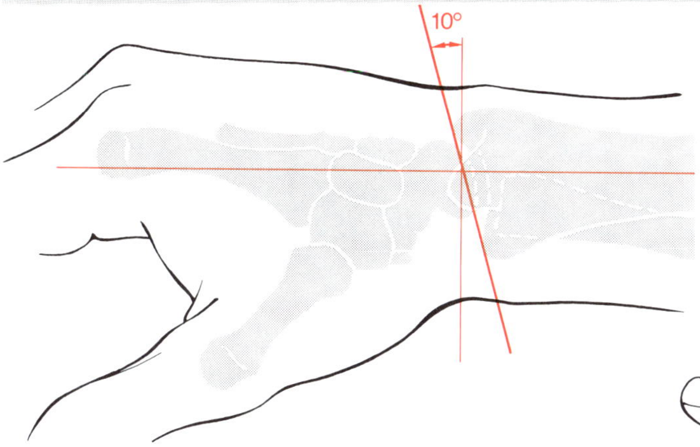

1

The articular surface of the radius is inclined about 10° to its volar side.

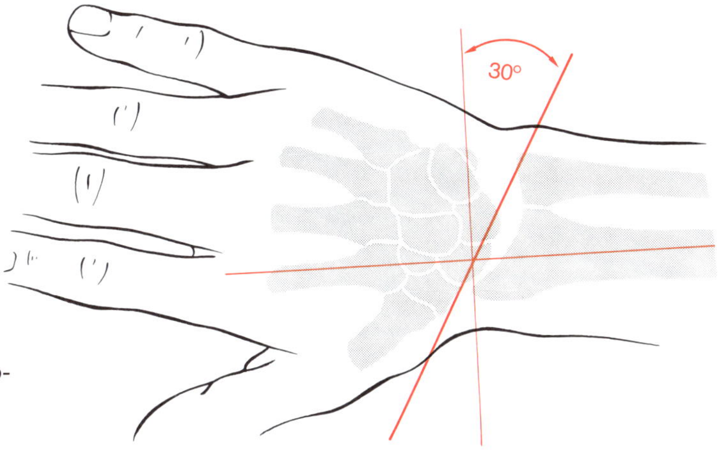

2

In the transverse plane the inclination amounts to about 30°.

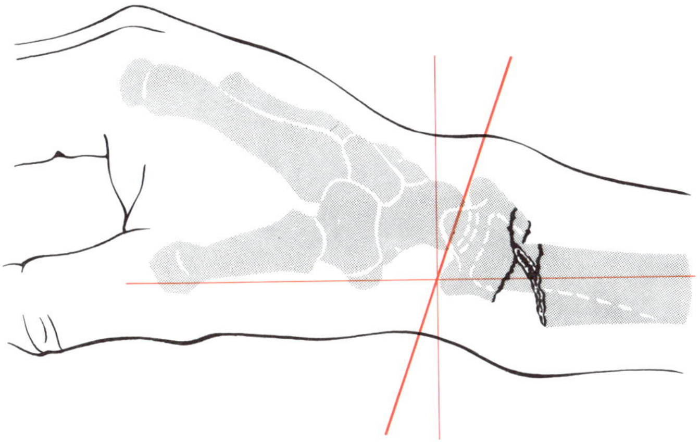

3

Hyperextension fracture, frequent. Treatment with use of a primarily split, circular plaster cast for the forearm. In comminuted fractures, a plaster cast is applied to the upper arm. Reduction through suspending the arm by the thumb for 20 to 30 minutes.

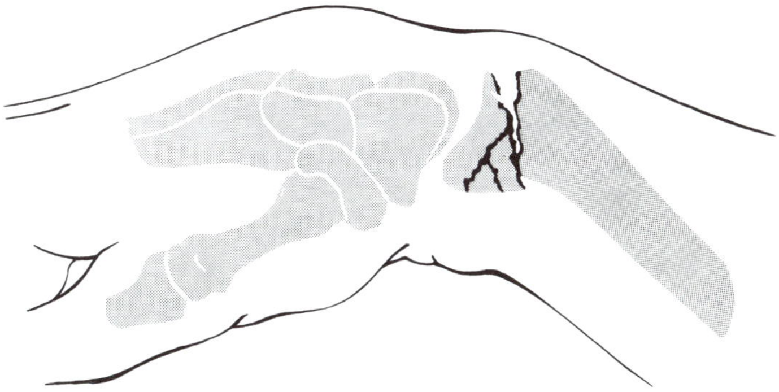

4

Flexion fracture. Conservative treatment. Adequate position of the fragments can, however, only be achieved in most cases by operation; this is particularly so in maintenance.

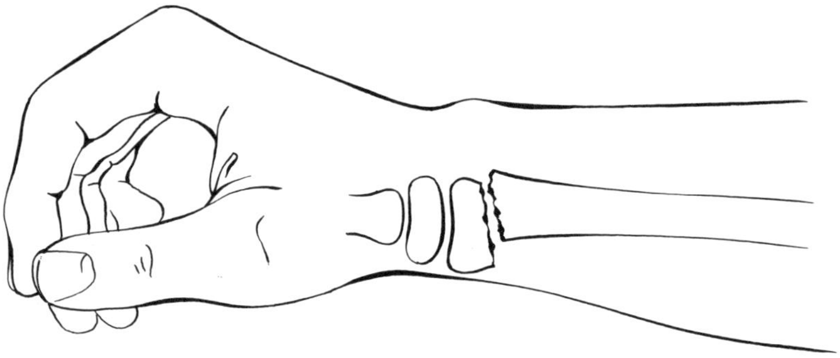

5

Flexion fracture: transverse, not intra-articular (type I).

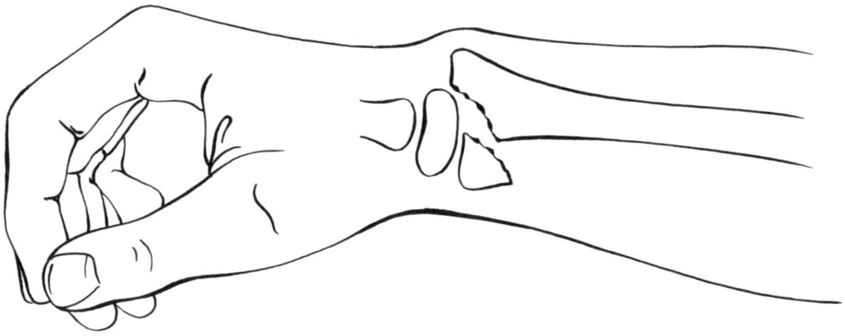

6

Flexion fracture: intra-articular, with subluxation of the carpus (type II).

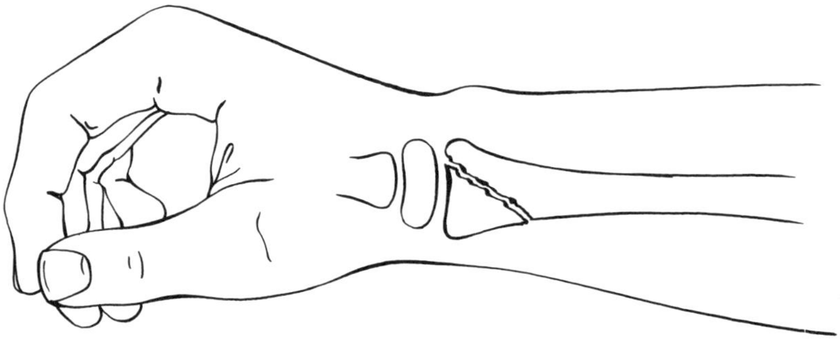

7

Flexion fracture: oblique (type III).

Indication

Conservative treatment for type I, often also for type II. Operative treatment for unstable fractures of type II, and without exception for type III.

Volar approach

For dorsal approach, see Figs. 119–1 ff.

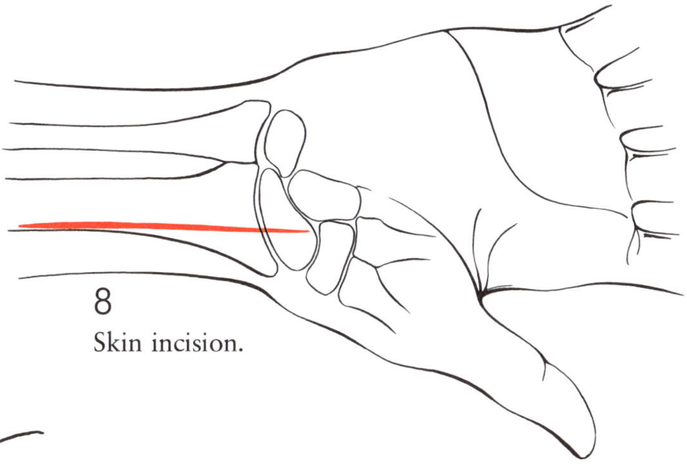

8
Skin incision.

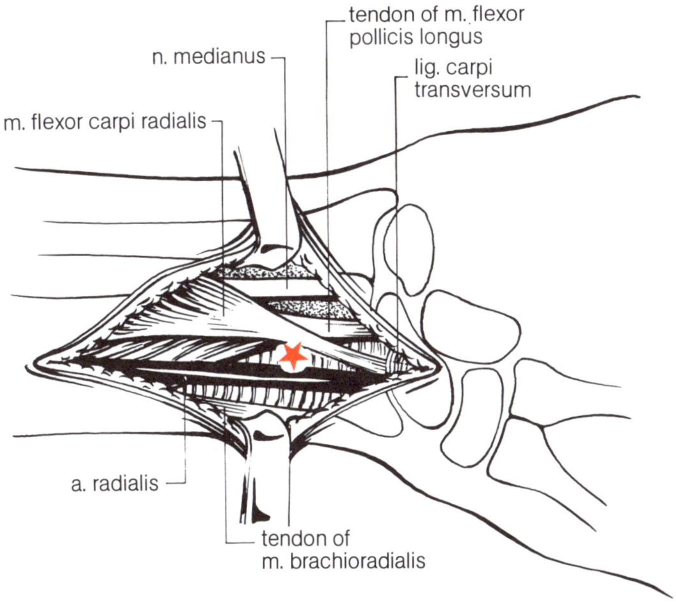

9
Anatomical situation following division of the subcutaneous tissues: median nerve, flexor carpi radialis and flexor pollicis longus muscles, radial artery and brachioradialis muscle are visible and remain on the radial side. The tendons of the flexor carpi radialis and flexor pollicis longus muscles are pulled toward the ulnar side.

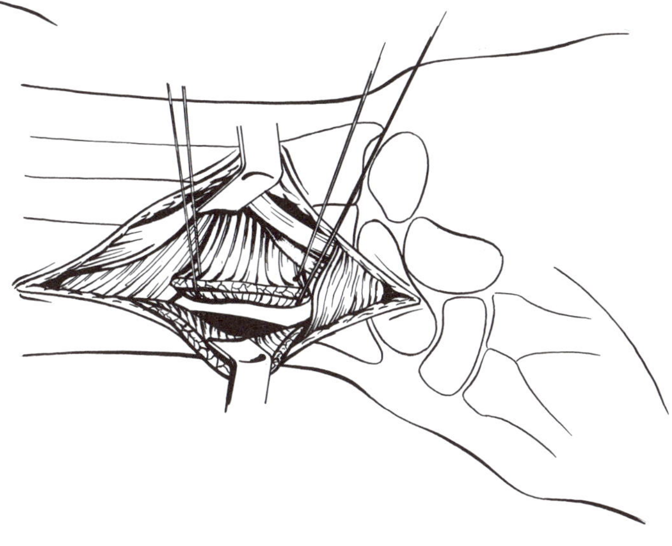

10
The pronator quadratus muscle is divided on the radial side and pushed toward the ulna.

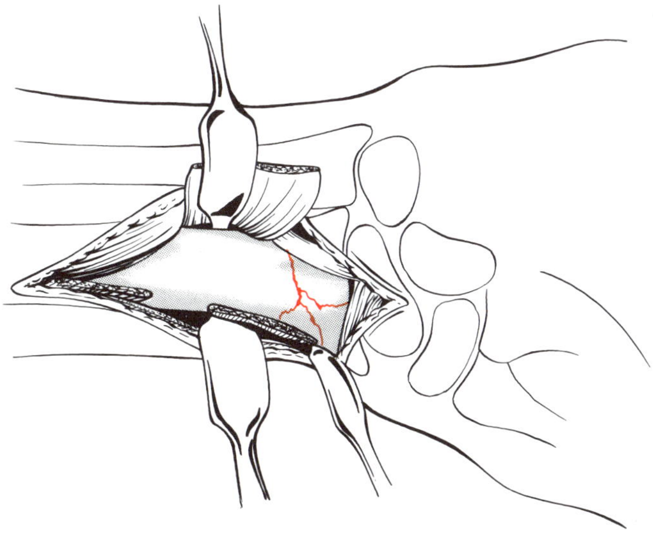

11
The distal volar surface of the radius is exposed.

Tactics

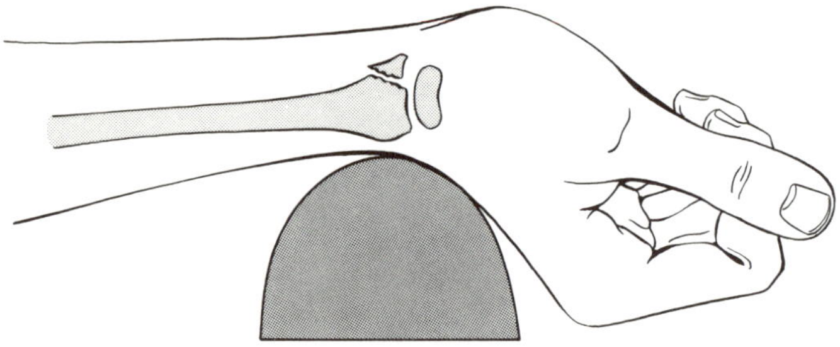

12

Reduction with traction over a fulcrum by hyperextension in the supinated position of the wrist.

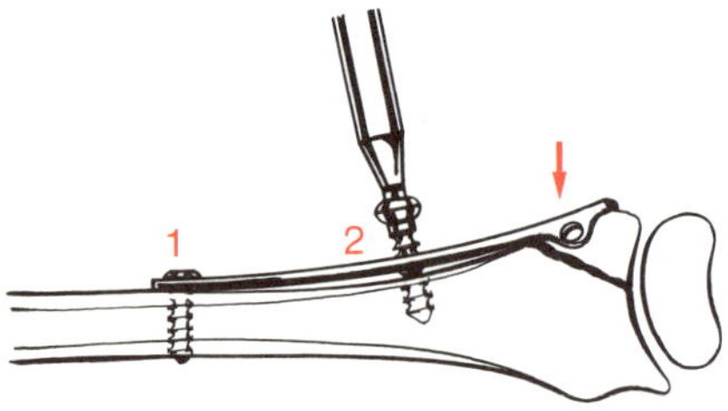

13

Preliminary bending of a small T plate. The first screw to be inserted (small-fragment cortical screw) is that in the most proximal hole of the plate.

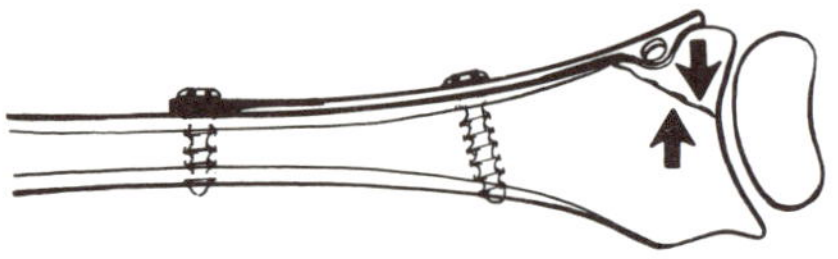

14

This alone suffices to develop interfragmental compression and to support the distal fragment.

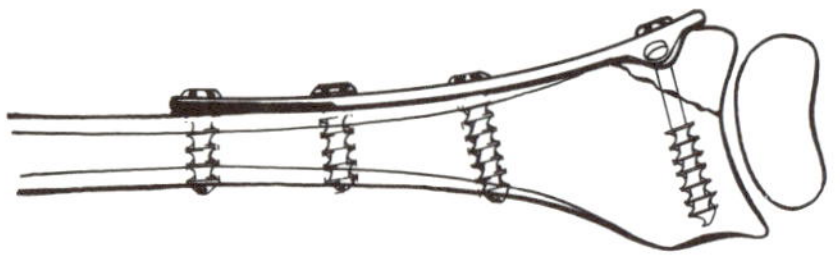

15

A cancellous screw is inserted through the distal fragment to increase interfragmental compression. When the bone is weak and osteoporotic this screw can be dispensed with.

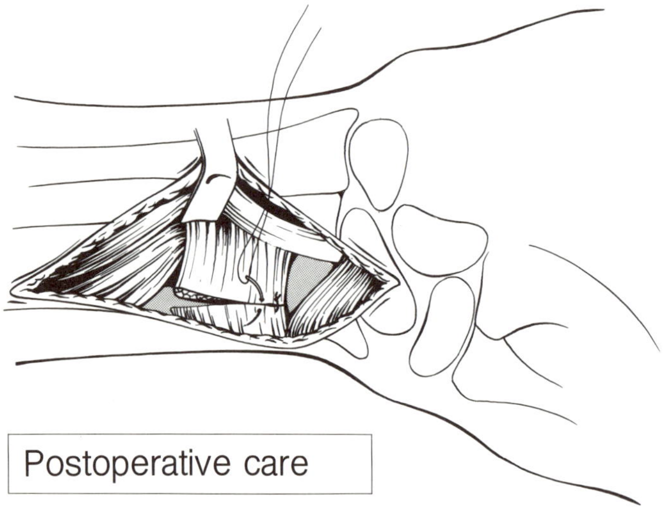

16

Closure of the wound: The pronator quadratus muscle is reunited by suture.

Postoperative care

A plaster cast or plaster shell is applied for a few days. The arm is suspended. Finger exercises are started immediately. Beginning on the third to fifth day, the fingers are actively exercised, with the plaster shell removed.

Monteggia's fracture

Anatomy

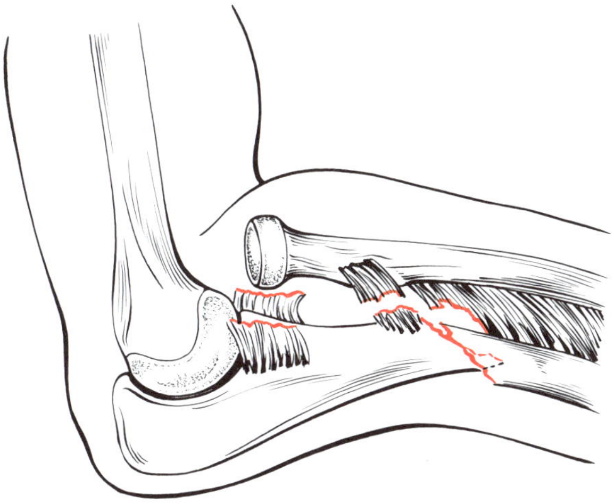

1
Anatomical situation.

Diagnosis

Clinical signs:
- Restriction of all movements at the elbow joint.
- The displaced head of the radius is readily felt.
- Tenderness over head of radius and fracture of ulna.

Roentgenologic findings:
- Anteroposterior view with the elbow extended as far as possible and the supinated forearm put on its dorsum.
- Lateral view with the upper arm on the roentgen table, the forearm flexed and supinated.
- The dislocation of the head of the radius can hardly be overlooked if one verifies whether the axis of the radius points in both planes to the center of the head of the radius.

Operative possibilities

- When the *difference in length of the ulna is appropriately corrected* by plate fixation, the head of the radius often undergoes spontaneous reduction.
- Intraoperative radiographic control.
- When osteosynthesis of the ulna fails to produce spontaneous reduction: the portions of capsule and ligaments that interfere with reduction are removed through a separate approach to the head of the radius (See Fig. 95–3 f.).
- The anular ligament of the radius does not as a rule require suturing; only the dorsal portions of the capsule may be reunited.

8. Pelvis – Acetabulum

Anatomy

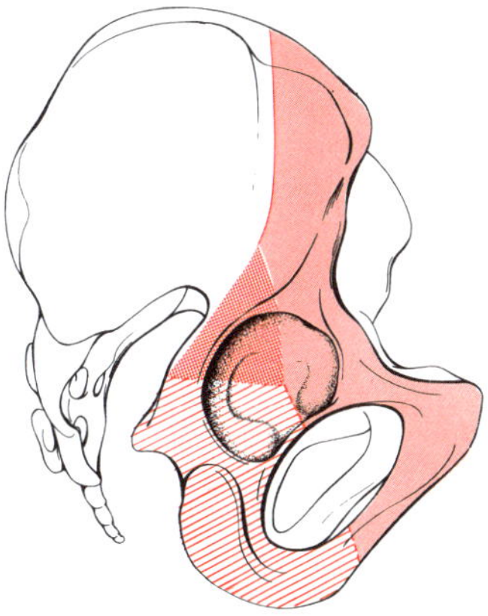

1
For the planning and tactics of operative interventions it is very helpful to conceive of the massive roof of the acetabulum as the keystone of an arch formed by the anterior and posterior pillars.

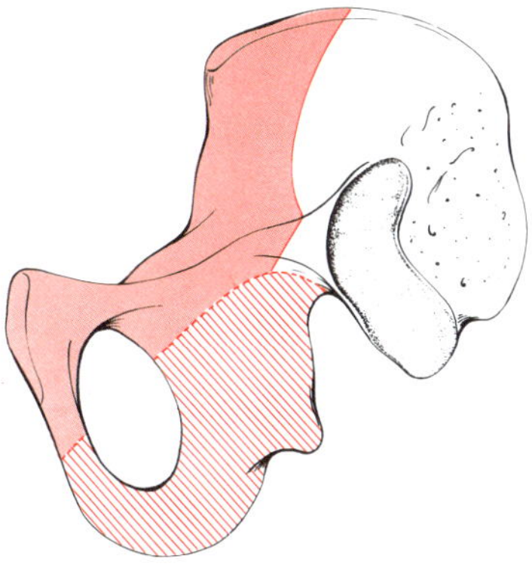

2
The most frequent fractures run along the borders of these pillars.

Types of injuries

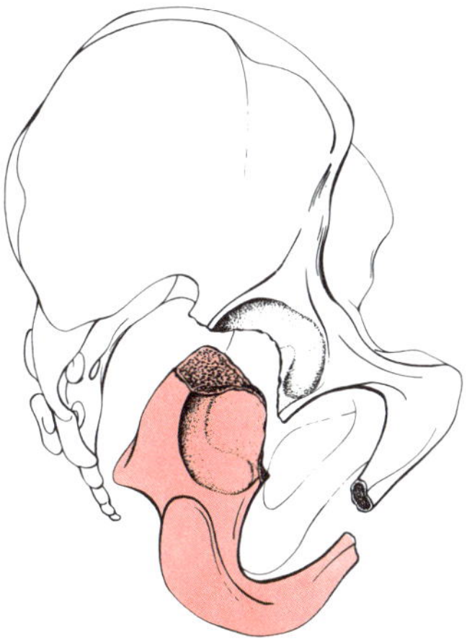

3
Break of the posterior pillar.

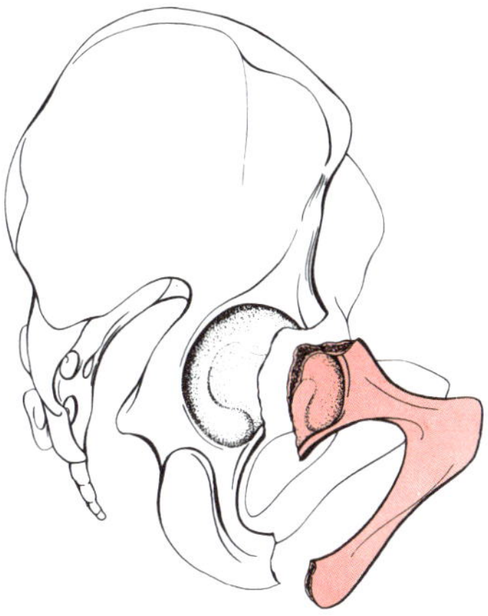

4
Break of the anterior pillar. With this isolated fracture, the fracture line does not as a rule extend as high into the iliac wing as might be expected from Fig. 127–1.

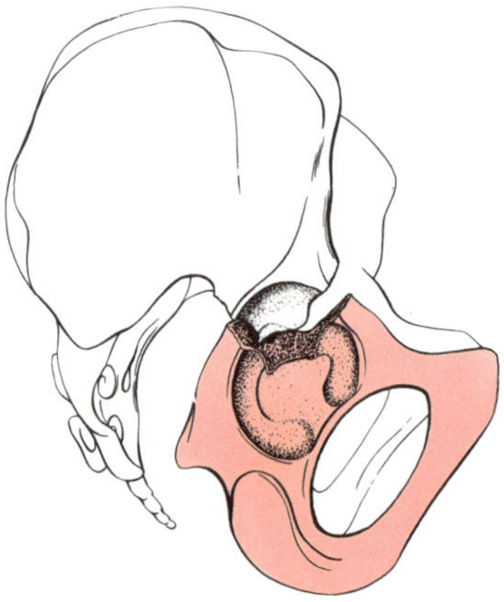

5

Transverse fracture. High transverse fractures may run above the acetabulum.

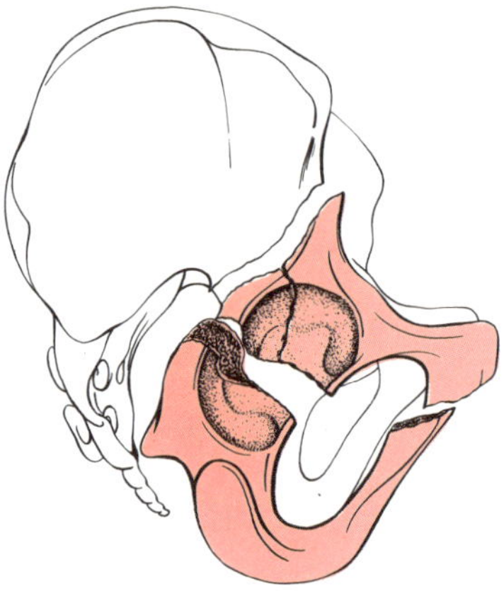

6

Combined fracture of the anterior and posterior pillars. Here the most cranial fracture line of the anterior pillar lies higher than in an isolated fracture of this pillar and thereby corresponds to the border of the pillar.
Particular feature: there is always an additional fracture in the acetabular region.

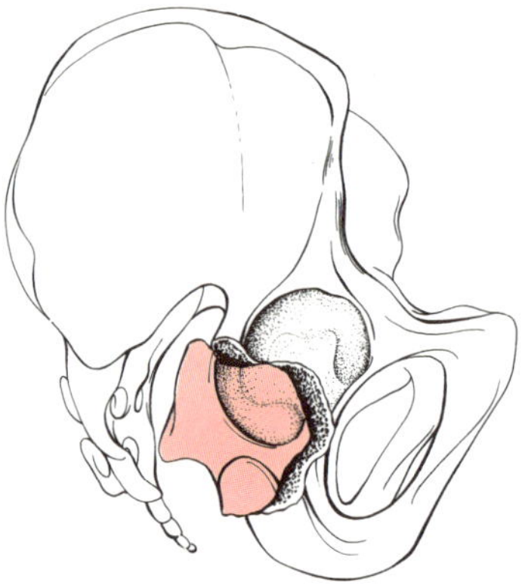

7

Fracture of the posterior wall, i.e. fracture of the posterior rim of the acetabulum.

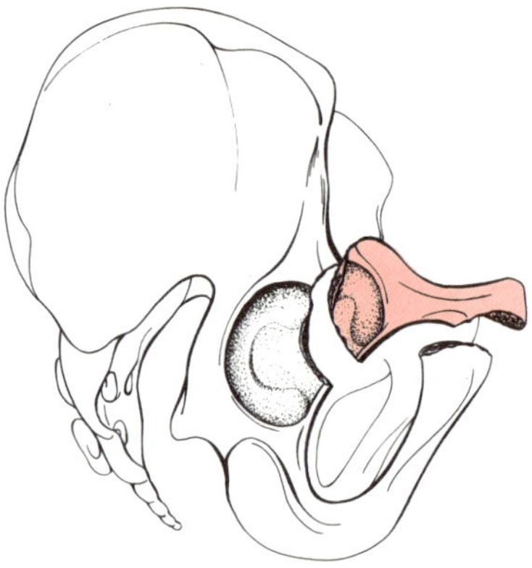

8

Fracture of the anterior wall of the acetabulum.

Diagnosis

Only the subsequent *combined interpretation of three different roentgenograms* allows one to form an adequate idea of the real extent of the acetabular injury.

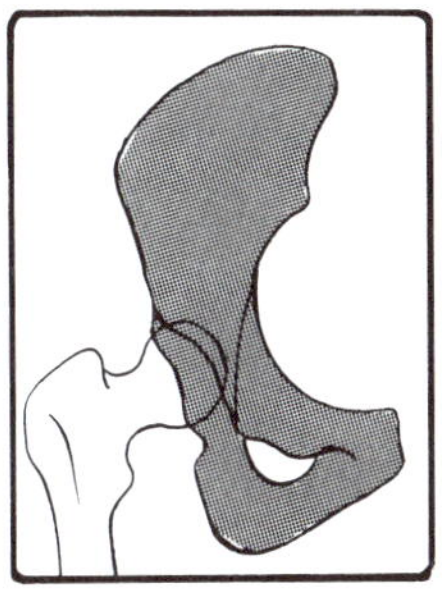

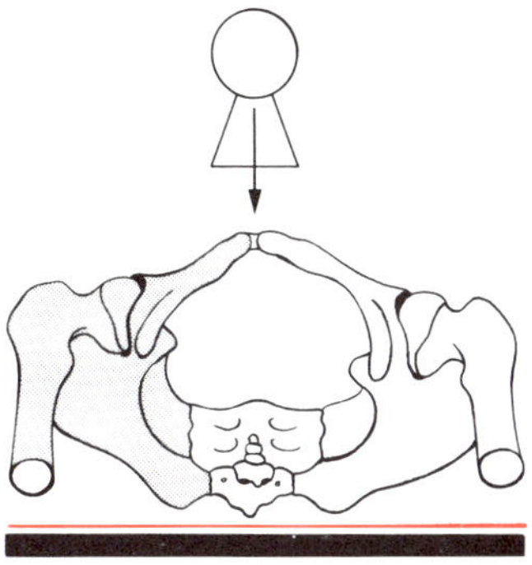

9
Standard anteroposterior view of the entire pelvis to exclude a bilateral injury.

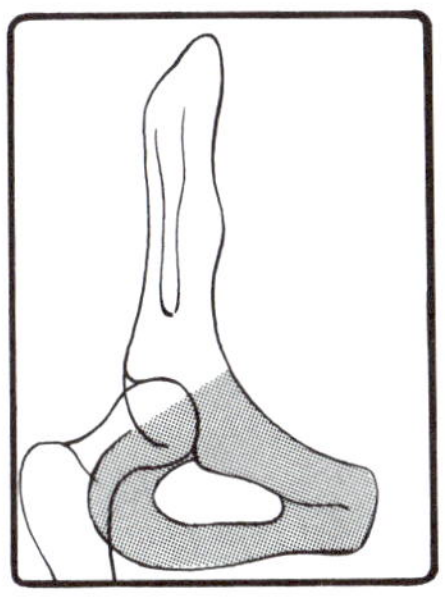

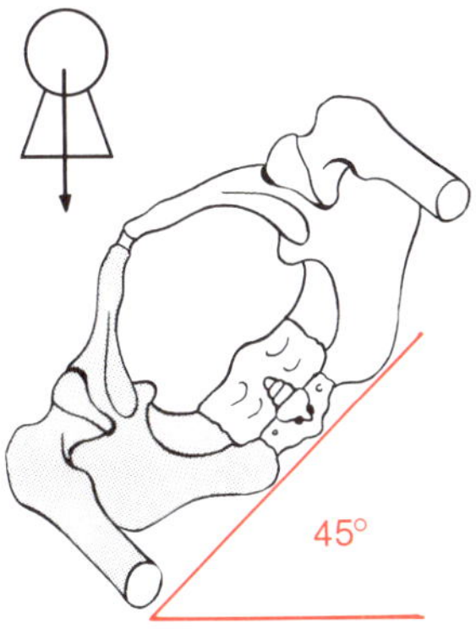

10
An *obturator view* shows the conditions in the posterior region of the acetabulum.

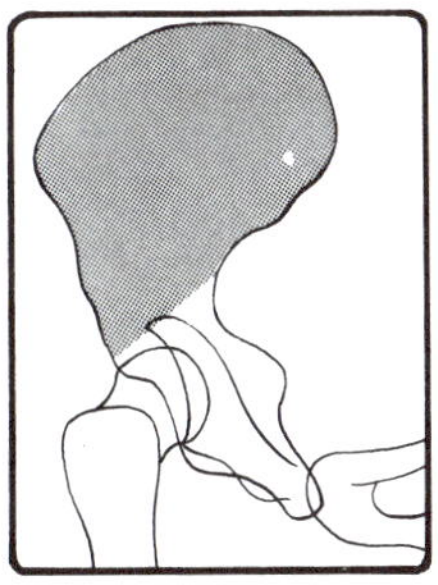

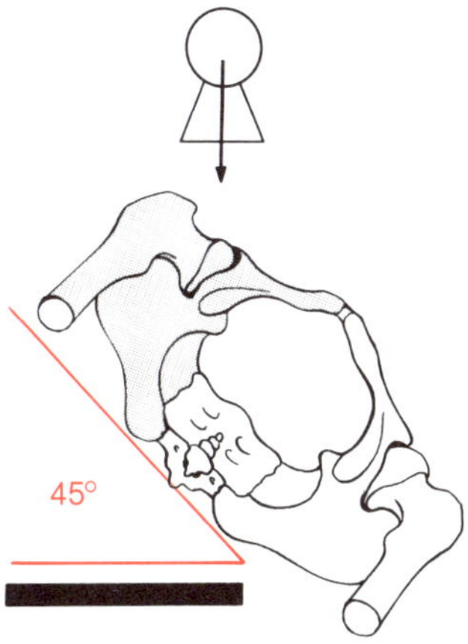

11
A *left anterior view* shows the conditions in the floor of the acetabulum and in the anterior pillar.

Timing of the operation

Operation should be performed at the earliest possible moment (within 24 hours), as soon as the circulatory conditions are stabilized. After a week, massive periarticular calcification must be anticipated.

Operative possibilities

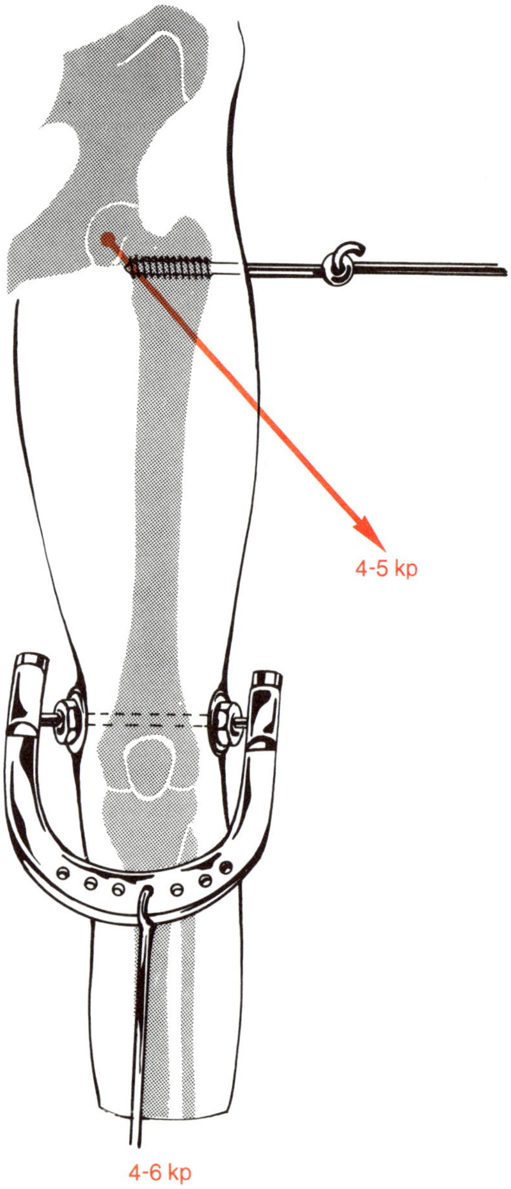

12
Conservative management with traction. By applying double traction and by adequate distribution of the weights, one can produce a traction vector along the femoral neck.

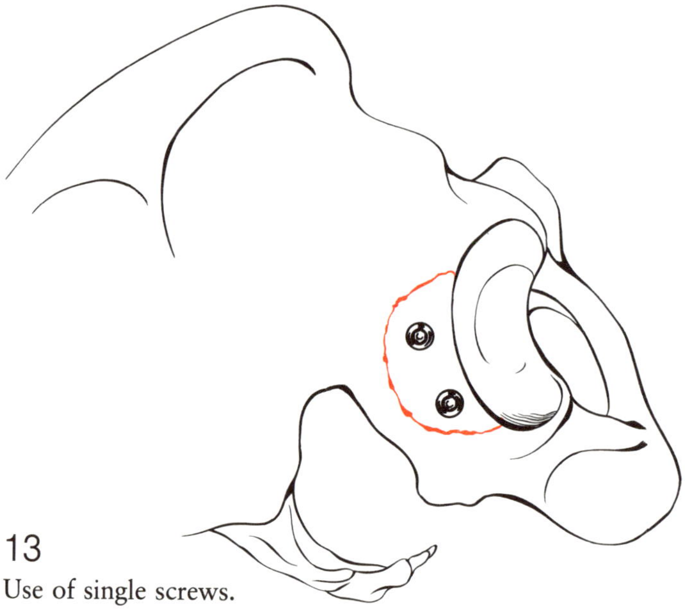

13
Use of single screws.

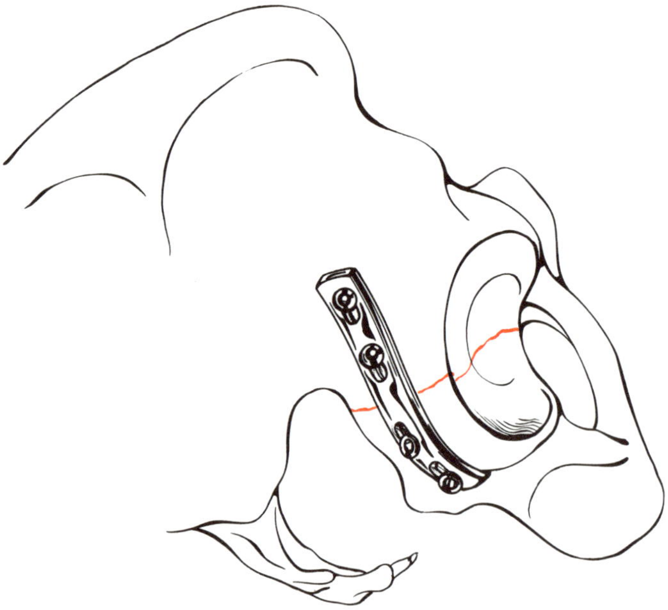

14
Dorsal plate fixation.

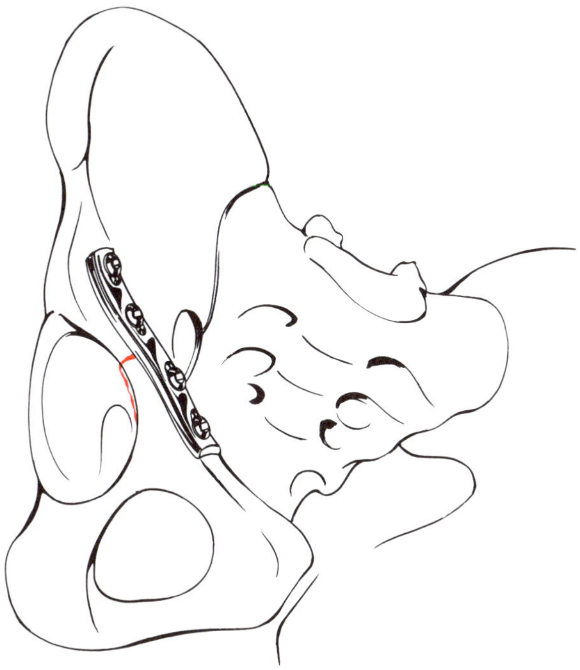

15
Plate fixation along and cranial to the linea terminalis. Front view.

Positioning, sterile draping

See Fig. 142–5. Lying position on the side allows concomitant approach from the anterior and from the dorsal. Sterile draping is applied to the freely movable leg.

Posterior approach See Figs. 142–1 ff.

Anterior approach

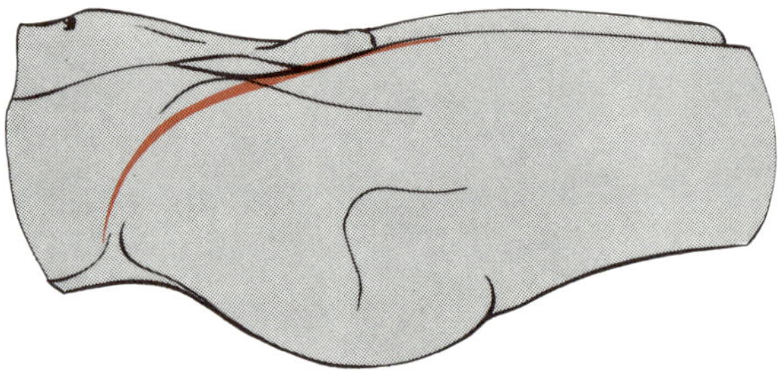

16
Skin incision along the iliac crest...

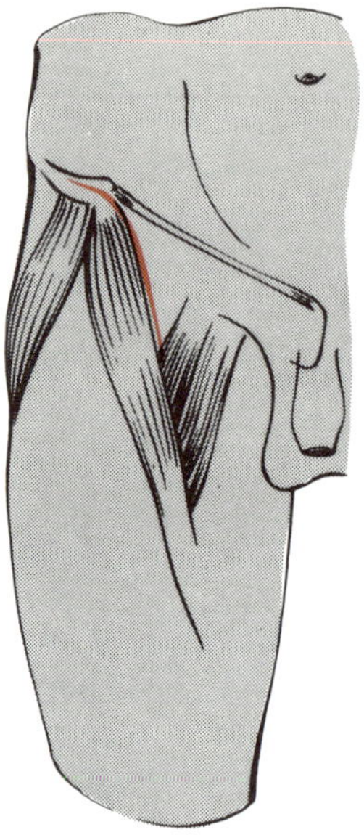

17
... and, turning caudally, along the inner border of the sartorius muscle. With this approach, the lateral cutaneous nerve of the femur cannot be spared.

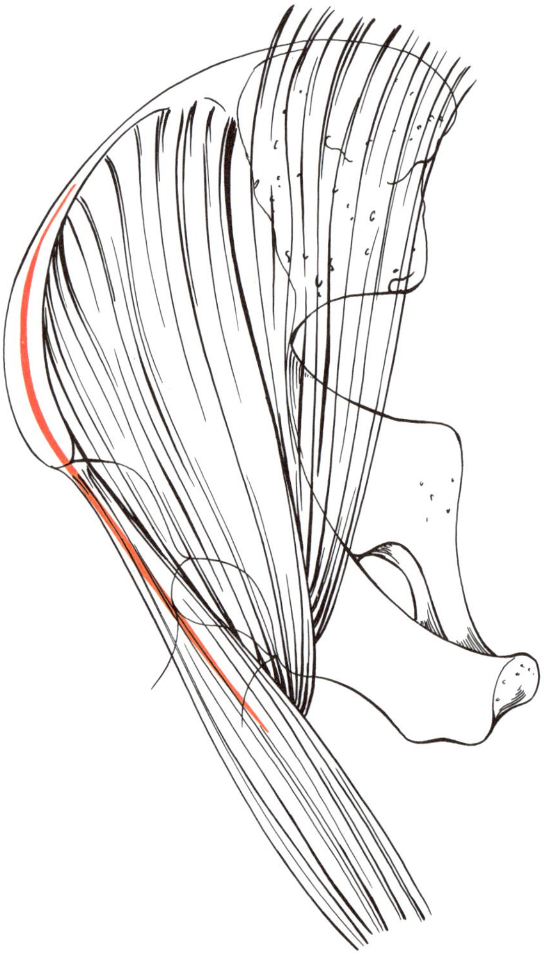

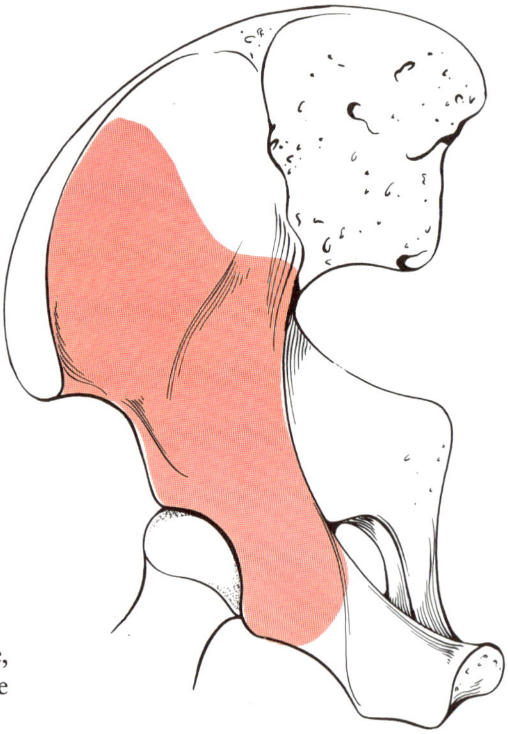

18
This area of the inner side of the pelvis becomes accessible. Here, practically all the fractures requiring operative management are found.

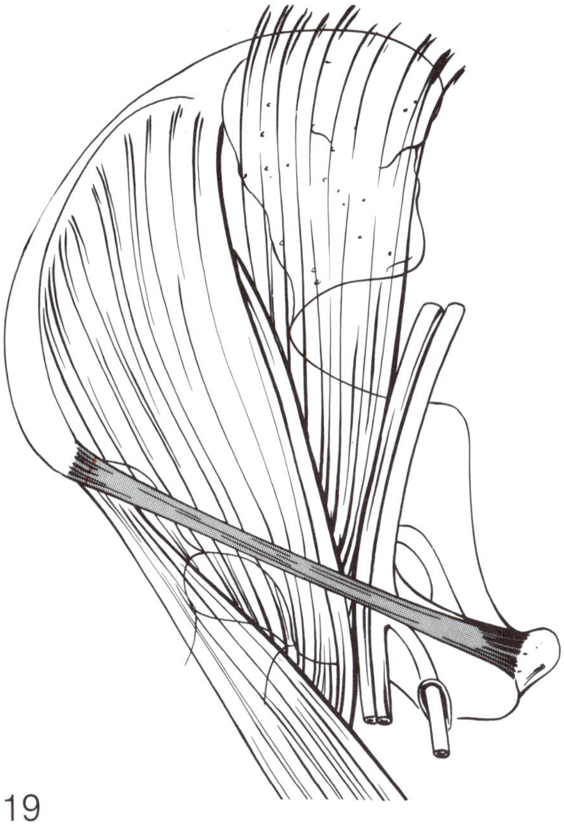

19

Topographic relationships. The inguinal ligament is divided laterally, with a small stump left for reinsertion. The sartorius muscle can, as a rule, remain.

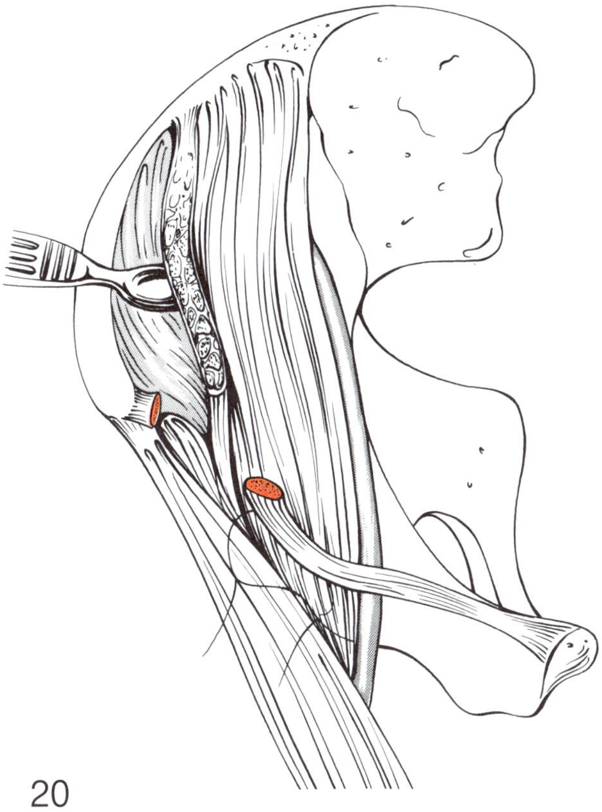

20

Starting from the iliac crest, one detaches the iliac muscle with a sharp raspatory from the inner aspect of the iliac wing, keeping close to the bone.

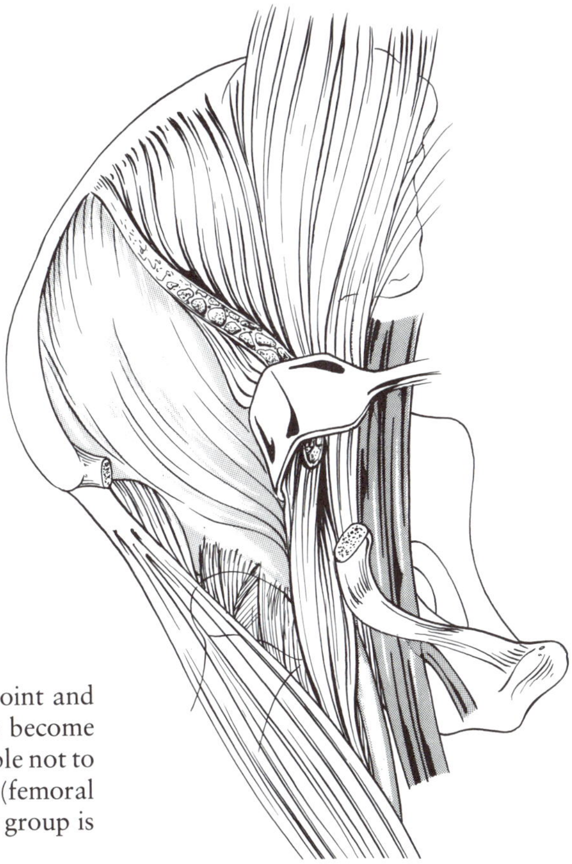

21

Under the muscle, the capsule of the hip joint and the insertion of the rectus femoris muscle become visible. Toward the medial side it is advisable not to apply elevators but exclusively retractors (femoral nerve!). By flexing the hip joint the muscle group is relaxed.

22

The iliopsoas muscle can be pushed aside in such a way that a finger may be put into the superior sciatic notch (See Fig. 135–25).

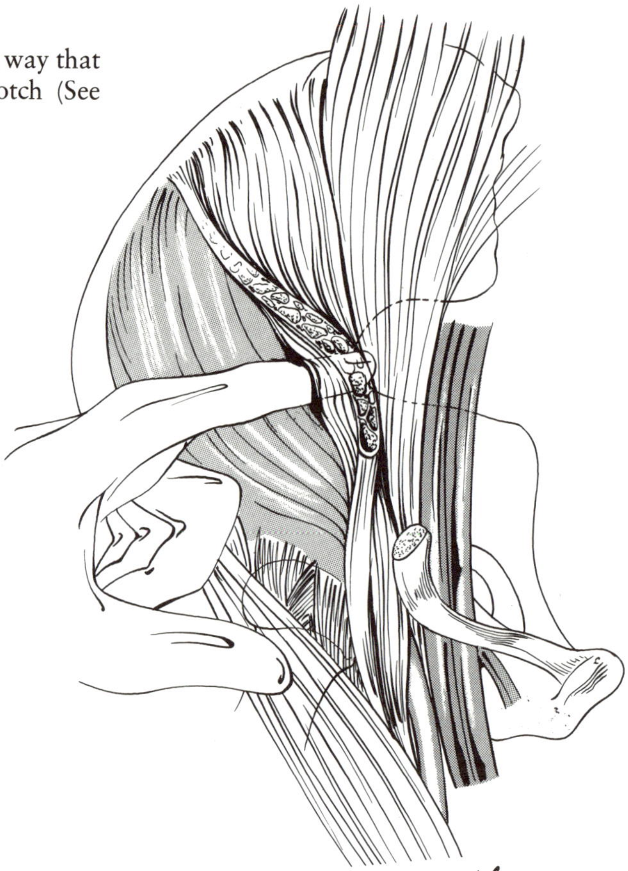

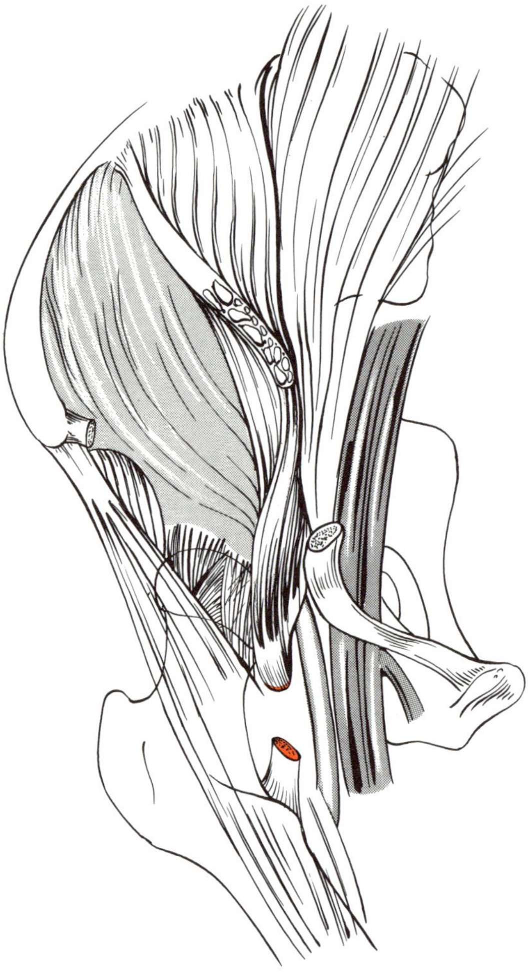

23

When the iliopsoas muscle interferes too greatly with an adequate approach, its insertion in the region of the lesser trochanter can be divided.

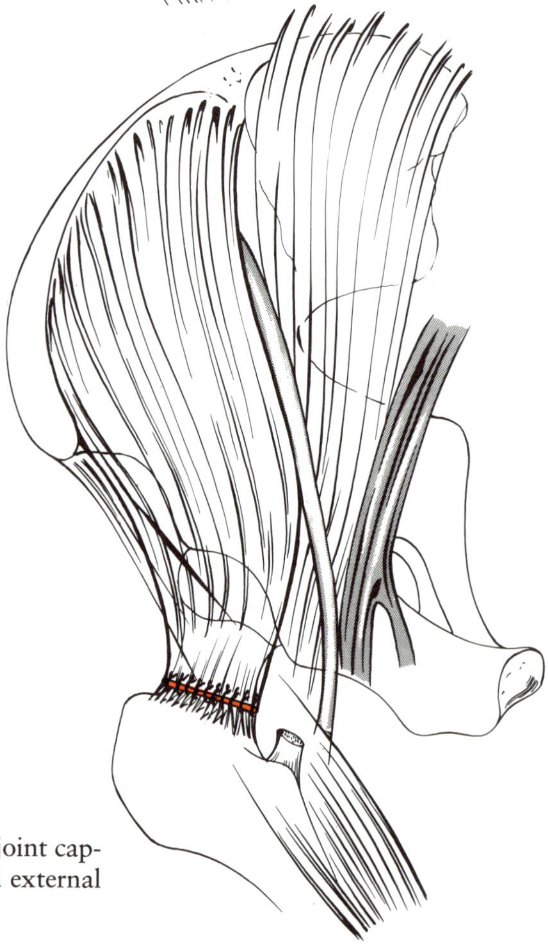

24

If necessary, the muscle can be reinserted into the joint capsule; this is facilitated by concomitant flexion and external rotation at the hip joint.

Tactics

Typical operative techniques can hardly be used in these cases.

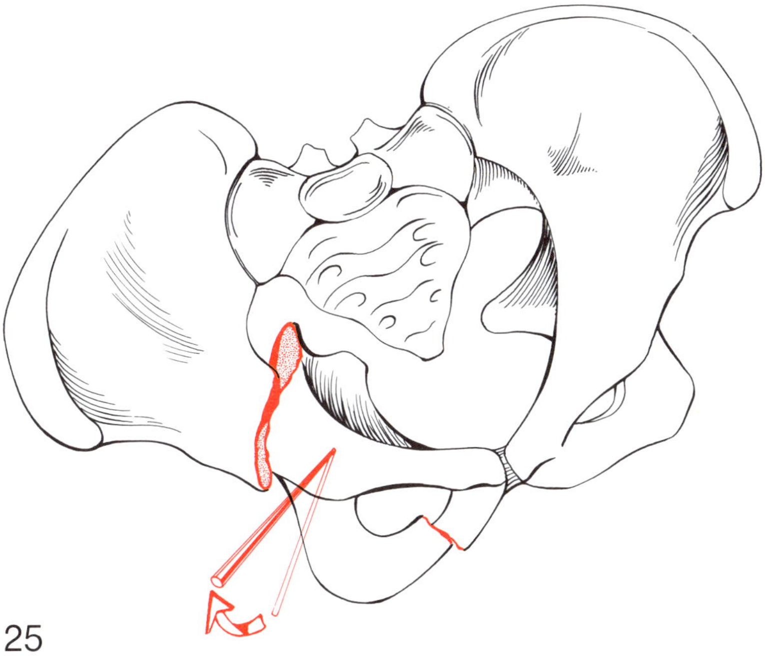

25

When one is faced with a transverse fracture, it should be kept in mind that the proximal and the distal portions of the pelvis are practically always *rotated against each other*. Adequate reduction can only be checked by feeling in the superior iliac notch to ascertain whether the fragments have been reduced without forming a step (See also Fig. 134–22). Safer, still, is a direct visual control at that point.

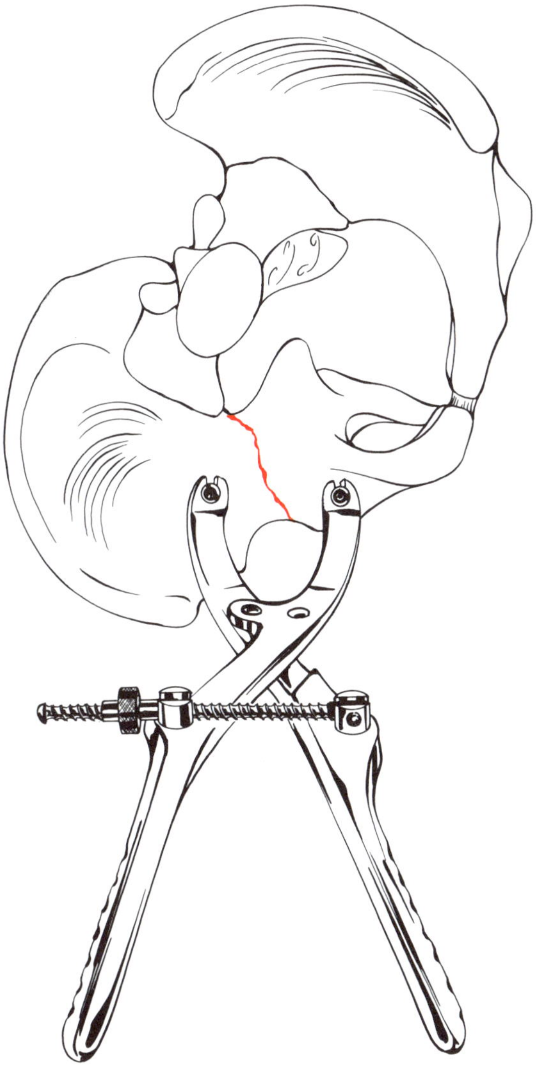

26

Reduction often can be achieved only with the aid of a special instrumentarium. Traction on the leg, assisted by adequate rotational movements in the hip joint, facilitate performing the reduction.

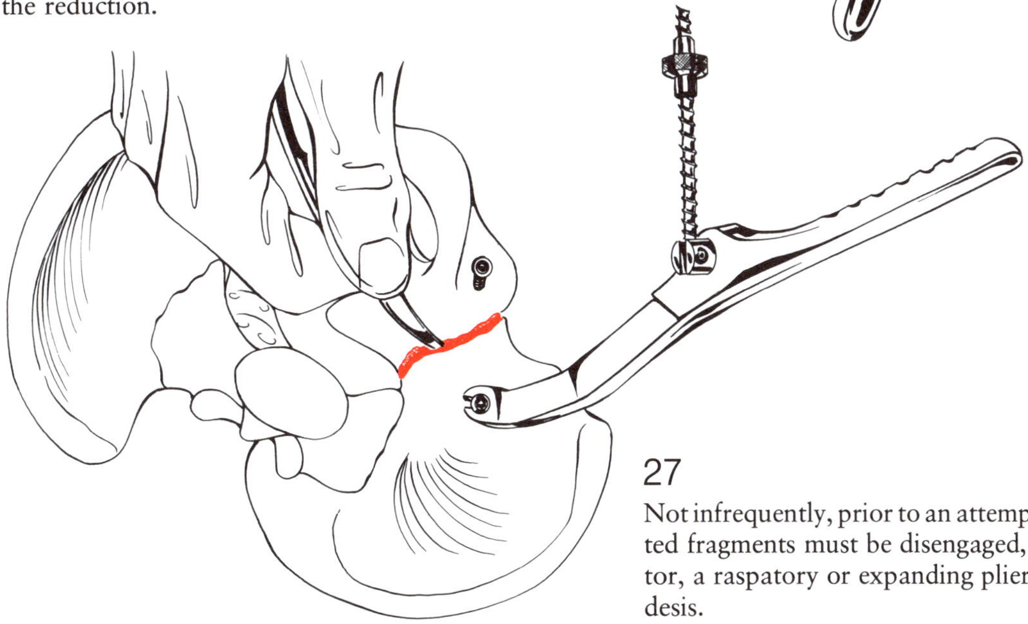

27

Not infrequently, prior to an attempt at reduction, the impacted fragments must be disengaged, using a periosteal elevator, a raspatory or expanding pliers as employed in arthrodesis.

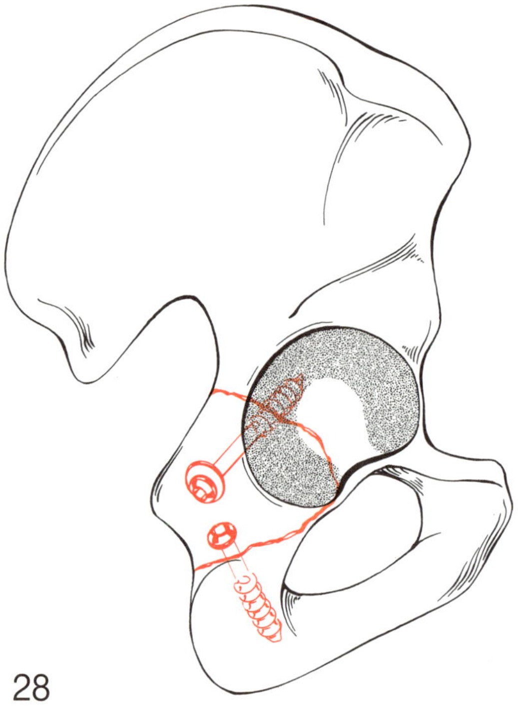

28

Dorsal fragments mut usually be protected against rotation by a second screw. Often, reduction is only practicable after sufficient disengagement of the fragment farthest displaced cranially.

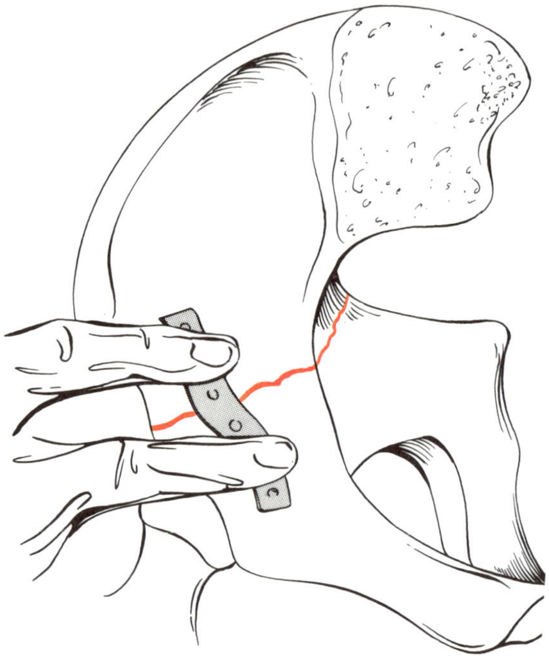

29

Proper bending of the plate can be achieved with use of a molding plate which,...

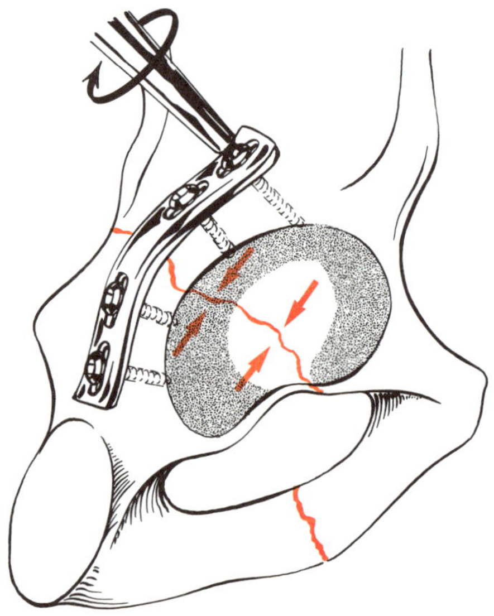

31

The DC plate provides interfragmental compression.

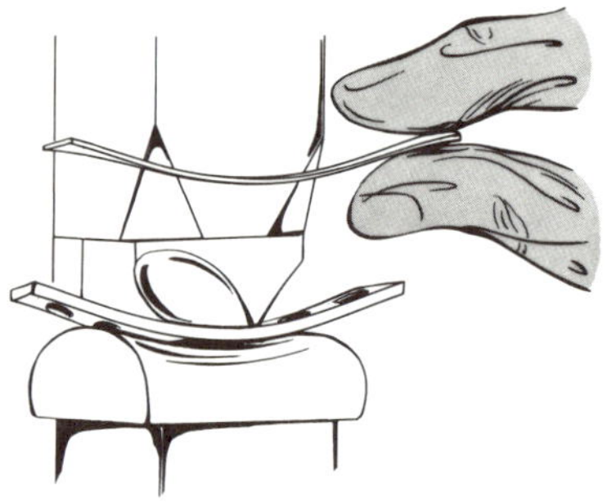

30

... on being bent with the press, serves as a model.

9. Symphysis – Sacroiliac Joint

Device for external fixation

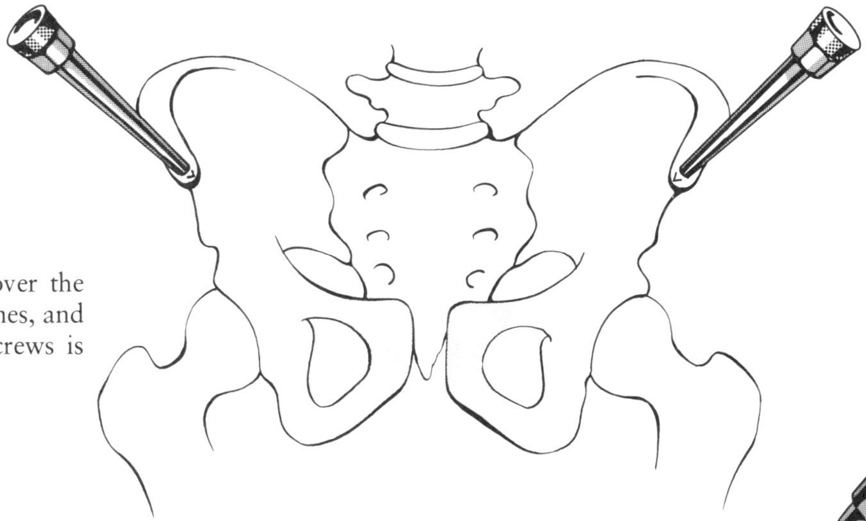

1

Small incisions are made in the skin over the readily palpable anterosuperior iliac spines, and the centering sleeve for the traction screws is attached.

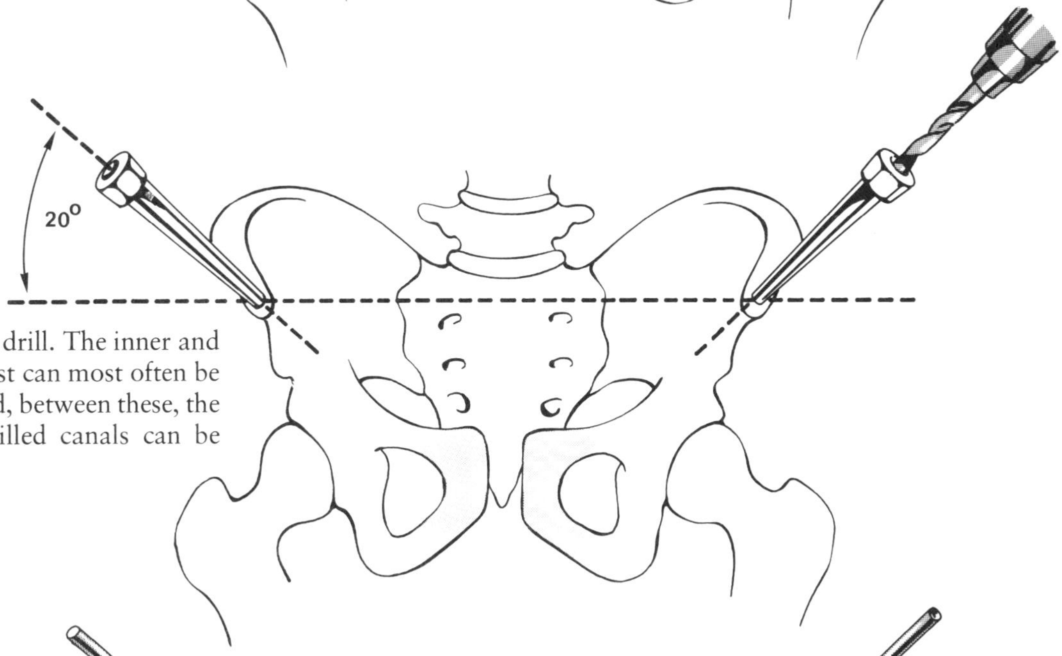

2

Predrilling with the 3.2 mm drill. The inner and outer aspects of the iliac crest can most often be grasped with two fingers and, between these, the correct direction of the drilled canals can be estimated.

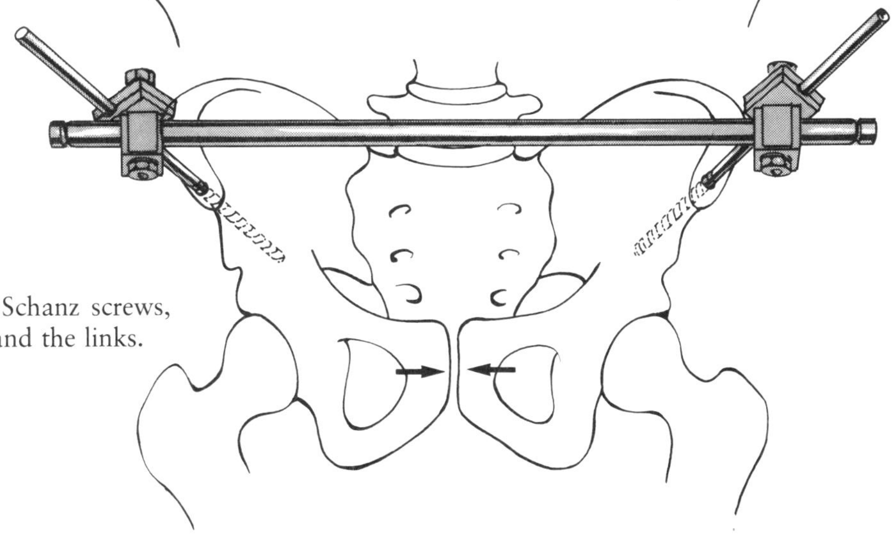

3

After insertion of the first two Schanz screws, they are connected to the tube and the links.

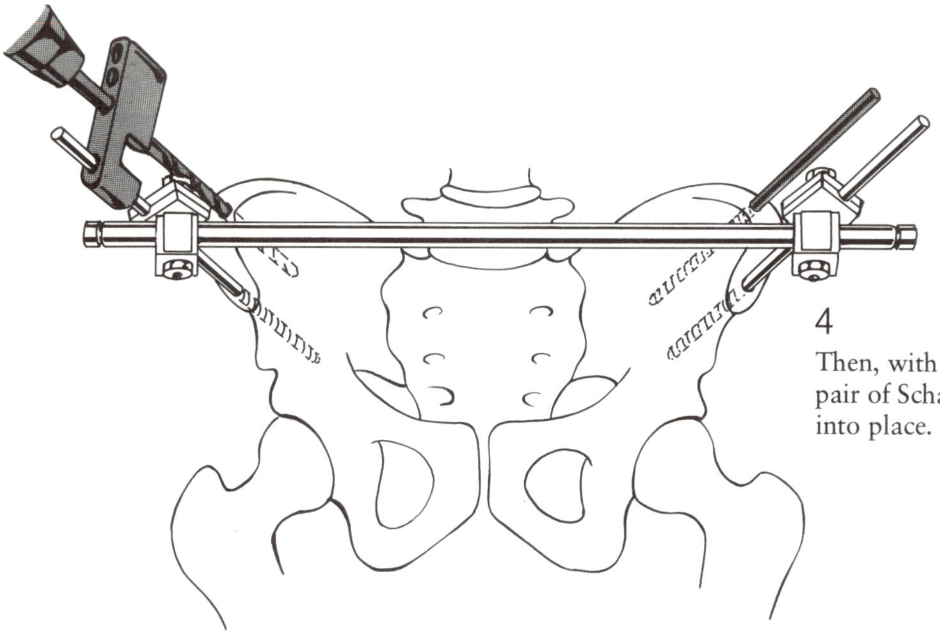

4

Then, with use of the drill sleeve, the second pair of Schanz screws can be readily brought into place.

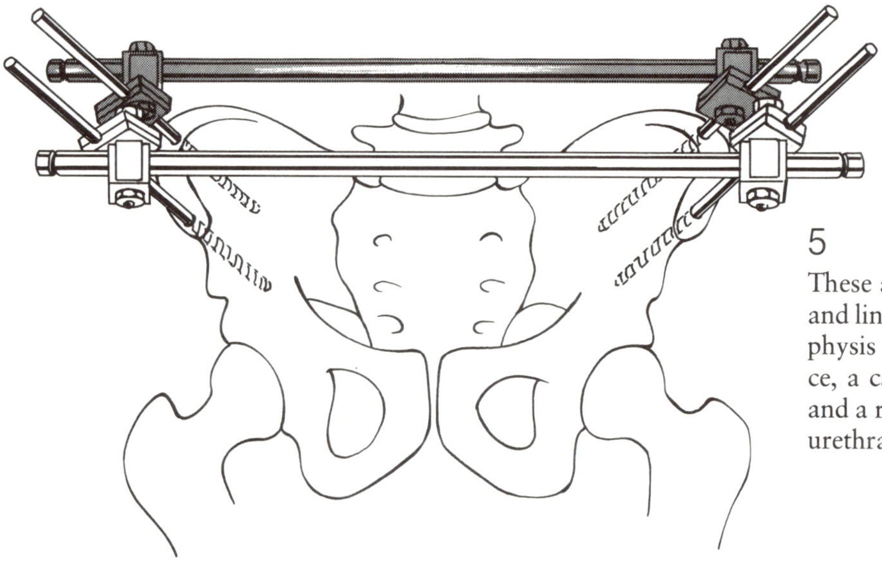

5

These are also connected by means of a tube and links, and now the two halves of the symphysis are joined together. *Caution:* In advance, a catheter must be placed in the bladder and a radiograph taken to make sure that the urethra is not nipped within the symphysis.

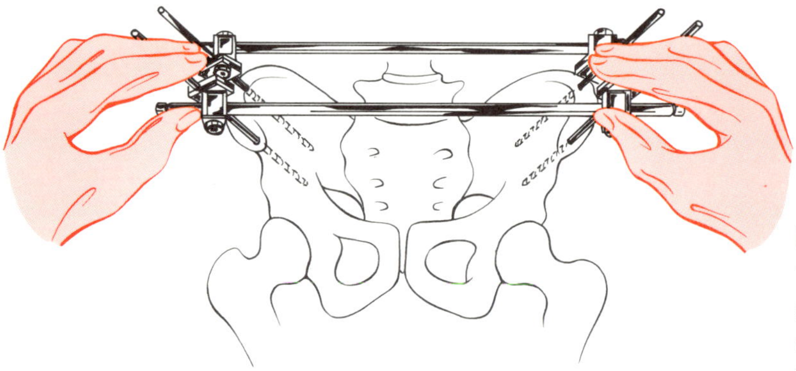

6

The two halves of the pelvis can be approximated by means of a tightener. Here, however, and by way of exception, no interfragmental pressure should develop!

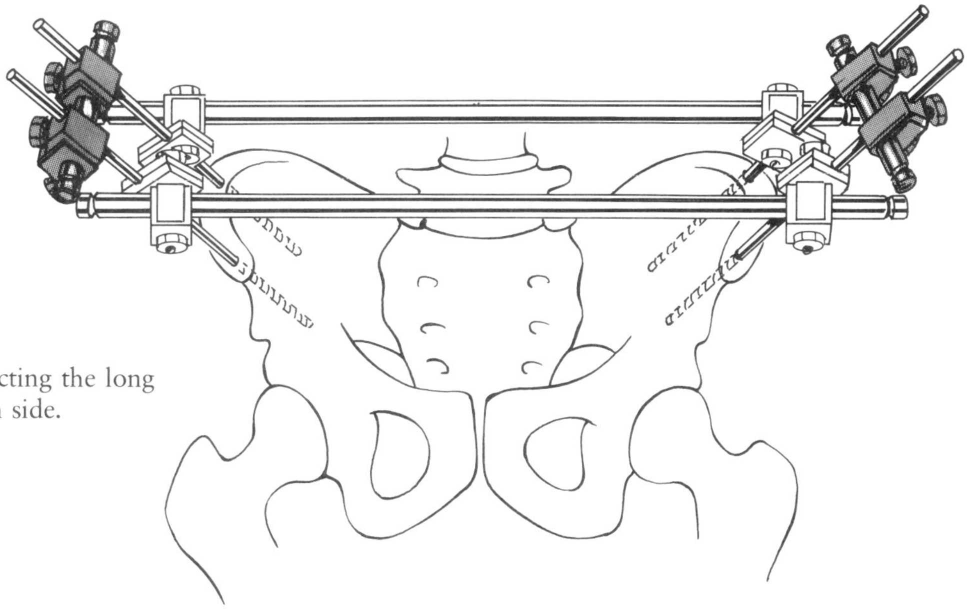

7
Stability is increased by connecting the long tube with a short tube on each side.

Fixation

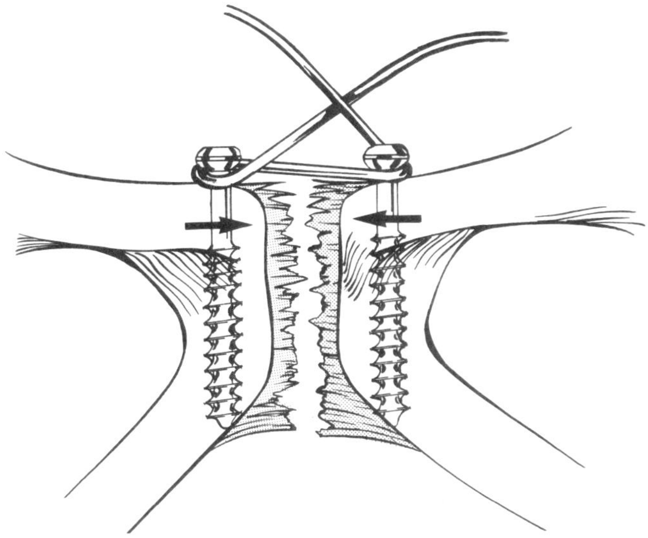

8
Rigid osteosynthesis and compression plate fixation meet with little success in the symphysis because both are easily liable to break or loosen. Should, instead of a device for external fixation, a technique of internal fixation be chosen, traction wiring over screwheads as anchors provides sufficient stability.

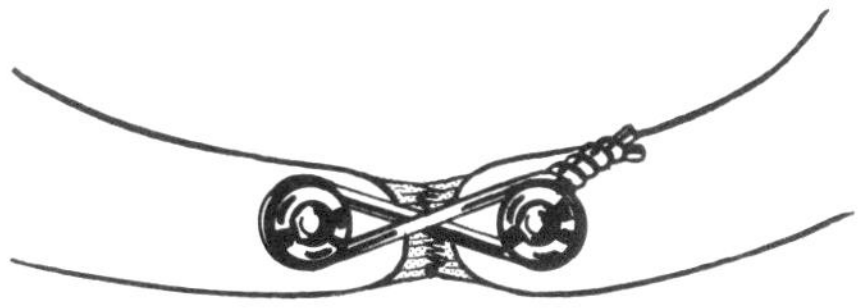

9
The wire should, however, be tightened only by hand. Any compression between the two halves of the symphysis must be avoided.

10. Hip Joint

Anatomy

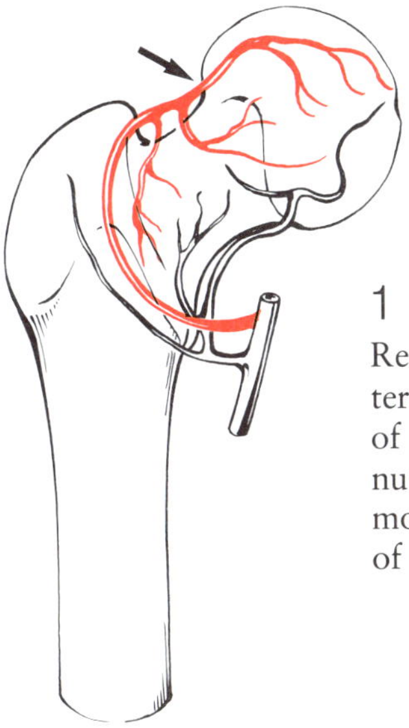

1

Red: territory supplied by the deep branch of the medial femoral circumflex artery. In elderly individuals, interruption of that branch usually leads to necrosis of the femoral head. The arrow points to the site of entrance of the principal nutrient vessel into the bone. The vessel possesses the least movability and is most liable to tear at this site. Fractures in this region are fraught with a high rate of necrosis.

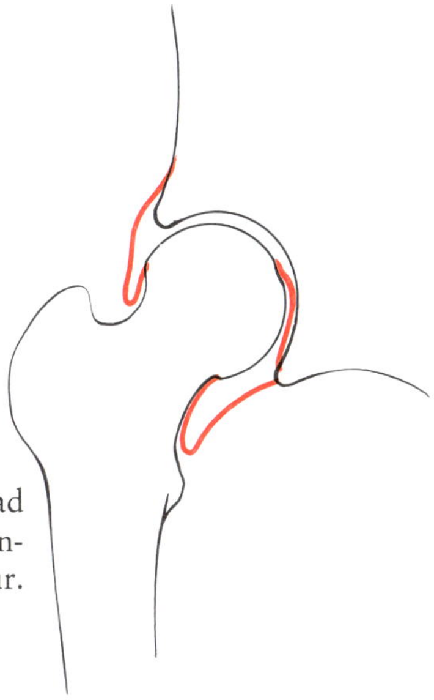

2

The vessels course on the periosteum to the head of the femur, enclosed by the portion of the synovium which is adjacent to the neck of the femur.

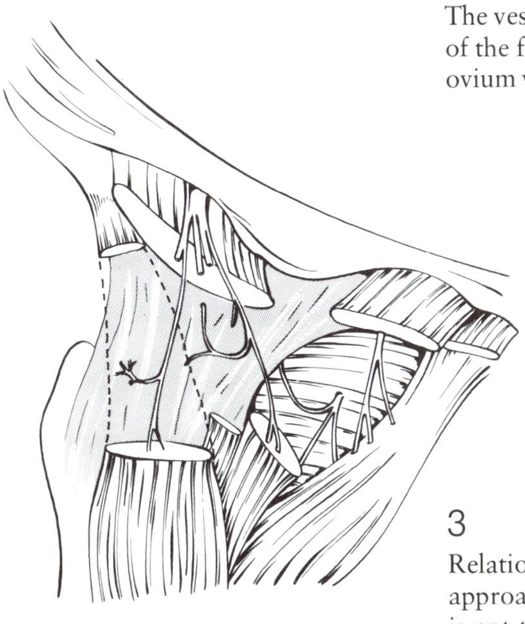

3

Relationship of the nerves to the hip joint. When, in the anterior or anterolateral approach, Hohmann elevators are improperly applied, femoral nerve paralysis is apt to supervene. (See also Figs. 15–1 ff.)

Diagnosis

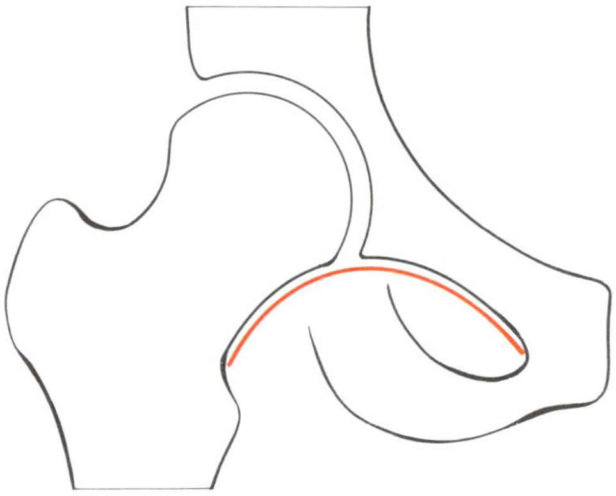

4

Distortion of the arch formed by femoral neck and os pubis ("Adam's arch"), visible in the roentgenogram, often gives a clue to the presence of fracture or dislocation. X-ray examination as shown in Figs. 128–9 ff.

Positioning

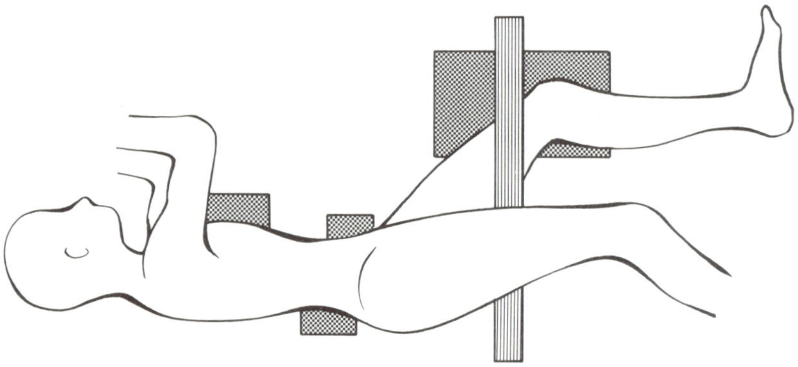

5

Side-lying position. The supports for back and symphysis must not be too high since, otherwise, sterile conditions in the area of operations are insufficient.

Posterolateral ("southern") approach

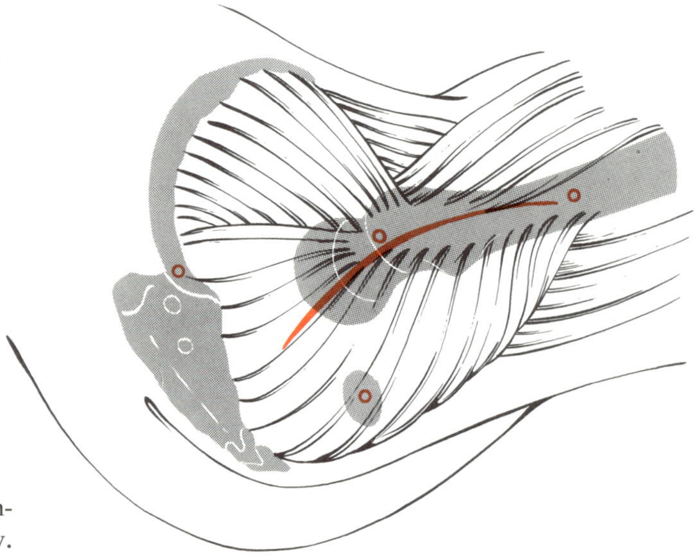

1

Skin incision. Reference points: greater trochanter, femoral shaft, posterosuperior iliac spine, ischial tuberosity.

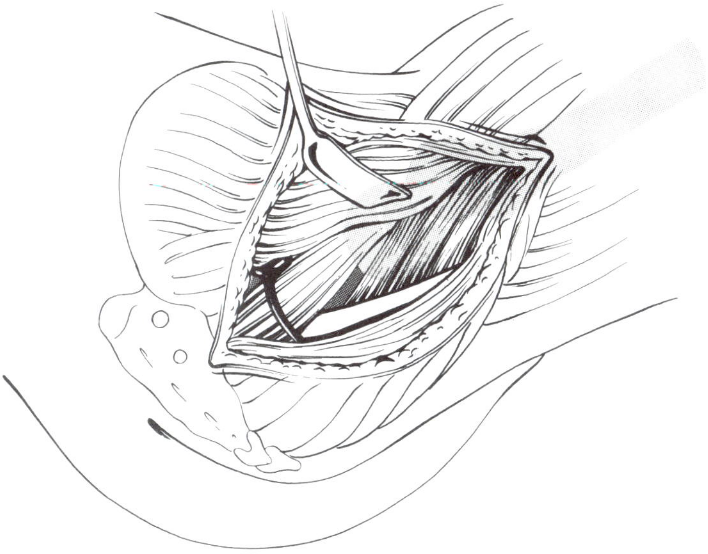

2

The insertion of the gluteus maximus muscle is detached from the iliotibial tract. Starting at the trochanter, one separates the muscle fibers as far as possible by blunt dissection until one comes upon the subjacent fatty tissue which also envelops the sciatic nerve.

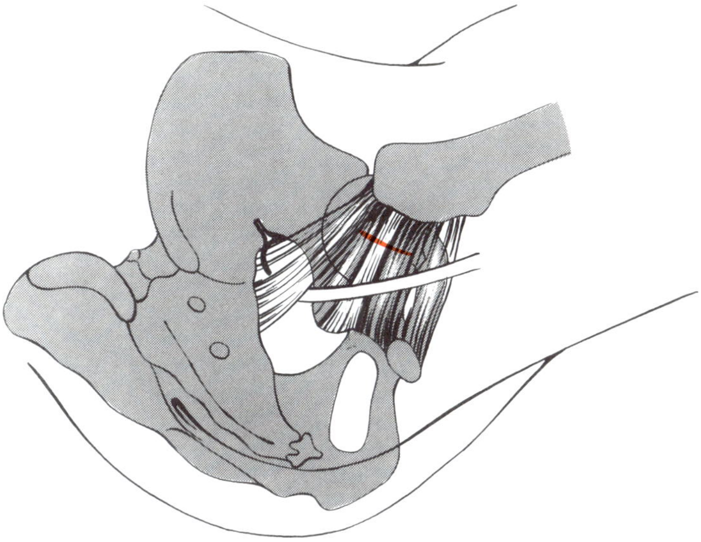

3

The sciatic nerve is relatively easily identified in the loose adipose and gliding tissue by palpation and dissection. The short external rotators are divided in such a way that...

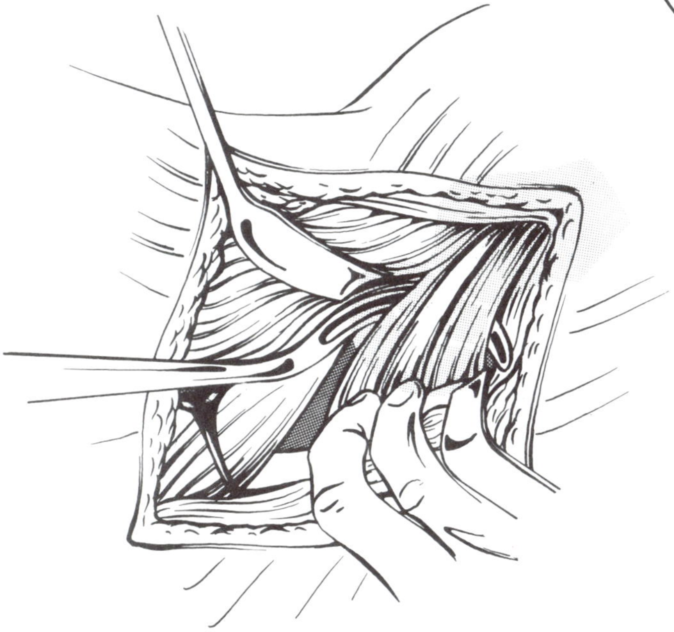

4

... small stumps for reinsertion remain behind the trochanter.

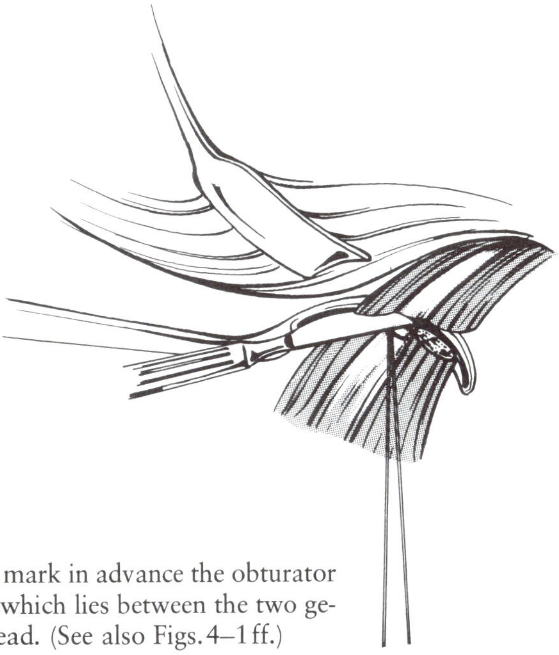

5

It is expedient to mark in advance the obturator internus muscle, which lies between the two gemelli, with a thread. (See also Figs. 4–1 ff.)

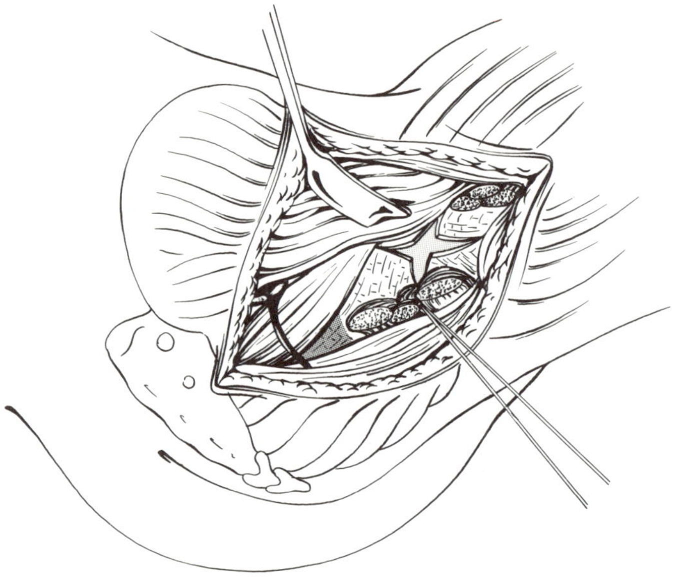

6

Part or all of the quadratus femoris muscle may be detached distalward, as well as the piriform muscle cephalad. In handling the piriform muscle, take care to spare the caudal gluteal artery!

Anterolateral approach

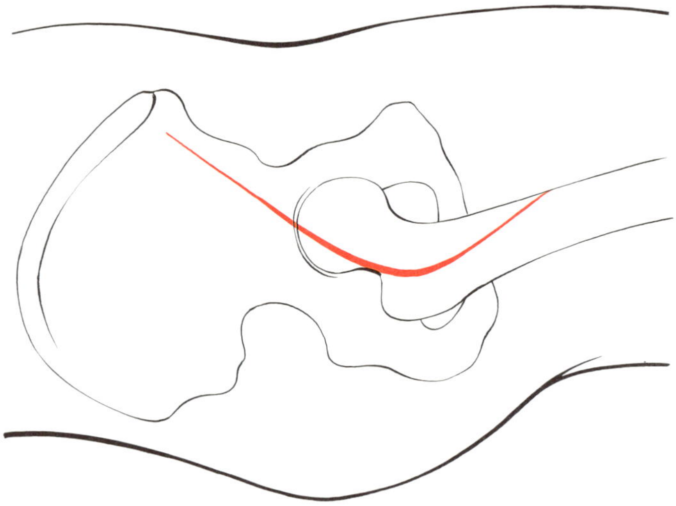

1

Skin incision. * = reference points (anterosuperior iliac spine and tip of the greater trochanter).

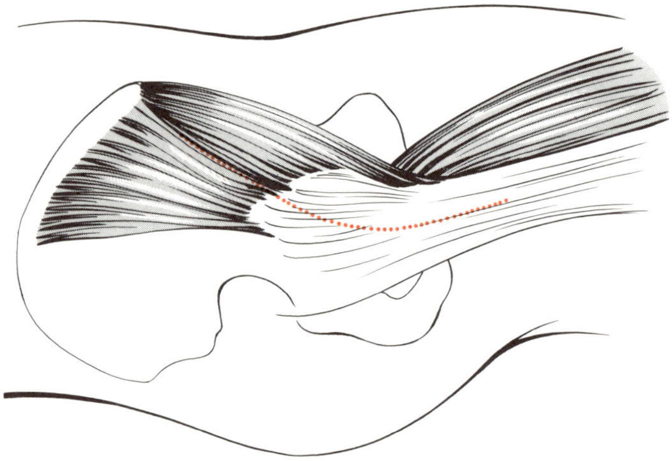

2

After splitting the fascia in the direction of its fibers over the cleft between the posterior border of the tensor fasciae latae muscle and the anterior border of the gluteus medius muscle, one penetrates between these muscles toward the joint capsule. The agglomeration of adipose tissue in this triangle can serve as a reference point.

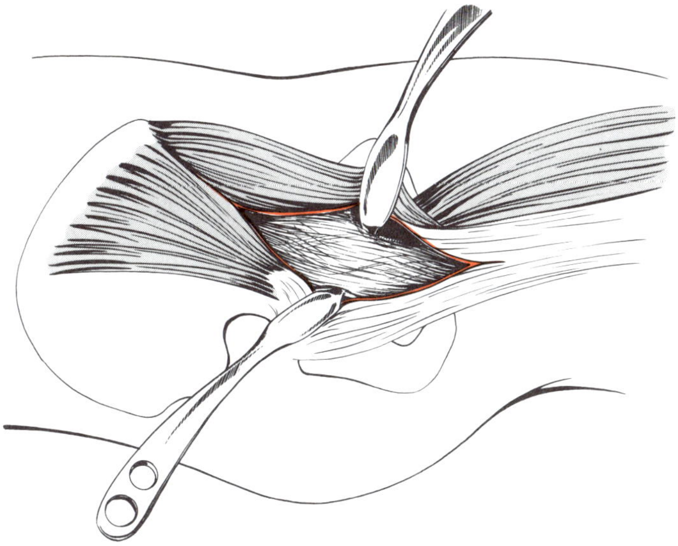

3
Hohmann elevators are applied caudally and cranially around the femoral neck.

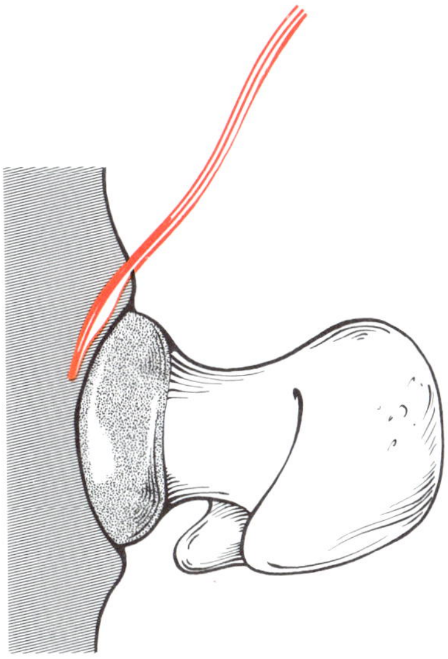

4
A third elevator is applied across the anterior rim of the acetabulum. The tip of this elevator should not be bent too forcefully because it may very easily be pressed through the bone.

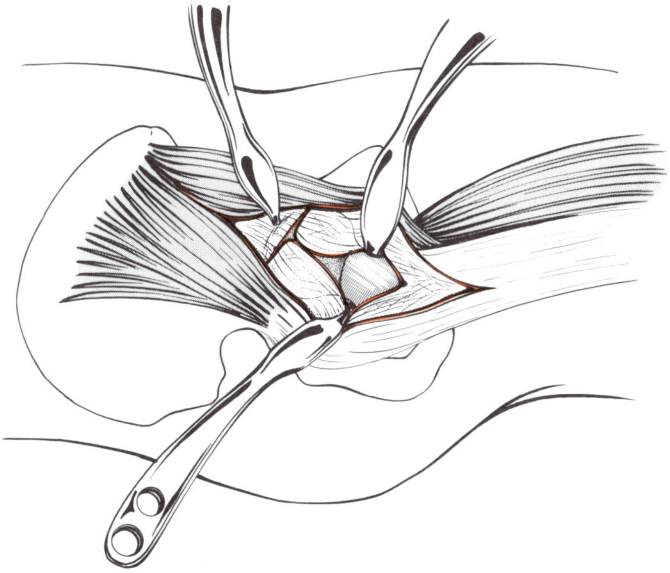

5
The capsule is opened. The caudal and the cranial Hohmann elevator are moved within the capsule around the femoral neck.

Anterior approach

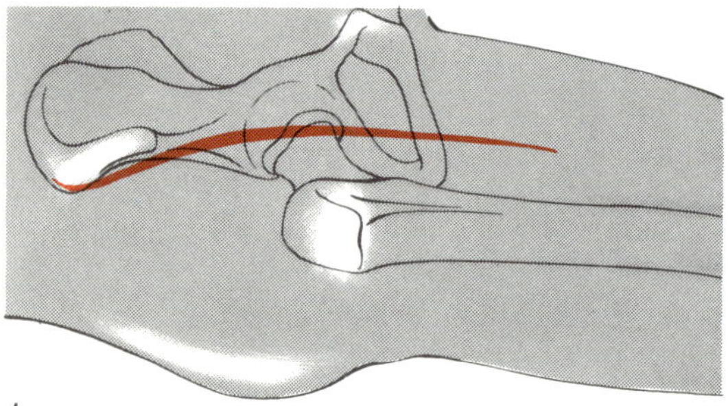

1
Skin incision along the outer border of the iliac crest.

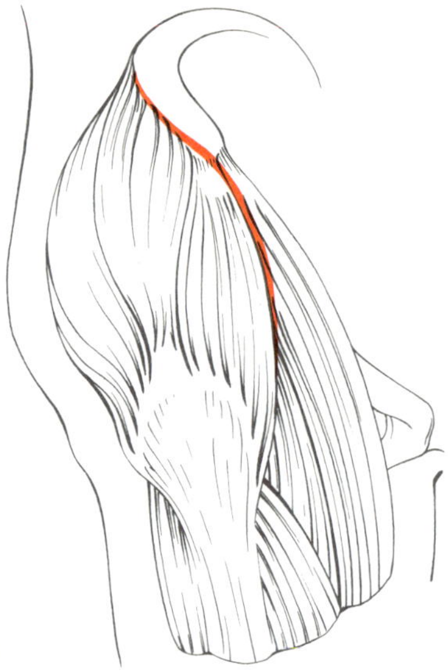

2
The gluteus muscle is detached from the lateral aspect of the iliac wing. First, the periosteum is cut through by scalpel down to the bone. Then, the muscles are pushed away from the bone with a sharp raspatory.
The sartorius muscle is pulled medialward.

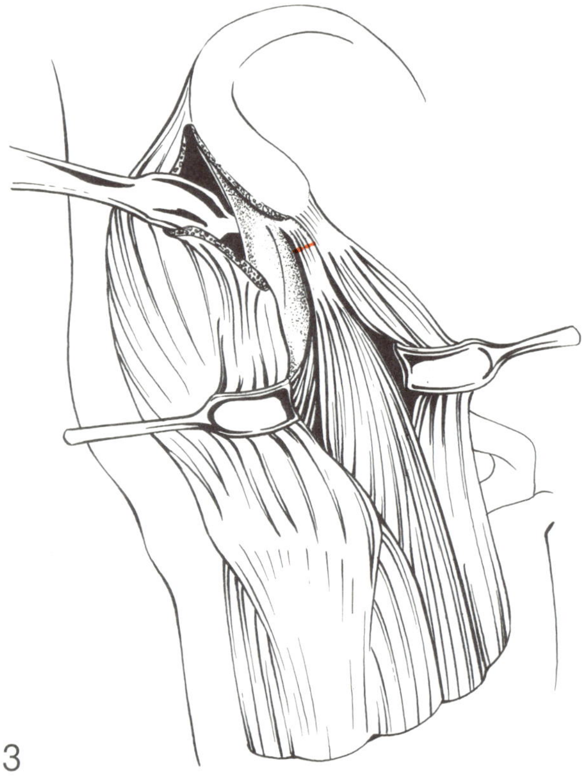

3
The rectus femoris muscle is detached from its insertion. A small stump remains for reinsertion.

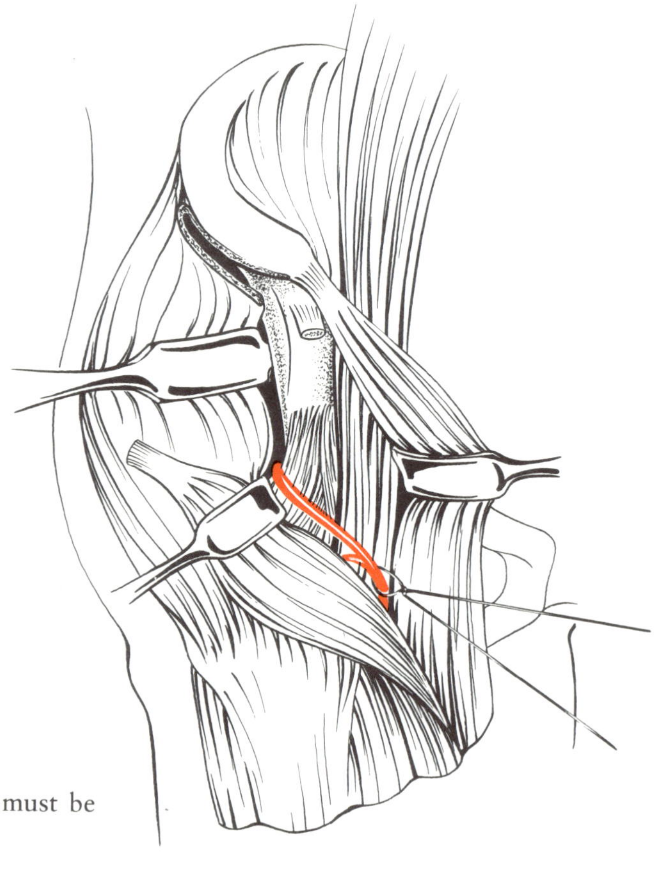

4
The circumflexa femoris artery must be ligated.

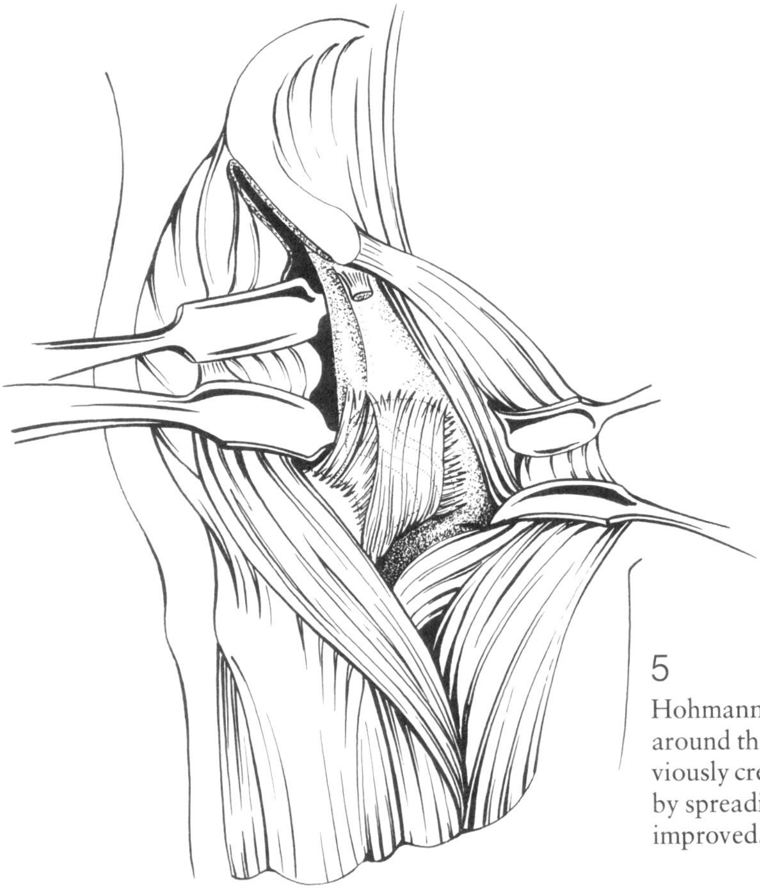

5
Hohmann elevators are inserted cranially and caudally around the joint capsule. This maneuver is facilitated by previously creating the necessary space – to a large extent bluntly by spreading a pair of scissors. The view is thus considerably improved.

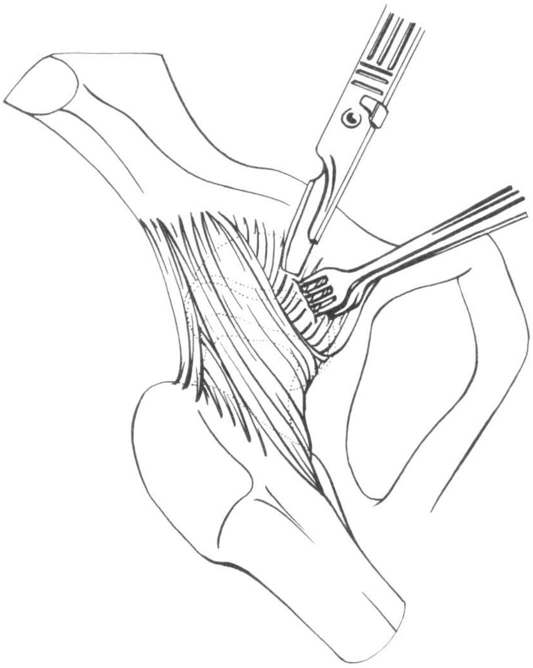

6
Only then is the capsule opened, beginning at the acetabulum if the head of the femur is to be preserved. (For the vascular supply, see Figs. 141–1 ff.)

11. Femur

Proximal part

Anatomy See also Figs. 141–1 ff.

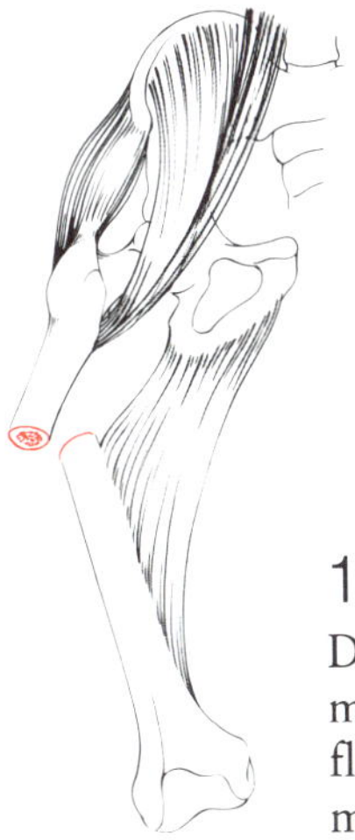

1
Displacement of fragments: proximal fragment externally rotated, flexed and abducted. Distal fragment adducted.

Types of injuries

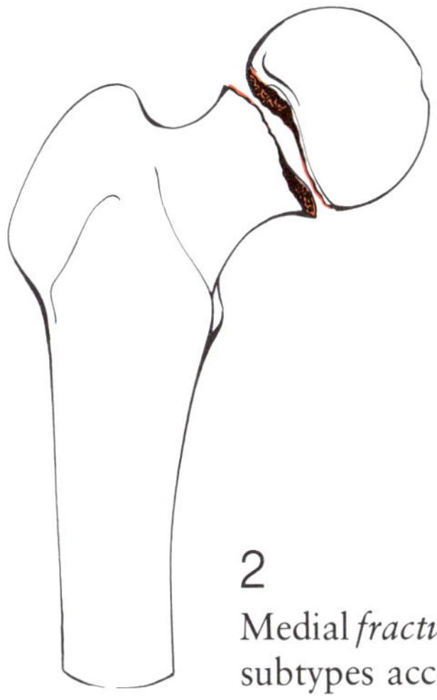

2
Medial *fracture of the femoral neck:* subtypes according to Pauwels.

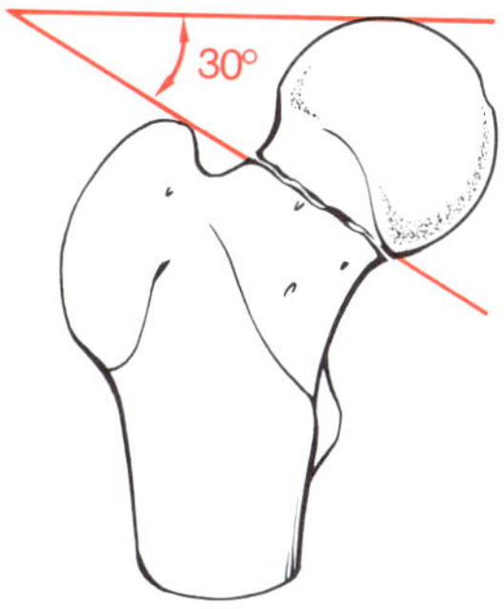

3
Pauwels type I.

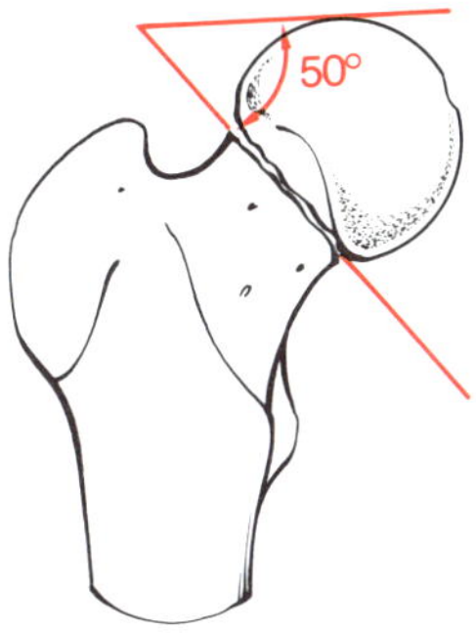

4
Pauwels type II.

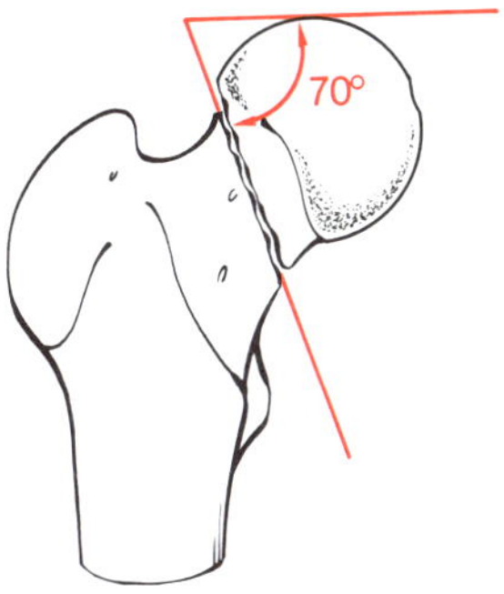

5
Pauwels type III. In this type, any head-preserving operation should be combined with an intertrochanteric, valgus-producing displacement osteotomy in order to approximate the fracture surface to the horizontal line so that the pressure effect is increased and the shearing effect deminished.

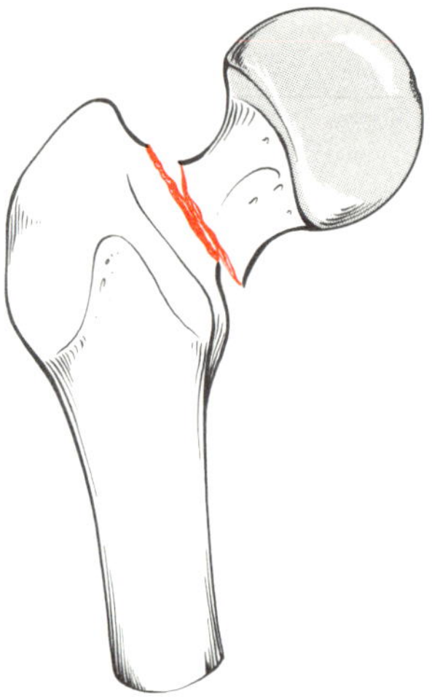

6
Lateral fracture of femoral neck.

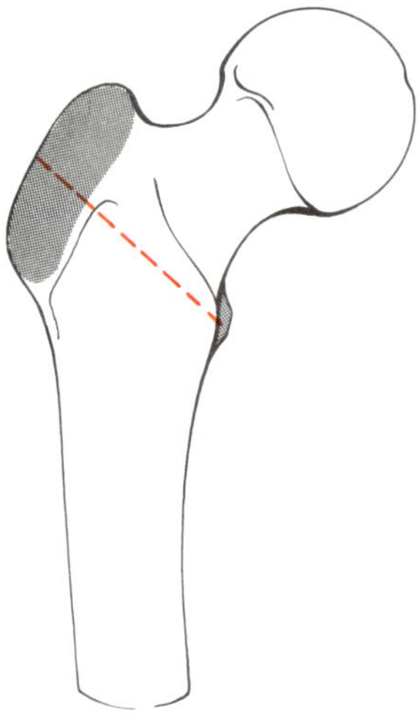

7
Pertrochanteric fracture of femur.

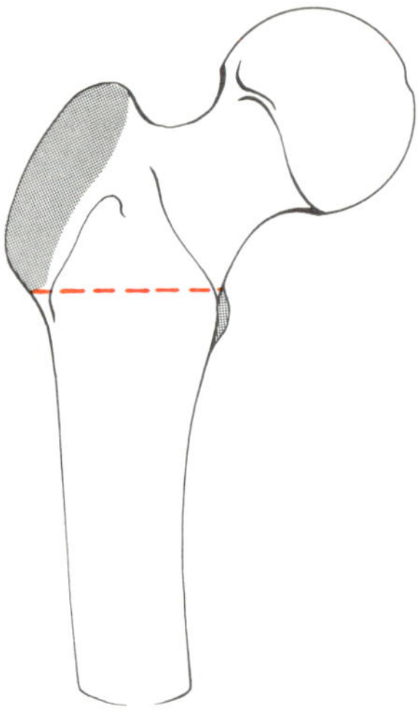

8
Intertrochanteric fracture of femur.

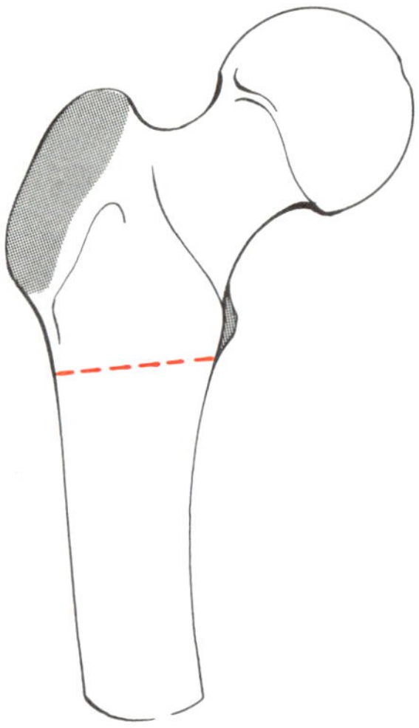

9
Subtrochanteric fracture of femur with the following subtypes: 3 to 4 types of bending fractures and 2 types of torsion fractures.

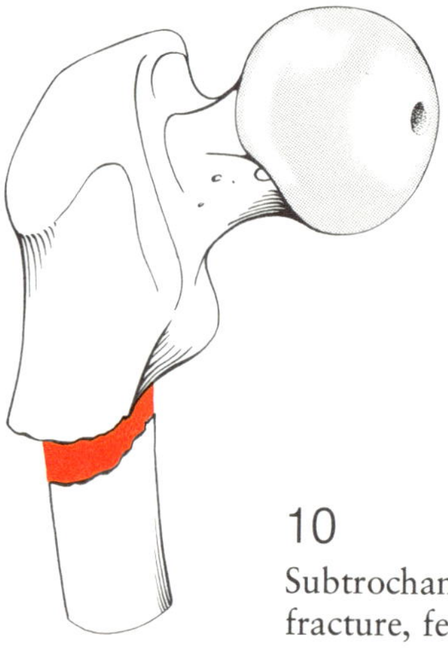

10
Subtrochanteric fracture of femur: simple transverse fracture, few complications.

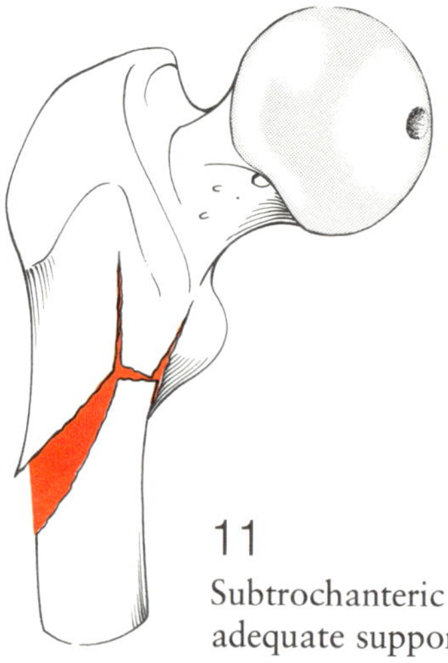

11
Subtrochanteric fracture of femur: "reversed fracture", adequate support, few complications.

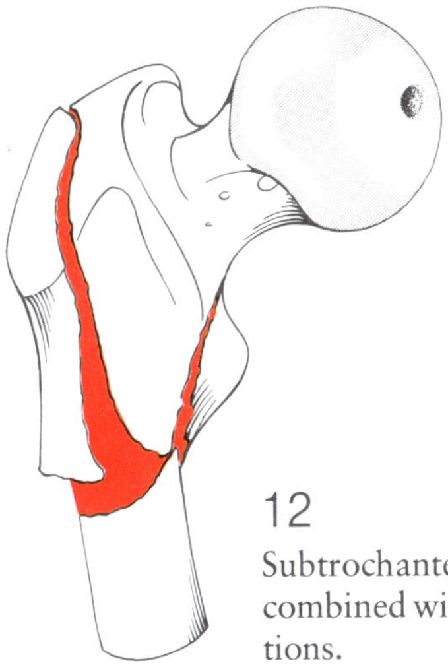

12

Subtrochanteric fracture of femur: transverse fracture combined with pertrochanteric fracture; few complications.

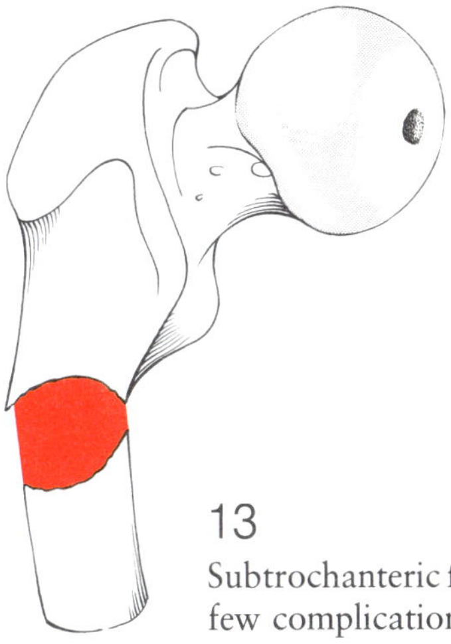

13

Subtrochanteric fracture of femur: pathologic fracture, few complications.

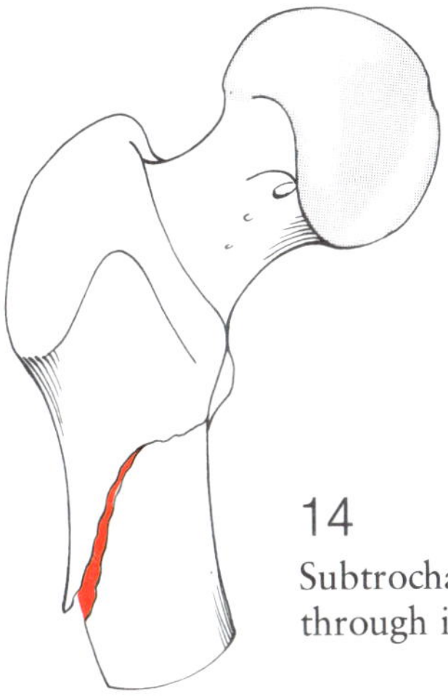

14

Subtrochanteric fracture of femur: torsion fracture through internal rotation. Reduction difficult.

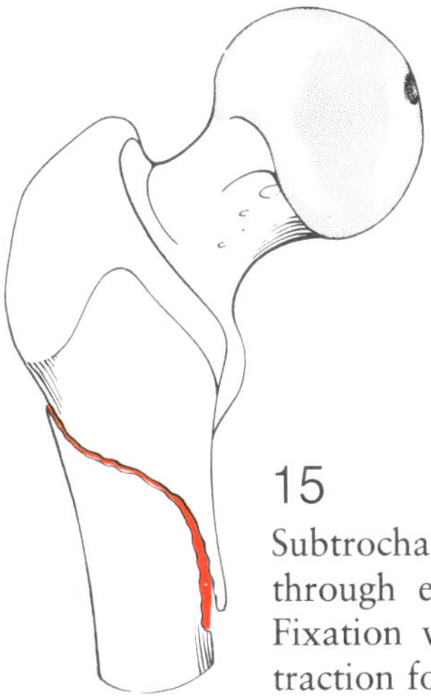

15

Subtrochanteric fracture of femur: torsion fracture through external rotation, tendency to shortening. Fixation with a spring nail may require additional traction for 3 weeks.

Principle

The further medial the fracture, the more internal rotation is required for reduction.

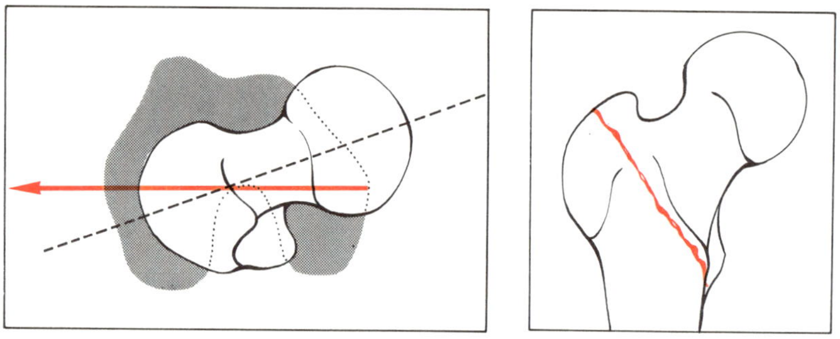

16
Pertrochanteric fracture of femur.

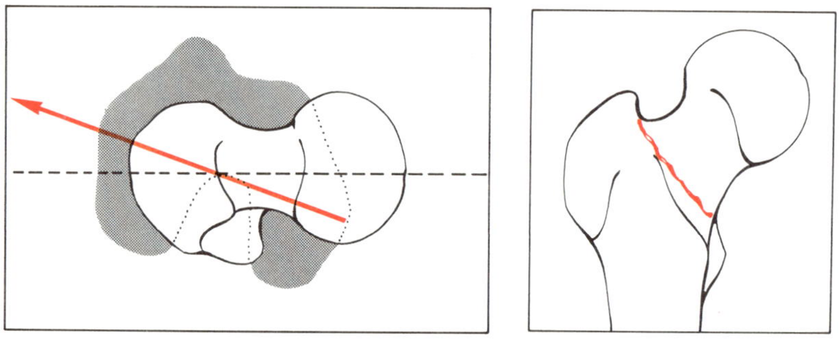

17
Lateral fracture of femoral neck.

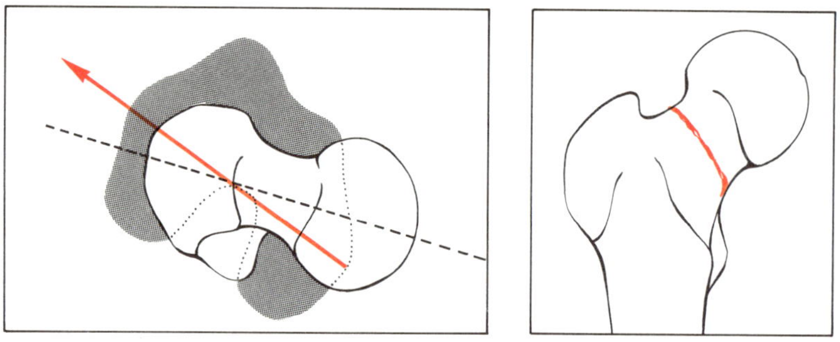

18
Medial fracture of femoral neck.

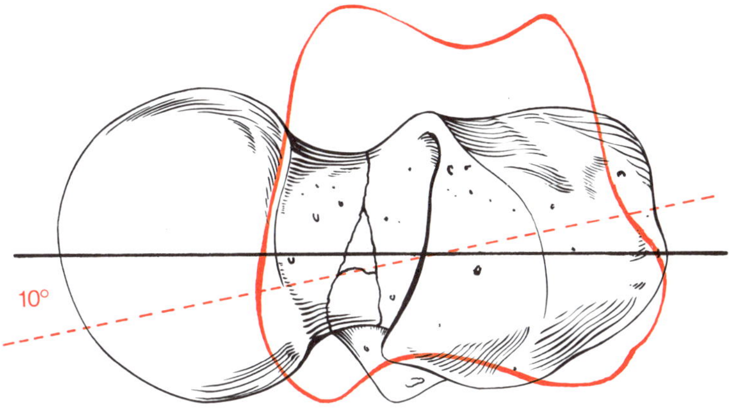

19

In the adult the femoral neck is directed about 10° ventrally. This means that, to reduce a fracture correctly, the direction of implants (nails, screws, plate blades) inserted from posteriorly into the femoral neck should always deviate by the same amount.

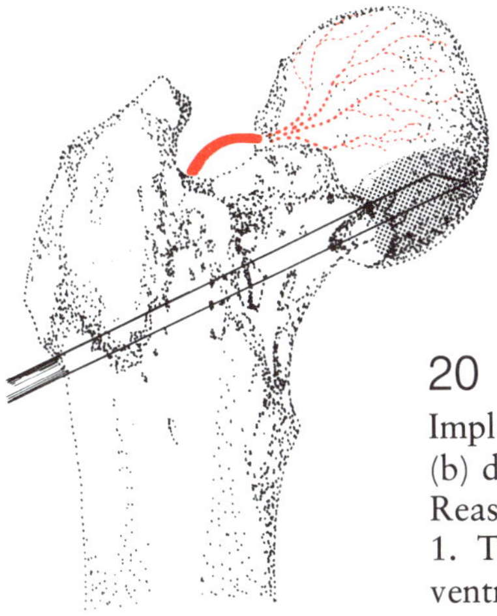

20

Implants inserted into the femoral neck and head should lie (a) caudal and (b) dorsal.
Reasons:
1. The main blood supply to the head, coming from the cranial and the ventral, must not be endangered.

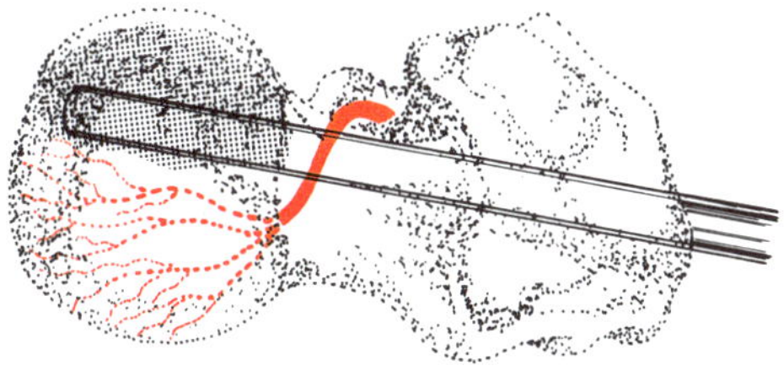

21

2. Cranially and ventrally, the cancellous bone is softest and the implants find little support.

Positioning

Supine position, standard operating table, see Fig. 192–6.
Traction table, image intensifier (only for screw, nail and spring nail).

Reduction

prior to reduction

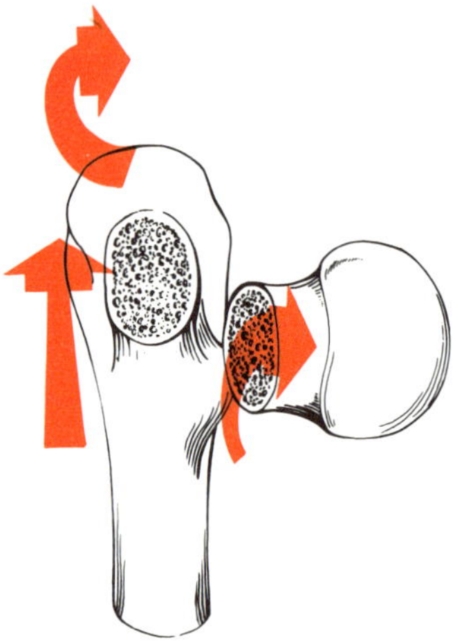

22
Shaft of femur: cranial, externally rotated
Head of femur: adducted, internally rotated
Reduction

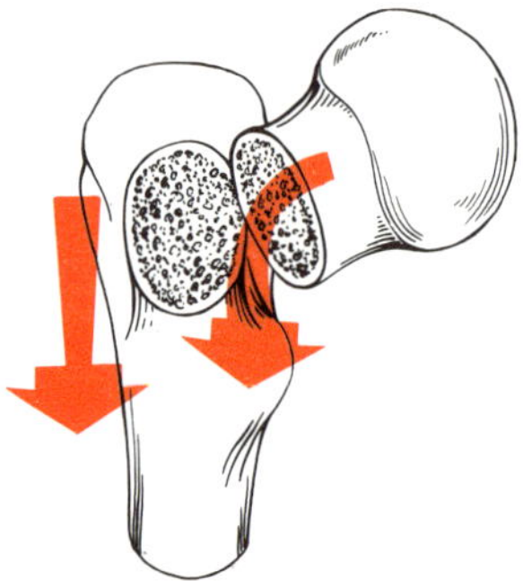

23
1st phase. Traction on shaft: the surfaces of the fracture are brought to the same level. Concomitant traction on the capsule eliminates the adducted position of the head.

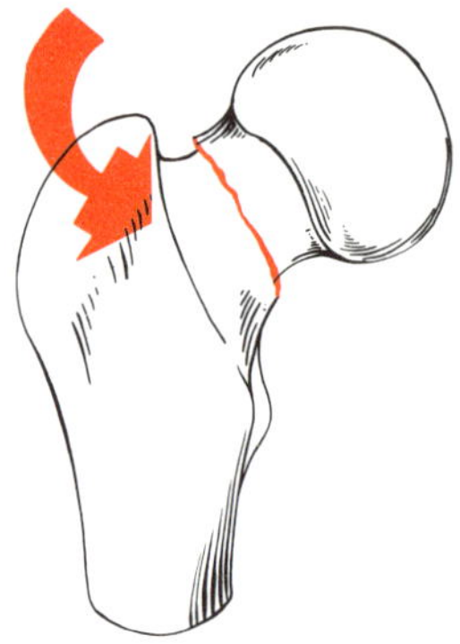

24
2nd phase: internal rotation of shaft. The separated surfaces of the fracture are joined together.

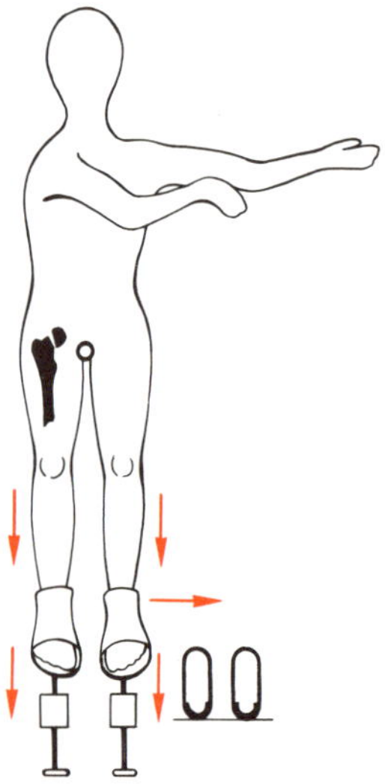

25
Traction is exerted caudally, concomitantly on both legs. It should be even, not jerky.

Check both planes with the image intensifier.

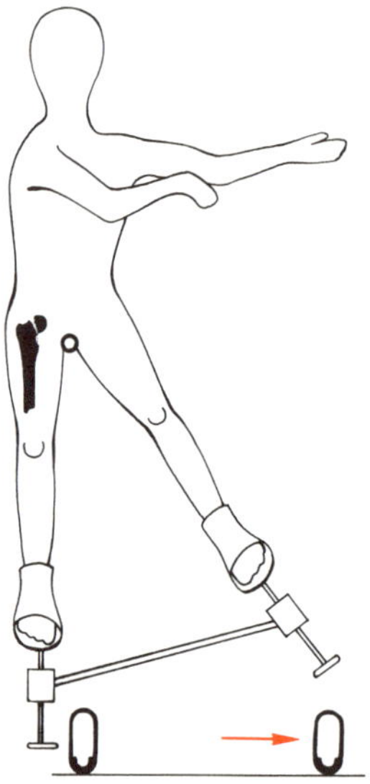

26
Sound leg abducted to allow transverse observation under the image intensifier.

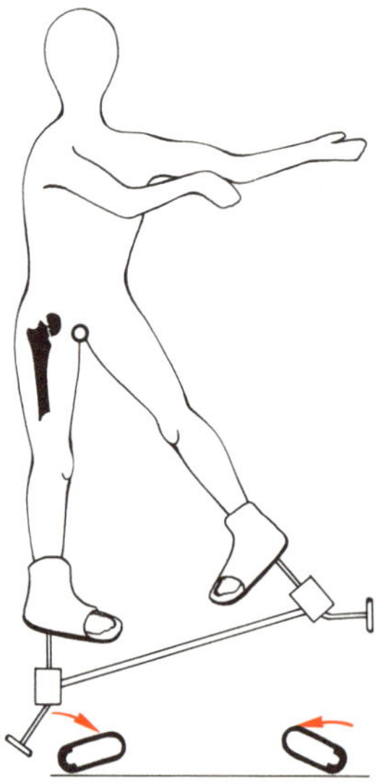

27
Bilateral internal rotation. In this way, tilting of the pelvis to the sound side is prevented.

Radiographic image intensifier

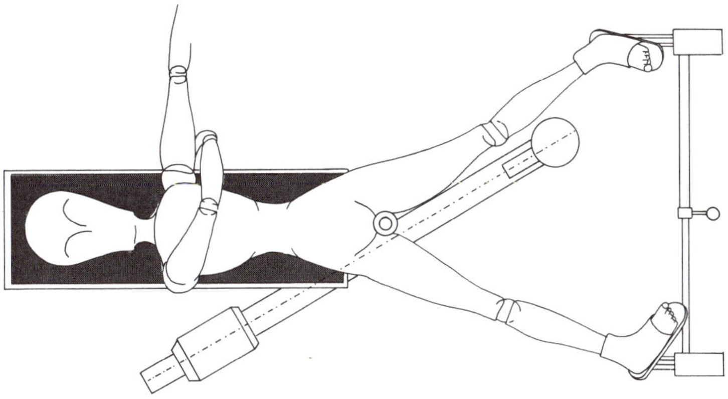

28

Before applying the sterile drapes, check the position and transillumination. The device is operated by a nonsterile person who follows the surgeon's instructions precisely.

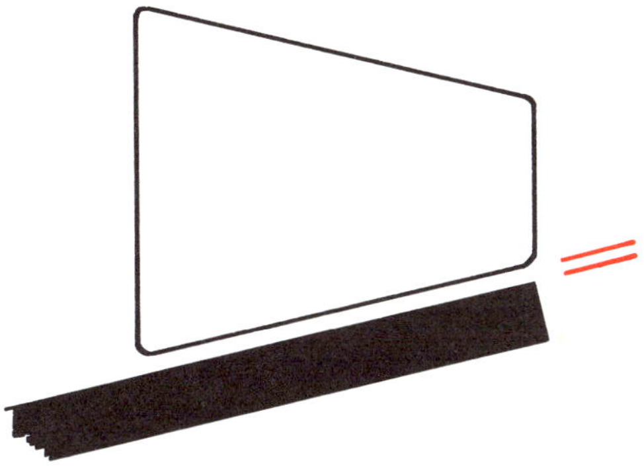

29

In positioning the image intensifier, it is best set up in such a way that its axis runs parallel to the lateral edge of the triangular traction table. This way of setting up the device allows transillumination in both planes simply by swinging the arc. Adhesive plaster markings on the floor help in repositioning the device precisely.

30

The device must be set up so that it can be swung from the vertical to the horizontal plane without displacing it and without touching the table or the patient. That is why the sterile drapes must be applied closely, with no loose corners dangling.

Note Figs. 8–1 ff.

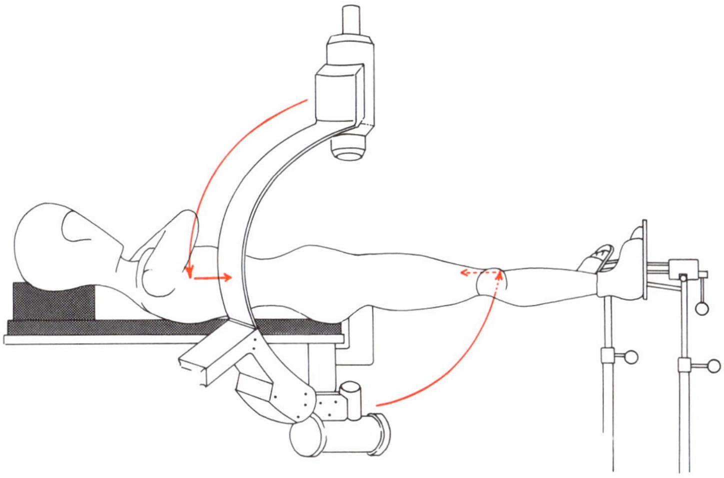

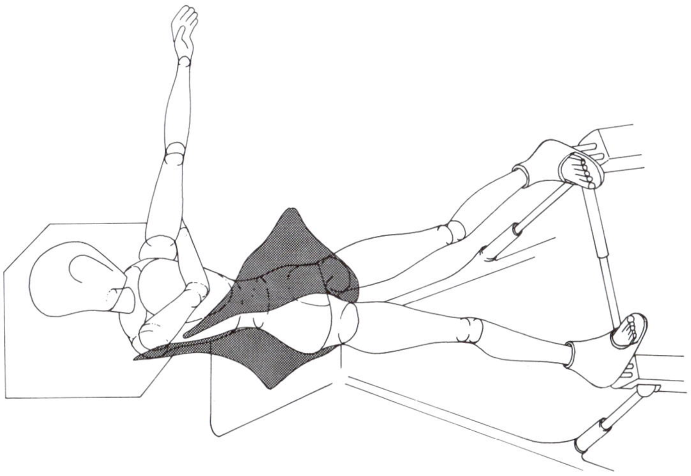

Sterile draping I

31

Drape size 3. Be careful to place the towel clips far enough cranially above the iliac crest because otherwise they will interfere with the axial ray path of the image intensifier.

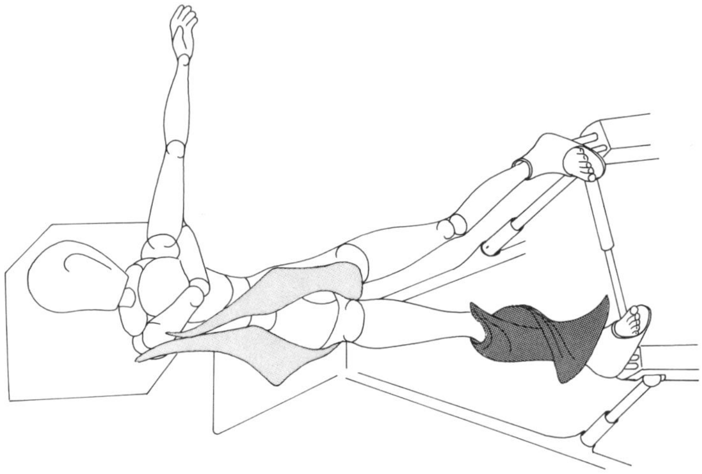

32
Drape size 4.

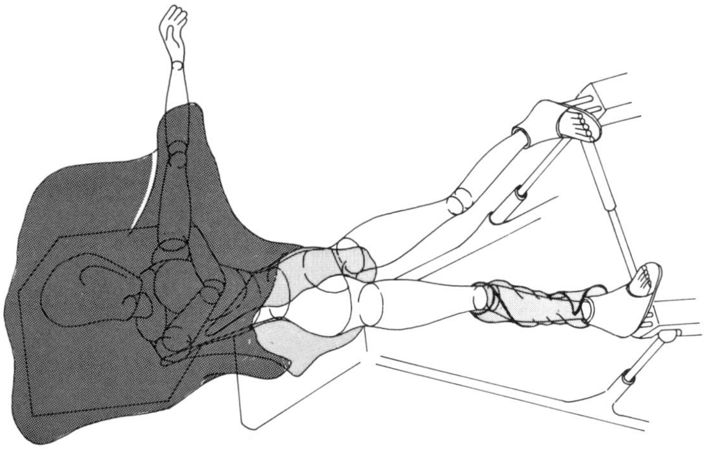

33
Drape size 1.

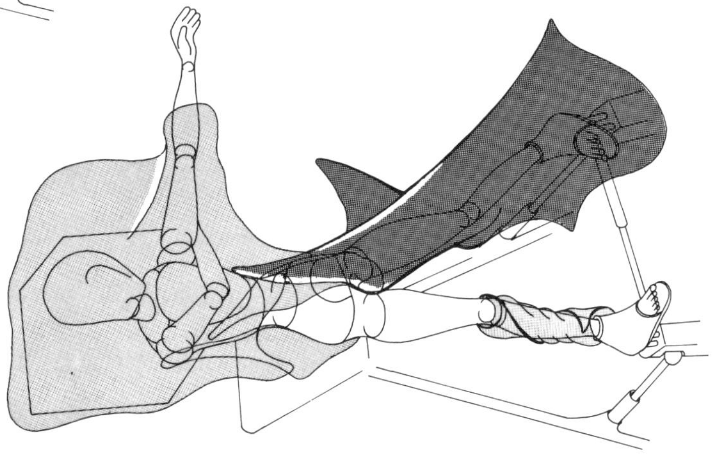

34
Using drape size 1, ...

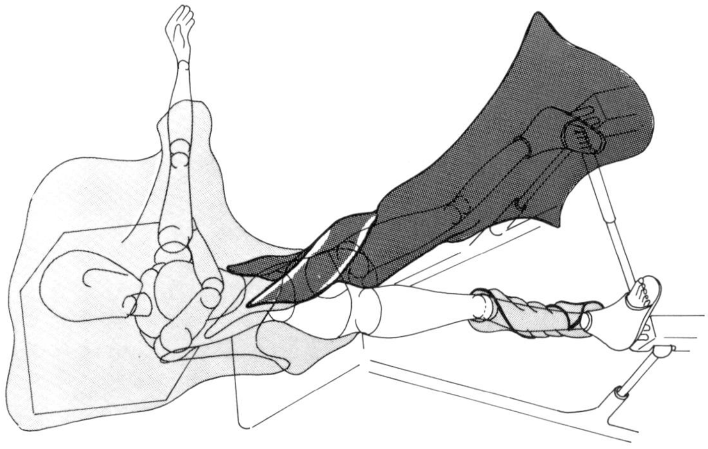

35
... apply the drape closely to the leg...

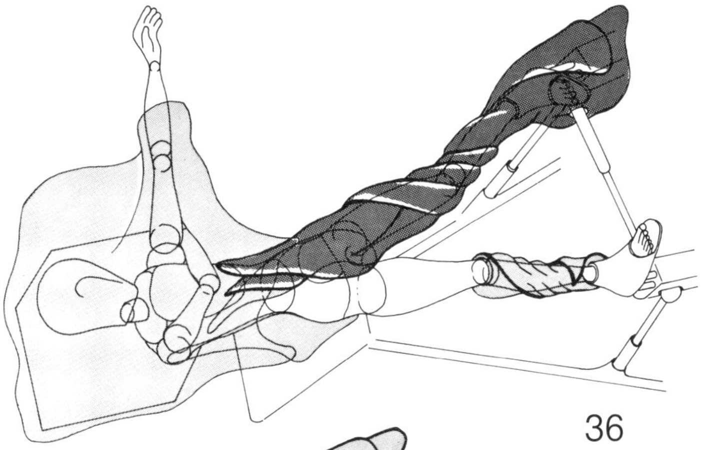

36

... so that the latter will not be touched on operating the image intensifier.

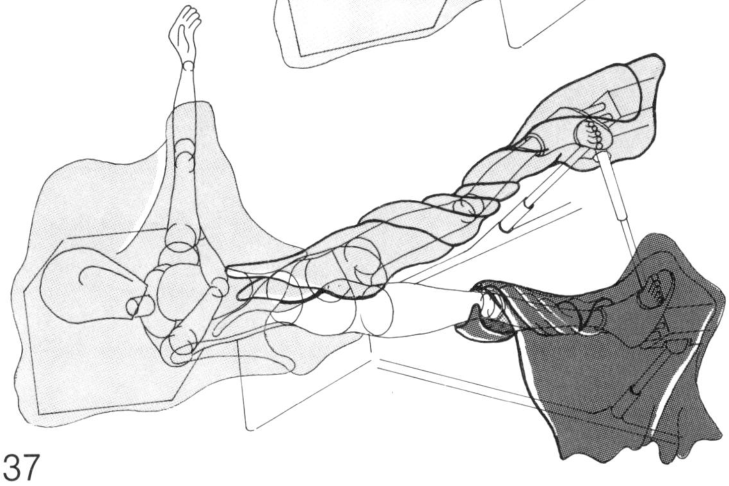

37

Drape size 1. Here, also, the drape...

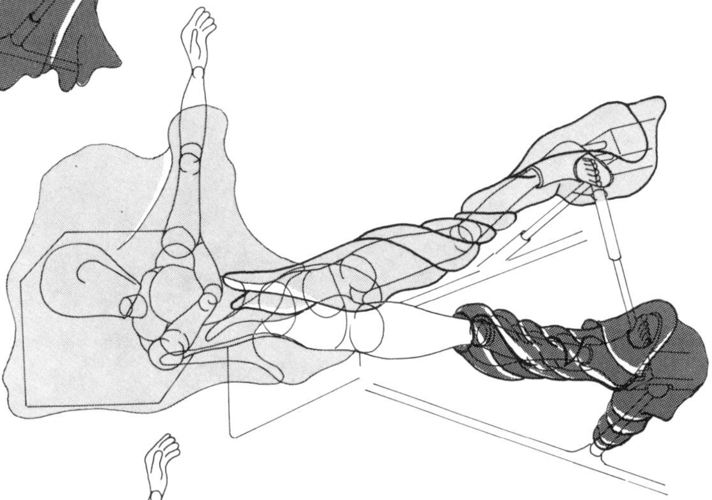

38

... should be applied closely to the leg and the pedestal.

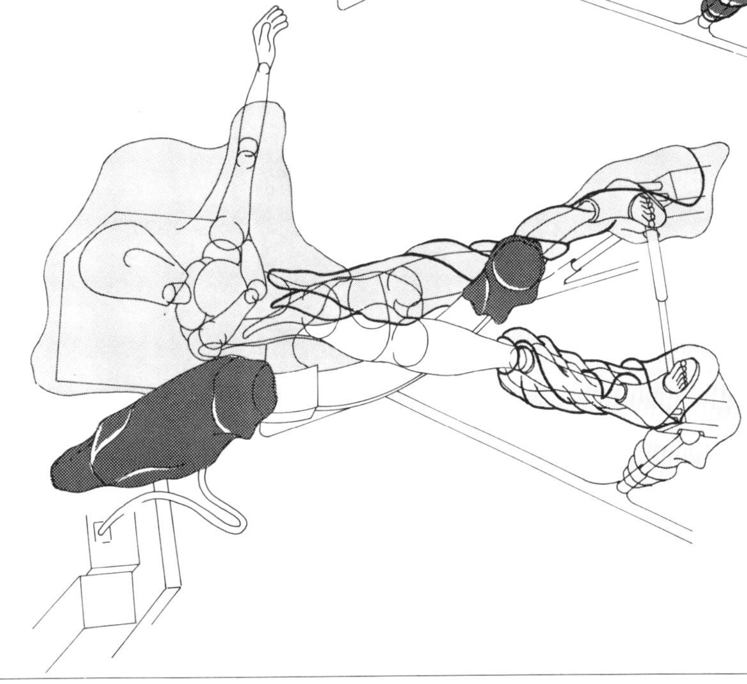

39

Sterile draping of the image intensifier. With this position of the device (See also Fig. 155–29), both planes of transillumination are accessible simply by tilting the arc without displacing the device.
When the image intensifier is not being used, it is moved back. Adhesive plaster markings on the floor make it possible to relocate the device in the correct position rapidly.

Sterile draping II

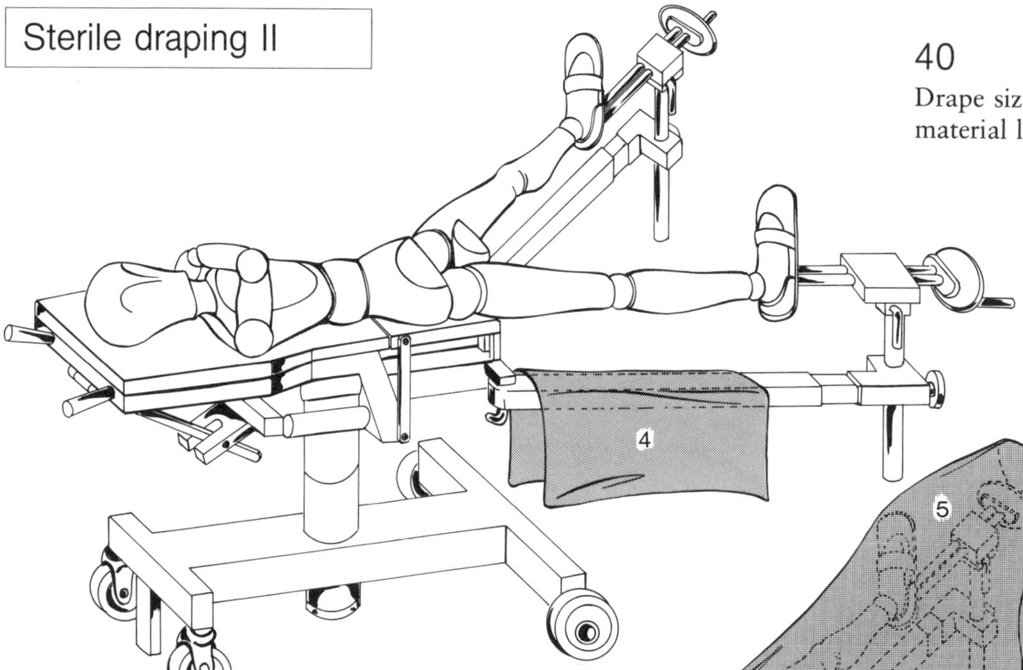

40
Drape size 4, with an impermeable material laid underneath.

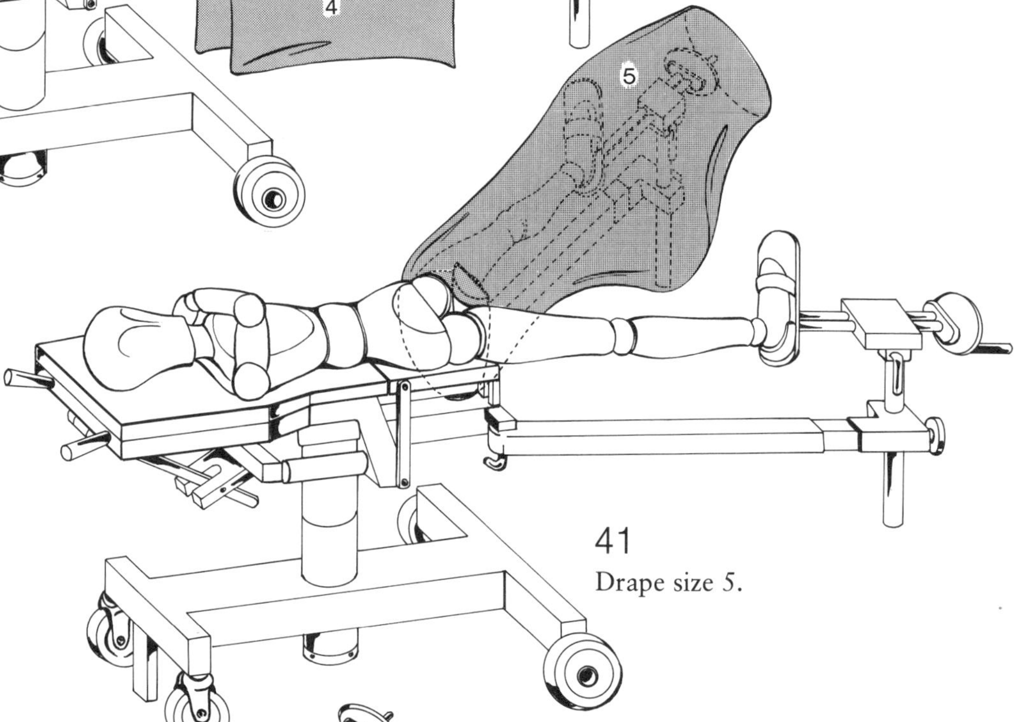

41
Drape size 5.

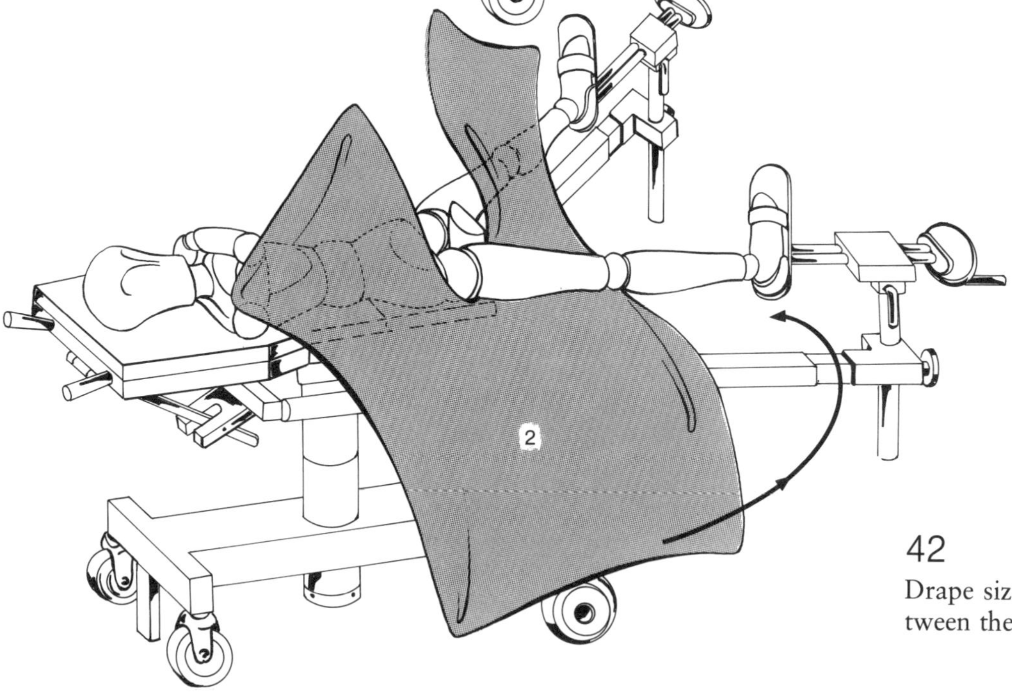

42
Drape size 2 is carefully pulled between the leg…

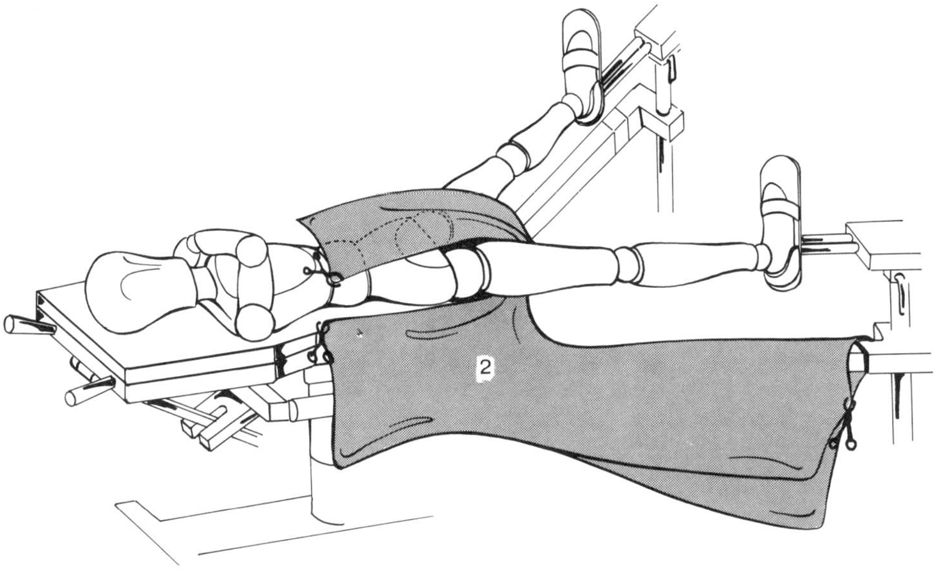

43
... and the traction arm.

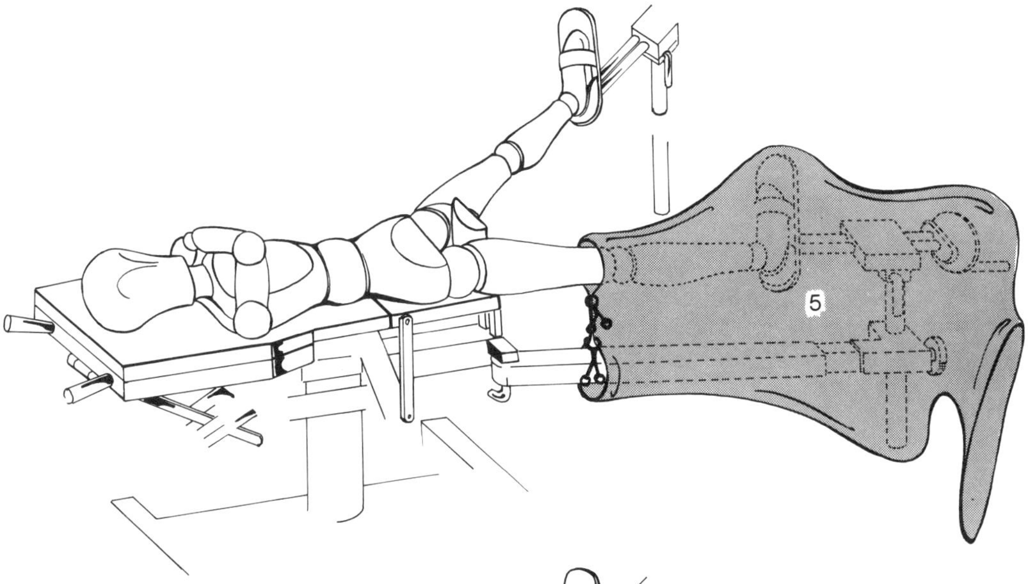

44
Drape size 5.

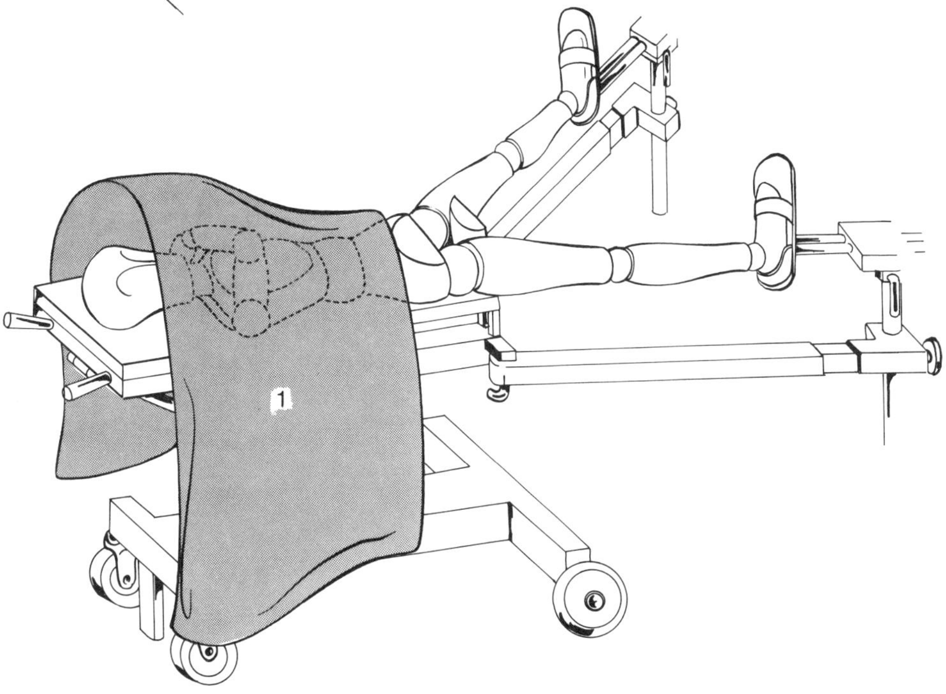

45
Drape size 1.

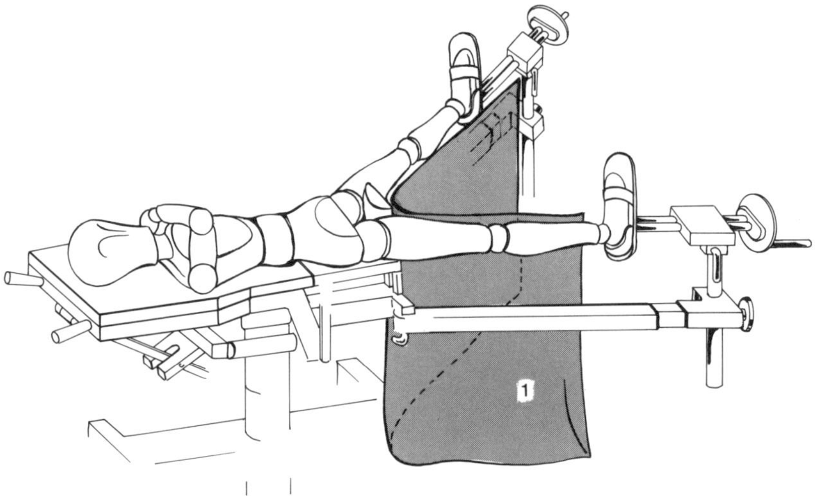

46
Drape size 1.

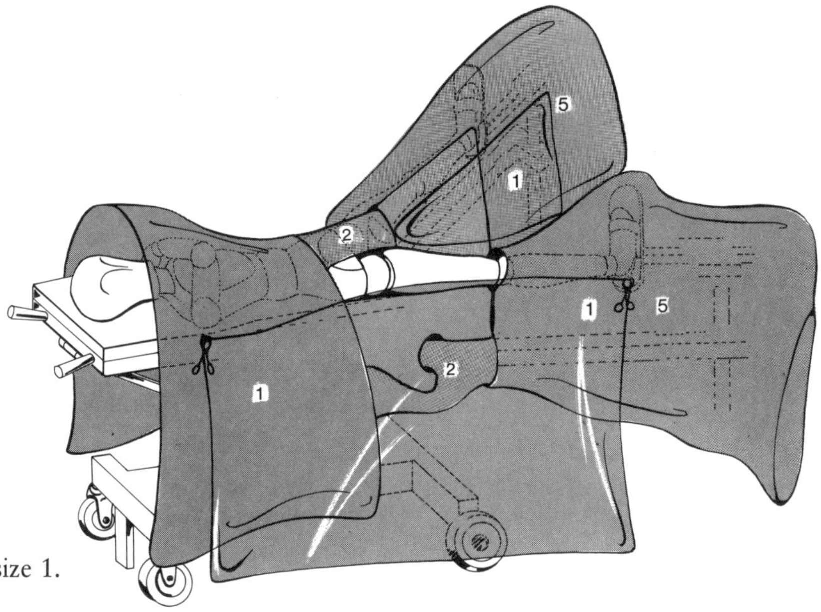

47
Drape size 1.

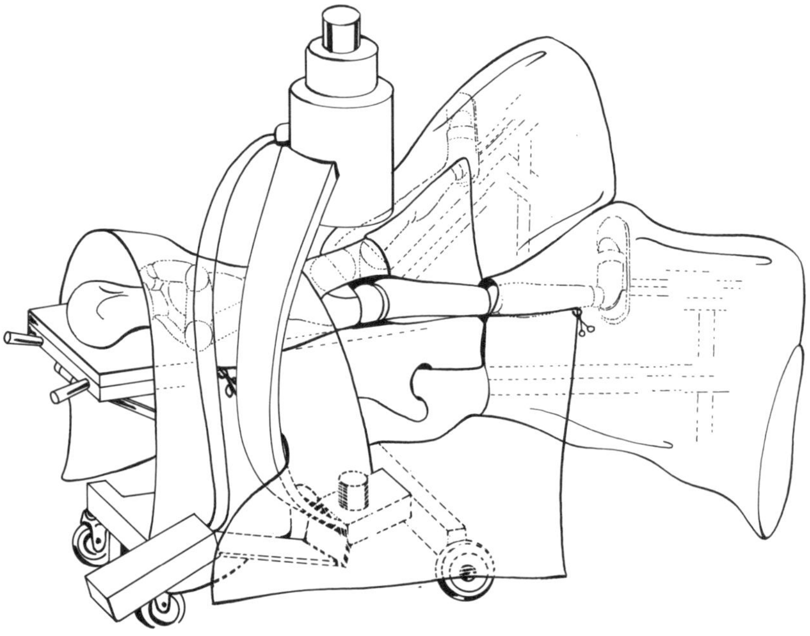

48
Setting up the image intensifier.

Approach

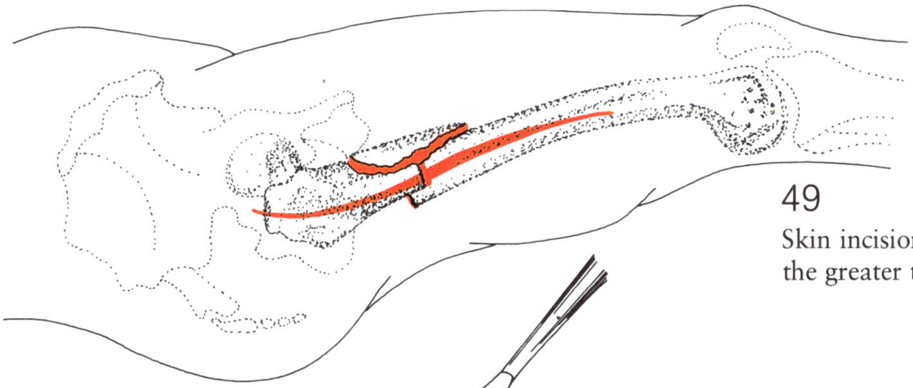

49

Skin incision *exactly lateral*, between the tip of the greater trochanter and the femoral condyle.

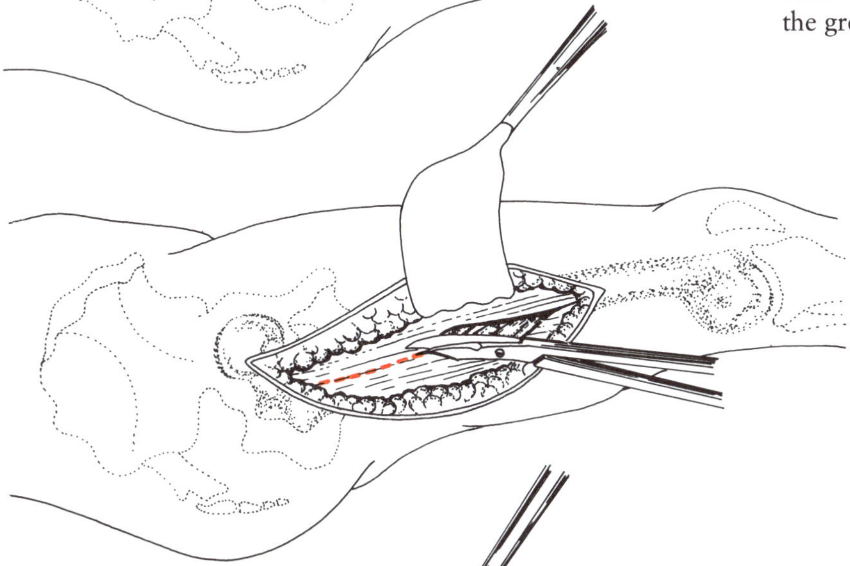

50

The fascia is split without injuring the subjacent muscular fascia.

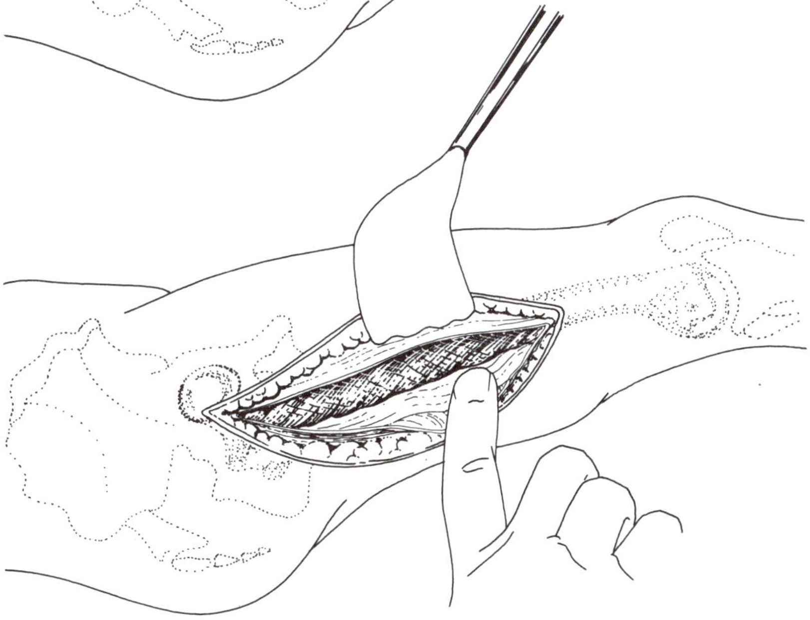

51

Blunt dissection of both fascias renders the posterior origin of the vastus lateralis muscle accessible.

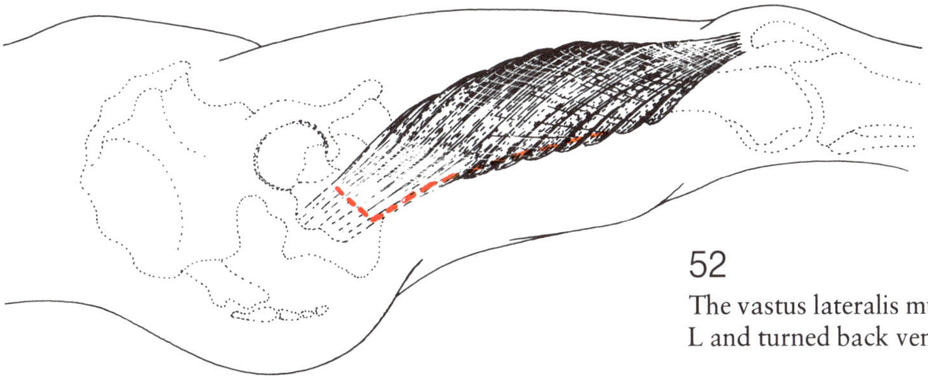

52

The vastus lateralis muscle is detached in the shape of an L and turned back ventrally.

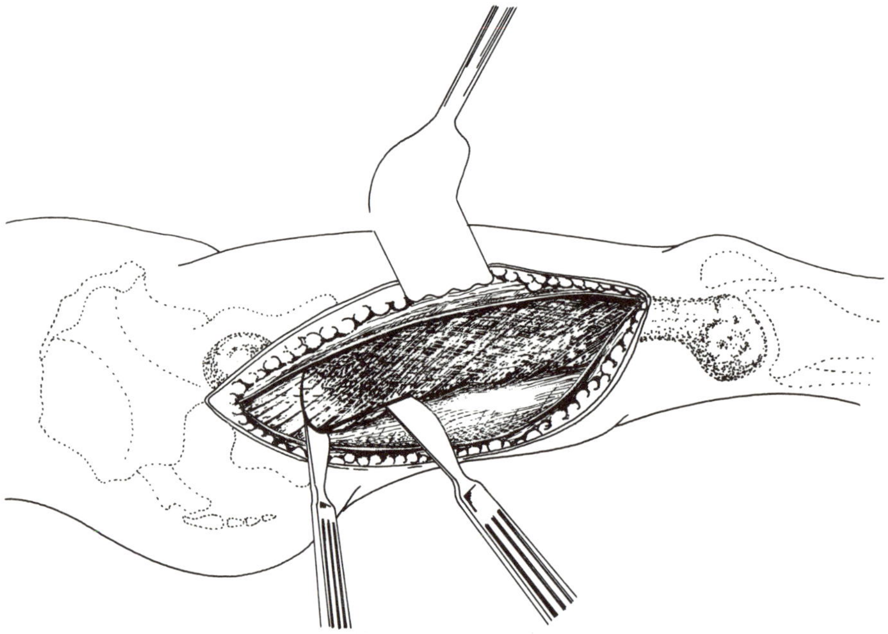

53

The proximal tendinous origin of the vastus lateralis muscle is divided transversely; by turning the incision dorsally in the distal direction, the dorsal muscular origin of the vastus lateralis is divided longitudinally. By leaving a small fascial border in the posterior origin, good readaptation can be obtained later on with use of a suture.

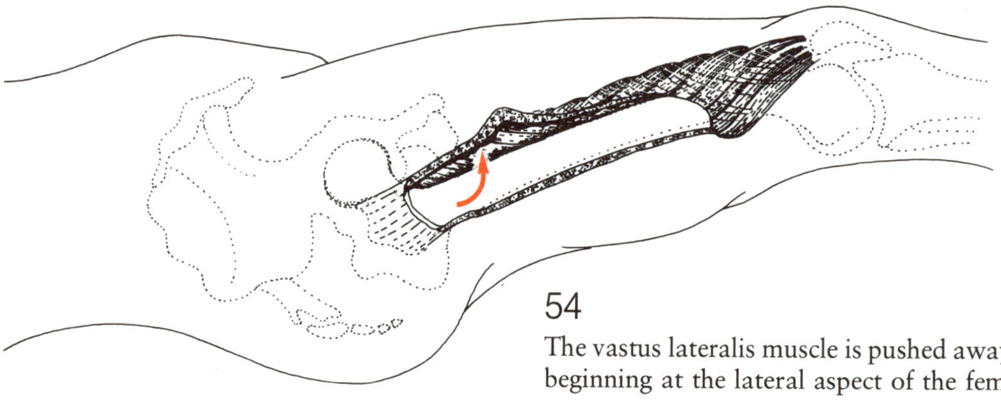

54

The vastus lateralis muscle is pushed away from dorsally to ventrally, beginning at the lateral aspect of the femur.

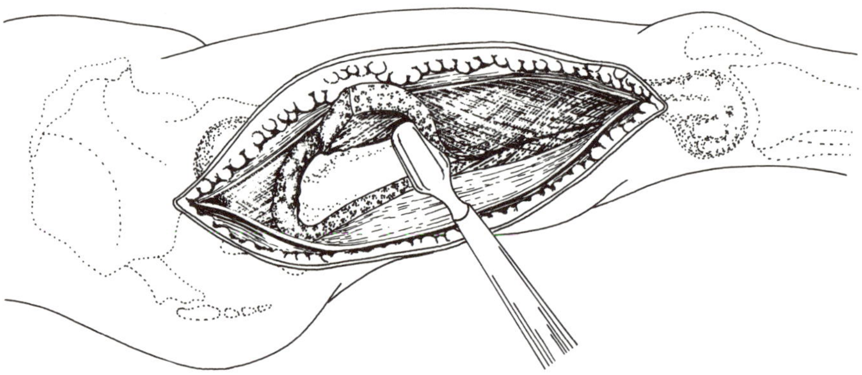

55

Pushing away the muscle from the lateral aspect of the femoral shaft with a raspatory. A bending wedge must stay in place touching the soft tissues.

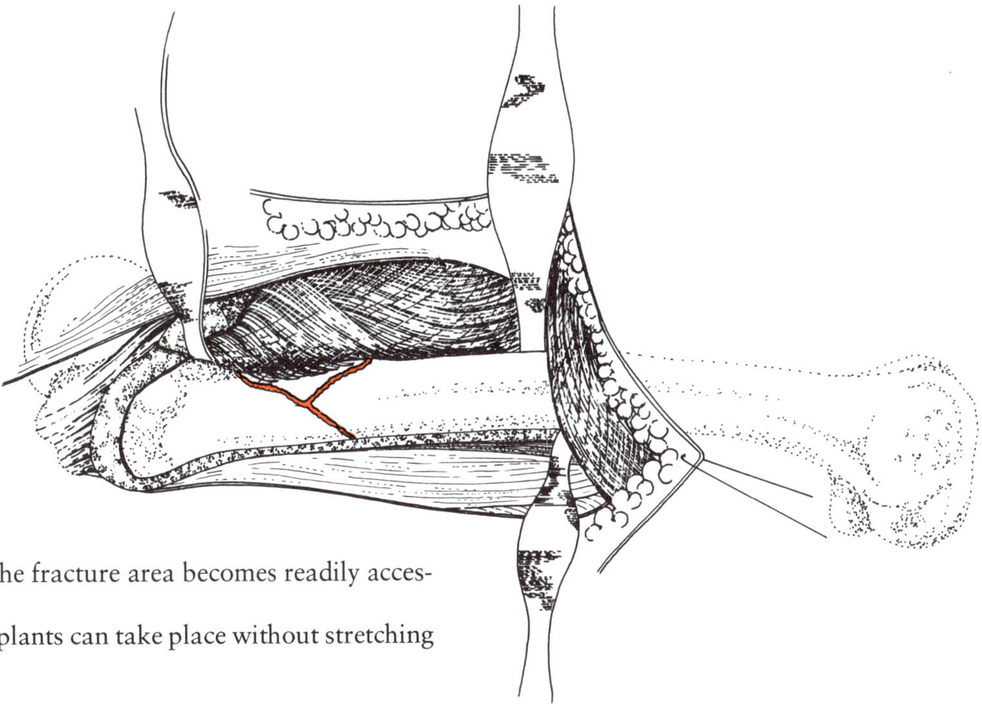

56
After applying the elevators, the fracture area becomes readily accessible.
Reduction and insertion of implants can take place without stretching the soft tissues.

Tactics

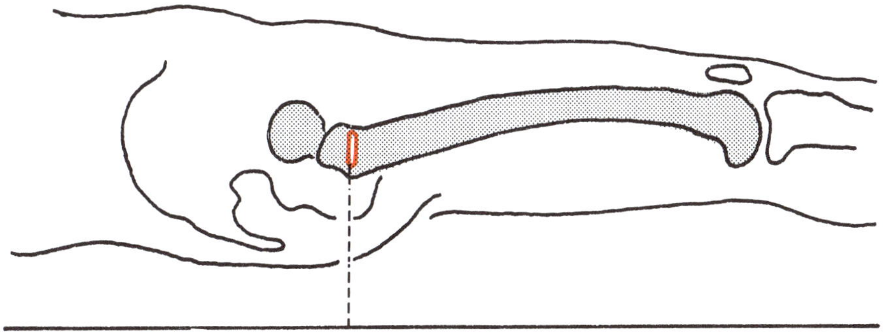

57
In drilling and cutting the slit in the plate, one runs the danger of its being fashioned vertical to the plane of the table (in the erroneous assumption that the femoral shaft runs parallel to the plane of the table or the floor).

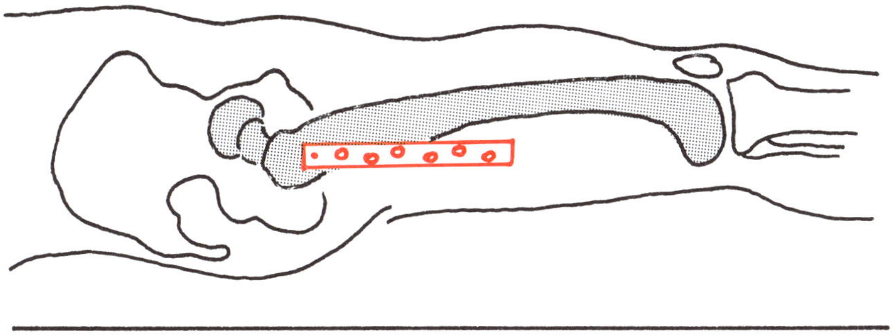

58
Only on driving the plate home does one notice that the holed part of the plate cannot be applied to the shaft of the femur. Correction is laborious and takes a great deal of time. Use of the caliper rule guards against this error.

Medial fracture of the femoral neck

Types of injuries See Figs. 149–2ff.

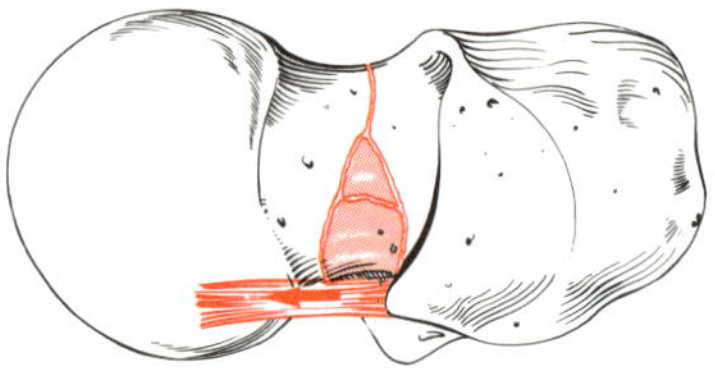

1
Right femoral neck, cranial view: fracture with characteristic area of comminution following reduction.

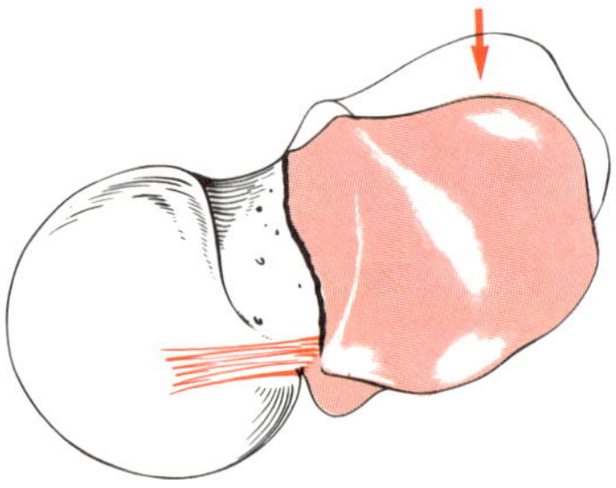

2
Right femoral neck, cranial view: typical backward tilting of the fragment through "wasting of the femoral neck" and pull on the small and the large external rotators.

Indication and operative possibilities

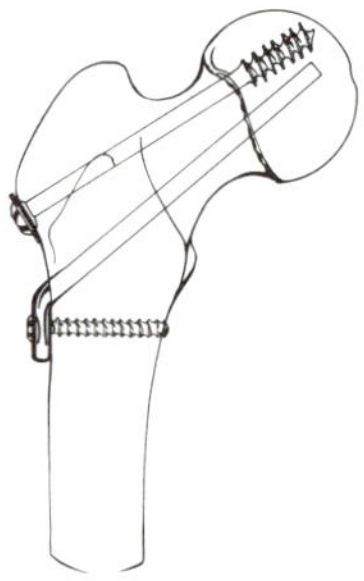

3
AO nail for femoral neck
Technique:
see Figs. 182–7ff.
Advantages: broad contact surface, stability; image intensifier not required
Disadvantages: difficulties when hard cancellous bone is present, can have a blocking effect, delicate technique, danger of necrosis of the femoral head
Preferential indication: patients under 65.

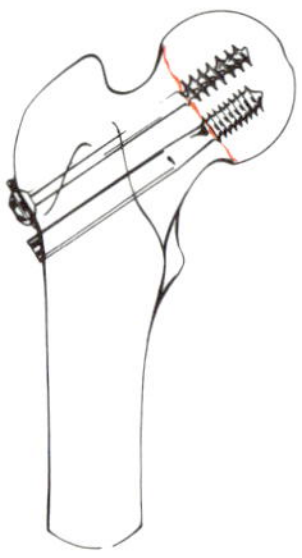

4
Sliding compression screw
Technique:
see Figs. 169–1ff.
Advantages: cannot have a blocking effect, no shock to the femoral head by hammer blows
Disadvantages: little resistance to shearing forces, delicate technique, danger of necrosis of the femoral head, requires image intensifier
Preferential indication: patients under 65.

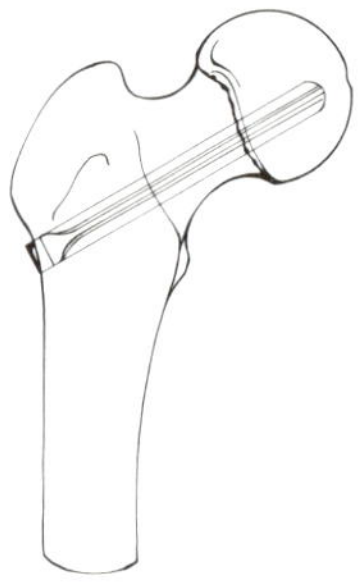

5
Triflanged nail
Technique:
see Figs. 173–1ff.
Advantages: simple technique
Disadvantages: little support in bone, danger of necrosis of the femoral head
Preferential indication: fractures in elderly patients which are impacted in valgus position.

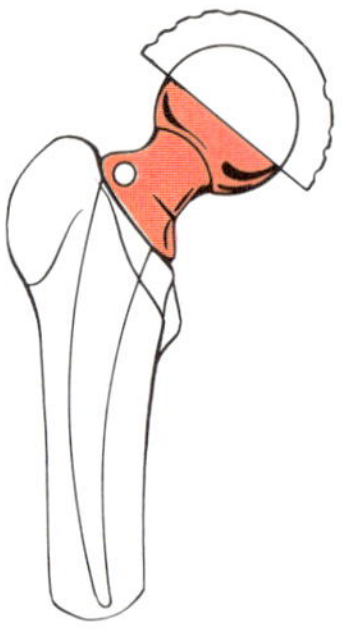

6
Total replacement arthroplasty
Advantages: very rapid rehabilitation, resistant to weightbearing, no necrosis of the femoral head
Disadvantages: delicate technique, prosthesis, anchoring problems over the long run
Preferential indication: very old patients.

Principle

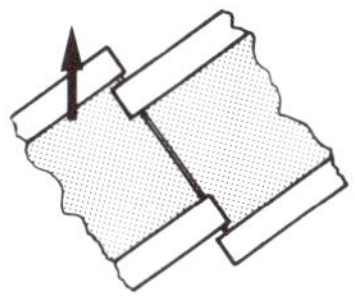

7
If the fragments are left in the *varus position*...

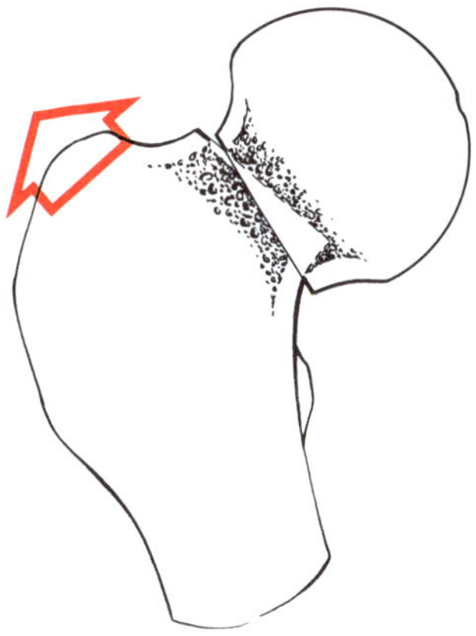

8
... the cranial pull of the abductors and adductors leads to displacement of, or dangerous strain on, the implants.

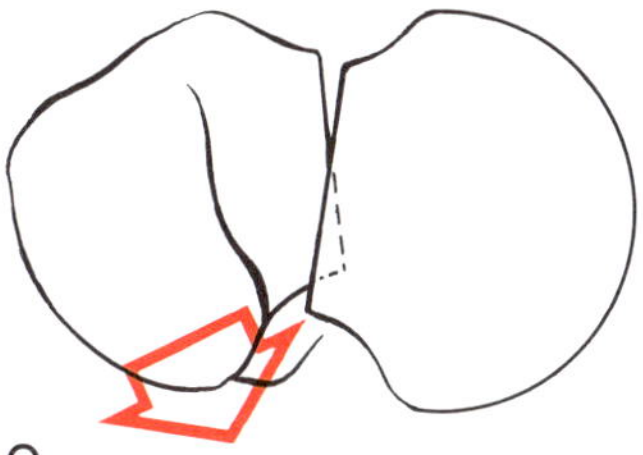

9
In the axial direction there is also insufficient support against the externally rotating pull.

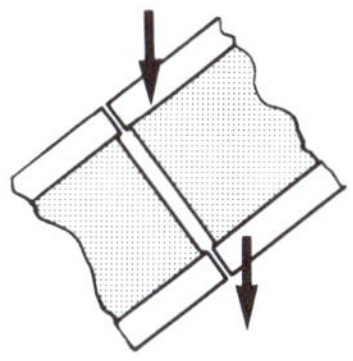

10
A sufficient degree of *accurate reduction* can only be obtained by performing an osteosynthesis that ensures interfragmental compression.

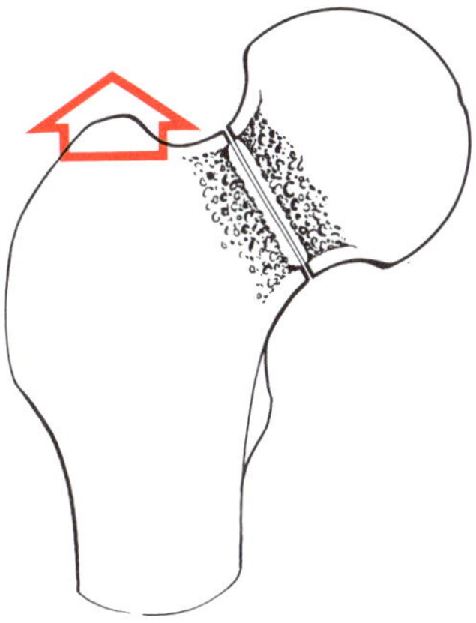

11
The pull of the abductors and...

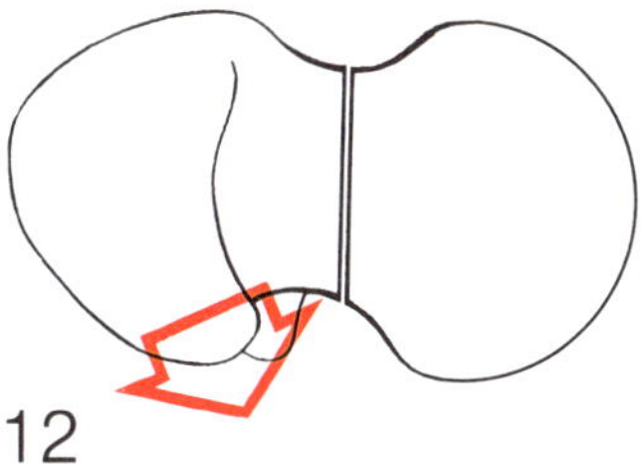

12
... the external rotators can lead to secondary displacement, particularly when bone resorption takes place in a comminuted area.

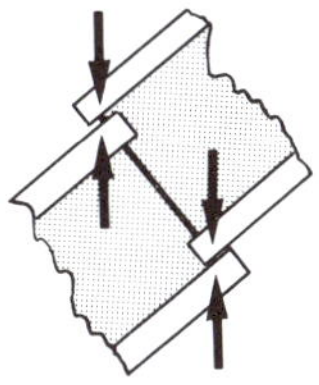

13
Only overcorrection producing a *valgus position* offers sufficient protection against secondary displacement.

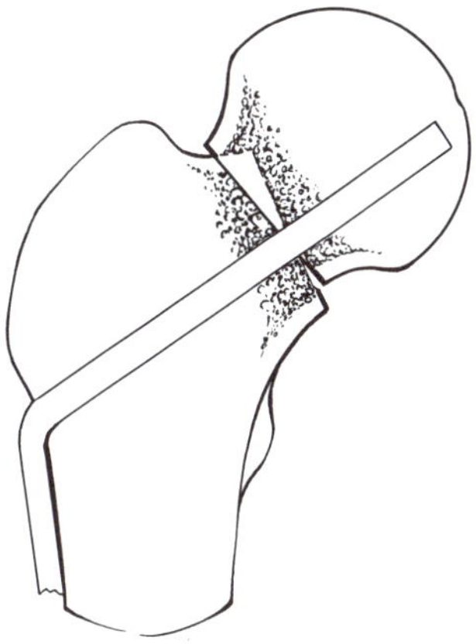

14
The head should be fitted to the femoral neck "like a hat hanging on a peg".

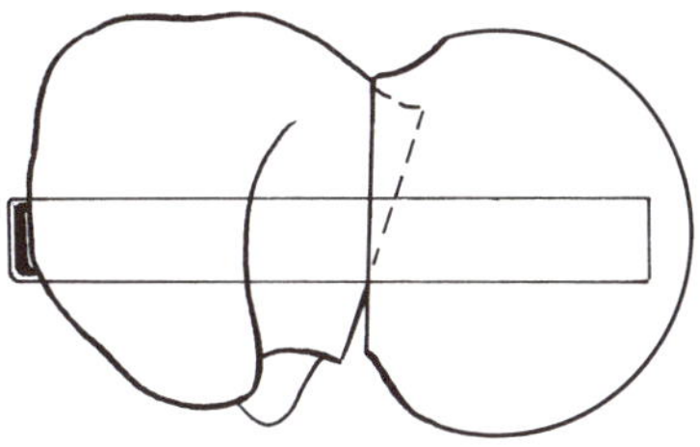

15
This adjustment, shown in the axial view, prevents secondary displacement in external rotation through strain.

Positioning: See Figs. 154–25 ff.

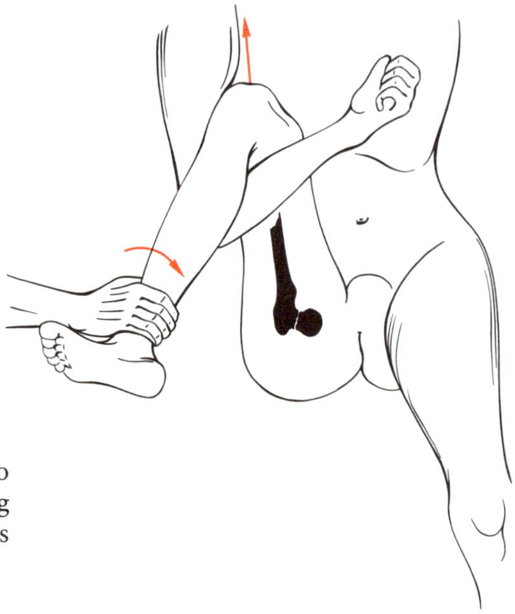

16

When, despite the measures depicted in Figs. 154–25 ff., no satisfactory reduction can be effected, distinct repositioning maneuvers may be successful. (To effect this, the traction is removed.)
Repositioning maneuver I.

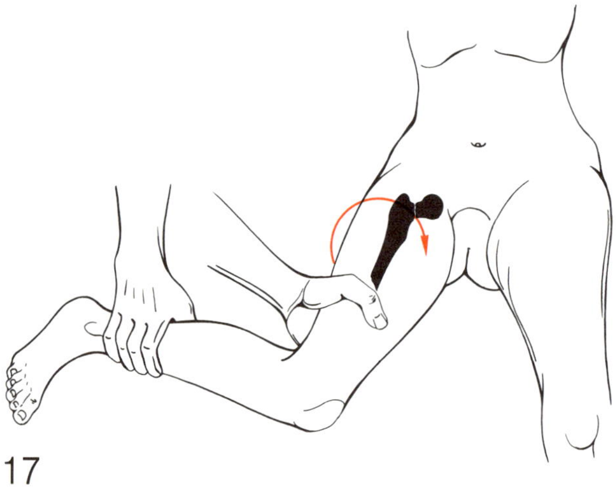

17

Repositioning maneuver II.

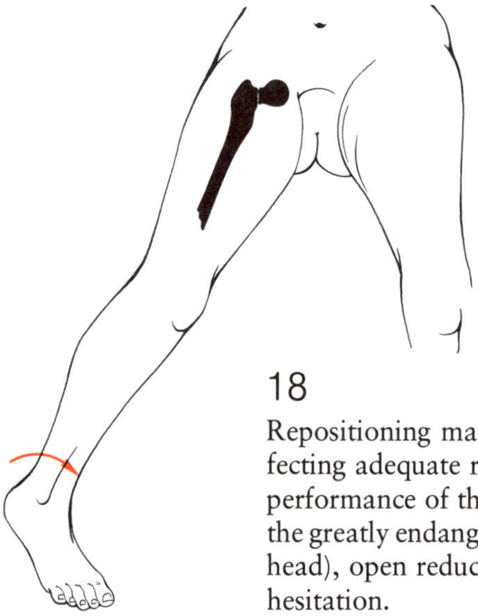

18

Repositioning maneuver III. If one does not succeed in effecting adequate reduction for closed nailing by *atraumatic* performance of these measures (bearing constantly in mind the greatly endangered nutrient vessels supplying the femoral head), open reduction should be done without the slightest hesitation.

Approach: See. p. 144.

Lateral and pertrochanteric fractures

Operative possibilities

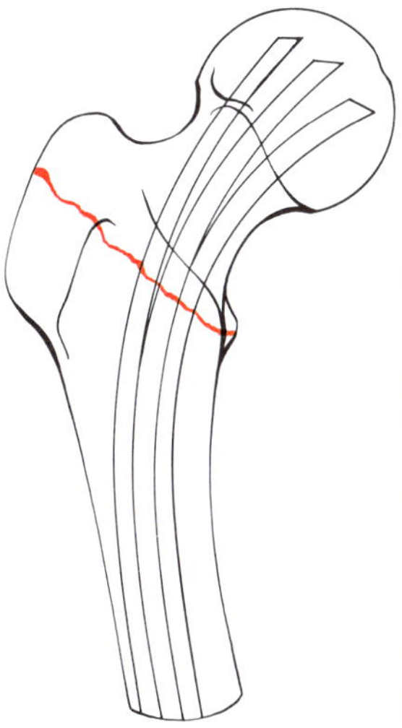

1

Spring nails

Technique: see p. 175

Advantages: wound remote from the fracture, a relatively unstressful intervention, immediate weight bearing generally possible

Disadvantages: traction table, image intensifier, no anatomical reposition

Preferential indication: patients over 60.

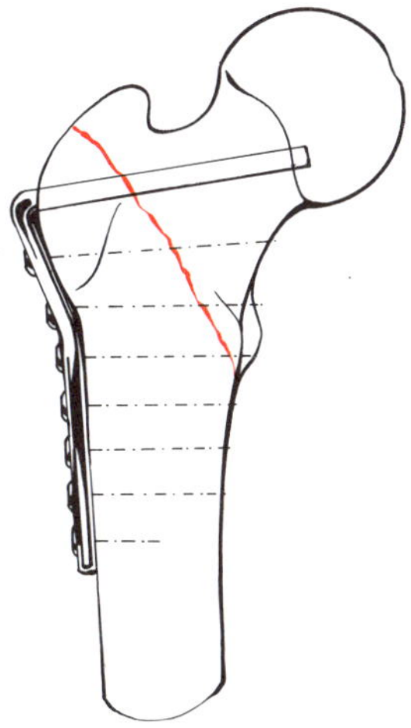

2

Condylar plate

Technique: see p. 186

Advantages: reduction stable, particularly in multifragment fractures; standard operating table, no image intensifier, accurate reposition

Disadvantages: delicate technique, no immediate weight bearing

Preferential indication: younger patients.

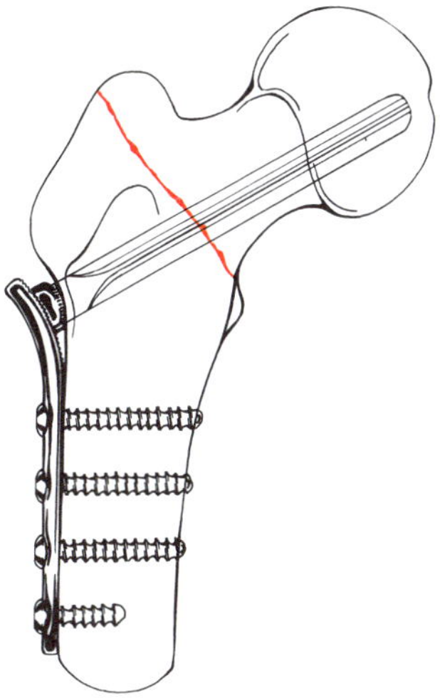

3

Mc Laughlin's nail with a side plate

Technique: see p. 173

Advantages:
simple technique,
minor intervention

Disadvantages:
little stability,
traction table,
image intensifier,
no immediate weight bearing

Preferential indication:
elderly patients.

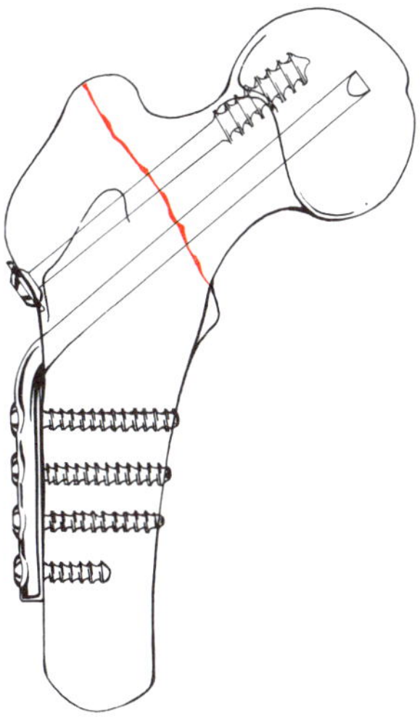

4

130° angular plate

Technique: see p. 181

Advantages:
stable, standard operating table, no image intensifier, anatomical reposition

Disadvantages: delicate technique, no immediate weight bearing

Preferential indication: younger patients.

Subtrochanteric fractures

Types of injuries

See Figs. on p. 150f.

Operative possibilities

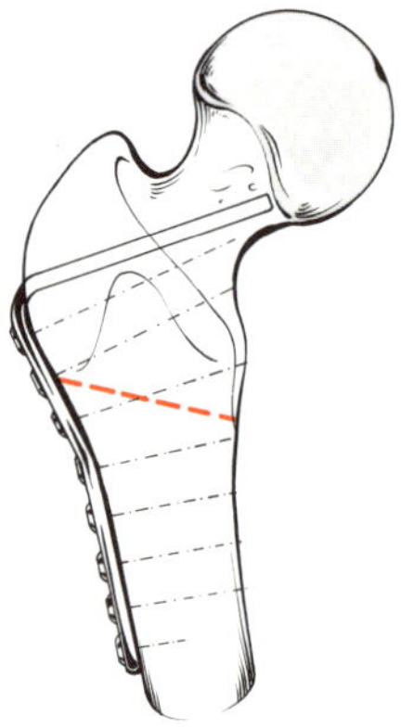

1
Condylar plate with cancellous graft (See p. 187).

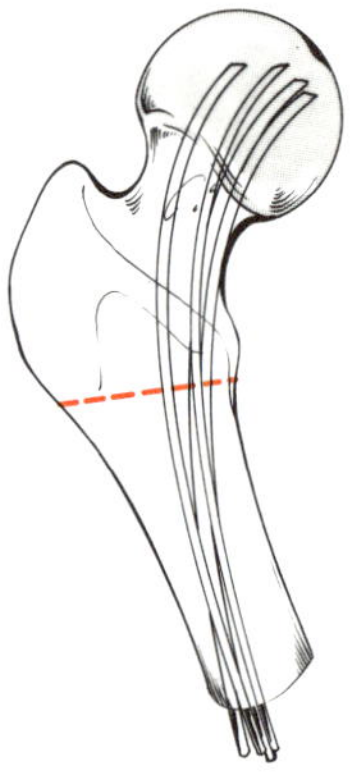

2
Spring nail (for aged patients): See p. 175.

Screw

Anatomy: See Figs. 141–1ff.

Types of injuries: See Figs. 149.

Indication: See p. 164.

Principle: See pp. 152 and 165.

Positioning: See pp. 192 and 154.

Tactics

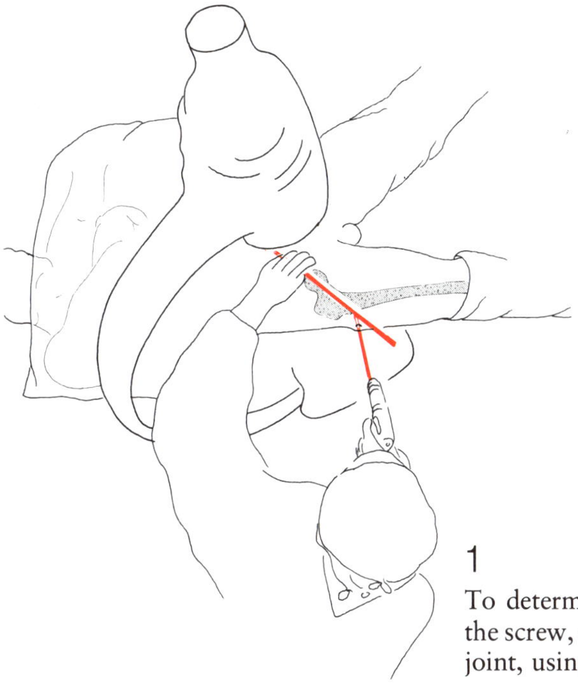

1
To determine the appropriate site for inserting the screw, a drilling wire is first placed on the hip joint, using the image intensifier.

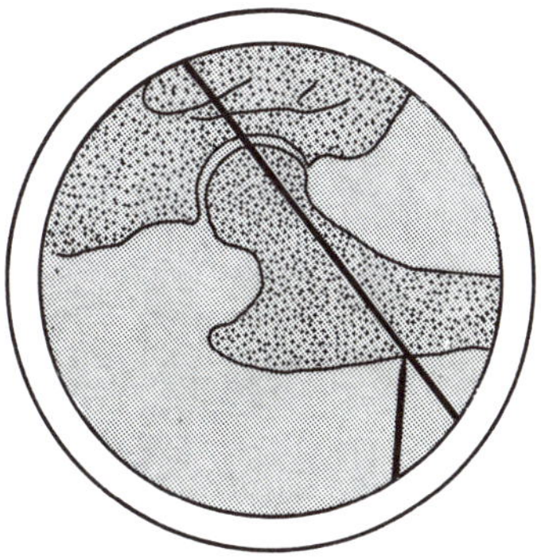

2
The direction can be established on the roentgenogram as shown in Figs. 153–19ff., and in this way the most favorable site for inserting the screw can be located.

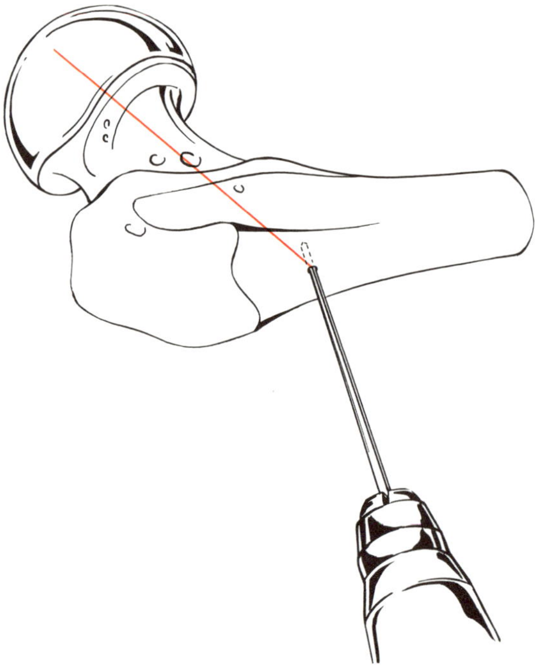

3

A Kirschner wire is inserted or knocked into place transcutaneuosly (one should first verify whether the projected implant with its bore hole can be pushed over the wire). Care must be taken to see that the site of insertion lies *exactly in the greatest diameter of the shaft.*

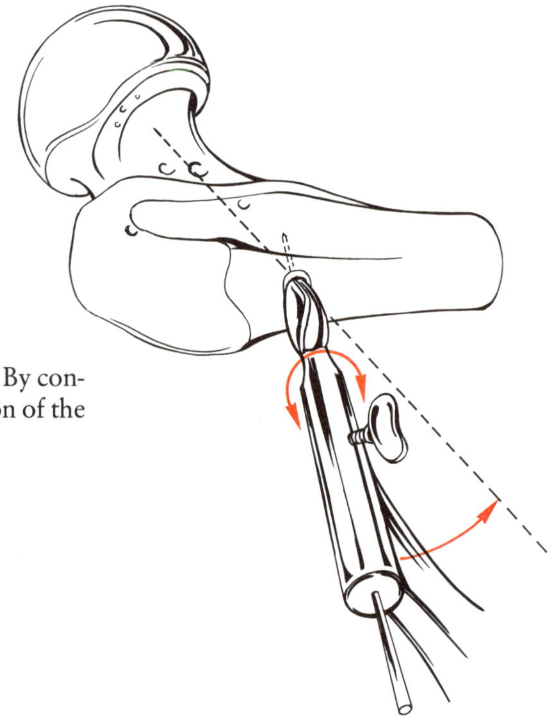

4

Incision. Drilling and widening of the cortex with a hand reamer. By continuous rotation of the reamer, the canal is tapered in the direction of the axis of the femoral neck.

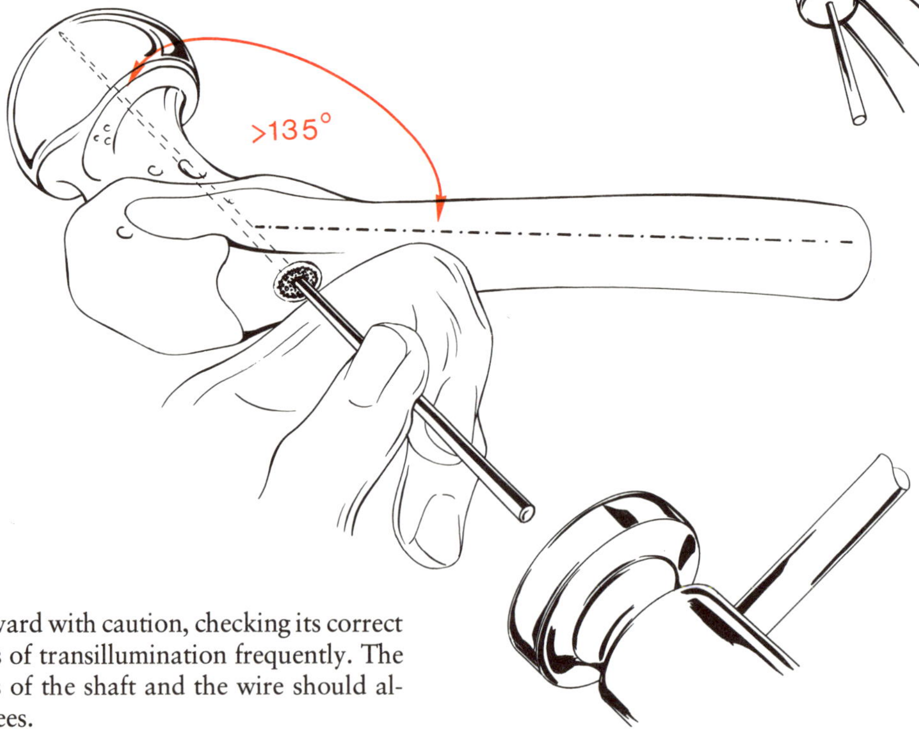

5

The wire is pushed forward with caution, checking its correct position in both planes of transillumination frequently. The angle between the axis of the shaft and the wire should always exceed 135 degrees.

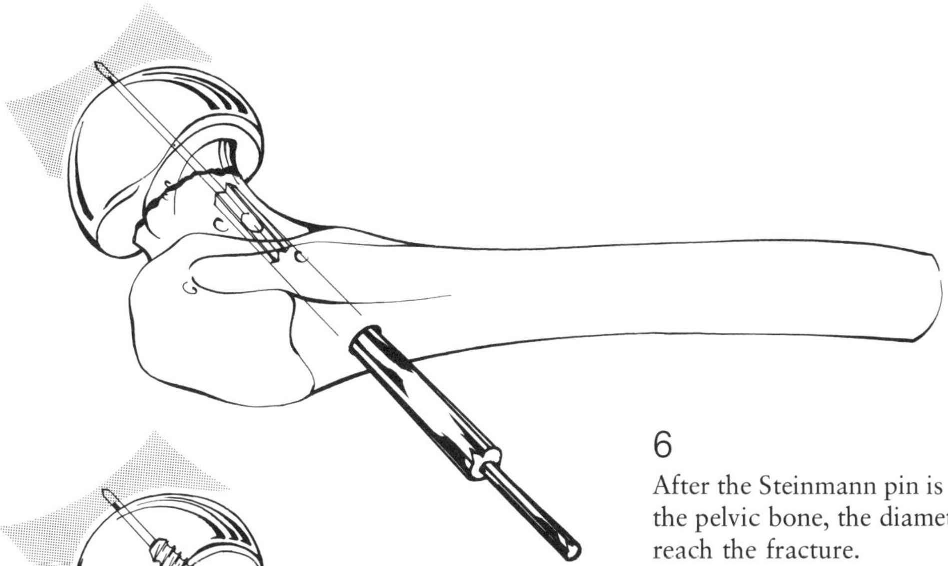

6

After the Steinmann pin is driven through the joint as far as the pelvic bone, the diameter of the screw body is drilled to reach the fracture.

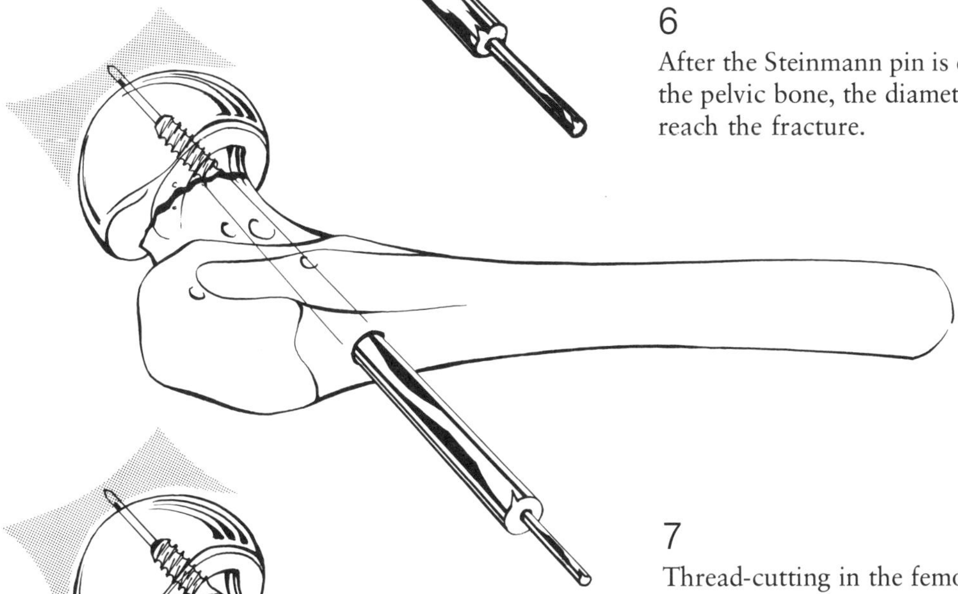

7

Thread-cutting in the femoral head.

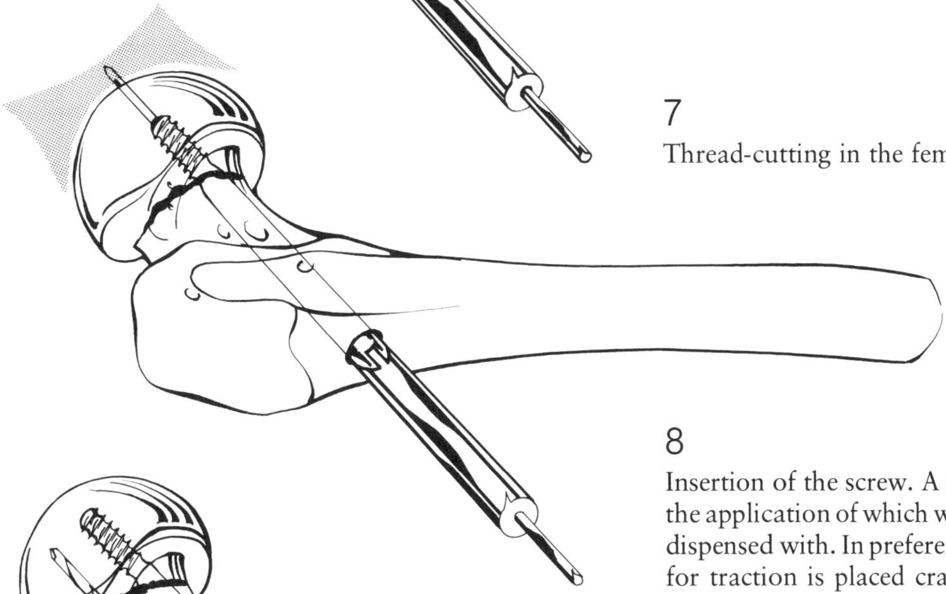

8

Insertion of the screw. A supporting plate or a lateral plate, the application of which would prolong the operation, can be dispensed with. In preference, an additional cancellous screw for traction is placed cranially, parallel to the Pohl screw.

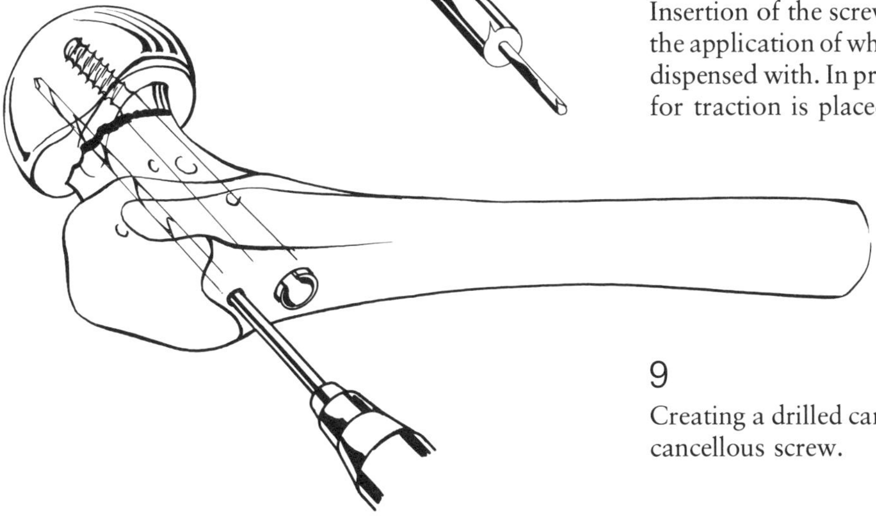

9

Creating a drilled canal with the 3.2 mm drill for a proximal cancellous screw.

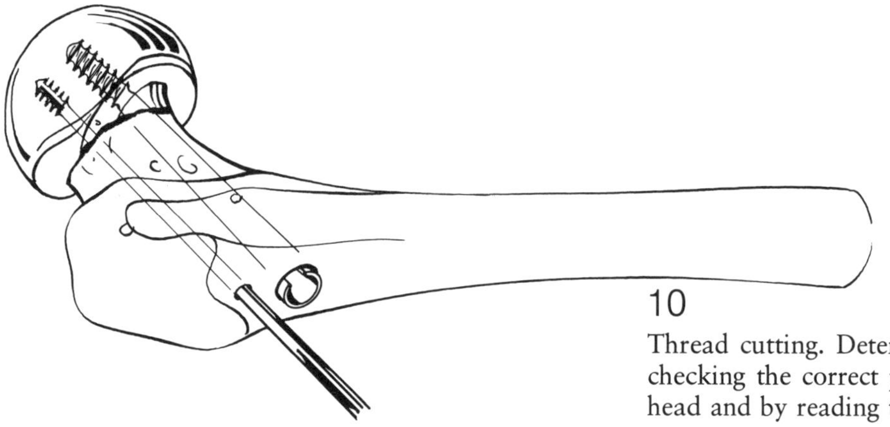

10

Thread cutting. Determination of the necessary length by checking the correct position of the thread in the femoral head and by reading the marks on the thread cutter.

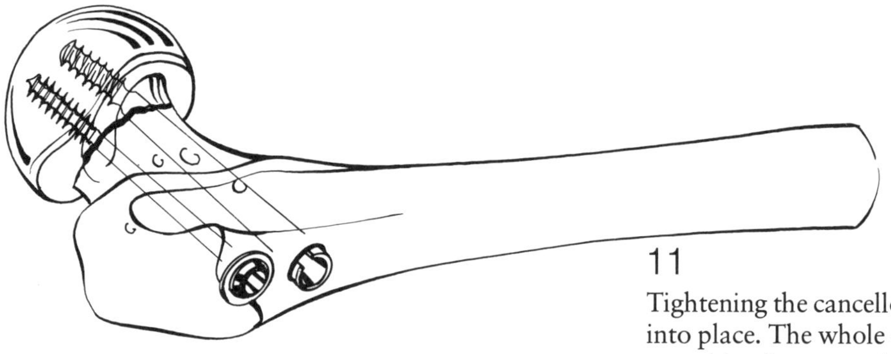

11

Tightening the cancellous screw fitted with a supporting disk into place. The whole cleft of the fracture must also be intersected by the screw thread.

3-L nail

Anatomy See p. 141.

Types of injuries See pp. 149 and 150.

Indication See p. 164.

Principle See pp. 152 and 165.

Positioning See pp. 192 and 154.

Tactics First see Figs. 169–1 and 169–5.

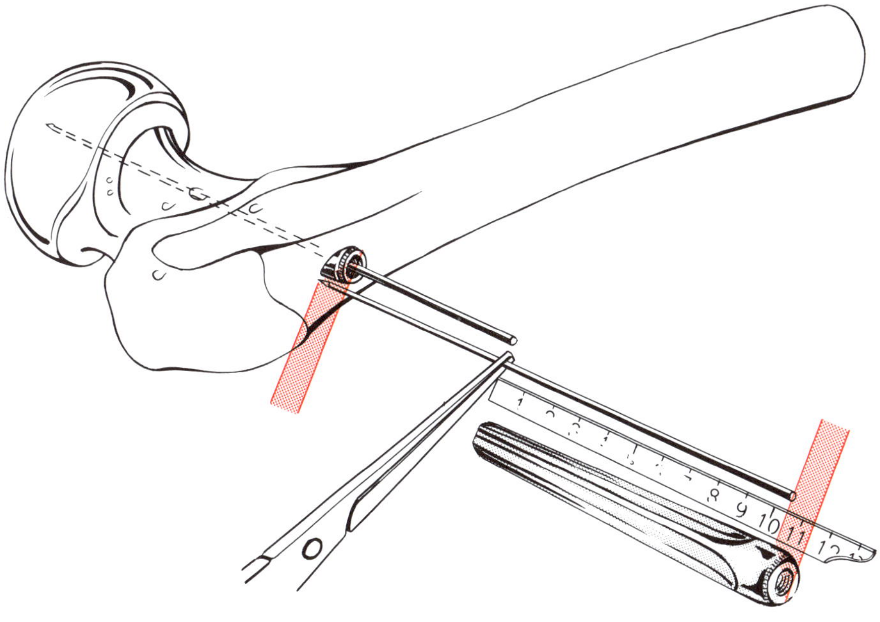

1
Measuring the nail length with the aid of a second wire of the same length. Owing to the slant of the drilled canal, about 0.5–1 cm should be added to the measured length.

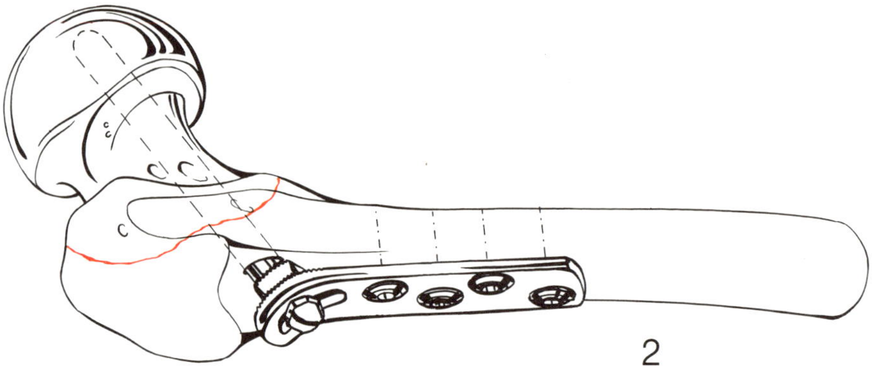

2

Such additional length is particularly of importance when a plate is to be screwed onto the nail.

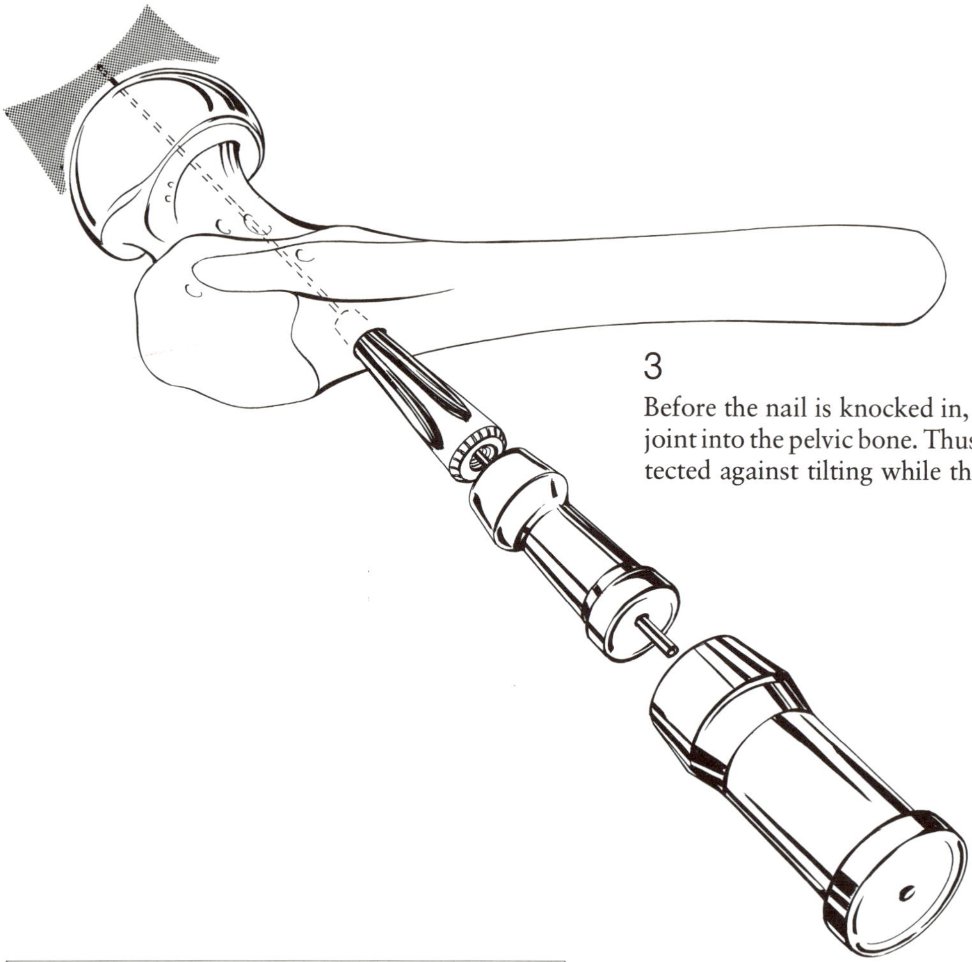

3

Before the nail is knocked in, the wire is driven through the joint into the pelvic bone. Thus the femoral head is better protected against tilting while the nail is being driven home.

Postoperative management See p. 9 ff.

Spring nail

Anatomy See p. 141.

Types of injuries See p. 150f.

Indication See pp. 167 and 168.

Principle See pp. 152 and 165.

Positioning See pp. 155 and 158.

Approach

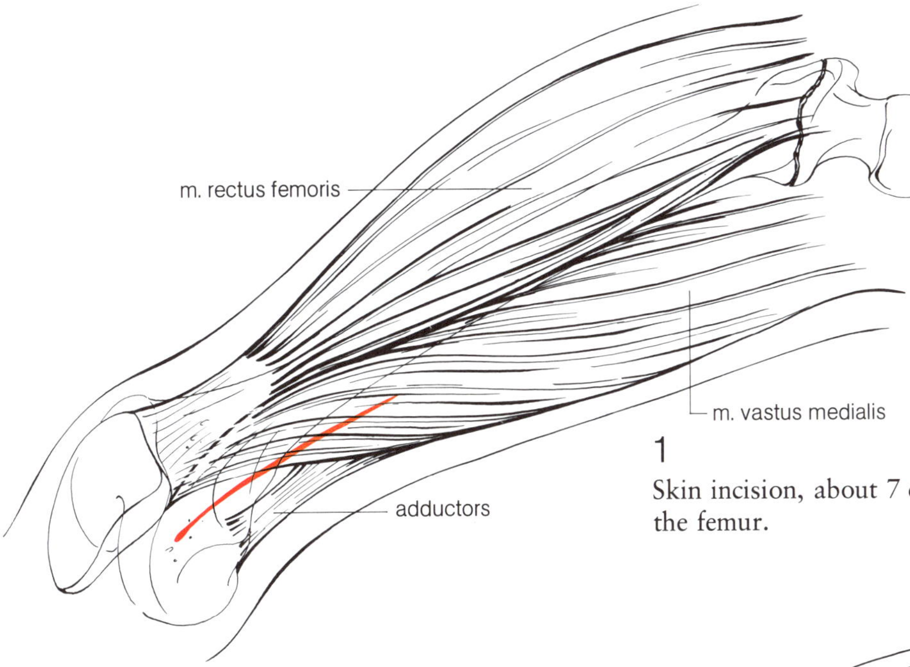

1
Skin incision, about 7 cm long, over the medial condyle of the femur.

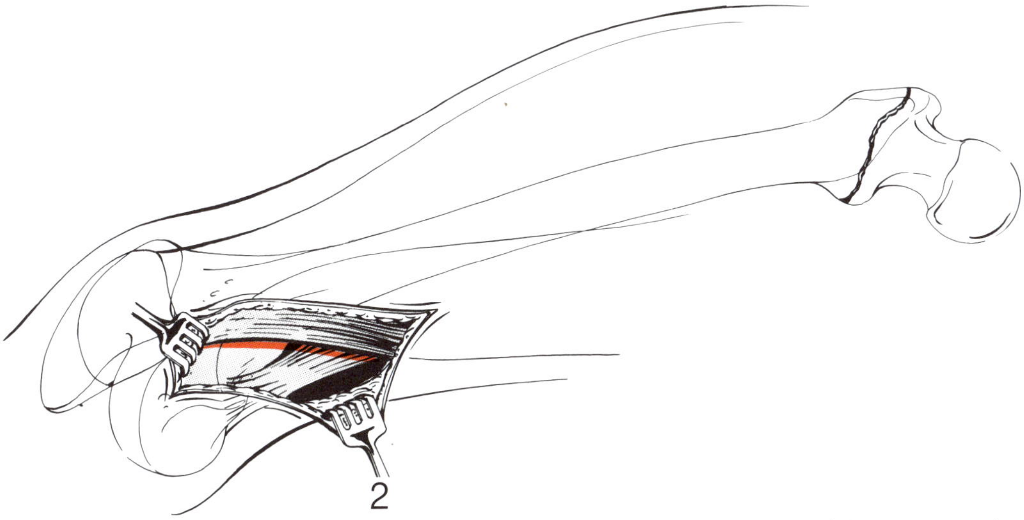

2
The fascia is split at the posterior border of the vastus medialis muscle.

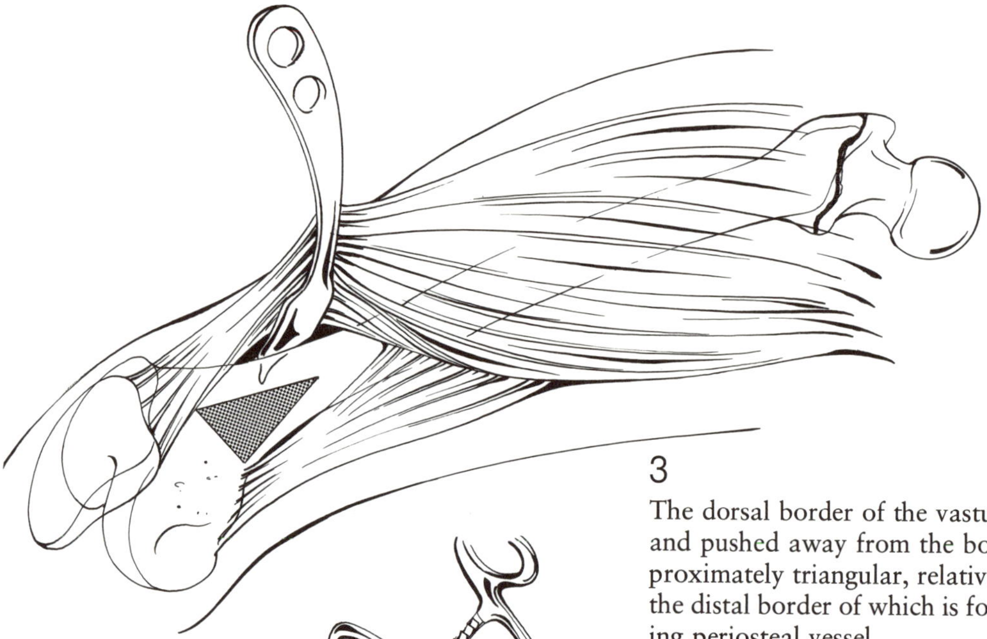

3

The dorsal border of the vastus medialis muscle is exposed and pushed away from the bone from rear to fore. An approximately triangular, relatively flat area comes into view, the distal border of which is formed by a transversely coursing periosteal vessel.

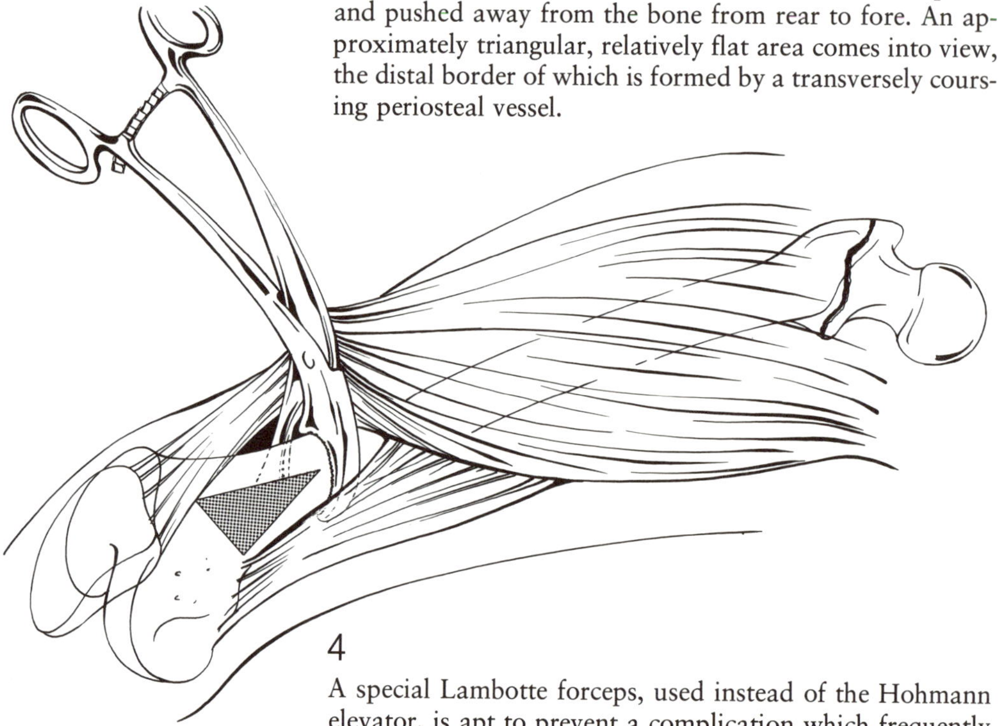

4

A special Lambotte forceps, used instead of the Hohmann elevator, is apt to prevent a complication which frequently supervenes in the further course of the operation, namely, breaking out of a cranial window in the cortex.

Tactics

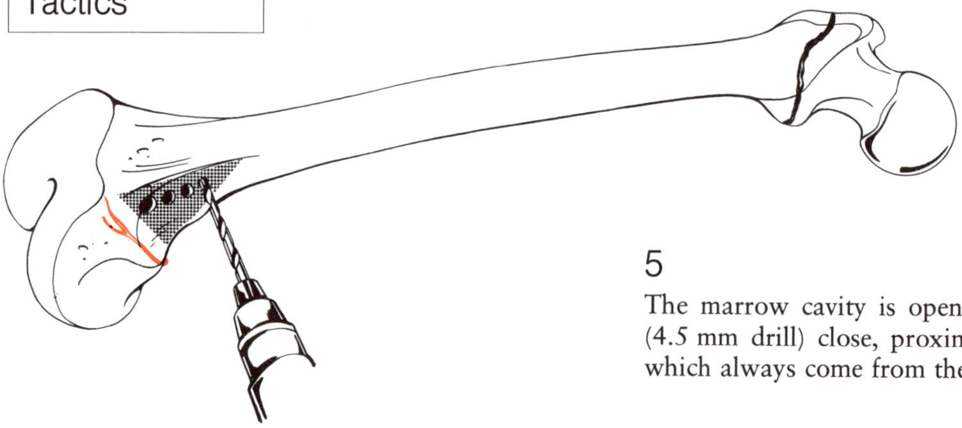

5

The marrow cavity is opened through several drill holes (4.5 mm drill) close, proximally, to the periosteal vessels which always come from the dorsal side.

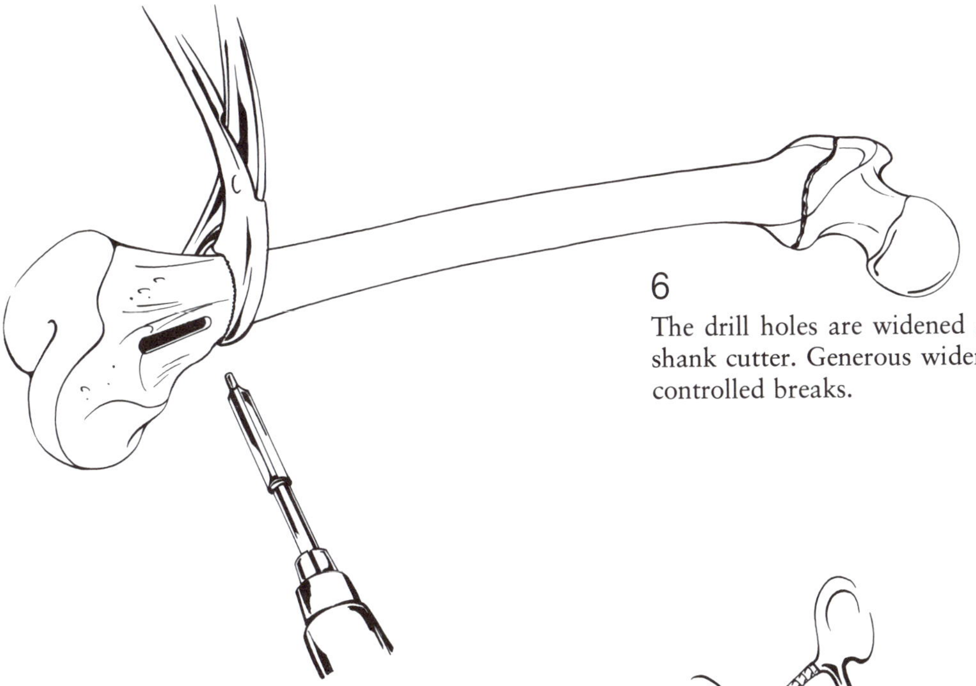

6

The drill holes are widened and connected by means of a shank cutter. Generous widening is expedient to avoid uncontrolled breaks.

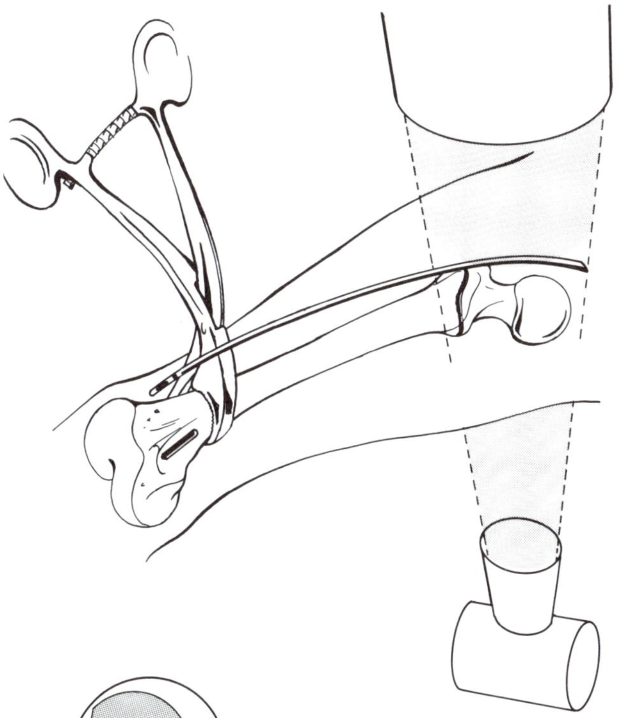

7

Determining the nail length: a nail is placed on the thigh, corresponding to its later position. To mark the distal end of the nail, a forceps is placed into the distal window. Under x-ray control with the intensifier, the point of the nail should be reflected within the joint space because its roentgenographic image is larger than that of the bone.

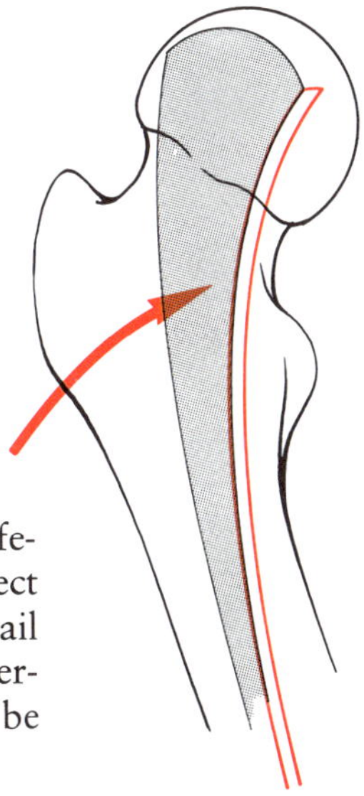

8

The *first nail* is passed medially along Adam's arc into the femoral head. It is possible, and generally necessary, to correct the curvature of the nail with a saw set. However, the nail should not be stretched or bent too strongly because otherwise its elasticity, which is essential to its hold, might be impaired.

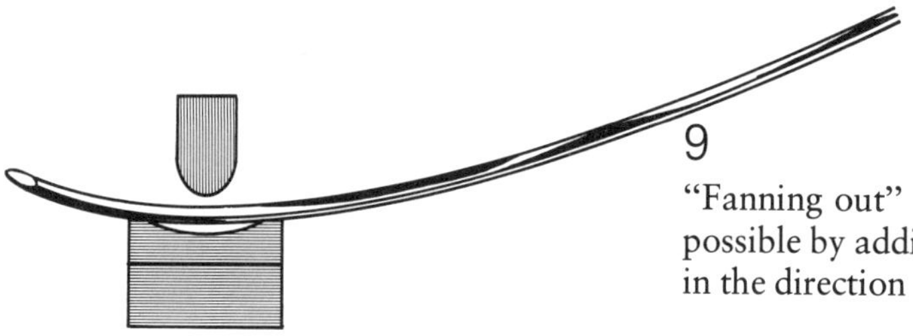

9

"Fanning out" of the nails in both planes of transillumination is made possible by additional bending of individual nails in the other plane (i.e., in the direction in which the femoral neck has suffered anterior torsion).

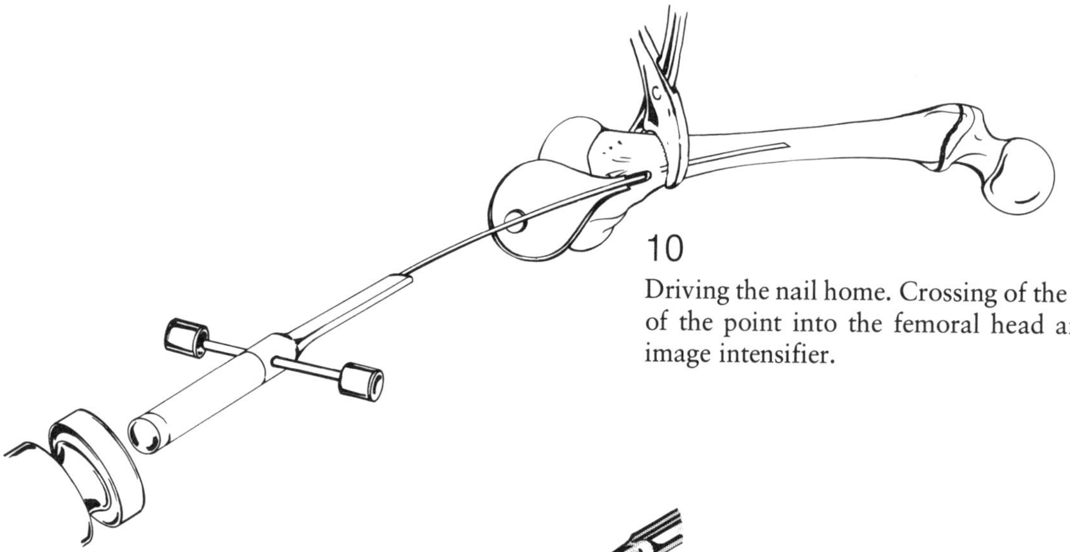

10

Driving the nail home. Crossing of the fracture and entrance of the point into the femoral head are checked under the image intensifier.

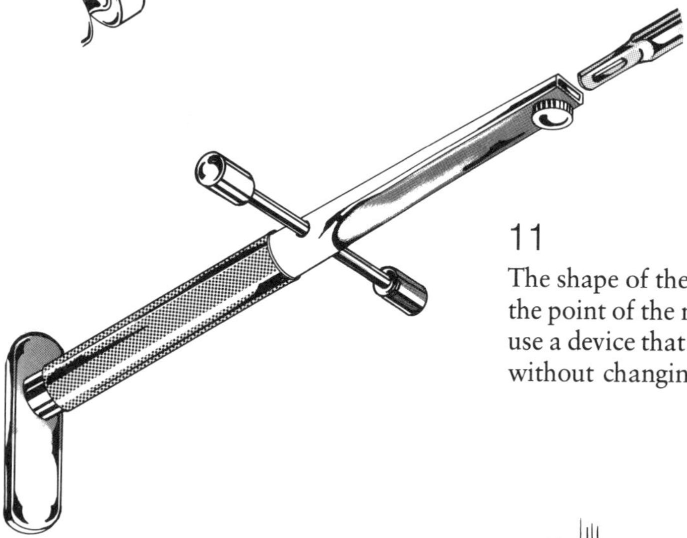

11

The shape of the end of the nail and of the impactor allows one to direct the point of the nail accurately by appropriate rotation. It is expedient to use a device that makes it possible to drive the nail in as well as pull it out without changing the instrument...

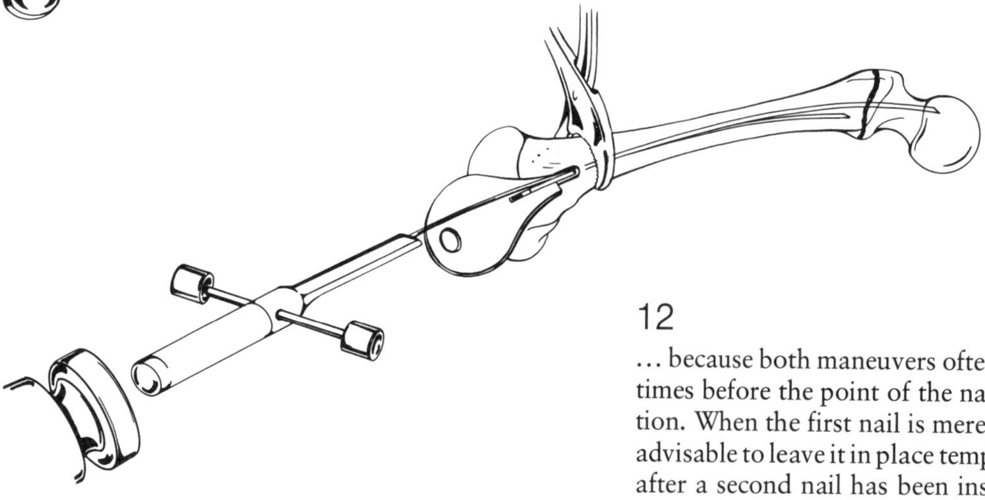

12

... because both maneuvers often have to be repeated several times before the point of the nail has found its correct position. When the first nail is merely too short or too long, it is advisable to leave it in place temporarily and to replace it only after a second nail has been inserted correctly.

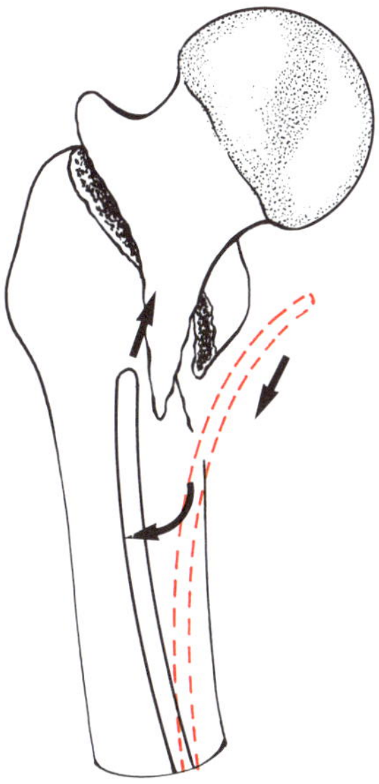

13
A nail which, through inadequate reduction, has run out of the fracture area...

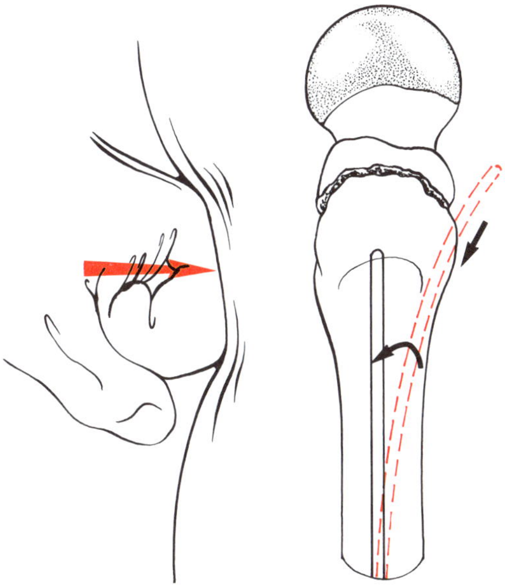

14
... can often be brought into its correct place by repositioning the fracture during surgery; the reduction then may become stable.

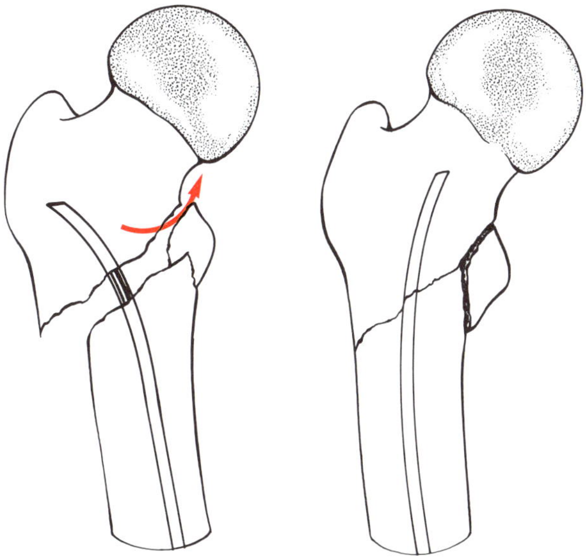

15
So, in certain cases, even repositioning is feasible *with use of the nail.*

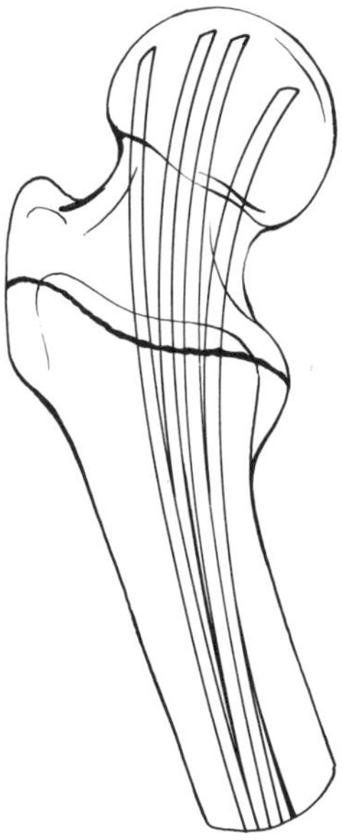

16

The nails should fan out in the head of the femur, in both planes of transillumination if possible.

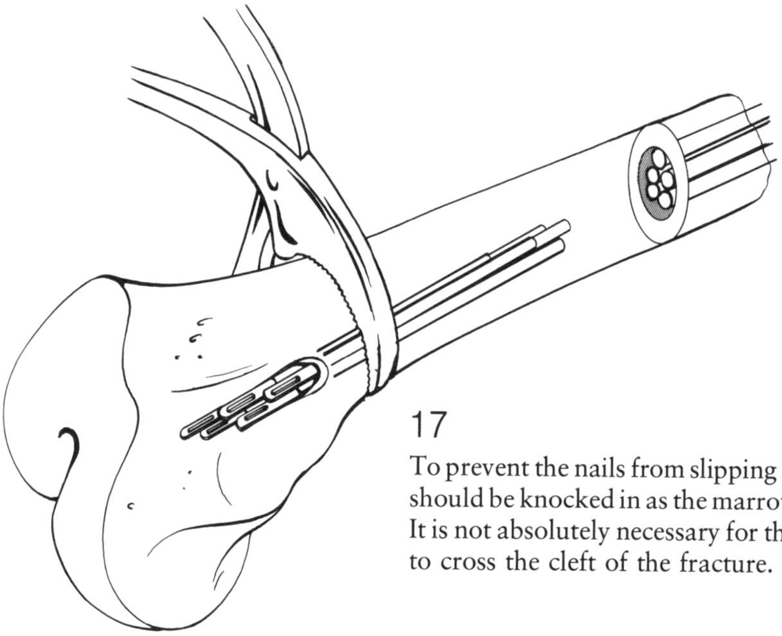

17

To prevent the nails from slipping out, as many nails should be knocked in as the marrow cavity can hold. It is not absolutely necessary for the last nail or nails to cross the cleft of the fracture.

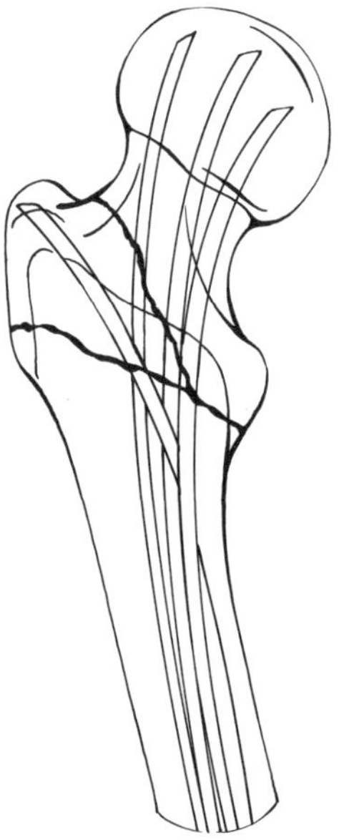

18

For some fractures, an additional spring nail can be inserted in the opposite direction of rotation through an incision at the lateral condyle.

Angular plate

Principle First see p. 153, Figs. 19–21.

Anatomy See p. 141.

Types of injuries See p. 150.

Indication See pp. 164 and 167.

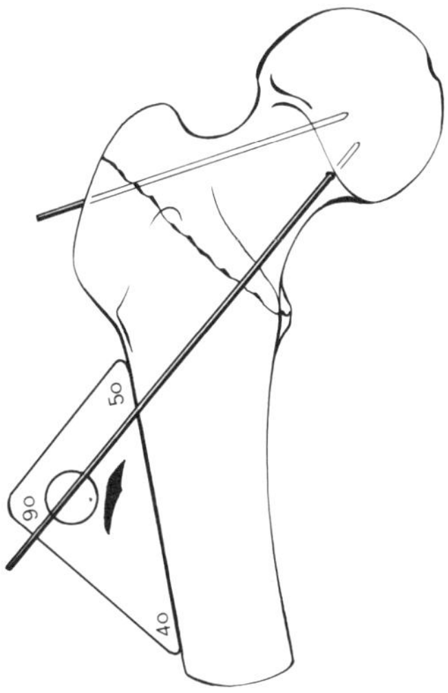

1

Following reduction and preliminary fixation of the fragments in the cranial area, a Steinmann pin at least 3 mm thick is inserted. The pin overlies the intertrochanteric line; its direction deviates from the axis of the femoral shaft by 130° and penetrates the femoral head at its border.

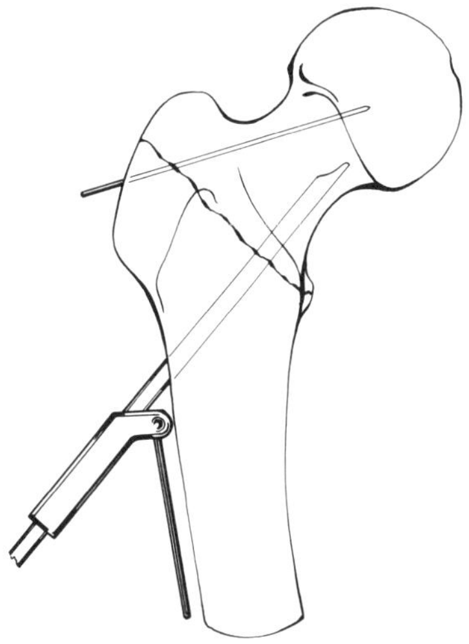

2

This pin is of the greatest importance for it indicates the correct direction, principally in the *frontal plane* as well.

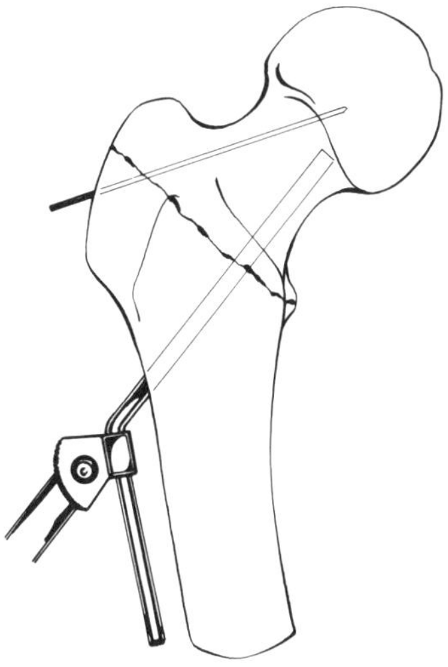

3

Before this stage is reached, the pin must be seated in the head firmly enough to indicate the direction unchangingly.

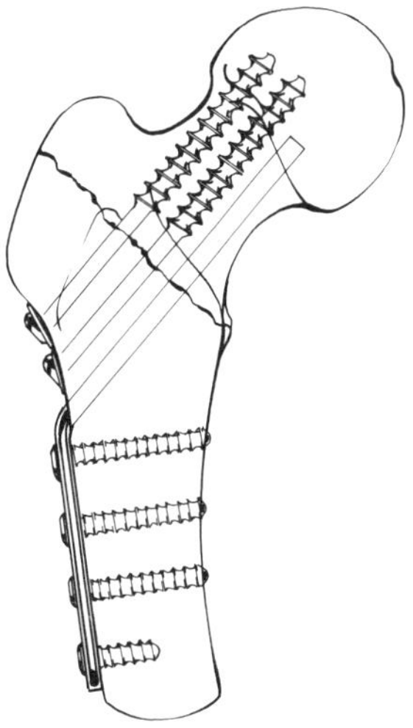

4

One or two cranial screws provide fixation and produce interfragmental compression.

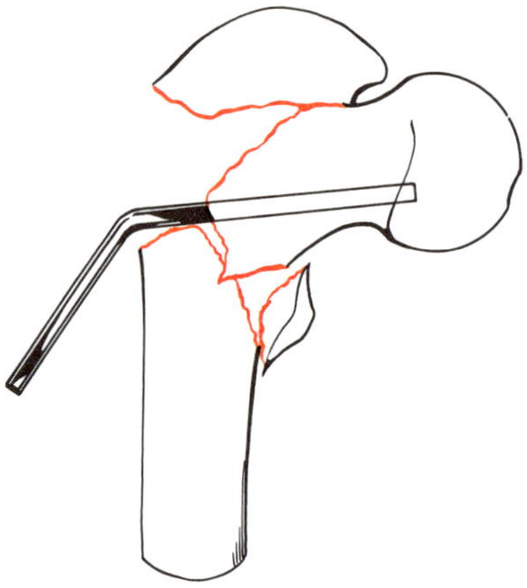

5
For multifragment or comminuted fractures, reduction with use of a plate is often advisable.

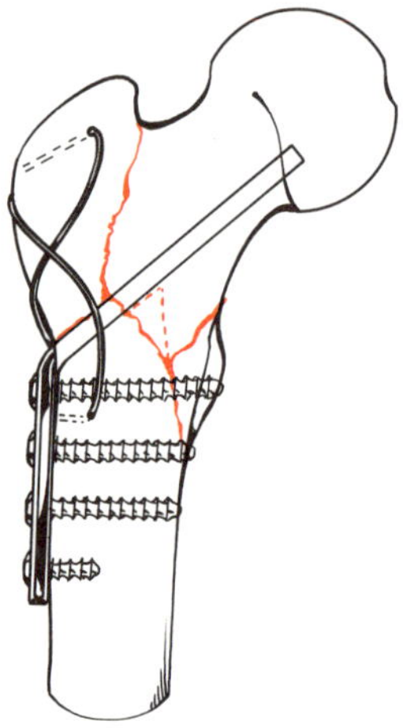

6
The trochanteric fragment is fastened by wiring.

Positioning See p. 207.

Approach See pp. 144 f. and 161 f.

Tactics

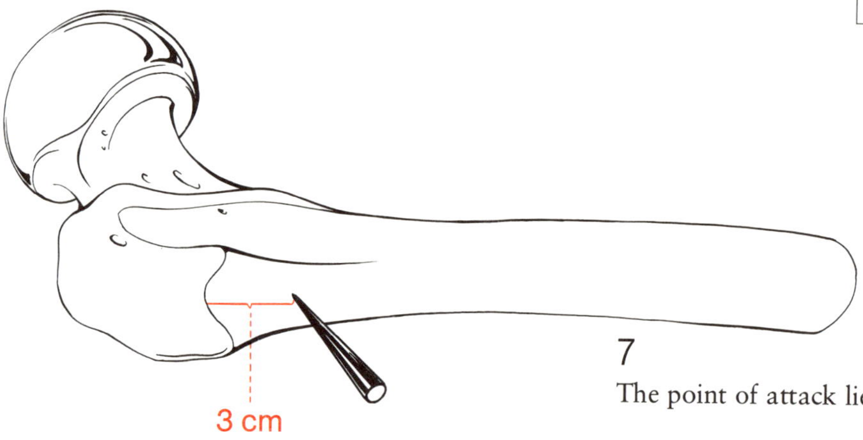

7
The point of attack lies 3 cm below the innominate tubercle.

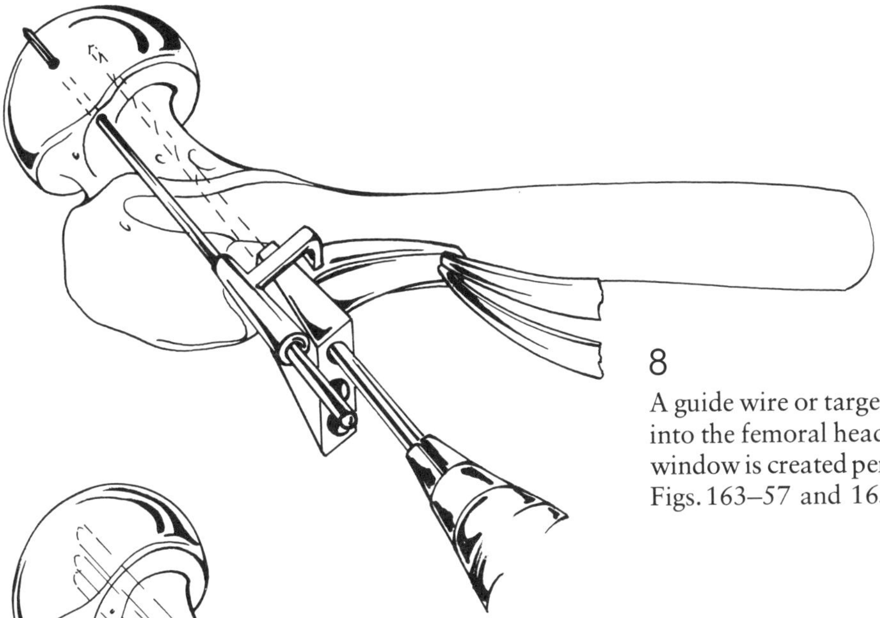

8

A guide wire or target wire is inserted along the femoral neck into the femoral head. Drill jig 130°, drill 4.5 mm. A cortical window is created perpendicular to the axis of the shaft (Note Figs. 163–57 and 163–58).

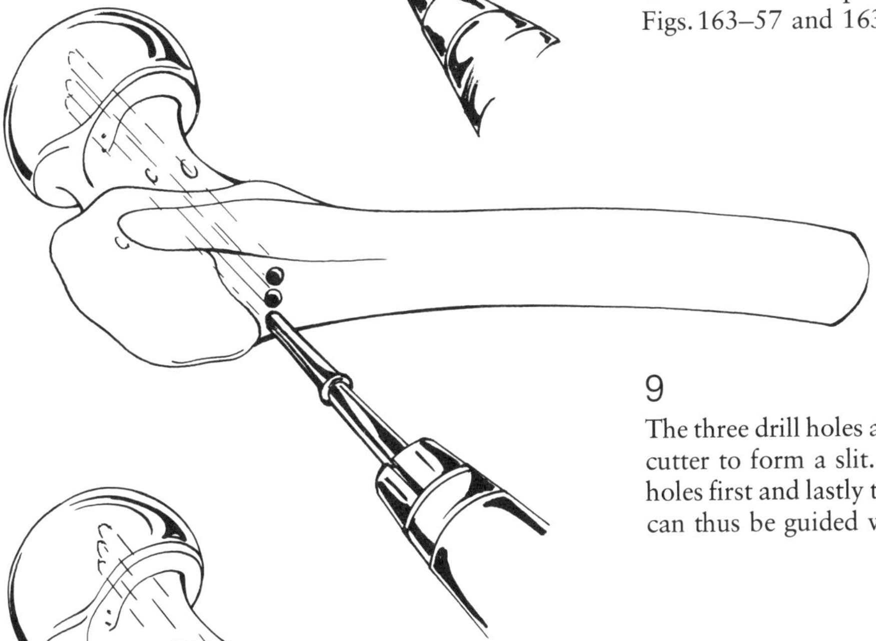

9

The three drill holes are widened and connected by the shank cutter to form a slit. It is advisable to widen the two outer holes first and lastly the middle one, because the shank cutter can thus be guided with grater ease.

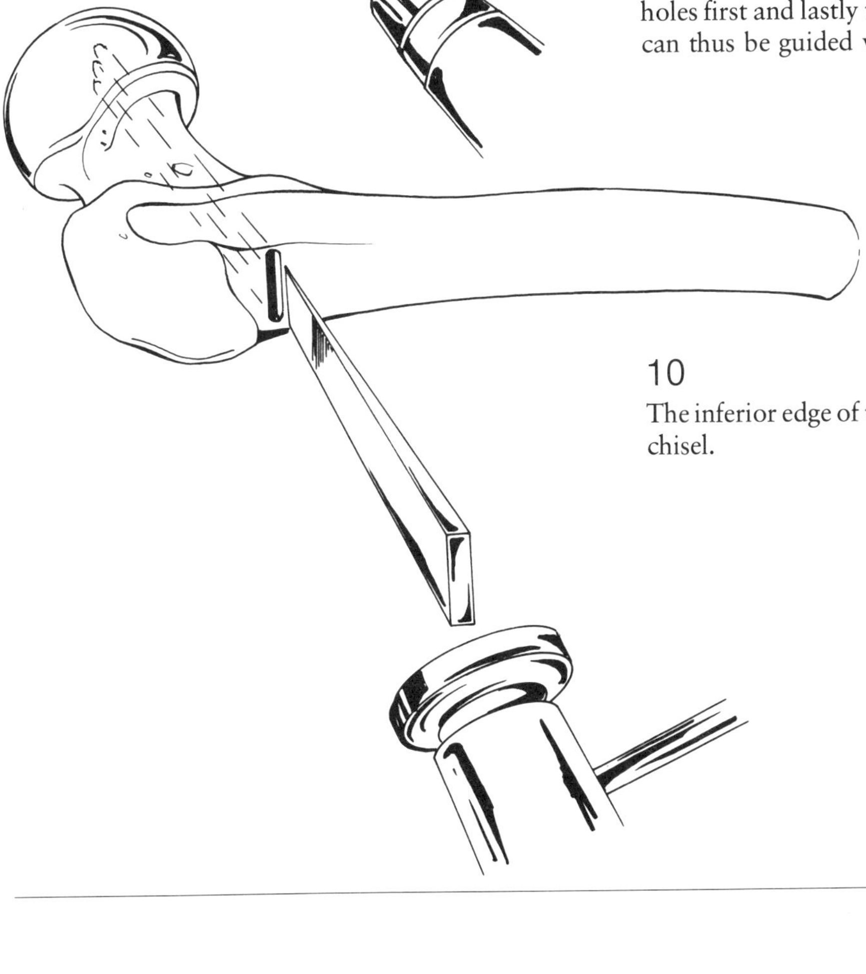

10

The inferior edge of the cortical window is rounded off with a chisel.

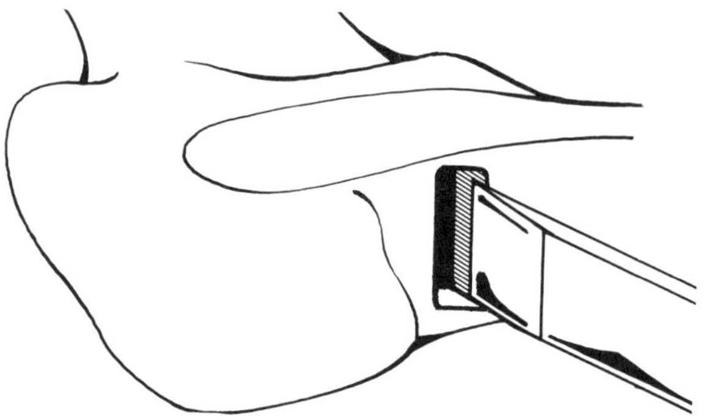

11

The slit must not be made too narrow since the blade needs room on all sides; otherwise it could easily cause the cortex to burst. This also facilitates the small corrections of direction nearly always necessary when knocking in the plate inserter.

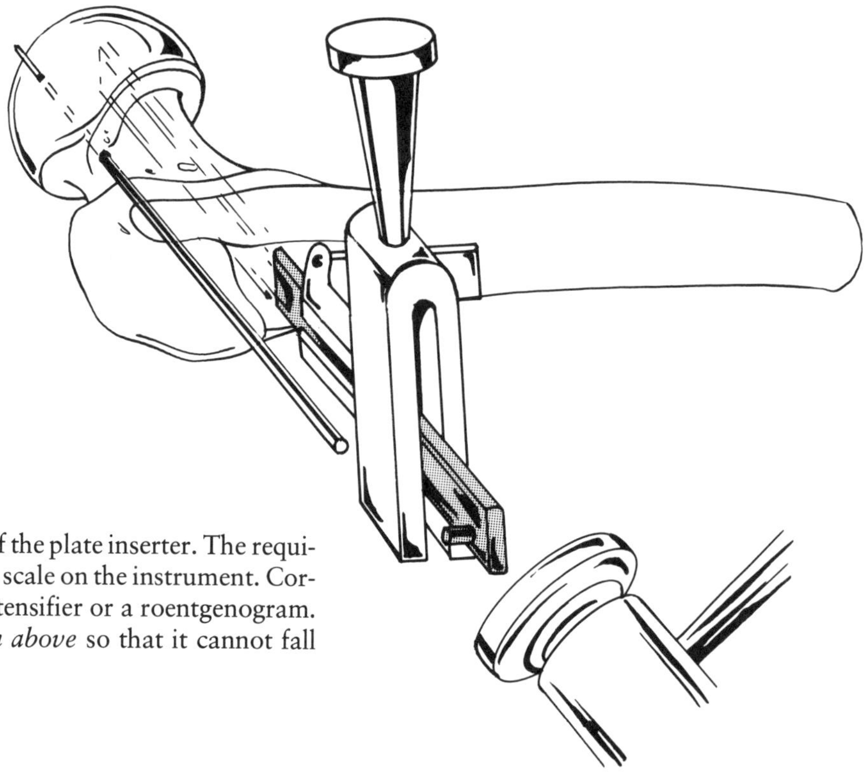

12

Preparing the seat of the blade with use of the plate inserter. The required length of the blade can be read on the scale on the instrument. Correct position is checked via the image intensifier or a roentgenogram. The slit hammer should be put on *from above* so that it cannot fall down inadvertently.

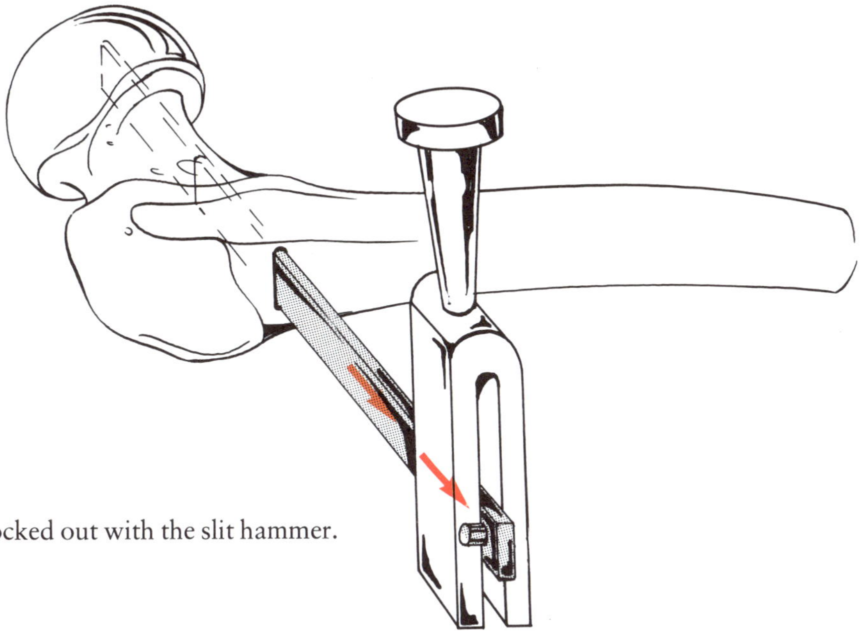

13

The plate inserter is knocked out with the slit hammer.

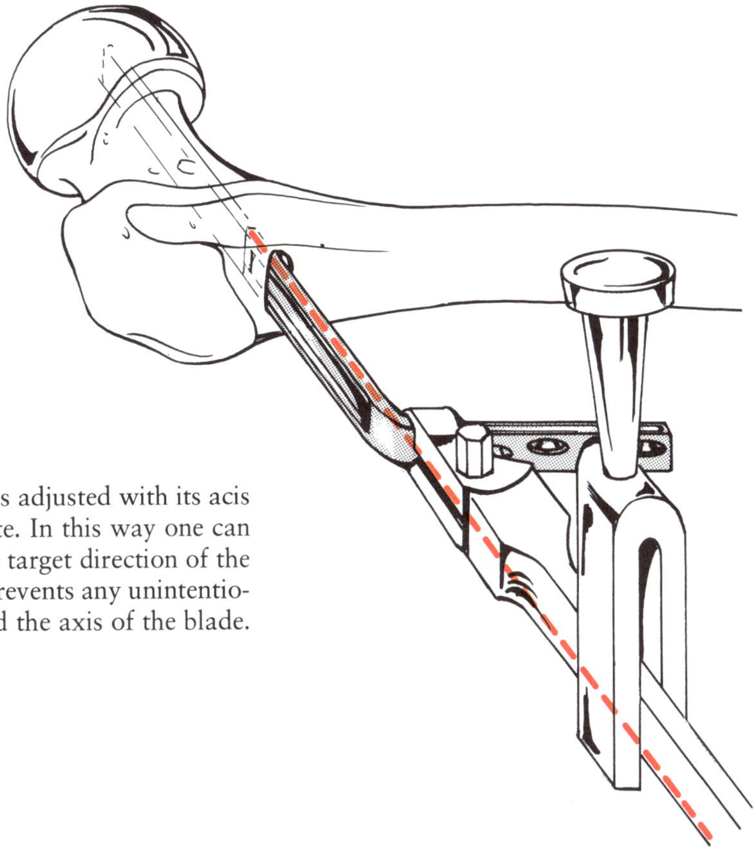

14

For angular plates the inserter is adjusted with its acis parallel to the blade of the plate. In this way one can always obtain a fair idea of the target direction of the blade. Use of the slit hammer prevents any unintentional rotation of the plate around the axis of the blade.

Condylar plate

Anatomy See p. 141.

Types of injuries See p. 150f.

Indication See p. 167 and p. 168.

Principle First see p. 153, Figs. 19–21.

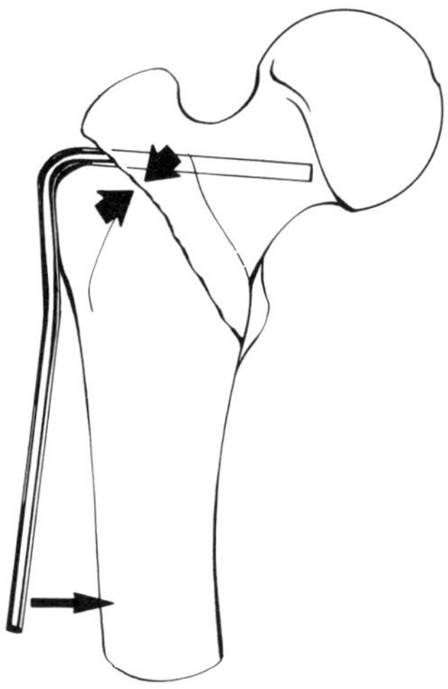

1
In using a condylar plate, a slightly craniocaudal course of the blade creates better conditions for impaction and development of compression in the fractured area.

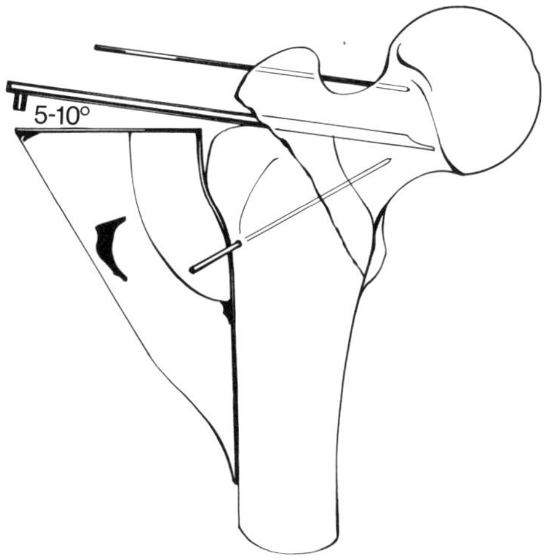

2
Therefore, the plate inserter is knocked in at an angle of 5 to 10 degrees from the cranial.

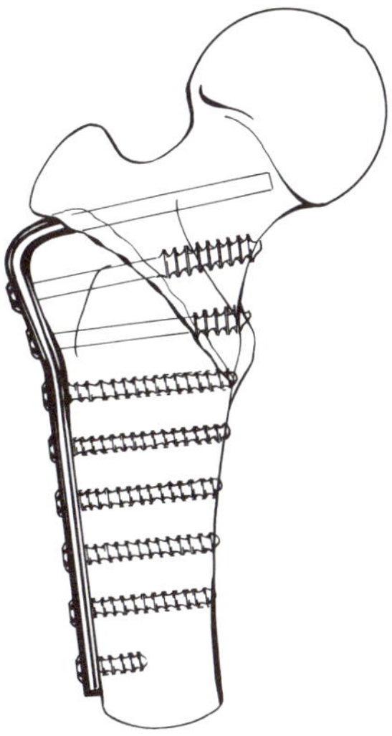

3
The two cancellous screws – or cortical traction screws – then cause the compression in the fracture cleft to be evenly distributed; nevertheless, the plate should be tightened distalward.

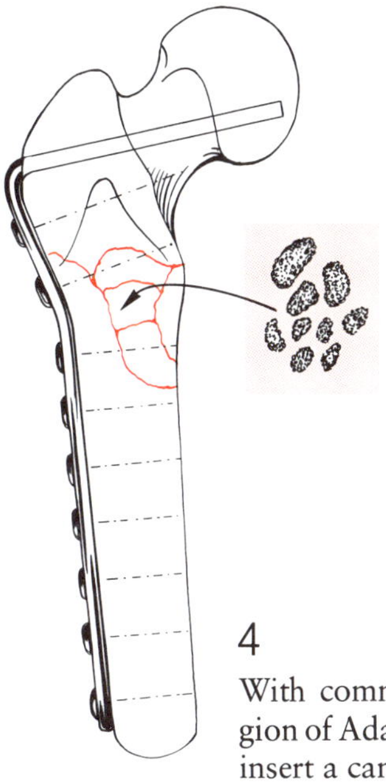

4
With comminuted fractures in the region of Adam's arc it is indispensable to insert a cancellous graft – in fresh fractures, e.g., from the bone bank.

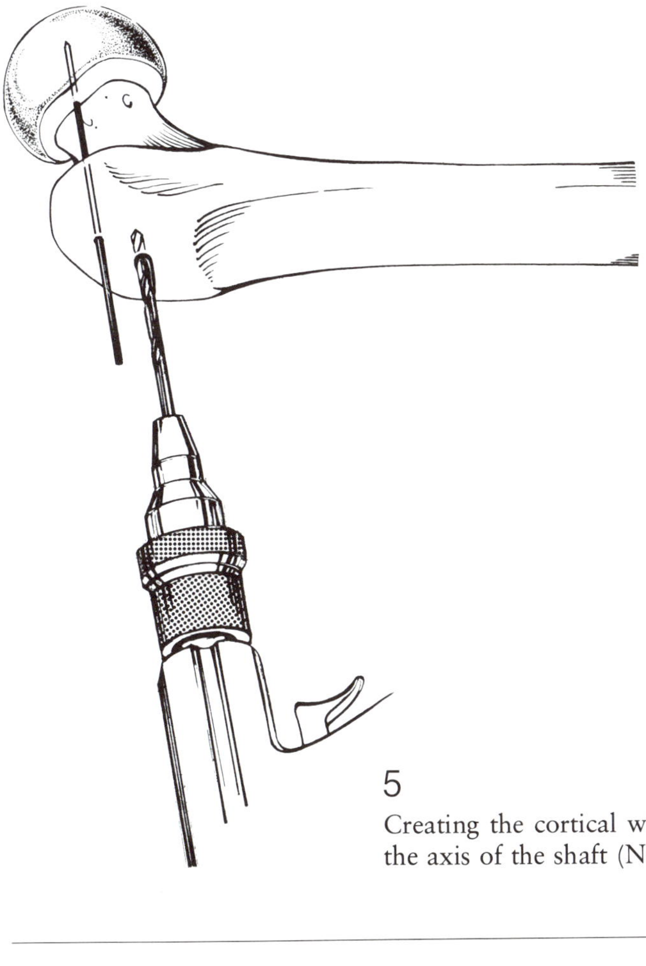

5
Creating the cortical window perpendicular to the axis of the shaft (Note p.163, Fig. 57f.).

Tactics

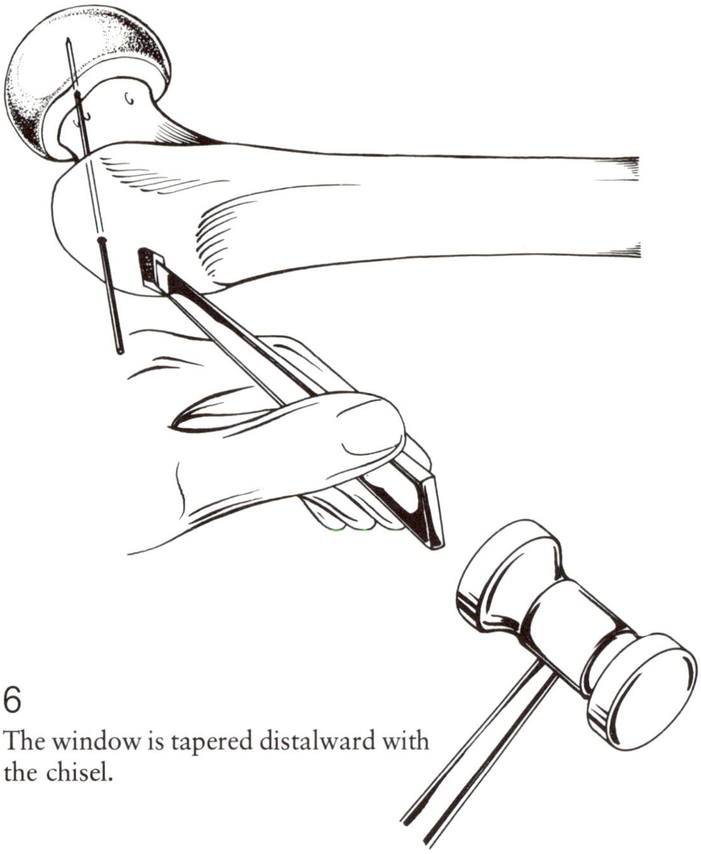

6
The window is tapered distalward with the chisel.

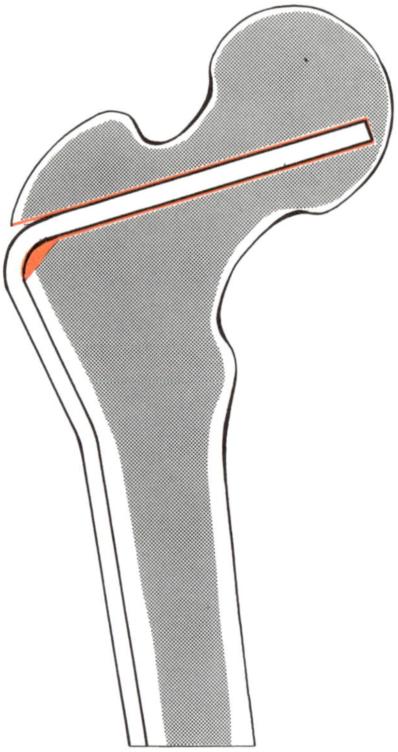

7
Tapering the inferior edge of the cortical window makes it possible to knock the plate insufficiently deeply and avoids having the angle of the plate burst the cortex open.

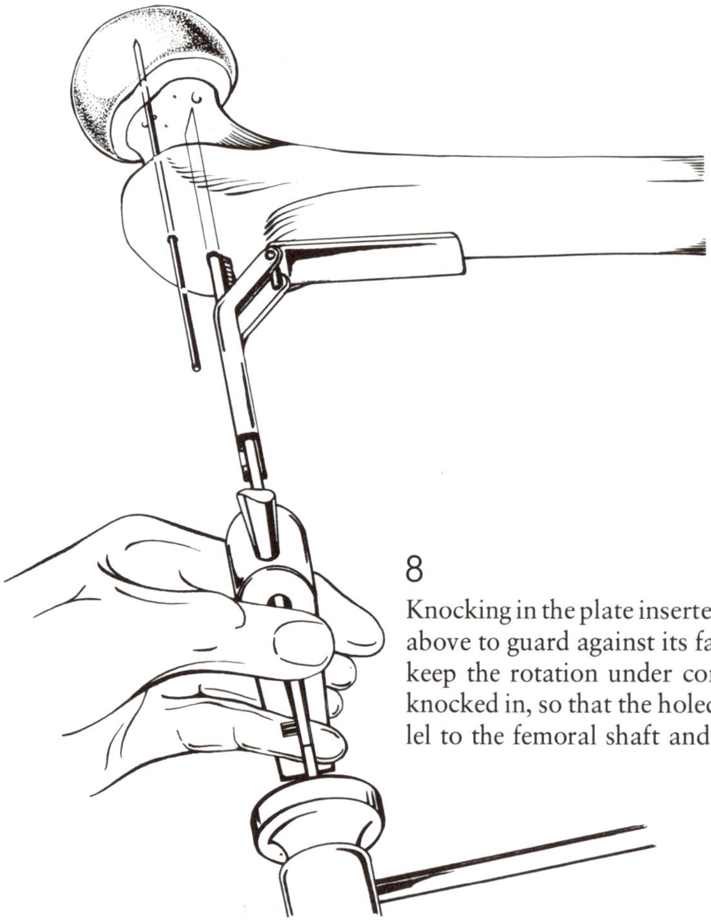

8
Knocking in the plate inserter. The slit hammer is put on from above to guard against its falling down inadvertently and to keep the rotation under control while the inserter is being knocked in, so that the holed part of the plate remains parallel to the femoral shaft and does not deviate backward.

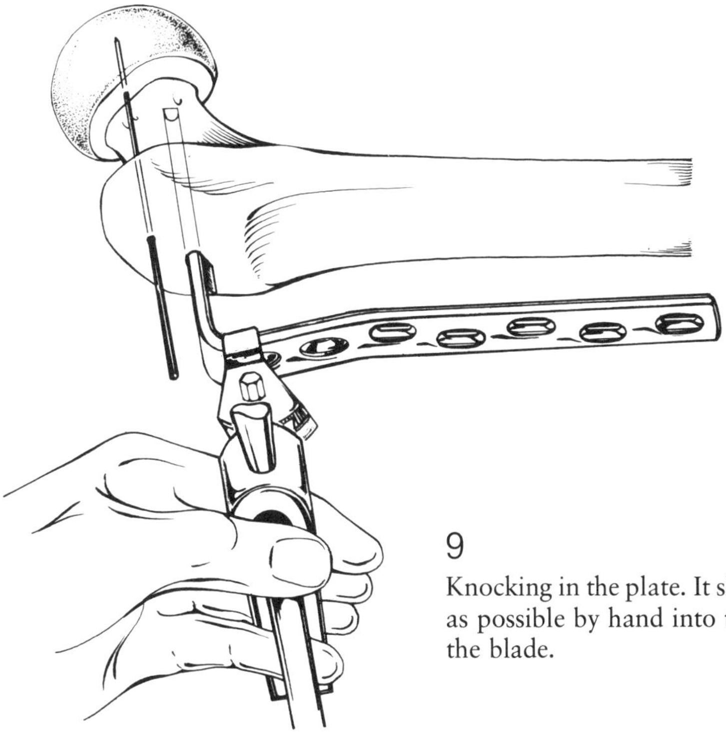

9

Knocking in the plate. It should be pushed as far as possible by hand into the canal prepared for the blade.

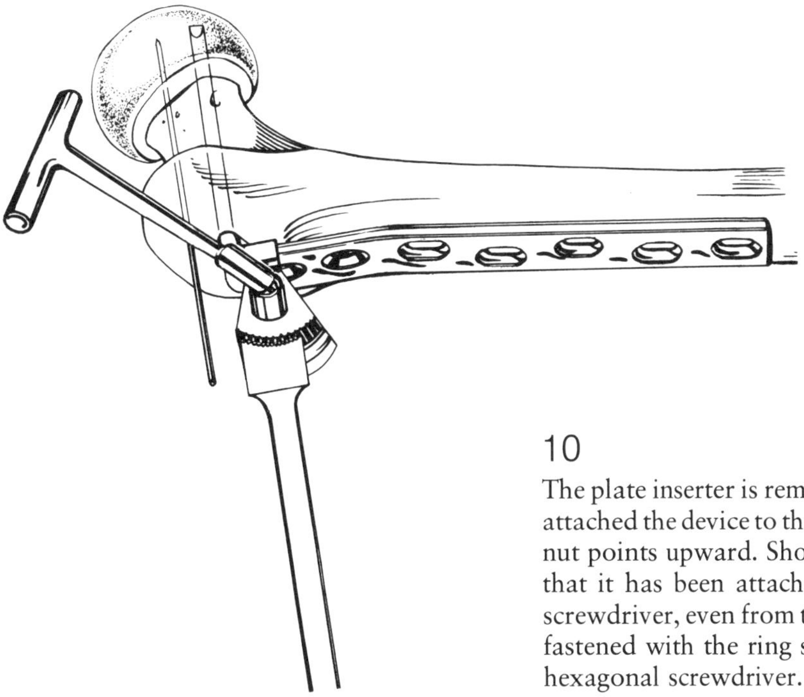

10

The plate inserter is removed. One should see that the assistant has attached the device to the plate in such a way that the corresponding nut points upward. Should one note only on removing the device that it has been attached incorrectly, it can be detached with a screwdriver, even from the wrong side. The inserter must always be fastened with the ring spanner, never with a cardan wrench or a hexagonal screwdriver.

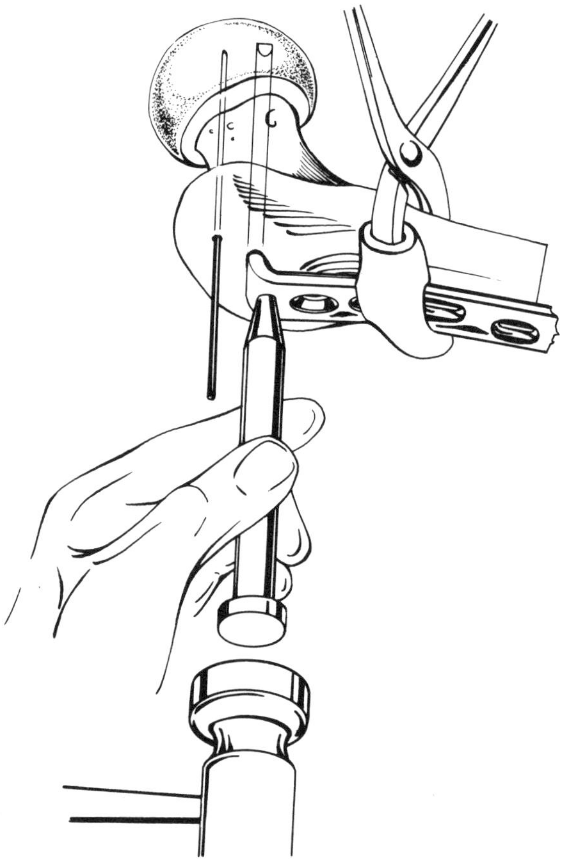

11

Knocking in is completed with a special impactor.

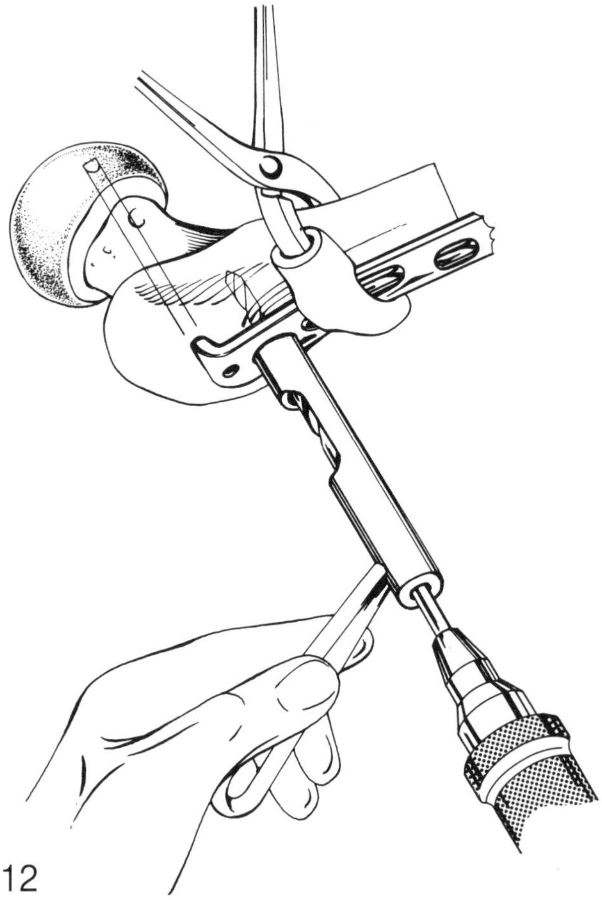

12

The screws are attached to the proximal fragment so that, on tightening the plate, the blade is not pulled from its bed.

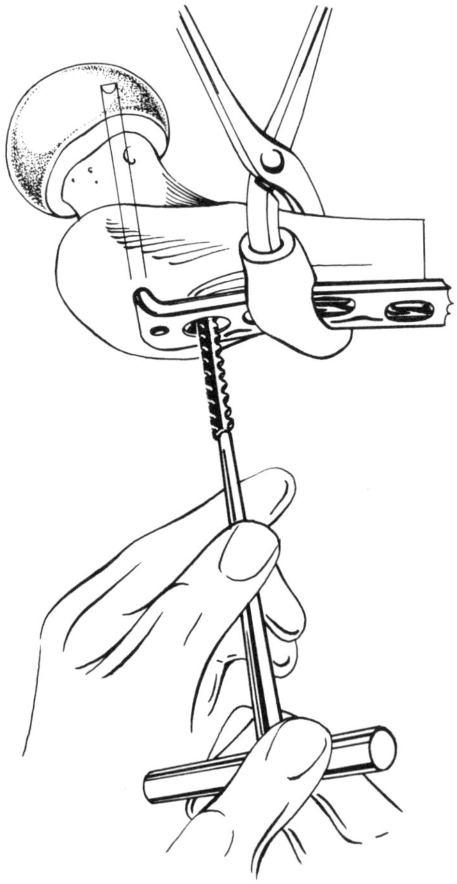

13

Cancellous screws fit into the screw holes near the blade; they may be useful in the presence of a thin cortex. However, in the proximal fragment, one should always try to anchor at least one cortical screw in the cortex of Adam's arc.

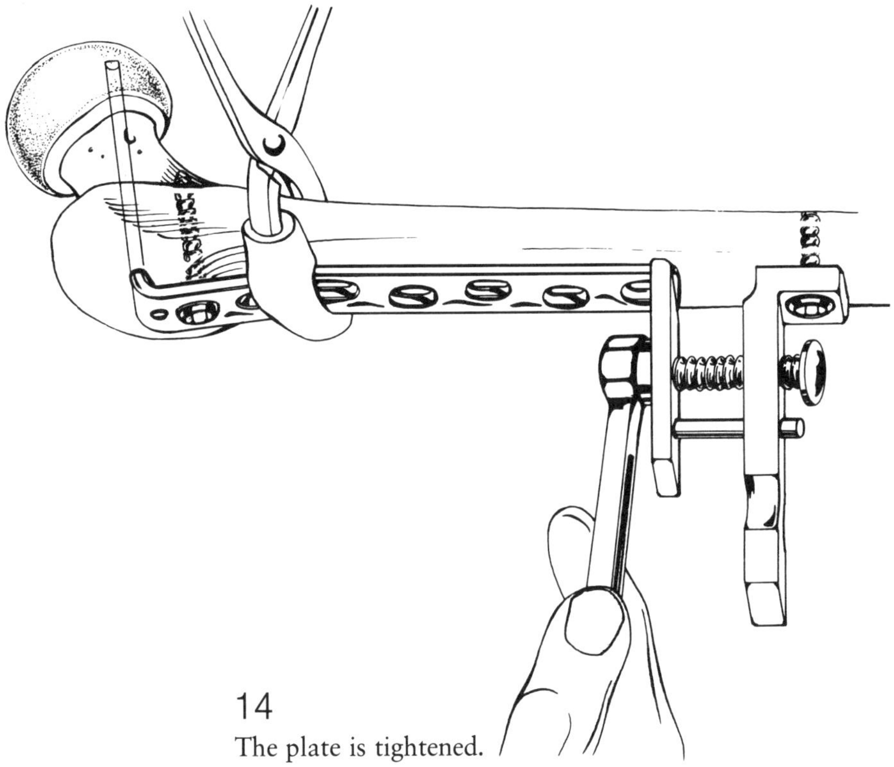

14
The plate is tightened.

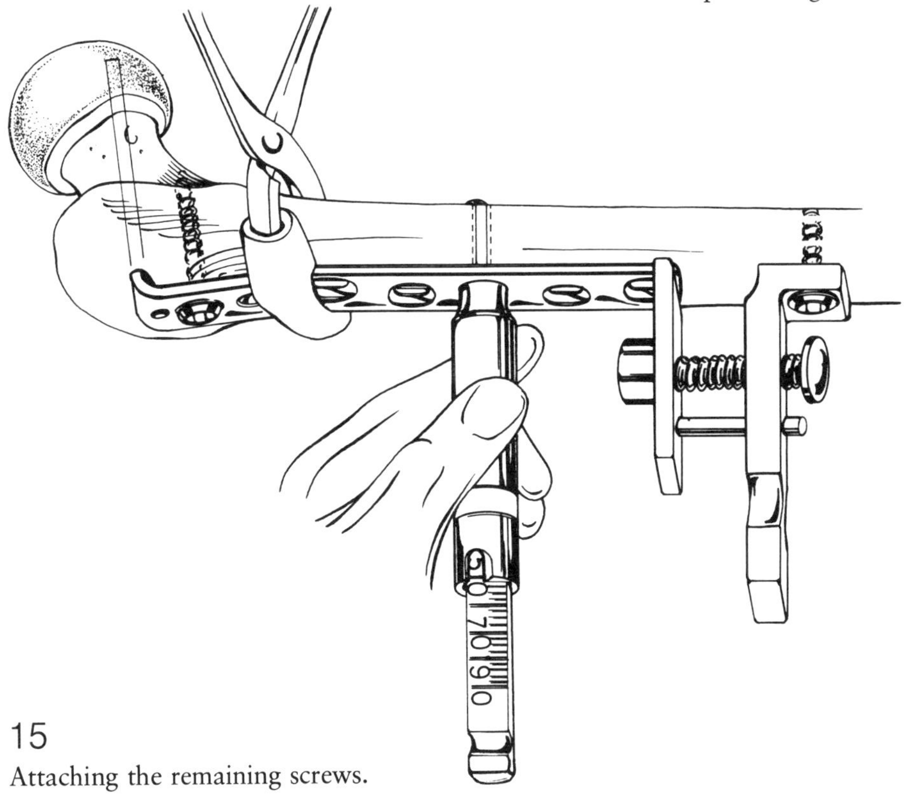

15
Attaching the remaining screws.

Aftertreatment See p. 9f.

Femur – middle part

Indication

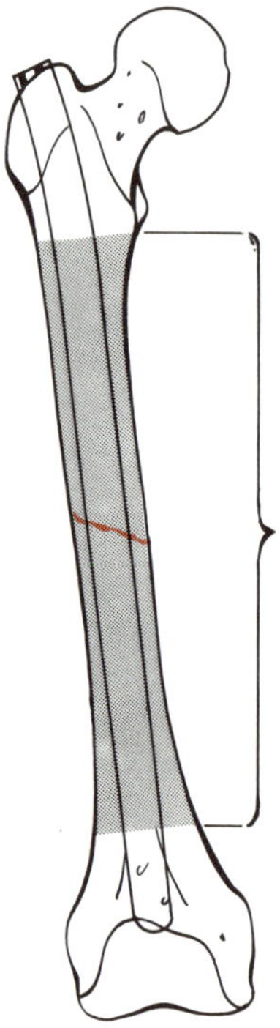

1

Simple fracture of the shaft: intramedullary nailing through the middle three-fifths of the length of the femur.

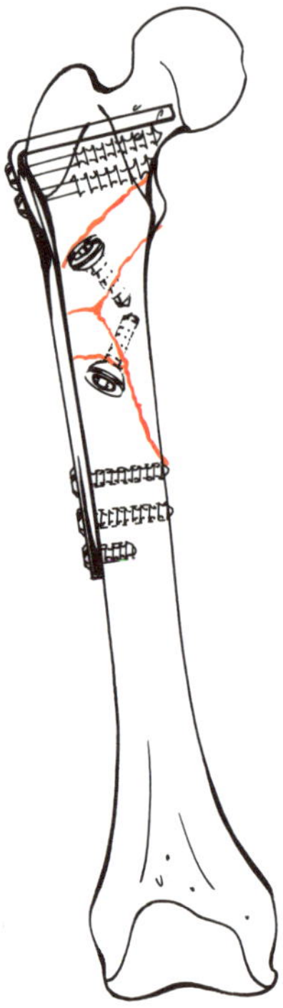

2

Fractures with multiple breaks and comminuted fractures: condylar plate.

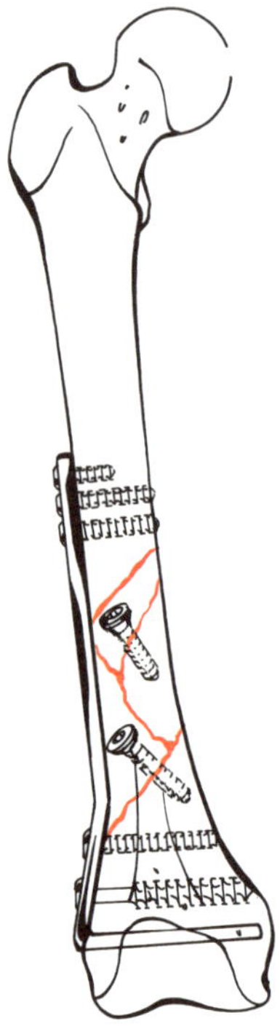

3

Fractures with multiple breaks and comminuted fractures: condylar plate.

Operative possibilities

Timing of the operation

As soon as satisfactory circulatory conditions have been definitely reestablished, i. e., generally after a few days. Until then, wire traction applied to the heel.

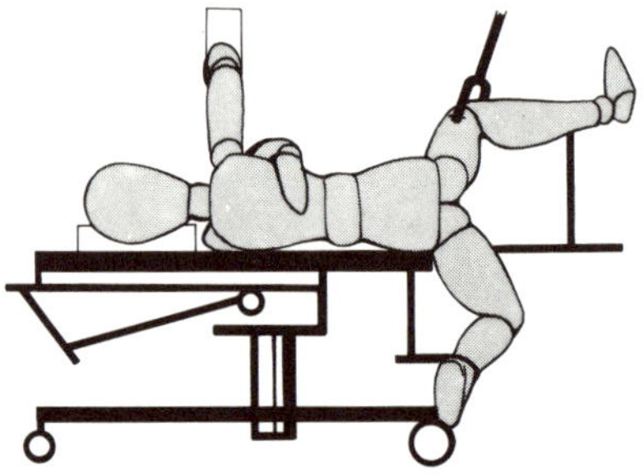

4

Closed nailing (traction table): see p. 193.

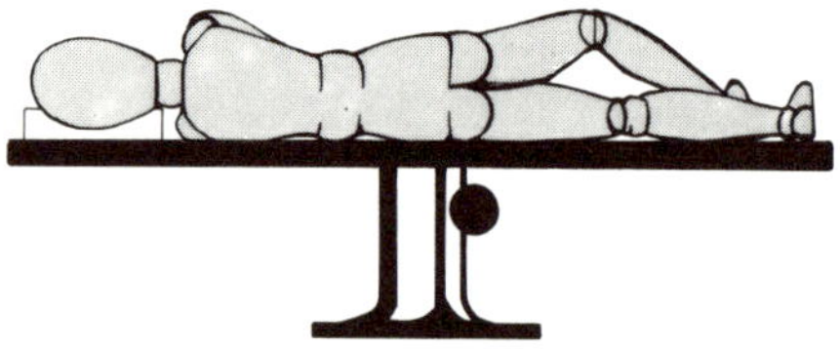

5

Open nailing (standard or traction table) when interposition of soft tissues or other obstacles to reduction exist.

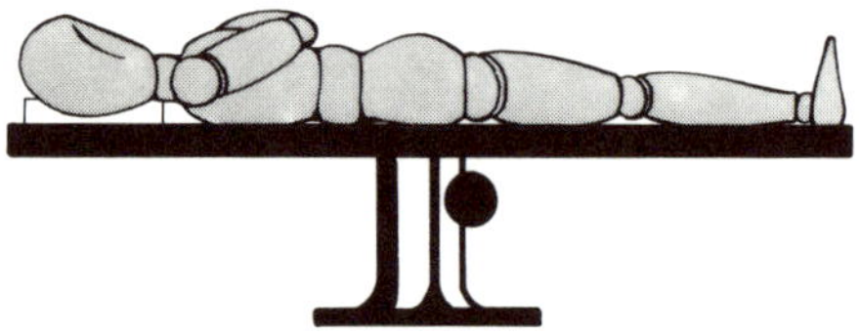

6

Condylar plate (standard table, supine position).

Nail

Positioning

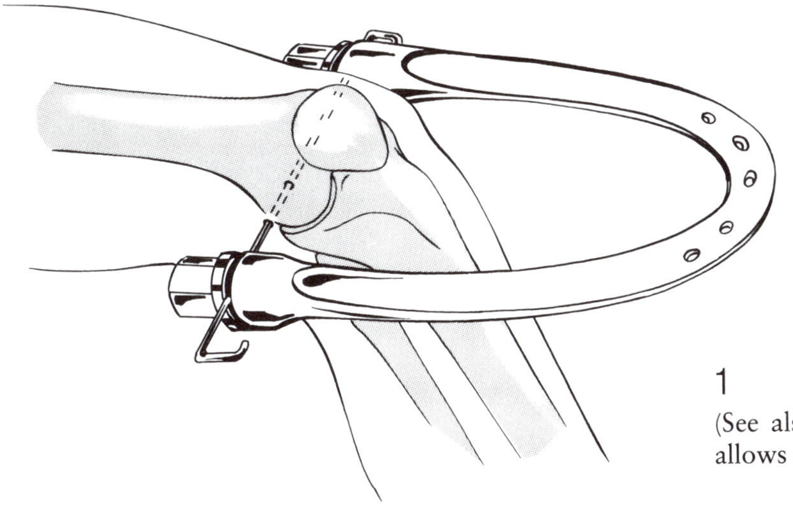

1

(See also Fig. 225–3.) Application of traction which allows control of the distal fragment.

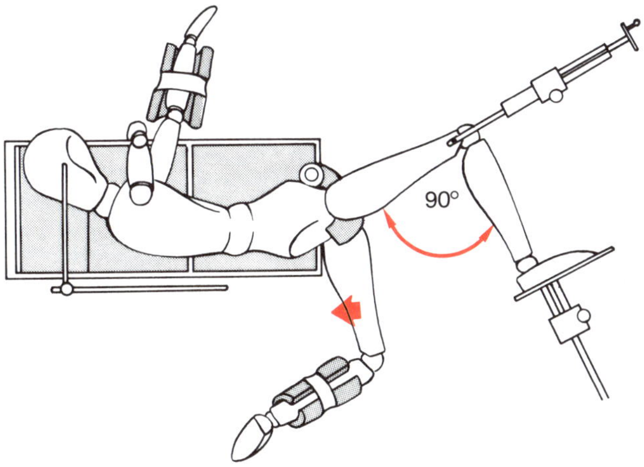

2

In placing the patient, unhindered positioning of the image intensifier requires

a) traction along the longitudinal axis of the femur,
b) 90° flexion at the knee joint,
c) maximal abduction and extension at the hip joint of the sound side,

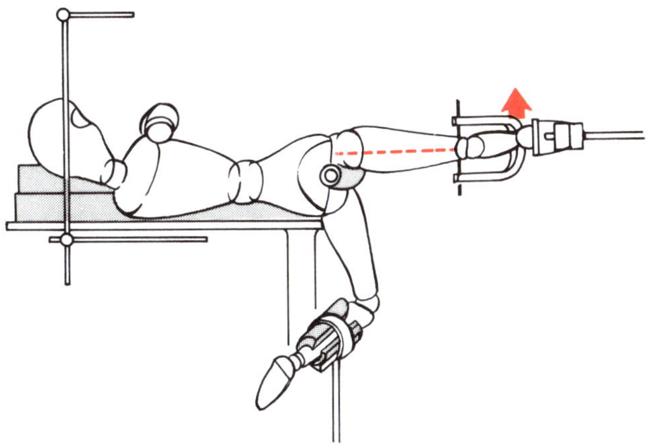

3

d) heel about 10 cm higher than the knee joint.

Sterile draping I

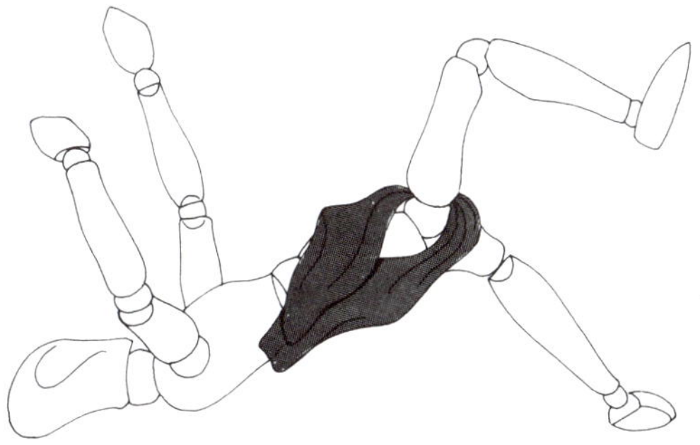

4

Here, sterile draping is simpler and less involved. Freedom of movement of the image intensifier is greater and sterility is less endangered than with use of a standard table. First drape: size 1.

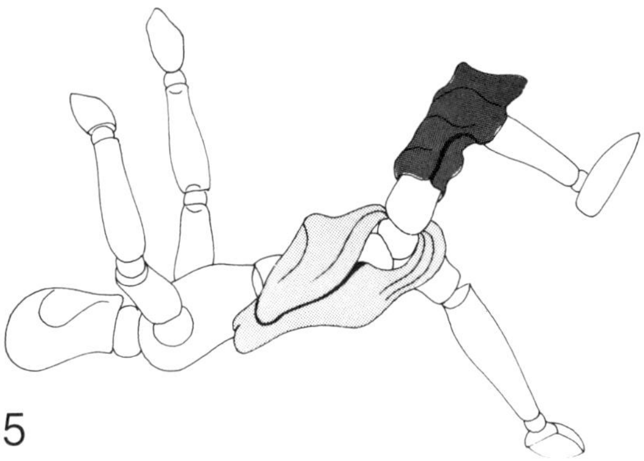

5
Drape size 4

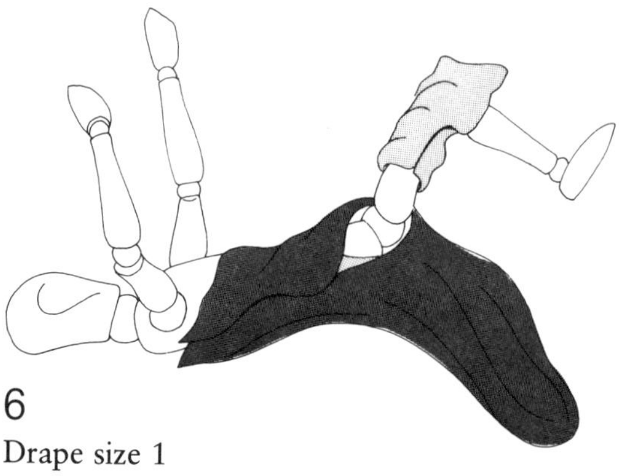

6
Drape size 1

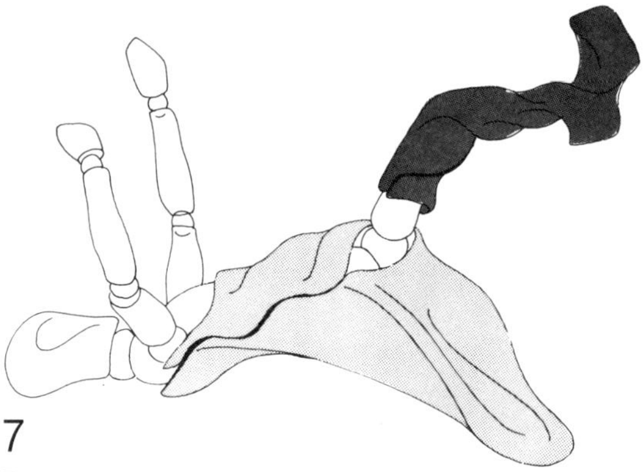

7
Drape size 1

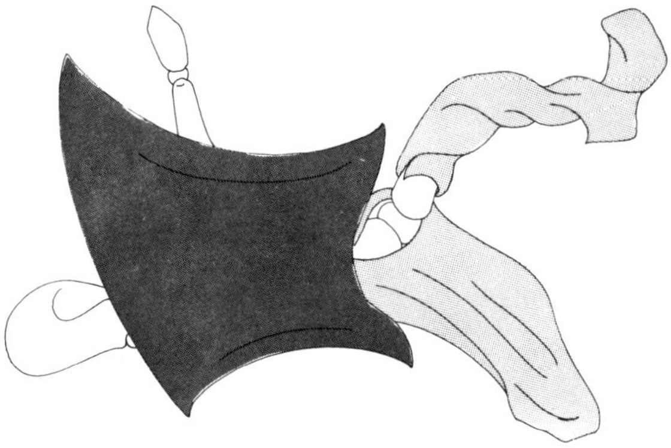

8
Drape size 1

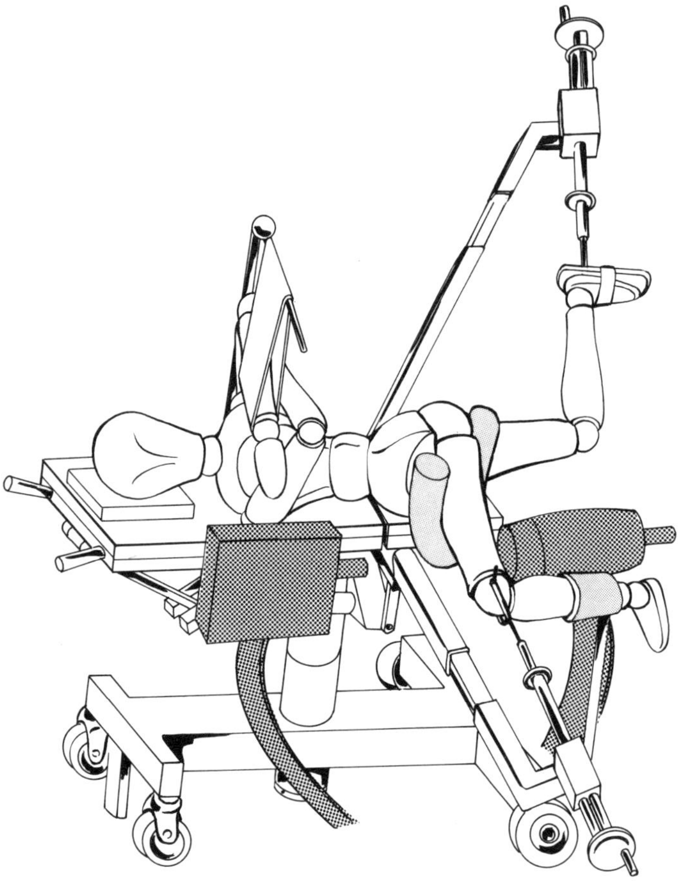

Positioning II

More involved than type I. Less freedom of movement of the image intensifier. Sterility more greatly endangered during draping as well as during the further course of the operation, owing to limited the freedom of movement of the image intensifier.

9
This mode of positioning is particularly unfavorable when the traction is mounted as depicted; access for the operator is greatly impeded. The following mode of positioning is to be preferred:

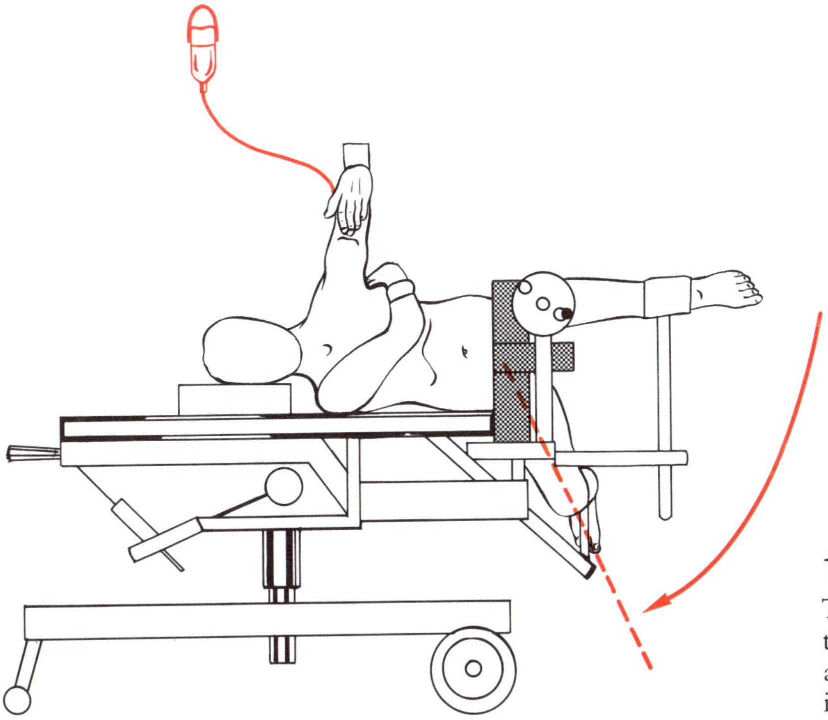

10

The sound leg is abducted as far as possible at the hip joint; the operator thereby gains better access to the area of operation. Infusion is instituted on the side that is to be nailed.

11

Axis of femur and traction must be in alignment. The arm on the sound side is pulled across the upper part of the body to the back of the patient with a loop.

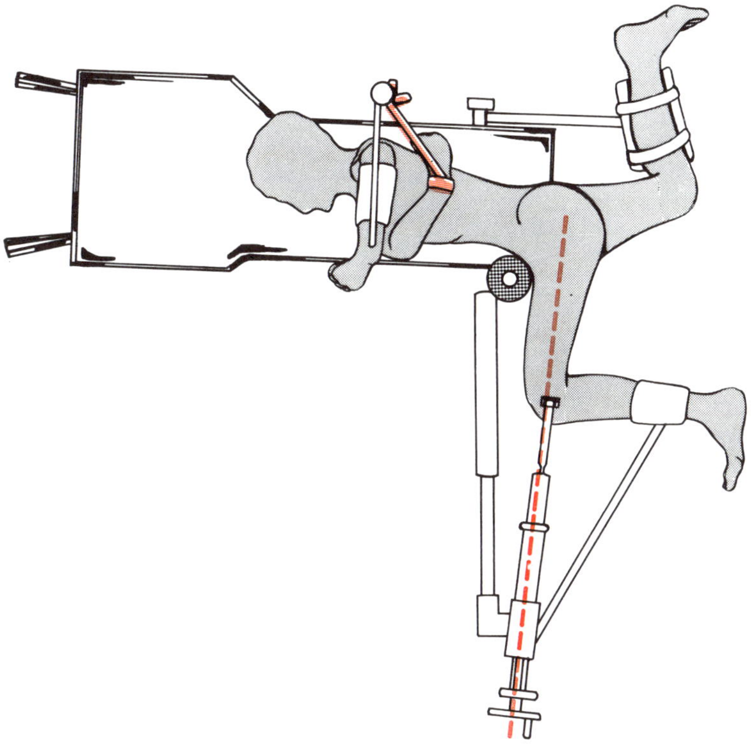

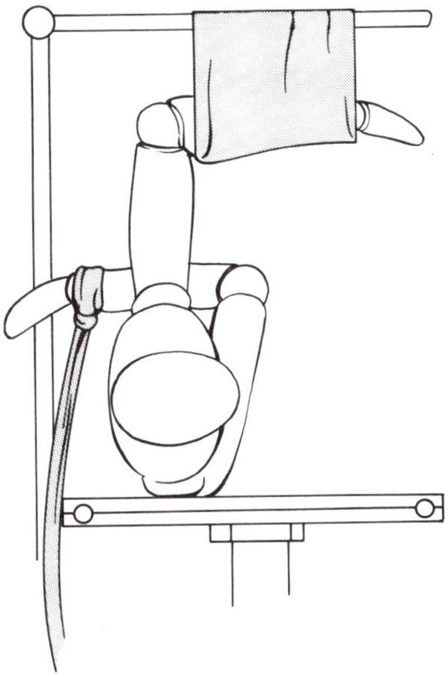

12

This kind of positioning and suspension provides sufficient room for the image intensifier.

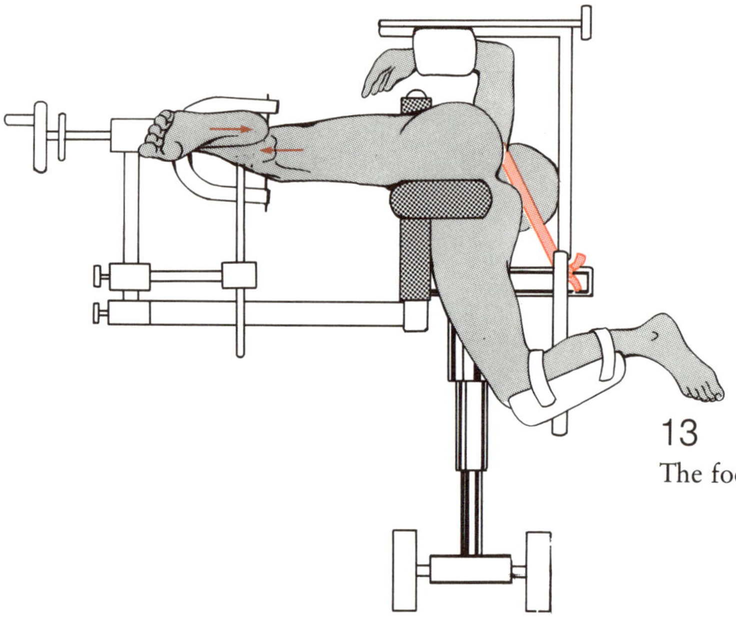

13
The foot is placed a little higher than the knee joint.

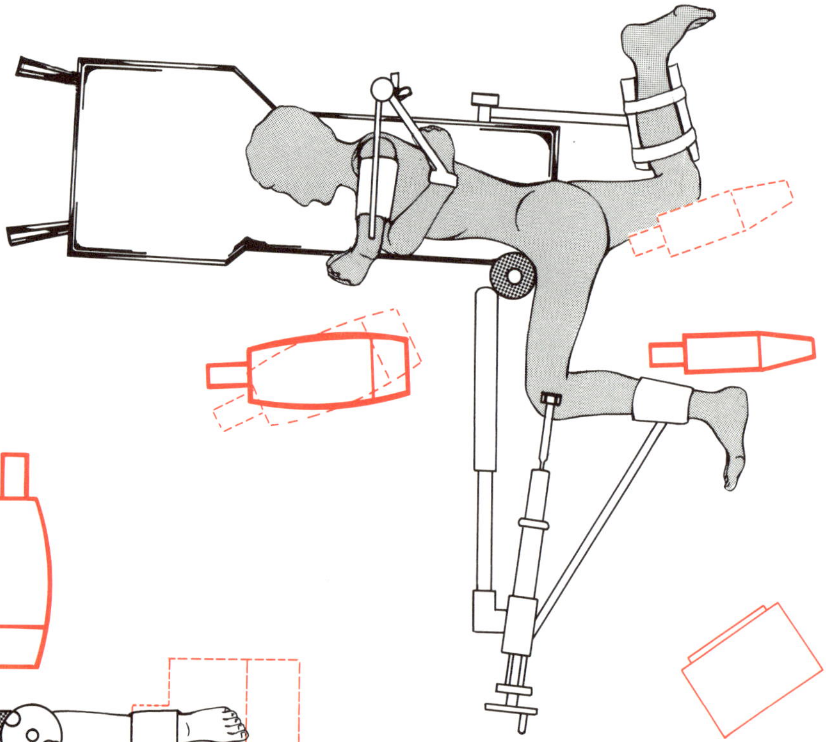

14
Test positioning of the image intensifier. It is expedient to mark the position of the wheels on the floor...

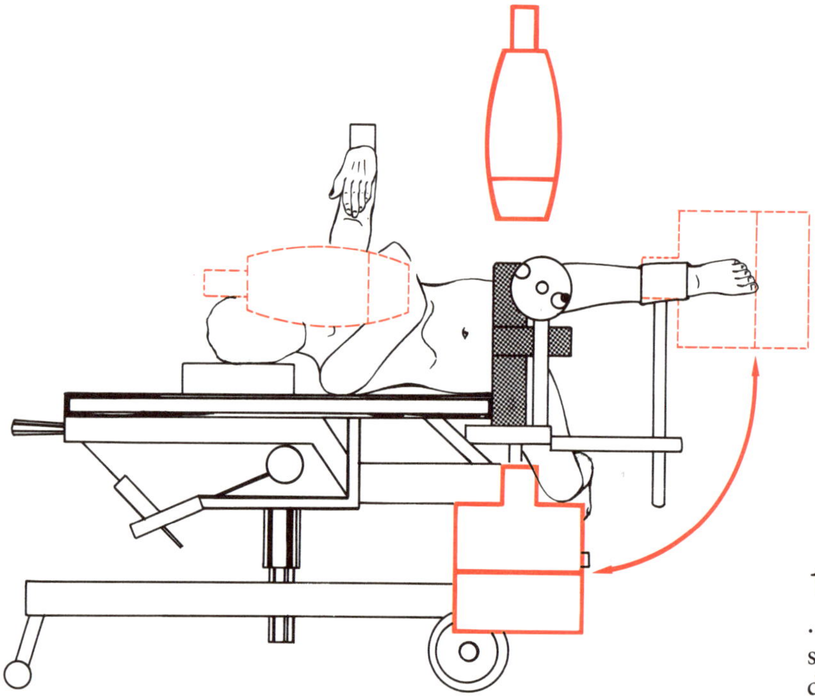

15
... by small strips of adhesive, and so to reposition the image intensifier easily after sterile draping.

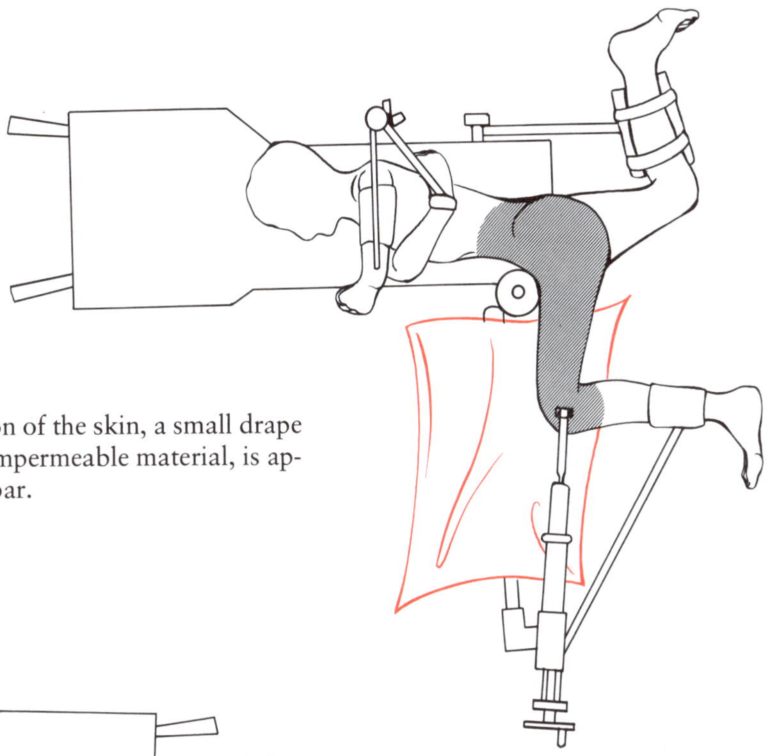

16

Following disinfection of the skin, a small drape (size 4), fitted with impermeable material, is applied over the crossbar.

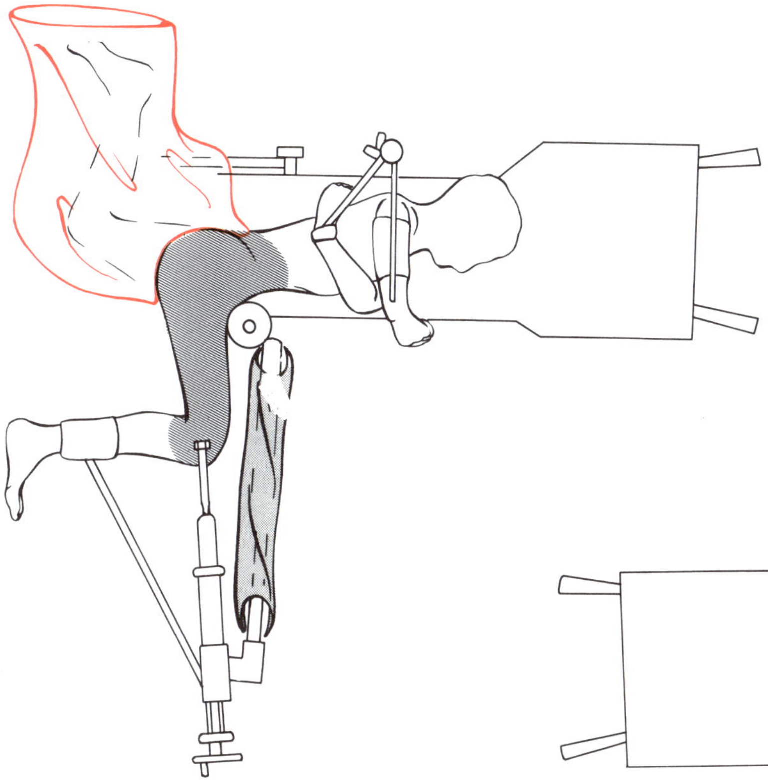

17

A bag (size 5) is placed over the sound leg. This bag is handed to the operator almost completely rolled up like a stocking, and then is unrolled over the leg and the frame.

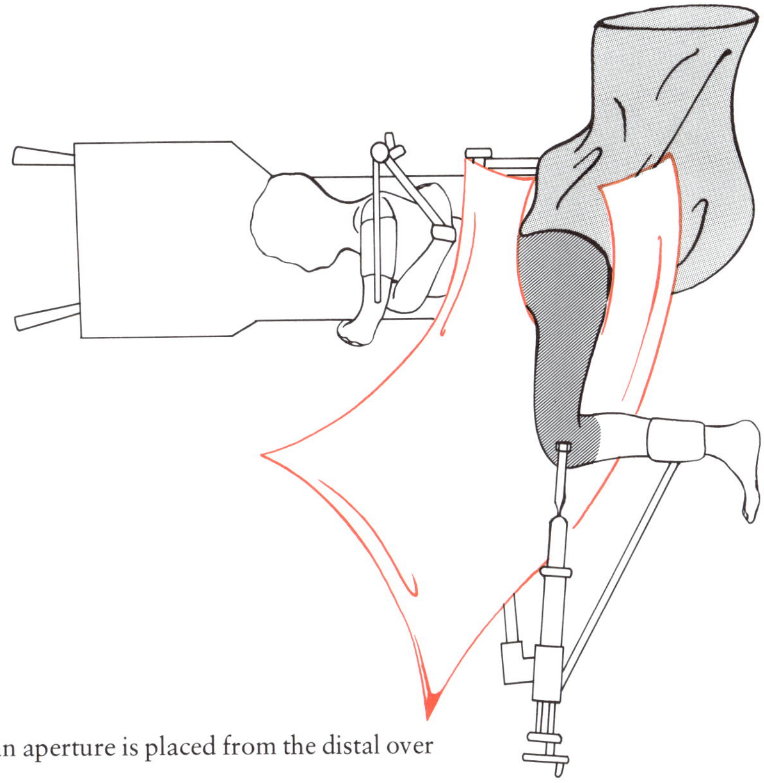

18

A size 2 drape with an aperture is placed from the distal over the crossbar.

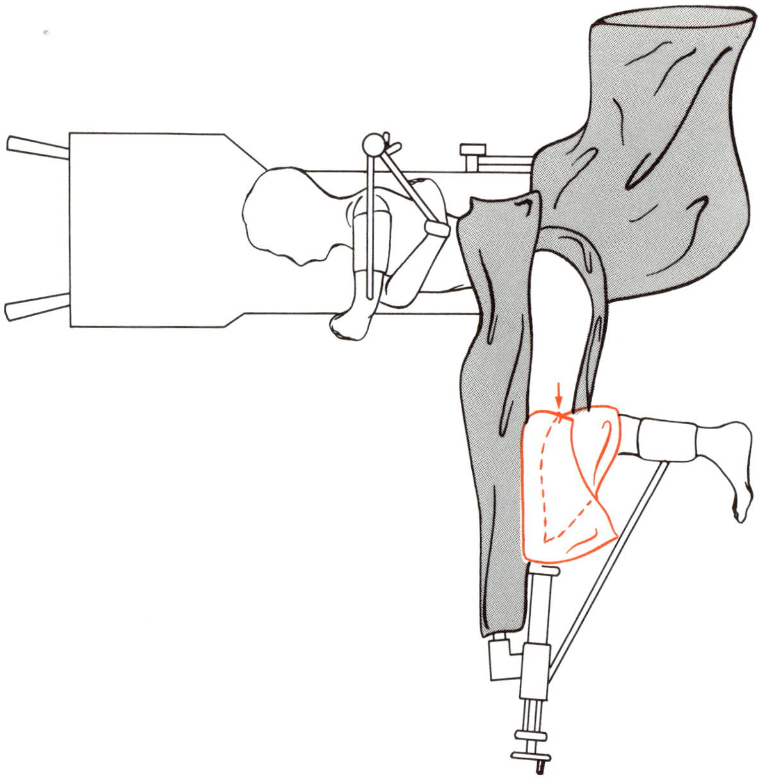

19

The traction frame and the knee are covered with a small drape (size 4). This drape is sewn on (arrow).

20

A size 1 drape is placed from underneath over the lower leg and the traction equipment.

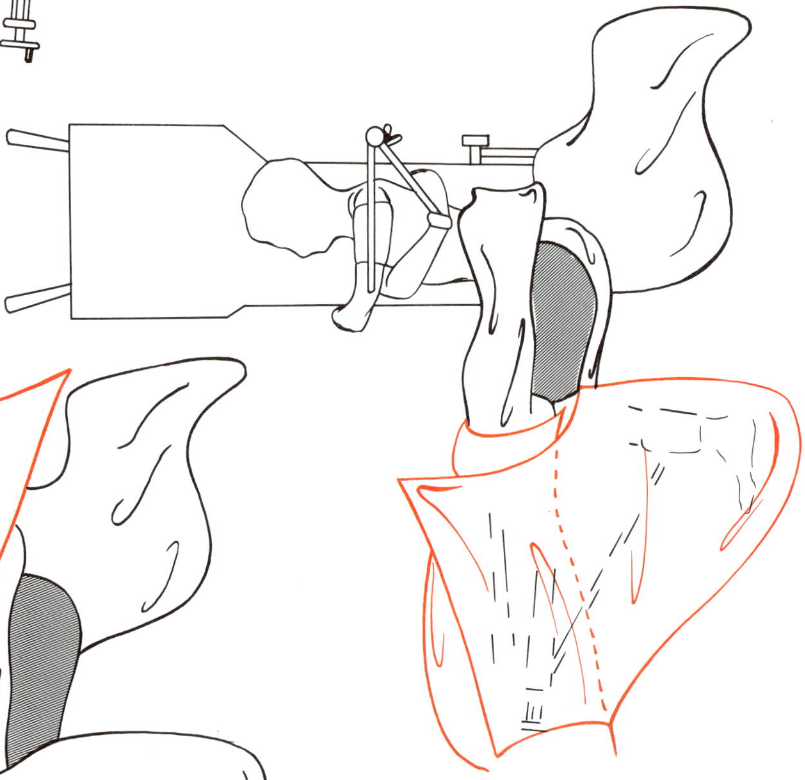

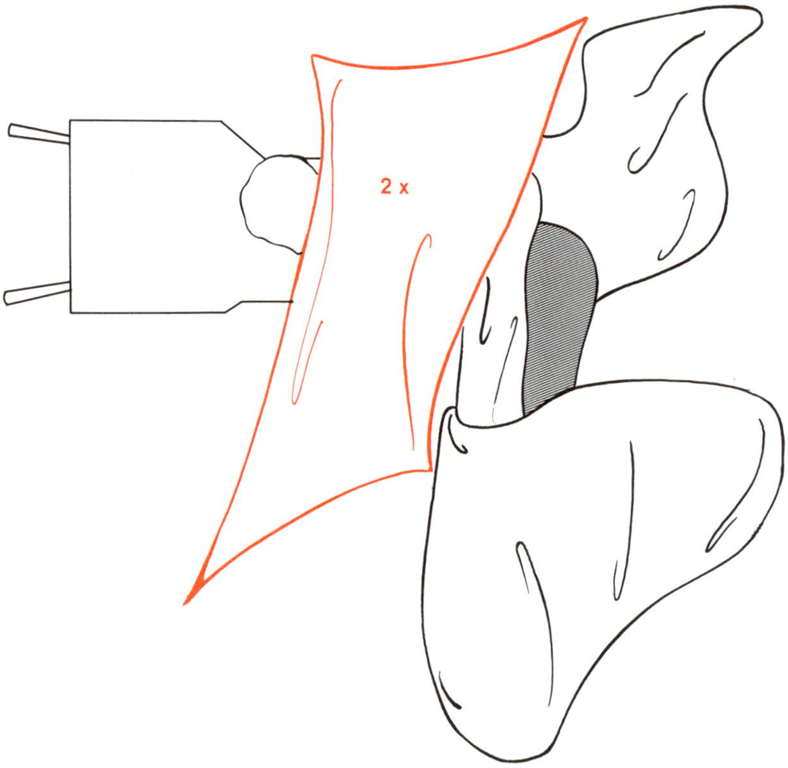

21

Two large drapes are placed cephalad transversely over the screen.

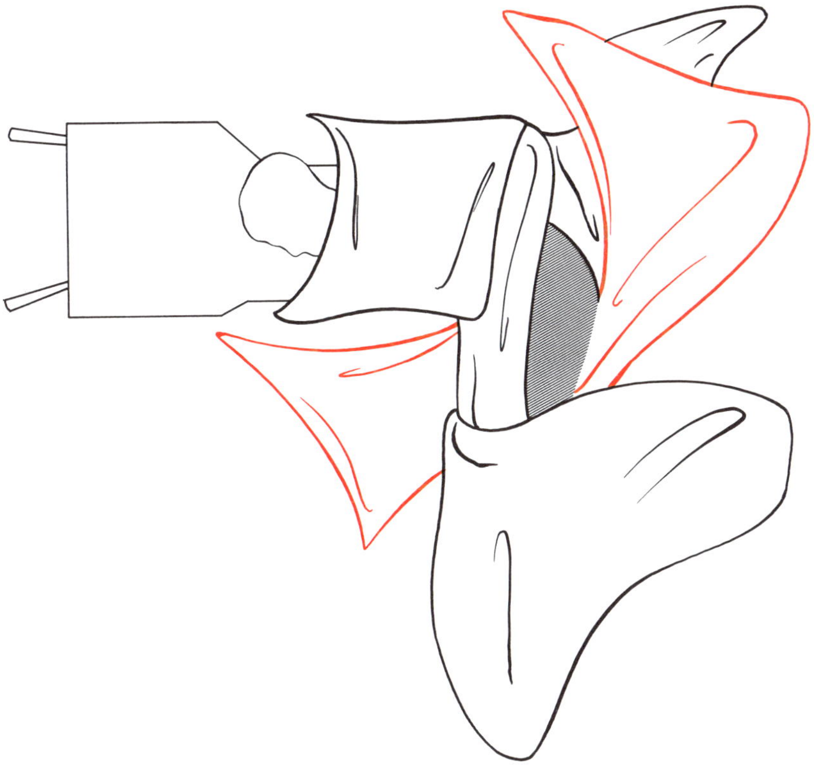

22

A size 1 drape is placed underneath the cross-bar. Adhesive foil.

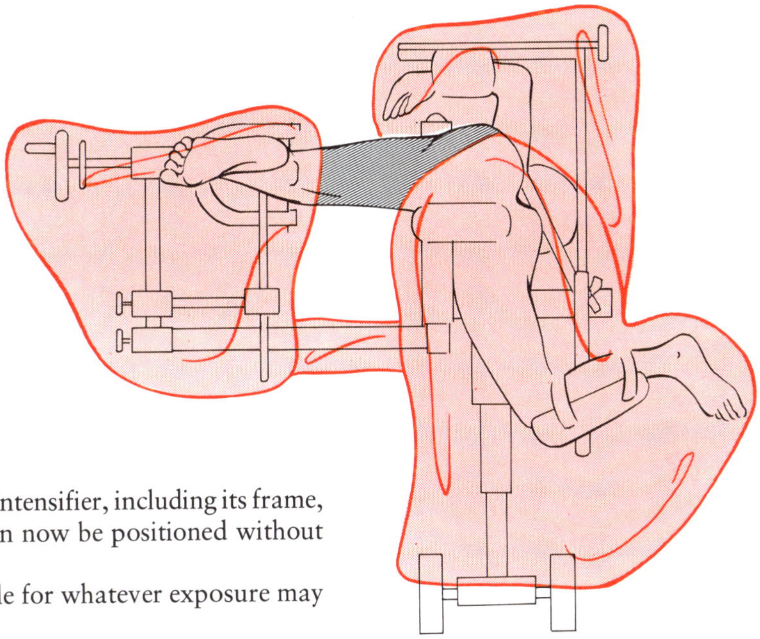

23

All the drapes are now snugly applied. The image intensifier, including its frame, has also been covered with sterile drapes and can now be positioned without touching the drapes (See also p. 8).
It is most important that the fracture be accessible for whatever exposure may become necessary during the operation.

Approach

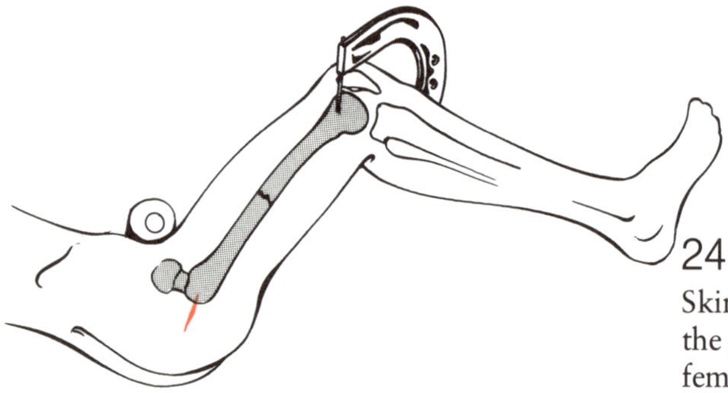

24

Skin incision 8 cm long, beginning at the level of the palpable tip of the greater trochanter and extended cranially in the direction of the femoral axis.

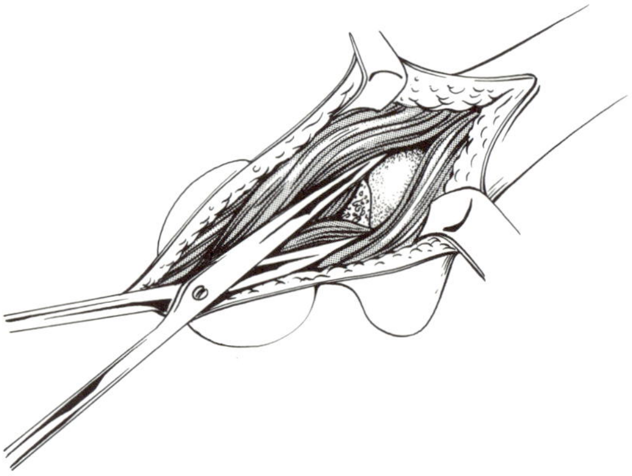

25

The fibers of the gluteus muscle are forced apart, transverse to their direction, by spreading the scissors until the outer aspect of the greater trochanter has been reached and Langenbeck retractors can be inserted.

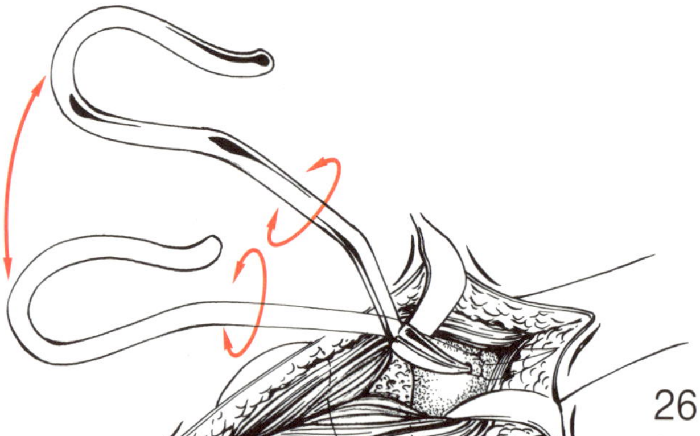

26

See also Fig. 56–6f. The marrow cavity is opened with the reamer. While the reamer is being turned, close watch must be kept on the axis of the femus so as not to perforate the bone laterally.

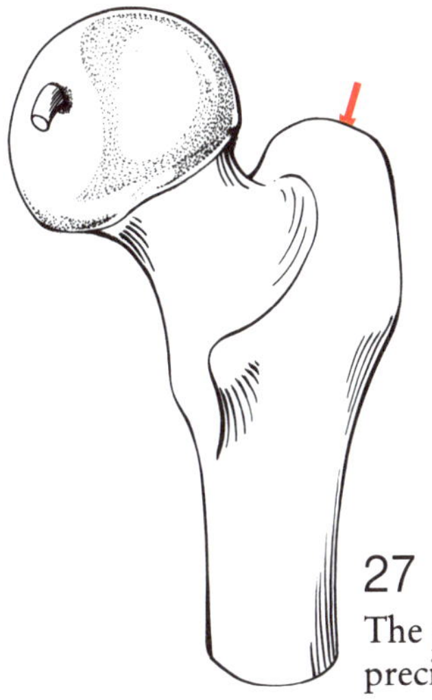

27
The point of entrance of the nail must not lie precisely over the tip of the trochanter, i.e....

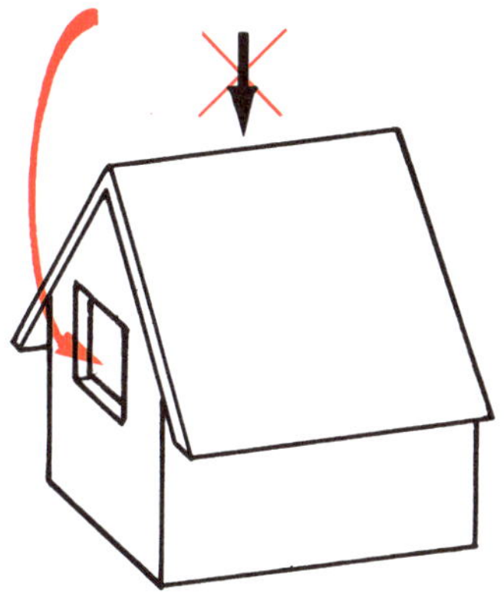

28
... the point of entrance should not lie on the "ridge" of the trochanter but in the region of the "gable window".

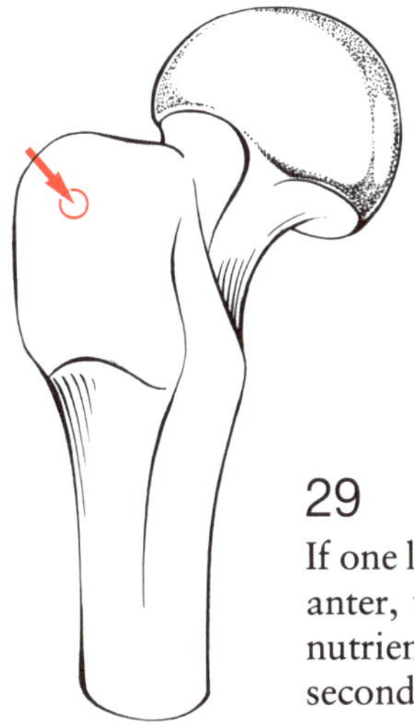

29
If one lands in the area of the trochanteric fossa – it is easy to slip off the trochanter, usually during drilling – the hip joint may be opened unnecessarily or nutrient vessels supplying the femoral head may be injured, with resultant secondary necrosis of the head.

Tactics

First see Figs. 56–6 to p. 57–13.

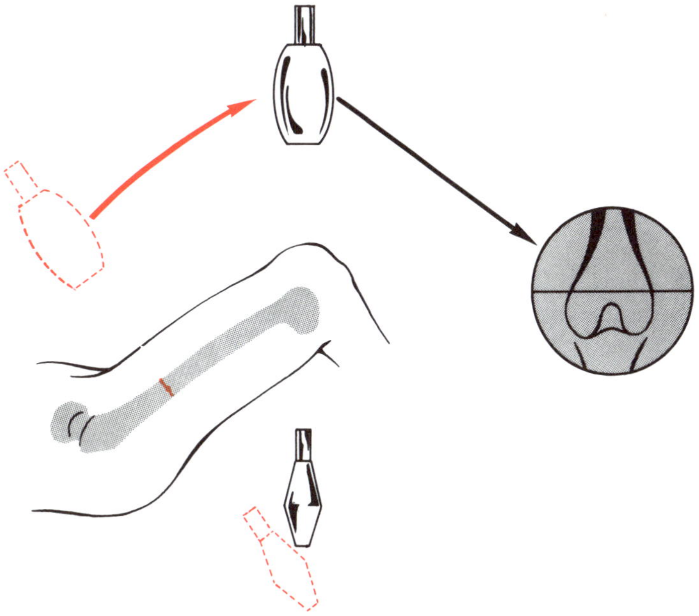

30
Insertion of the drill pin (See Figs. 56–8 to 57–13). To check whether the point of the drill pin or the guide staff lies exactly mesially, the image intensifier is moved a little distalward so that the intercondylar fossa comes into view. The correct length of the guide staff, by contrast, is checked in the lateral view.

31

Beginning with a 9.5 mm or 12 mm sharp drillhead, one drills the marrow cavity open, step by step, until contact is established with the cortex (See figs. 58–14 to 60–21). During this entire procedure, use of the image intensifier is normally unnecessary.

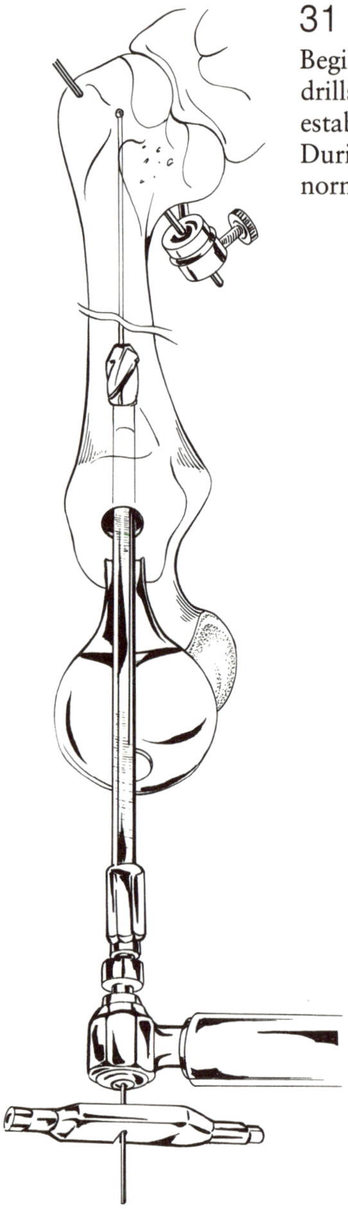

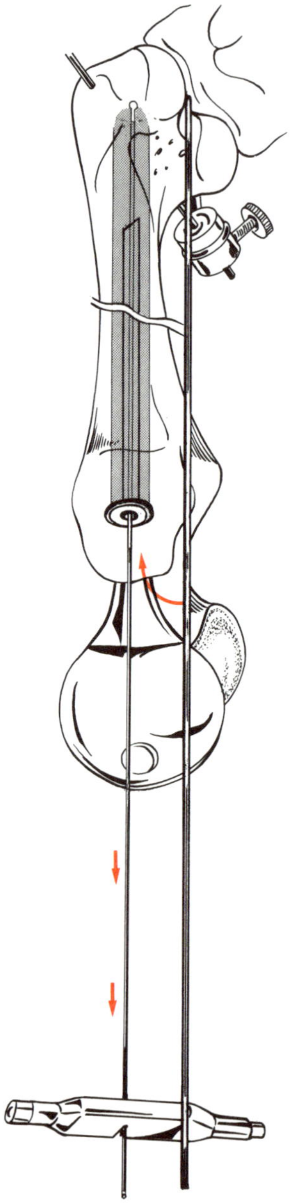

32

The drill pin is replaced by the stronger guide staff. Renewed checks via the image intensifier to see whether the tip of the staff is accurately centered distally in the anteroposterior plane and whether the staff has been sufficiently advanced distalward (See also Fig. 60–22f.).

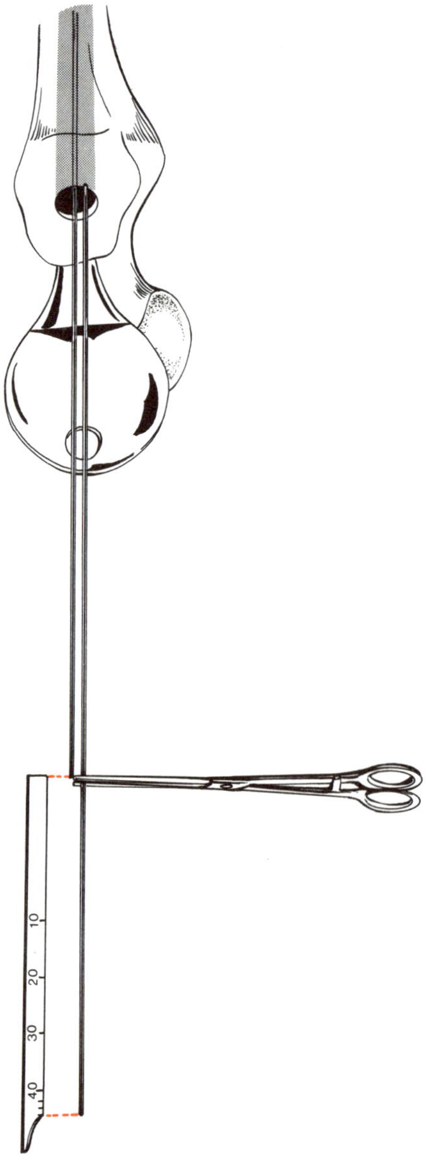

33

Measuring the nail length (See also p. 61.).

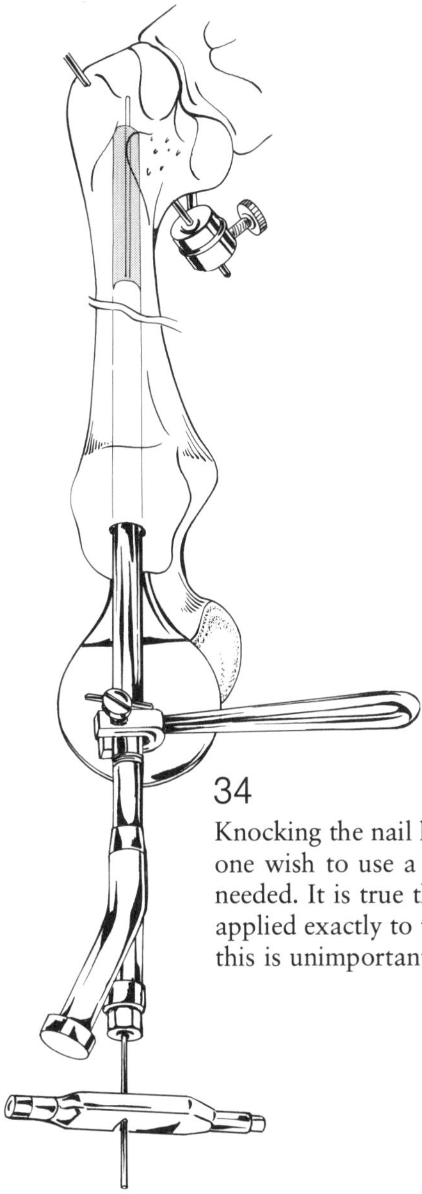

34

Knocking the nail home (See Figs. 61–25 to 62–30). Should one wish to use a hammer, an angular percussion piece is needed. It is true that thereby the hammerblows cannot be applied exactly to the axis of the nail. In practice, however, this is unimportant.

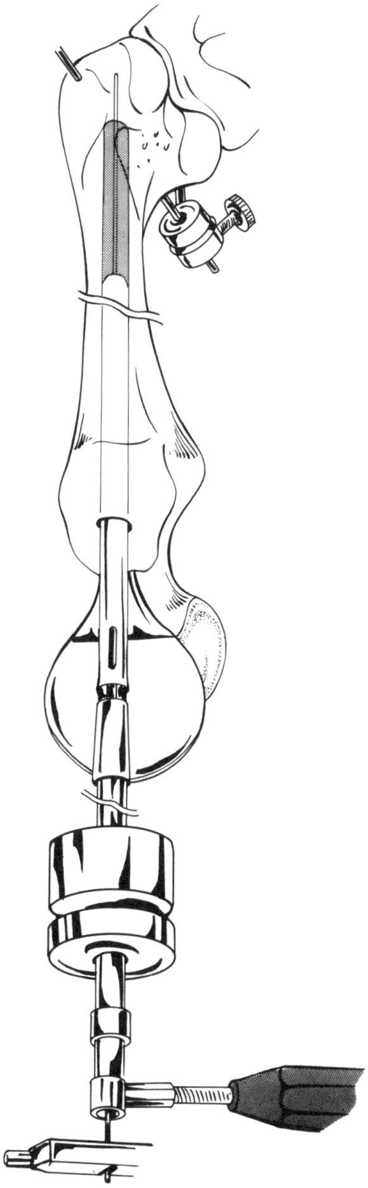

35

Use of the percussion weight on a perforated guide rod makes it possible to knock the nail back quickly when the latter, because of inadequate reduction, has run into the edge of a distal fragment. As soon as the nail enters the distal fragment, the image intensifier is needed again.

Femur – distal part

Anatomy

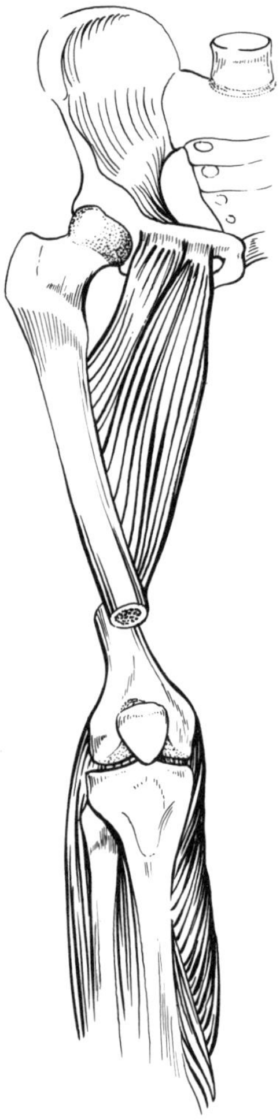

1

Typical displacement of fragments through pull of the adductors and the gastrocnemius muscle:
- proximal end of fragment displaced ventrally, distally and dorsally,
- proximal end of fragment displaced medially,
- proximal end of fragment externally rotated,
- mostly interposition of musculature,
- mostly considerable shortening.

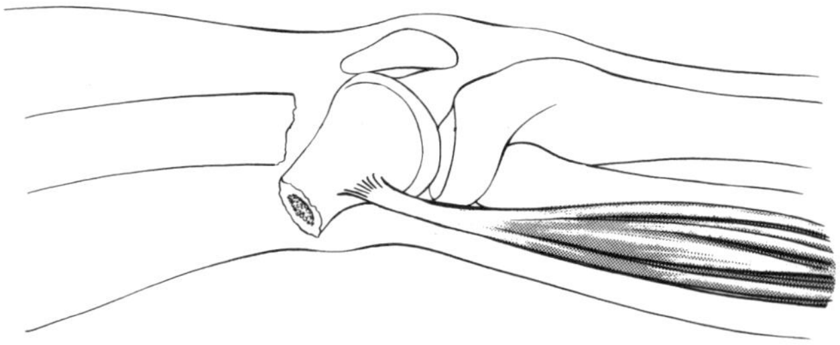

2

Angulation of distal fragment dorsally through pull of the gastrocnemius muscle.

Timing of the operation

As early as possible, i. e. within a few hours, immediately after the circulation has been stabilized with certainty, because then reduction can be most easily performed. If immediate management is not feasible, wire traction through the tibia should be instituted, paying due attention to correct positioning and direction of traction: See p. 1 first.

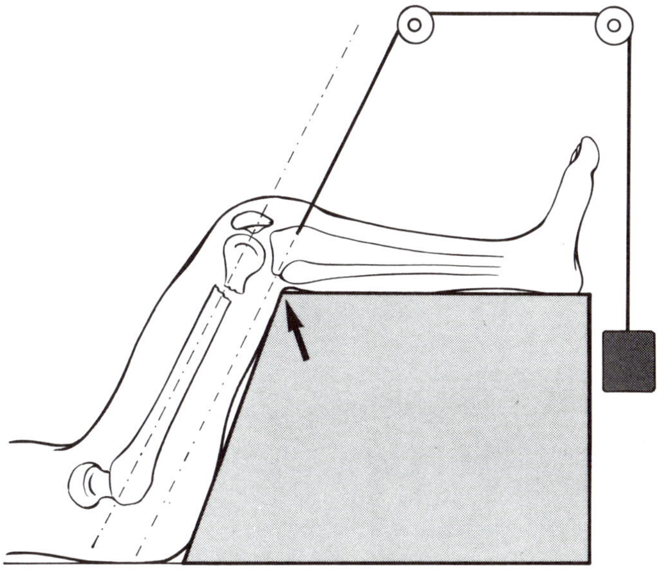

3

Traction on tibia, **wrong:** pull in the direction of the femur. Sharp bend of the supporting splint at the level of the popliteal space.

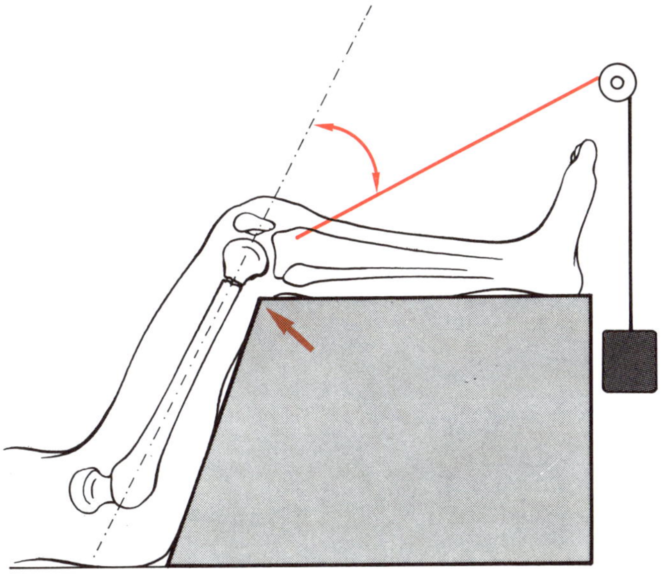

4

Traction on tibia, **correct:** pull more level than the longitudinal axis of the femur. Bend of the splint beneath the fracture. In this way the pull of the gastrocnemius muscle is neutralized and the fragments are aligned.

Principle

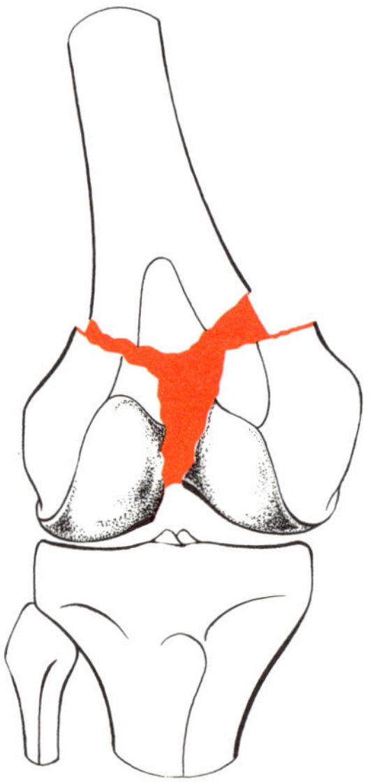

5
Displaced components of joint.

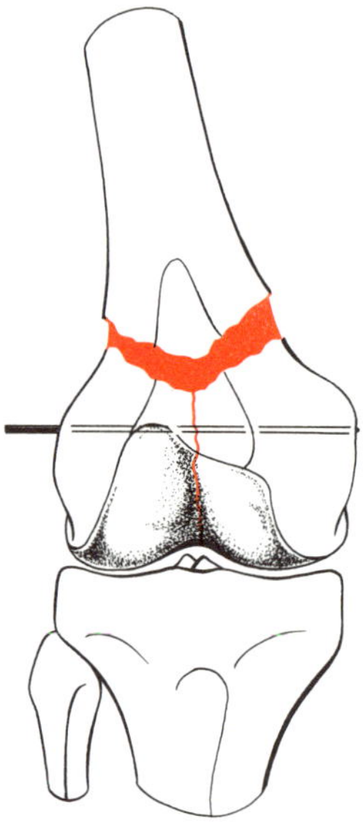

6
Reduction and preliminary fixation with drill wire.

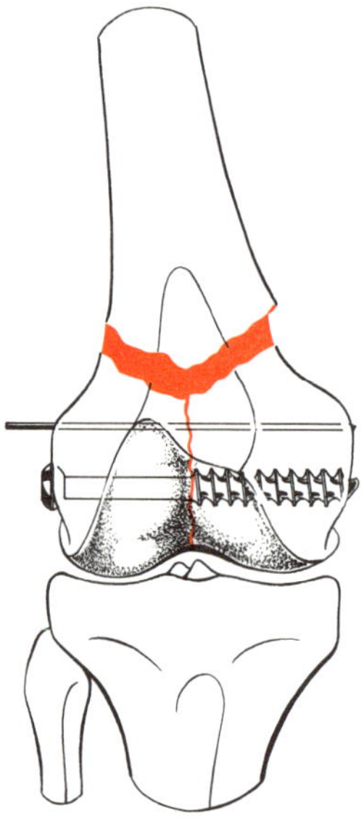

7
Stable connection by cancellous screws whose threads lie entirely beyond the fracture surface.

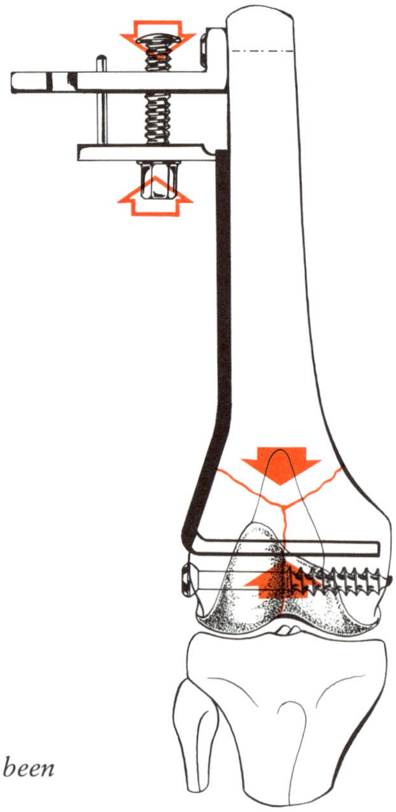

8
The condylar plate is mounted only *after the articular surface has been reconstructed.*

Positioning

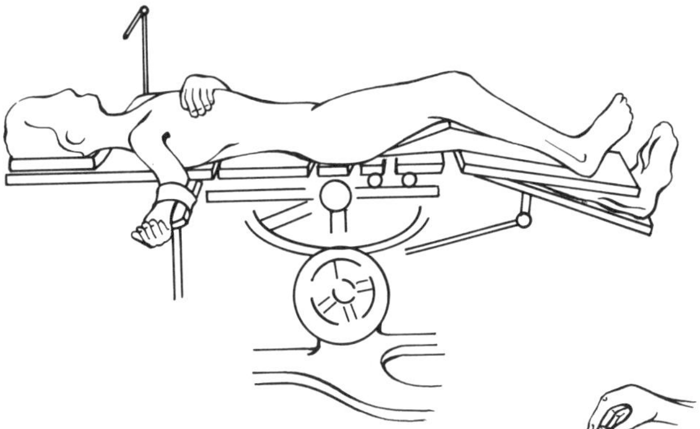

9

Two wedge-shaped cushions produce slight flexion at the knee joint.

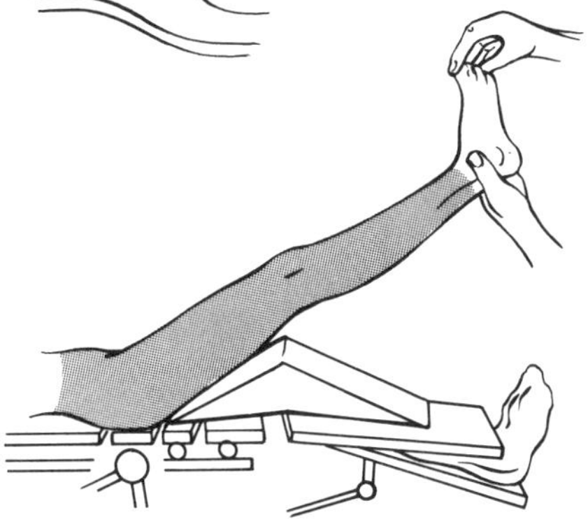

10

Painting with disinfectant; leg supported by a nonsterile person.

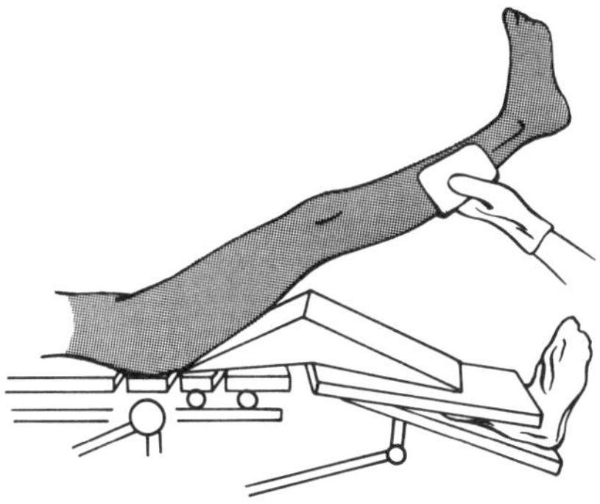

11

A sterile person takes over the leg; the foot can then be painted.

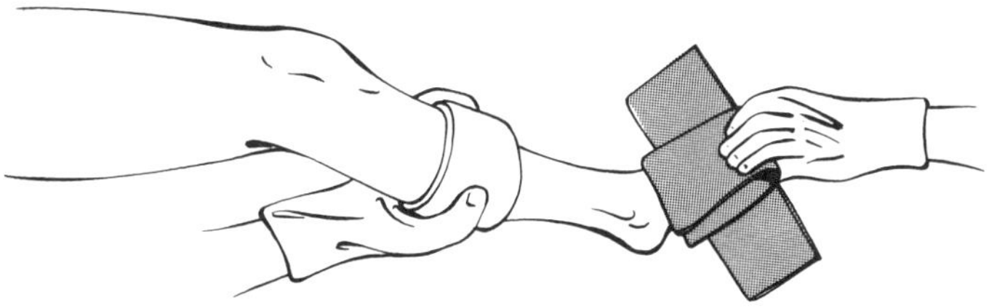

12

The toes are draped with sterile sponges.

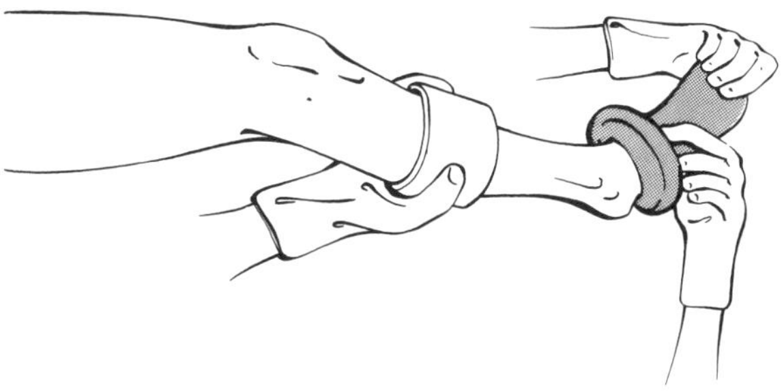

13

A sterile tube of stockinet is slipped on.

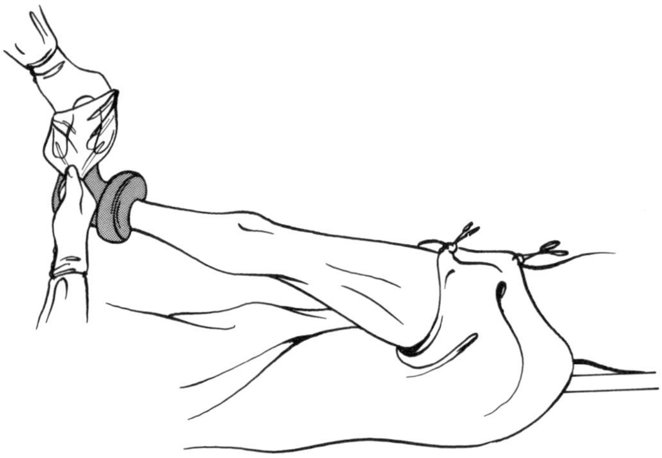

14
In addition, the toes and the foot are covered with a sterile glove.

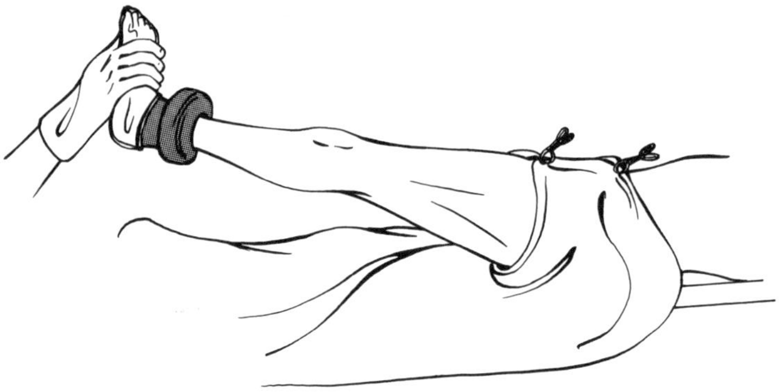

15
Covering with sterile drape, size 1.

16
The foil is glued on.

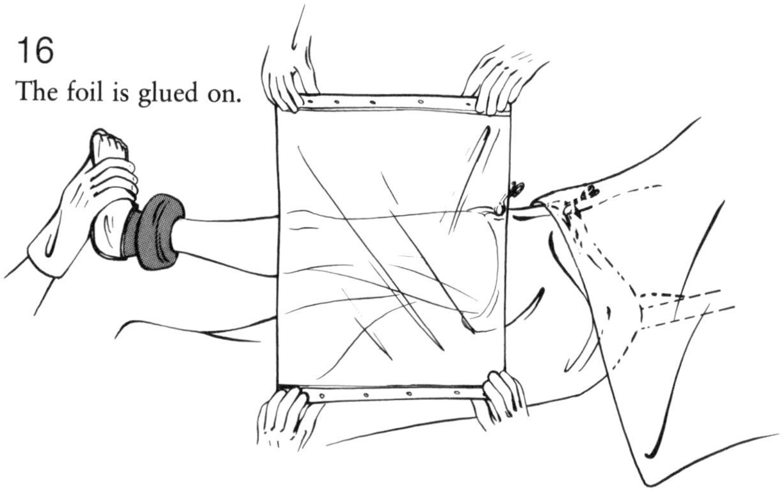

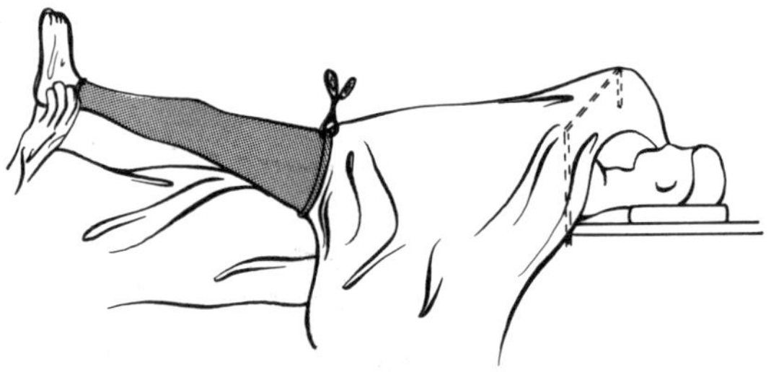

17
The tube of stockinet is pushed up completely.

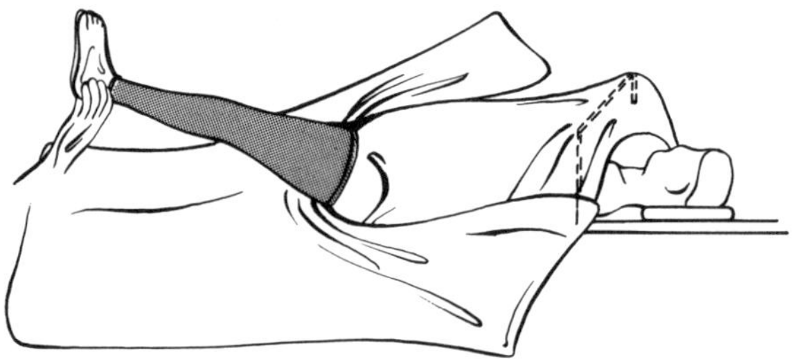

18
Drape with an aperture.

Lateral approach

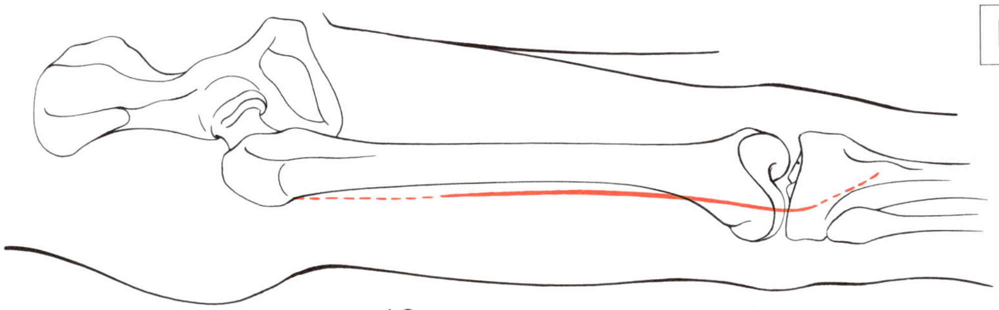

19
The skin incision is made in the middle of the lateral aspect of the thigh; beneath the knee joint it turns in the direction of the tibial tubercle.

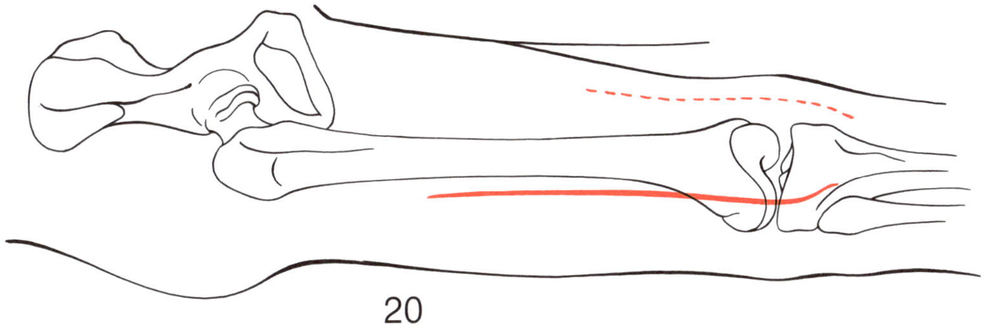

20
Occasionally an auxiliary incision is required to gain a better view and to perform the reduction. If needed, this incision is made subsequently, as shown in Figs. 175–1 ff.

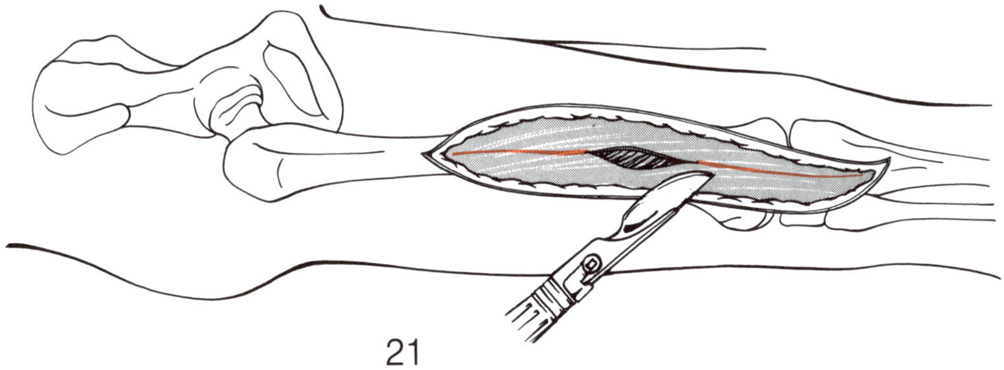

21
The superficial fascia is incised so as not to injure the subjacent muscular fascia.

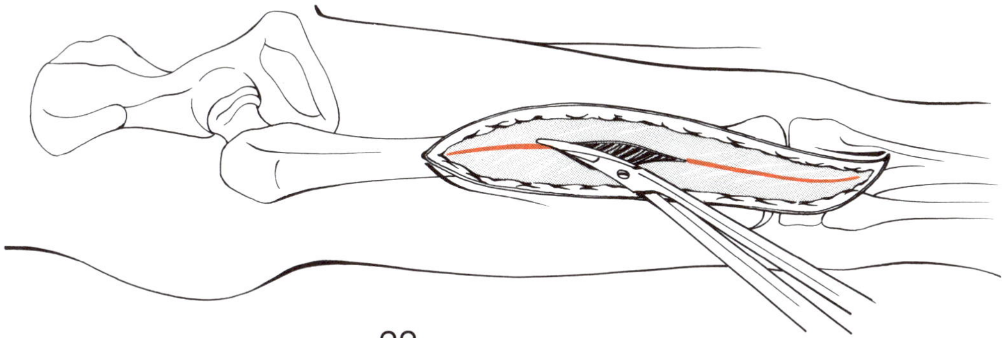

22
From a small incision, the superficial fascia is detached proximally and distally from the muscular fascia with closed scissors and then is incised.

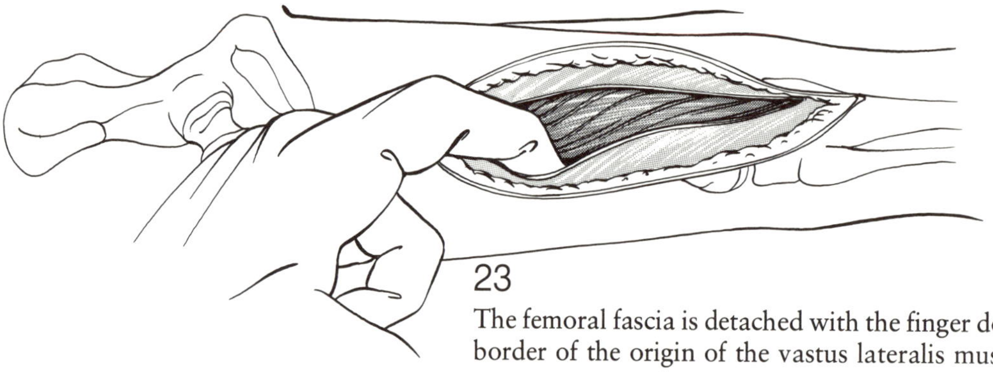

23

The femoral fascia is detached with the finger dorsally as far as the posterior border of the origin of the vastus lateralis muscle.

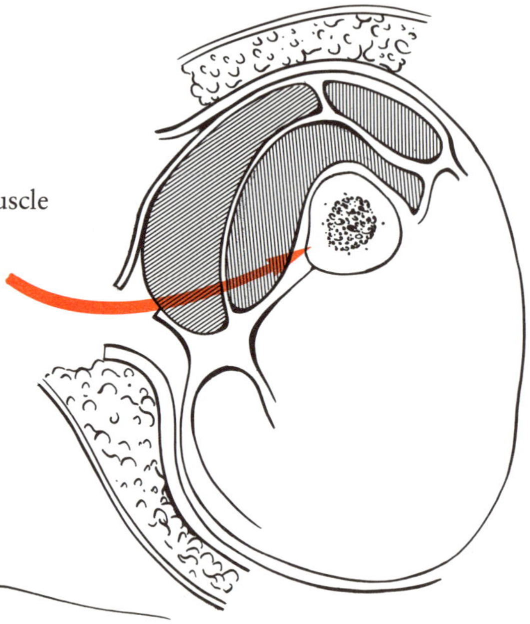

24

About 1 cm anterior to the border of the origin of the vastus lateralis muscle the muscular fascia is incised superficially by scalpel and then…

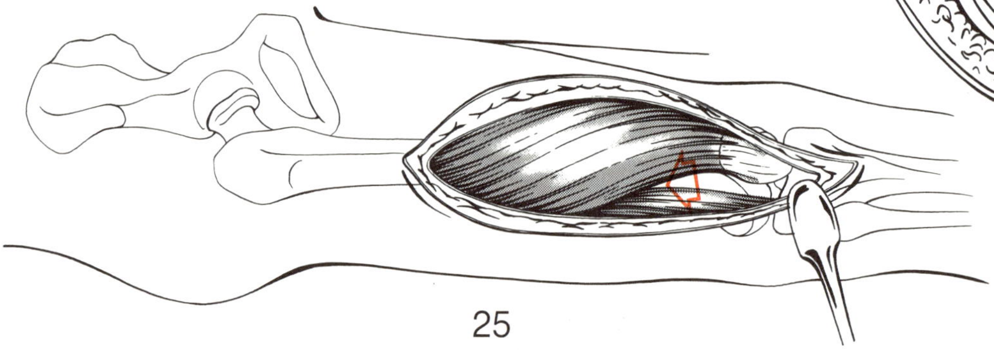

25

… the muscle is divided with a large, rounded raspatory as far as the bone and pushed away ventrally.

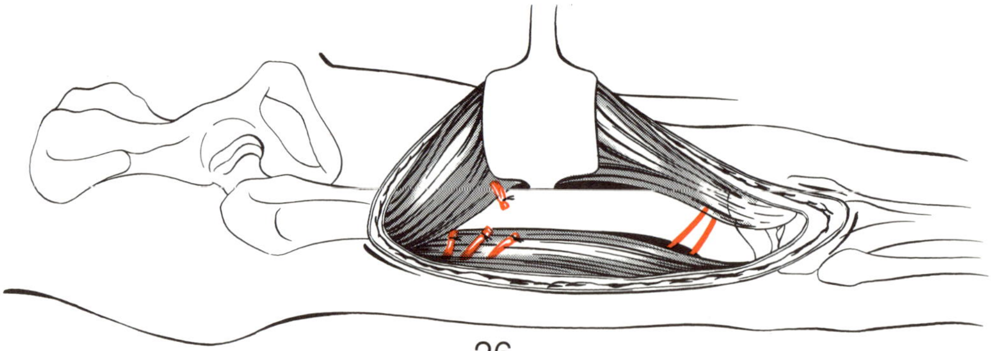

26

By proceeding in this way, the briskly bleeding branches of the second and third perforating artery as well as the superior and inferior genicular artery become visible in time so that they can be ligated ventrally and undersewn dorsally.

Medial approach See Figs. 175–1 ff.

Tactics

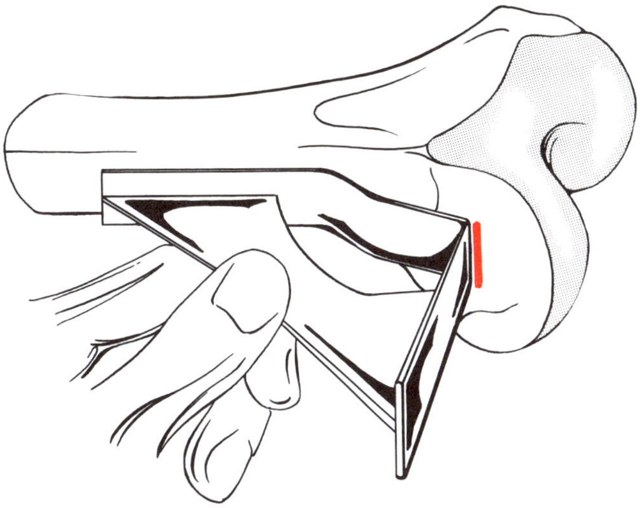

27
The site for driving in the blade is determined with the aid of the measured angle of the condyle.

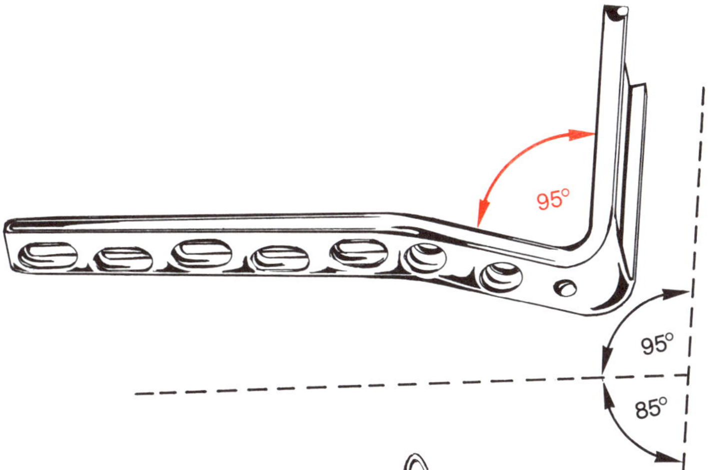

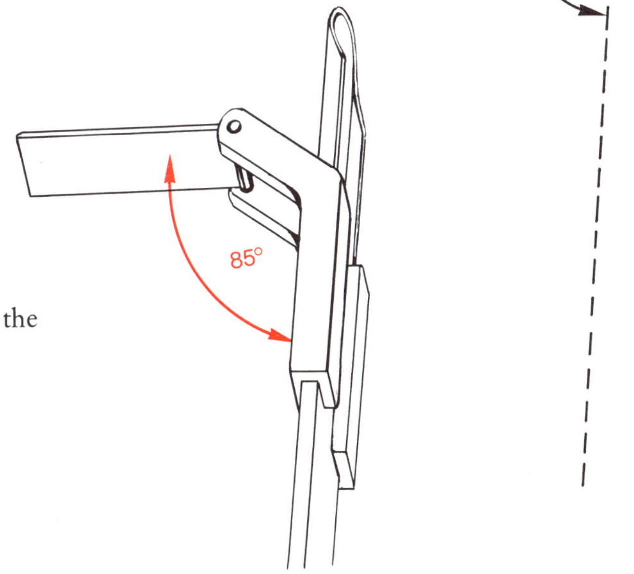

28
Another indication of direction is obtained by use of the caliper rule adjusted to the appropriate angle.

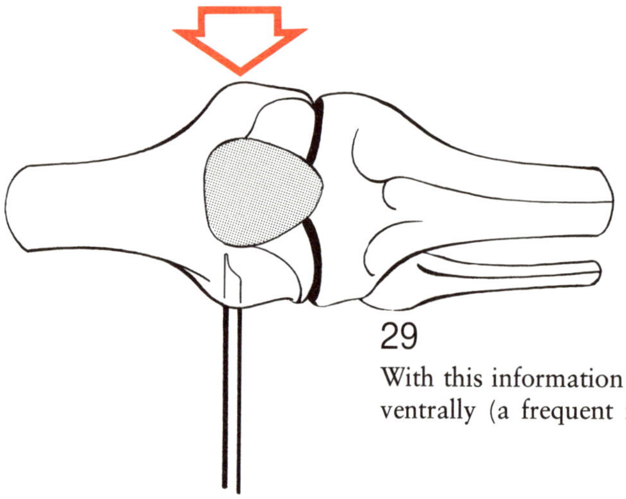

29

With this information one can prevent the tip of the instrument from lying too far ventrally (a frequent mistake), or from passing through the intercondylar fossa.

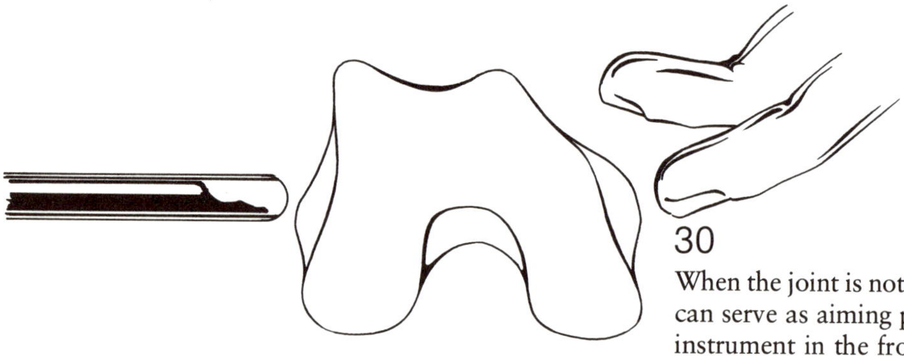

30

When the joint is not to be opened, the medial epicondyle can serve as aiming point for the correct insertion of the instrument in the frontal plane.

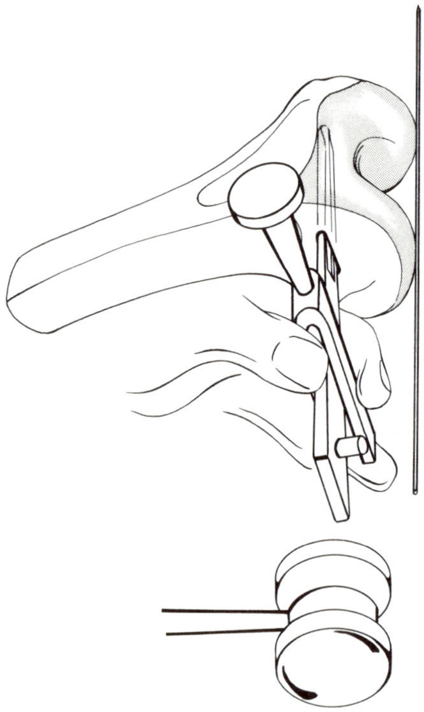

31

When, however, in cases of a short distal fragment, the axis of the shaft cannot be identified with certainty, the articular surface of the condyles must serve to indicate the right direction. A drill wire is then placed over the articular surface of both condyles and the plate inserter is knocked in parallel to the wire.

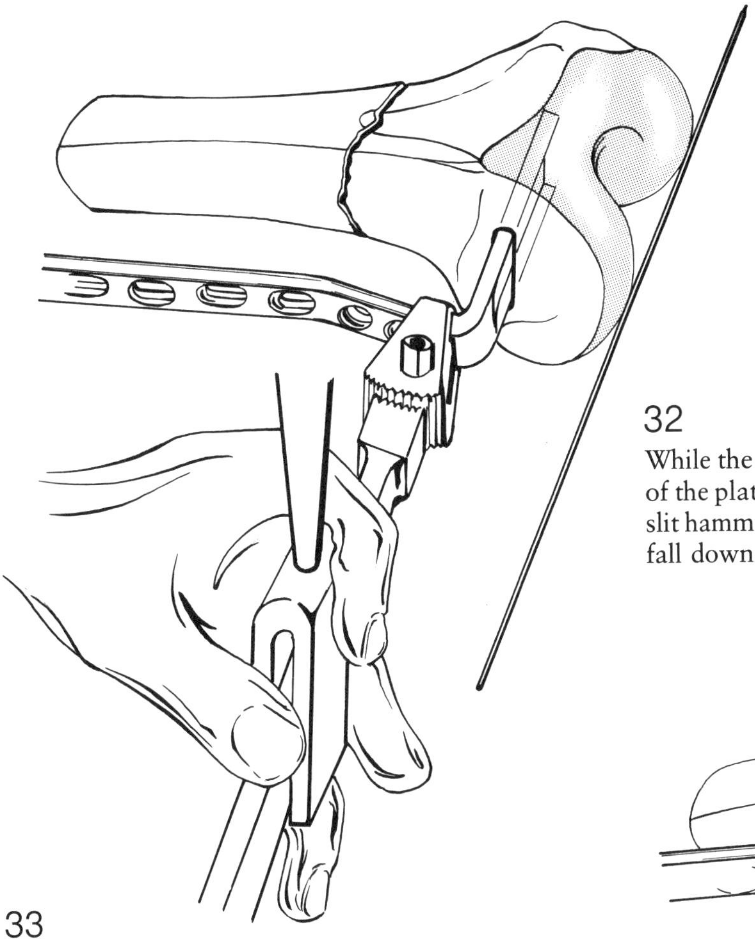

32

While the condylar plate is being knocked in, the holed part of the plate can be held parallel to the femoral shaft with the slit hammer. The latter is put on from above so that is cannot fall down.

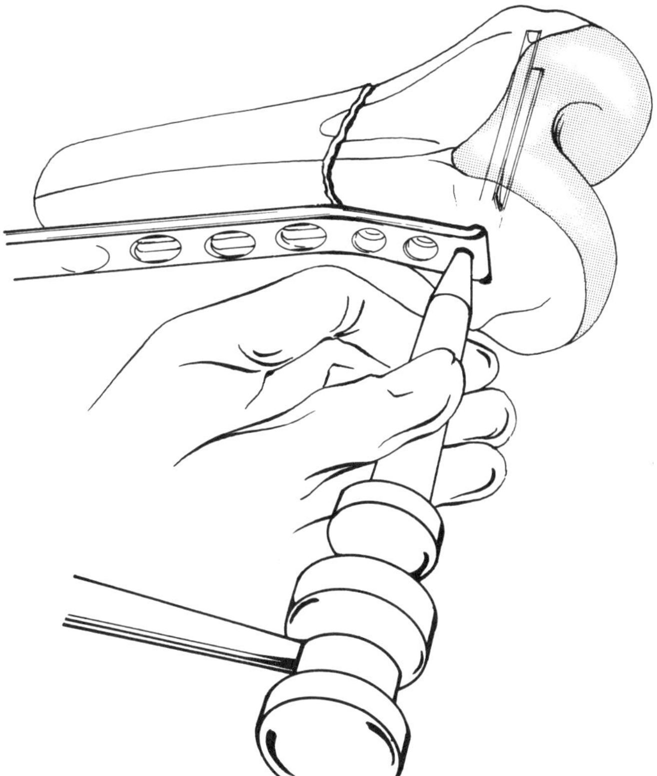

33

After removal of the plate inserter, the blade of the plate is knocked in completely with the percussion instrument.

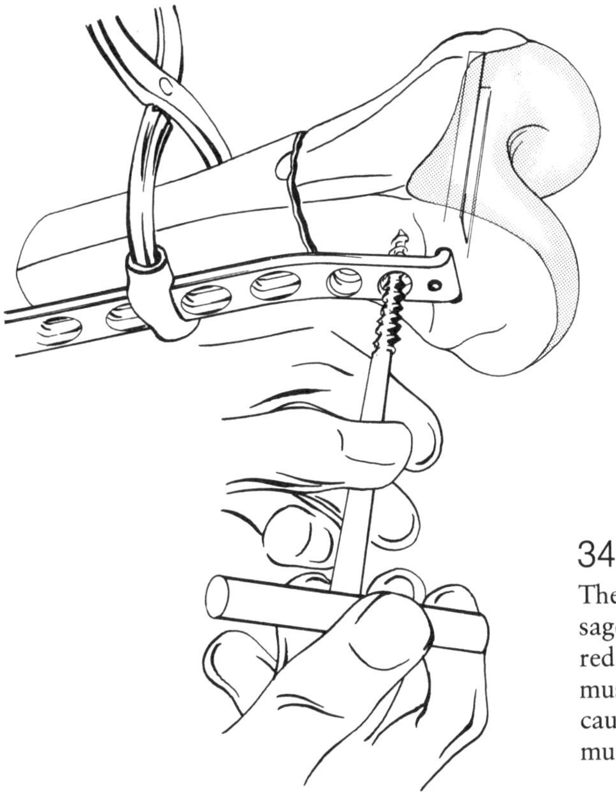

34

The two holes in each condylar plate near the blade allow the passage of cancellous screws which, in that region, are generally required. The screws should, if possible, just grip the opposite cortex, but must on no account protrude to a greater extent. They are sure to cause the patient great discomfort if they do. The blade of the plate must never protrude!

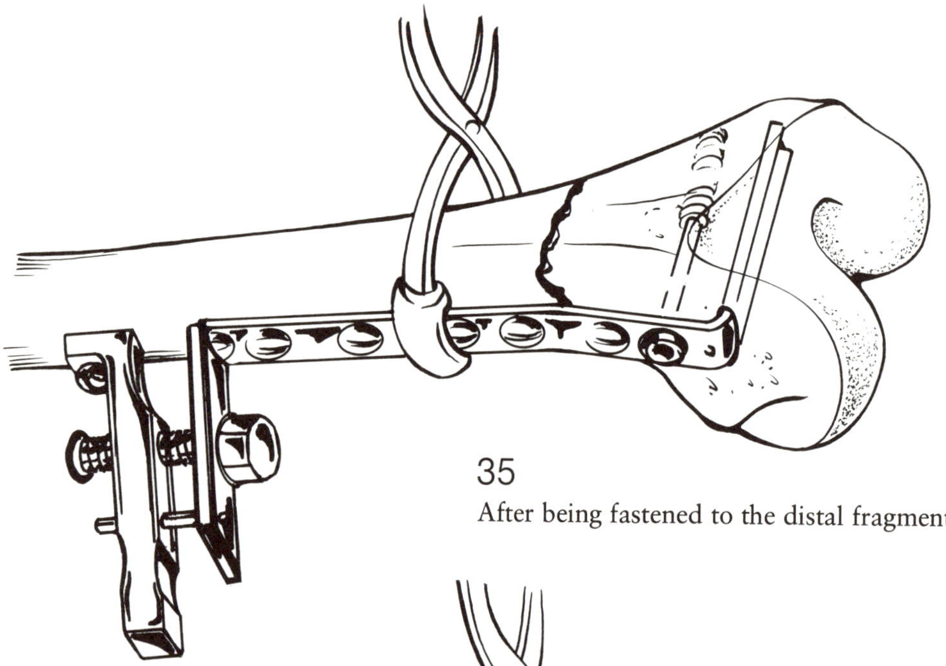

35
After being fastened to the distal fragment, the plate is tightened.

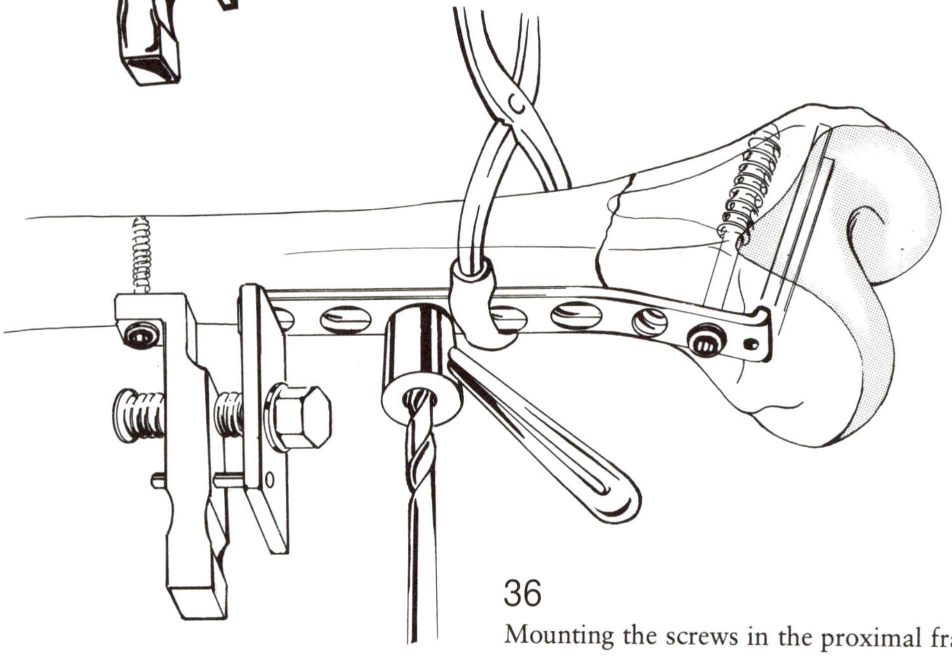

36
Mounting the screws in the proximal fragment.

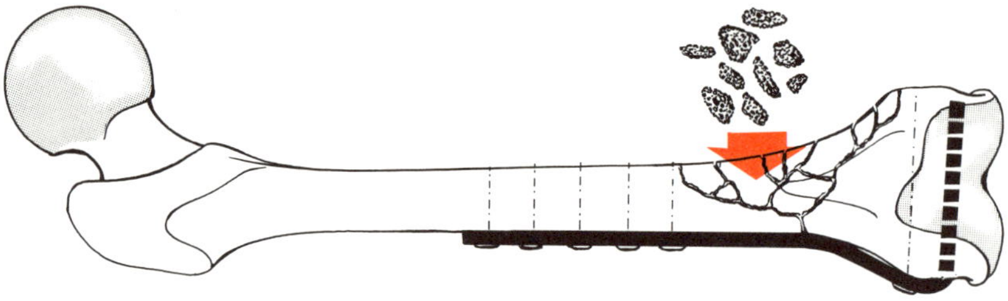

37
Since comminuted areas are frequently encountered in that region, one is strongly advised to appose, in addition, a generous quantity of autologous cancellous bone because, otherwise, the bony support cannot be expected to become sufficiently stable before the plate suffers fatigue fracture.

12. Patella

Types of injuries

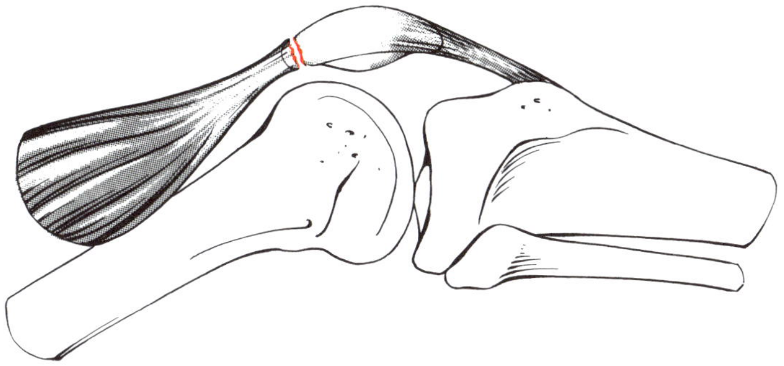

1

Small proximal fragment and quadriceps tendon.

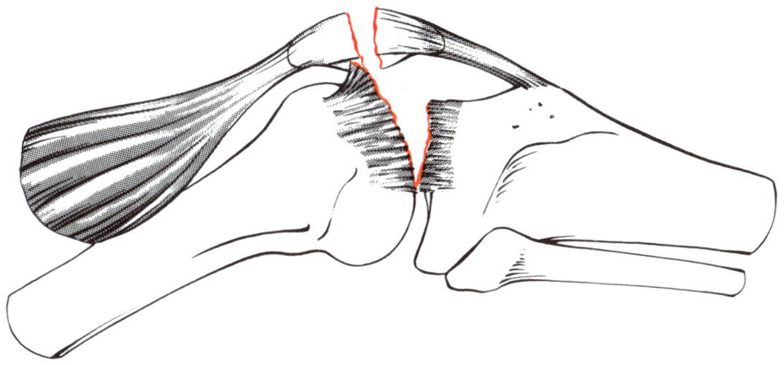

2

Transverse fracture.

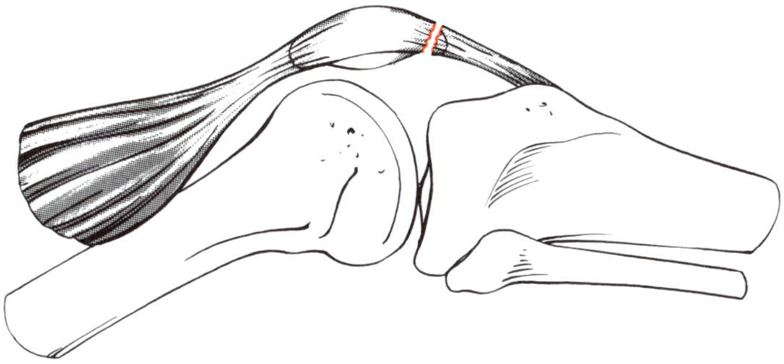

3

Small distal fragment.

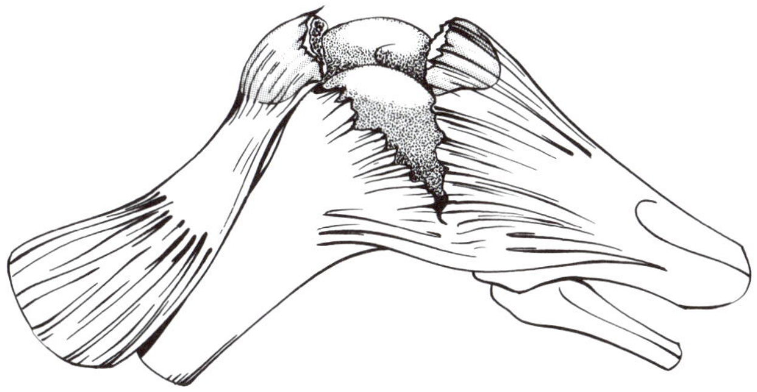

4

With nearly all strongly displaced fractures of the patella, the supplemental lateral set of extensor ligaments suffers extensive tearing and must be sutured.

Operative possibilities

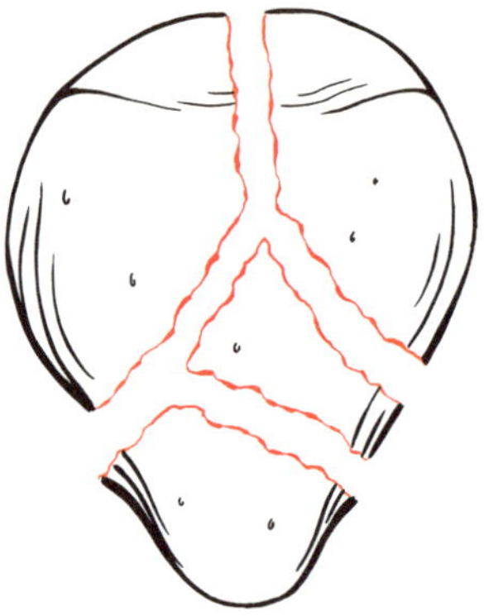

5
In the presence of fractures with more than one break, large fragments are, if possible, joined together...

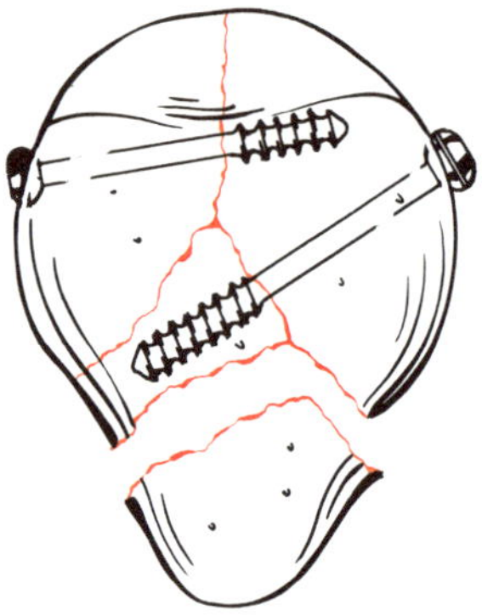

6
... with screws (not drill wires), until a transverse fracture has been created.

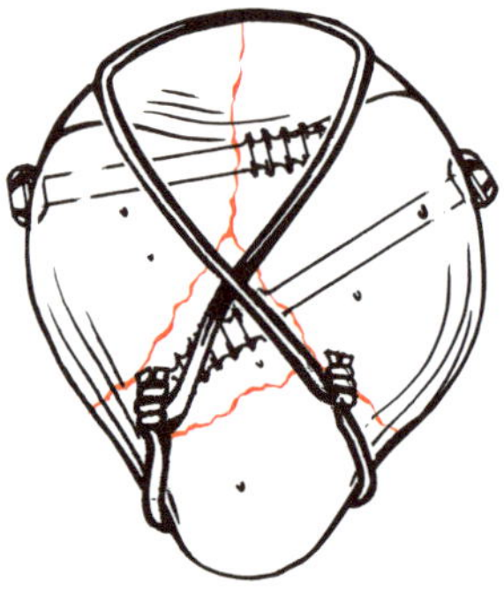

7
This transverse fracture is then cared for by external wiring fixation.

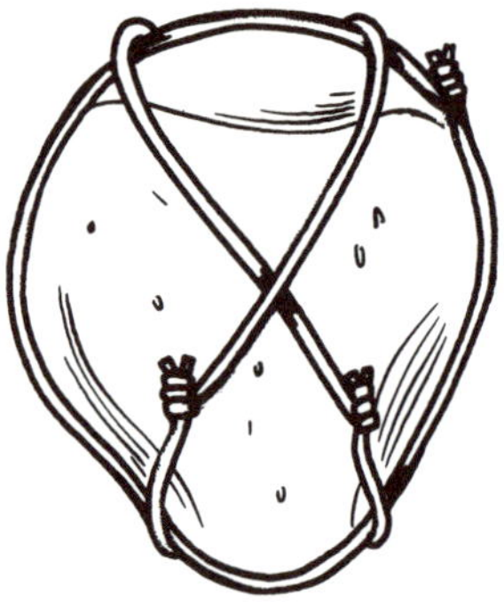

8
Stellar fractures often can better be managed by cerclage plus external wiring fixation. To this end, one should not previously separate the fragments too much, nor even loosen them from their connection which in most cases has been preserved.

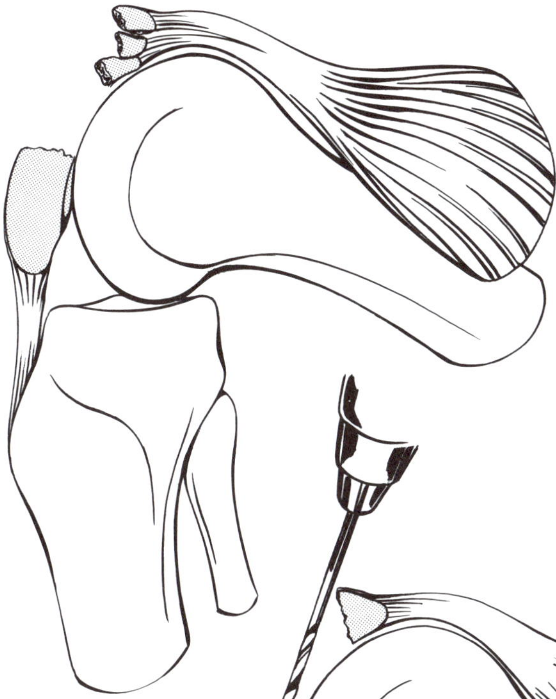

9

In fractures with more than one break, partial resections of the patella and fractures near the poles of the patella in which a small bony fragment has been preserved on the tendon or the ligament, reinsertion is undertaken in the following manner:

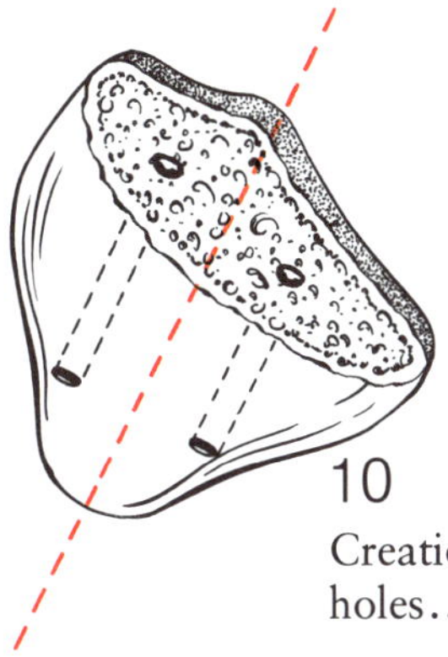

10

Creation of parallel drill holes…

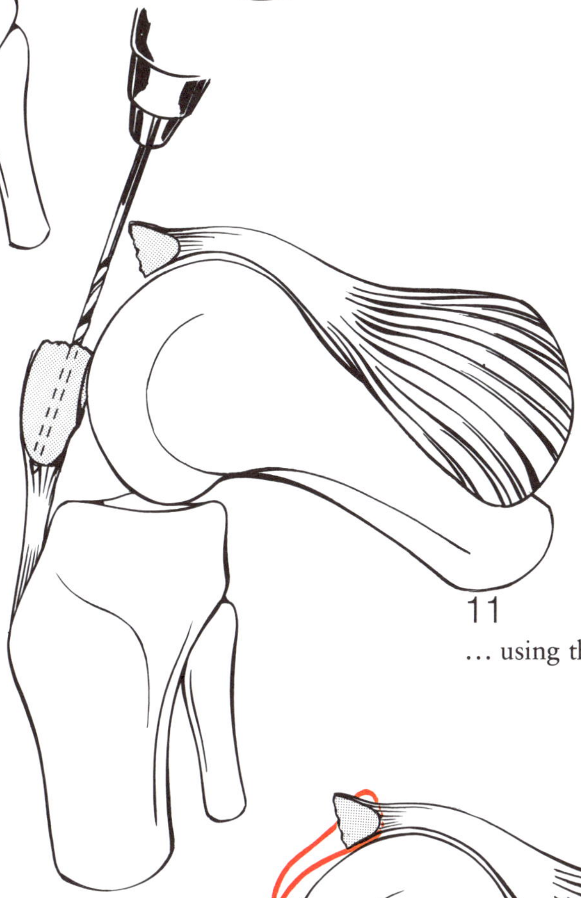

11

… using the 2.0 mm drill.

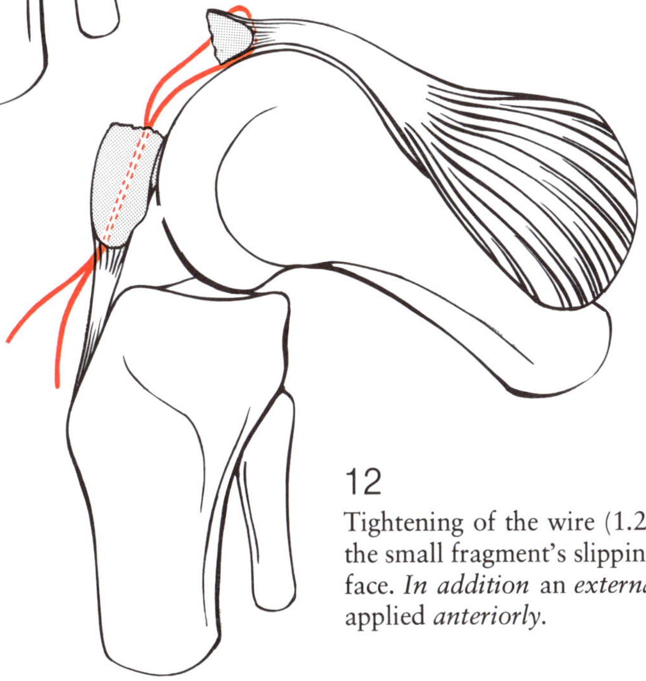

12

Tightening of the wire (1.2 mm, soft) insures against the small fragment's slipping toward the articular surface. *In addition* an *external wiring fixation* must be applied *anteriorly*.

Principles See pp. 52–3 ff.

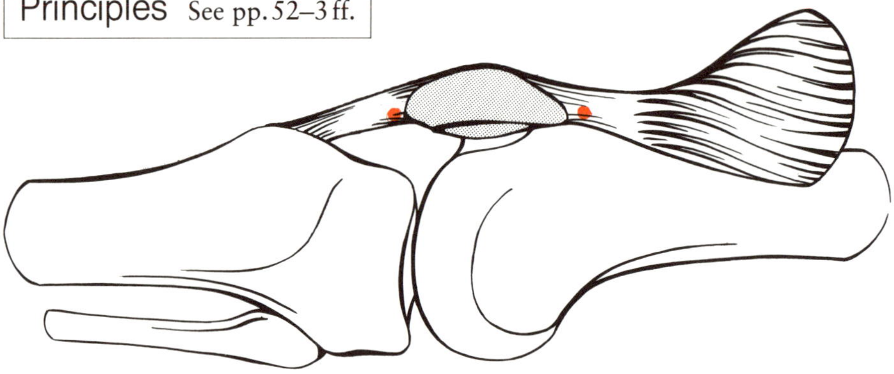

13

The wiring fixation is applied just above the superior border of the patella and beneath its inferior border. Posteriorly, the wire should lie in the tendon but not within the joint (See Fig. 221–24).

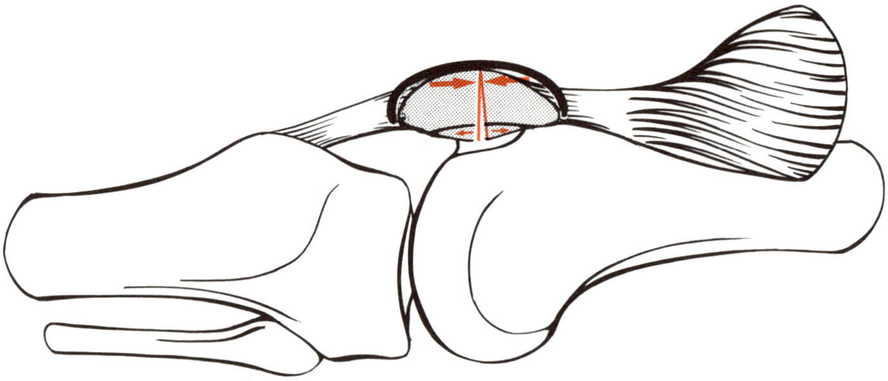

14

On tightening the wire, with the knee joint extended, the fragments gape dorsally.

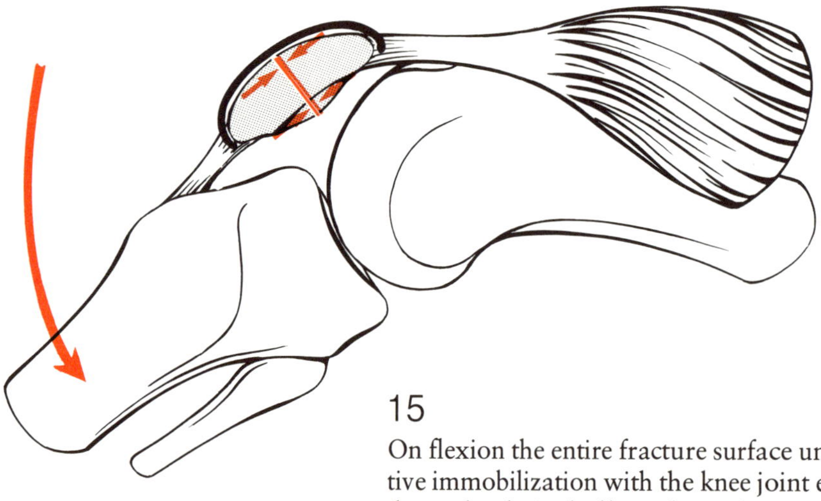

15

On flexion the entire fracture surface undergoes compression. Therefore, postoperative immobilization with the knee joint extended is not very useful. Only flexion produces the desired effect of interfragmental compression.

Positioning

16
It is expedient to place the uninjured extremity...

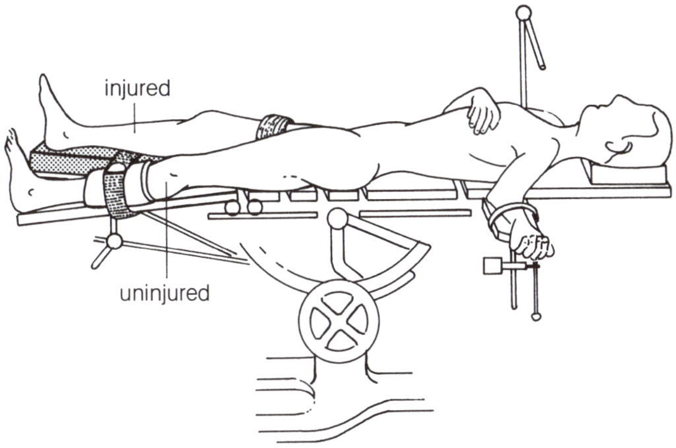

17
... a little lower than the one to be operated on.

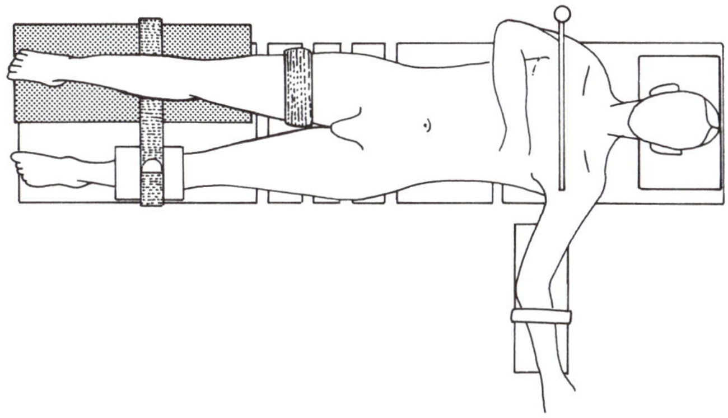

Approach

18
Skin incision over the center of the patella, coursing transversely. The subcutaneous tissues are divided down to the prepatellar tendon. In this layer the dissection proceeds, partly by scalpel and partly by spreading the scissors, to reach the palpable superior border of the patella.

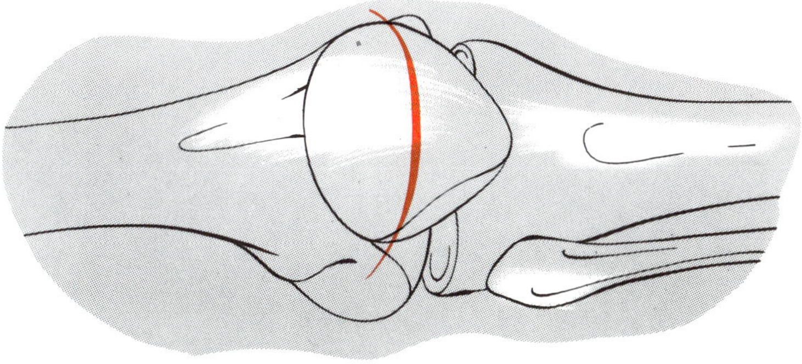

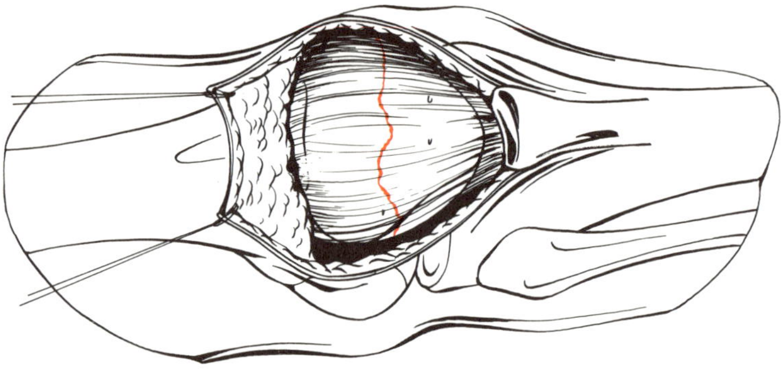

19

The flap consisting of skin and adipose tissue is held upward with two retention sutures (See Figs. 4–1 ff.). A small Roux hook is inserted distally.

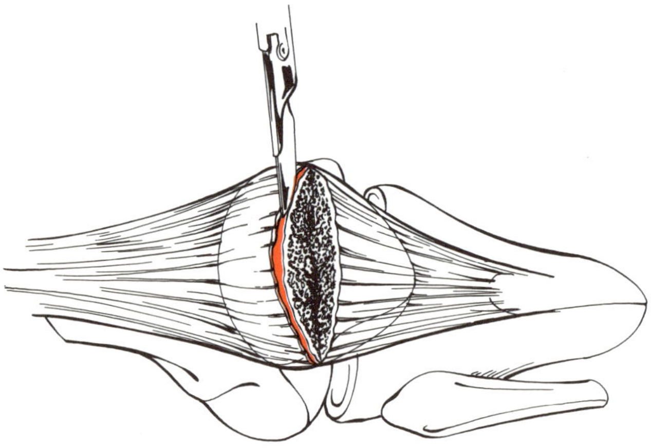

20

The periosteum and the stumps of the patellar tendon are pushed away by scalpel for a distance of about 1 to 2 mm from the border of the fracture. This maneuver enables accurate reduction of the fragments.

Tactics

21

Reduction is achieved through two strong, sharp single-pronged hooks inserted in opposite directions and temporary drill-wire fixation.

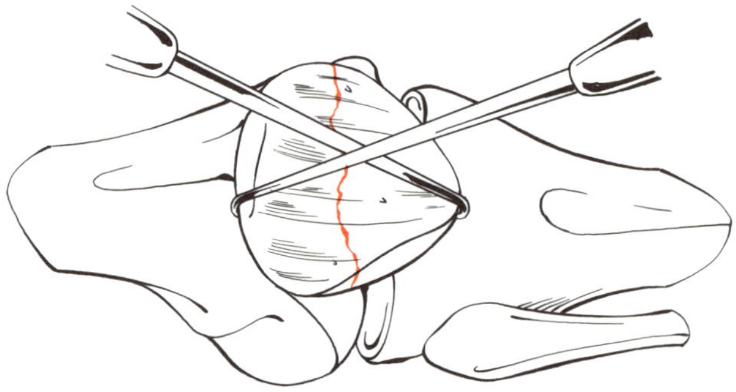

22

Good reduction of the fragments can also be effected with use of a large reducing forceps. In this case, (temporary) drill-wire fixation can usually be dispensed with.

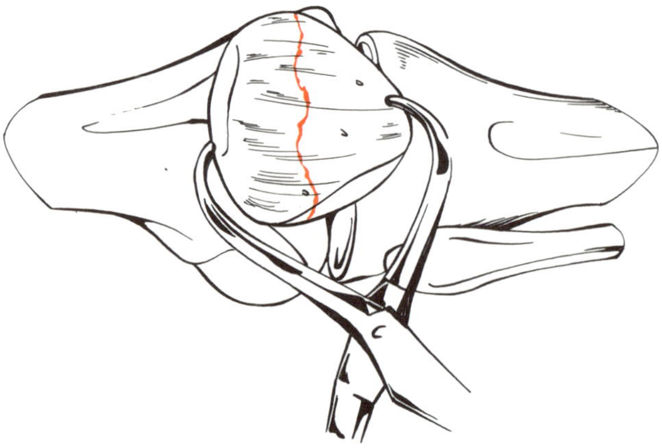

23

It is very helpful to nip off the end of the wire as obliquely as possible (See Fig. 52–1 f.) or to use a previously-bent thick cannula (See Fig. 52–3.). A thick, soft wire (1.2 mm) is carried around the upper pole of the patella, close to the bone. During this maneuver one verifies, with the finger in the joint, ...

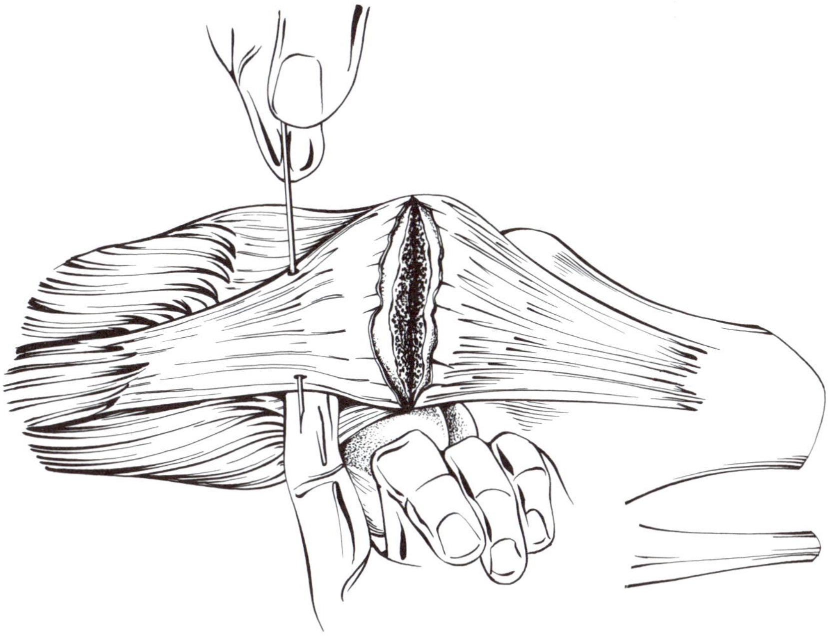

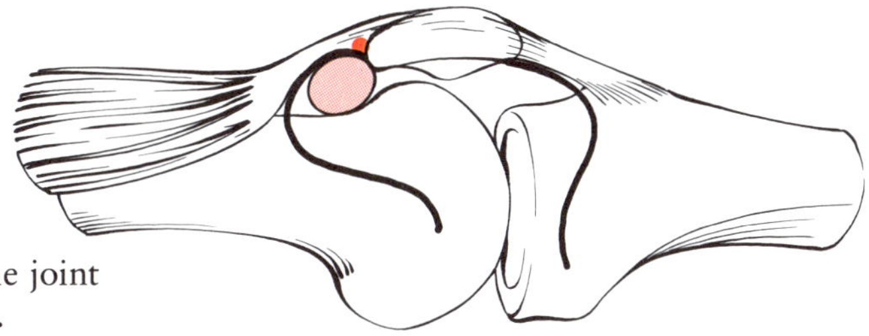

24

... whether the wire lies closely under the joint capsule without entering the joint cavity.

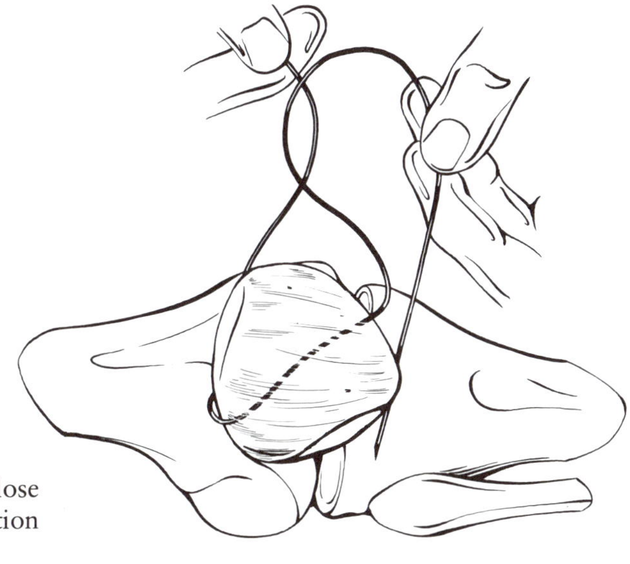

25

Also distally the wire should be carried so close to the bone as to pass under the distal projection without penetrating the joint.

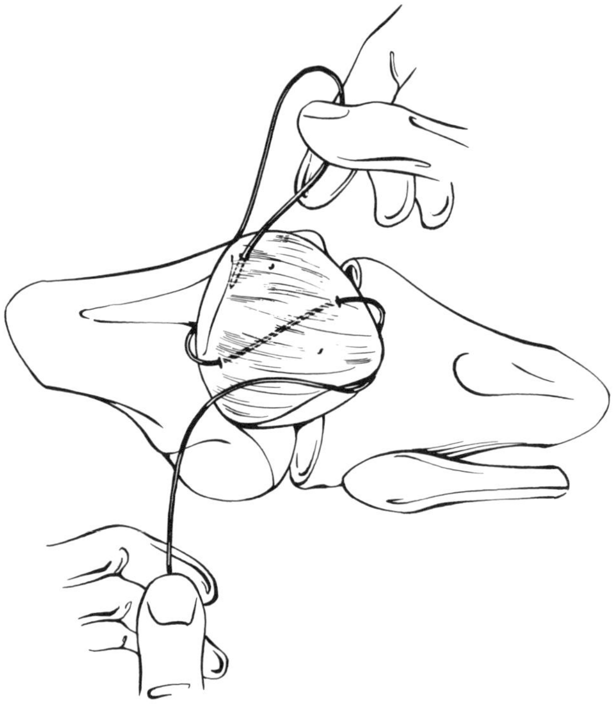

26

To avoid the development of a pressure necrosis, the wire should, as far as possible, be carried under the prepatellar ligament (i.e., right upon the bony surface of the patella).

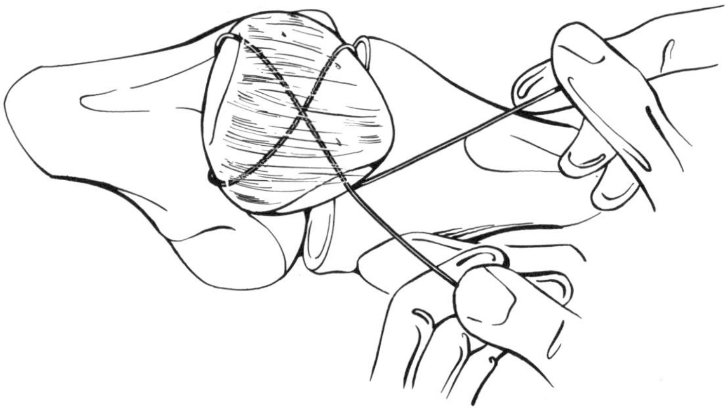

27

The fixing wire is tightened strongly enough to cause the cleft of the fracture to gape on the side of the joint. This can be effected by hand or, better, with use of a tightener.

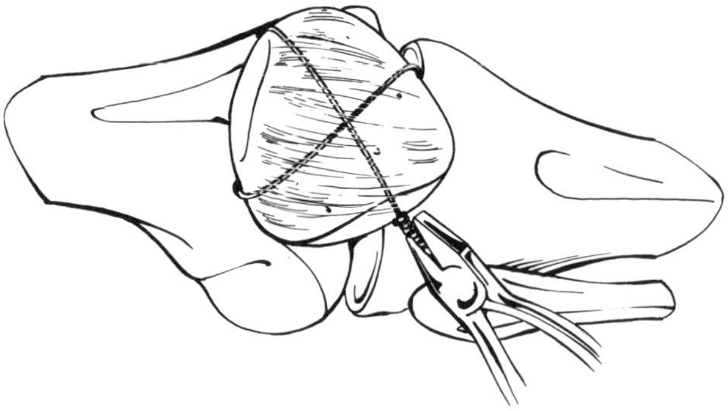

28

Finally, the wire is twisted together close to the bone (See also Figs. 52–7 ff.).

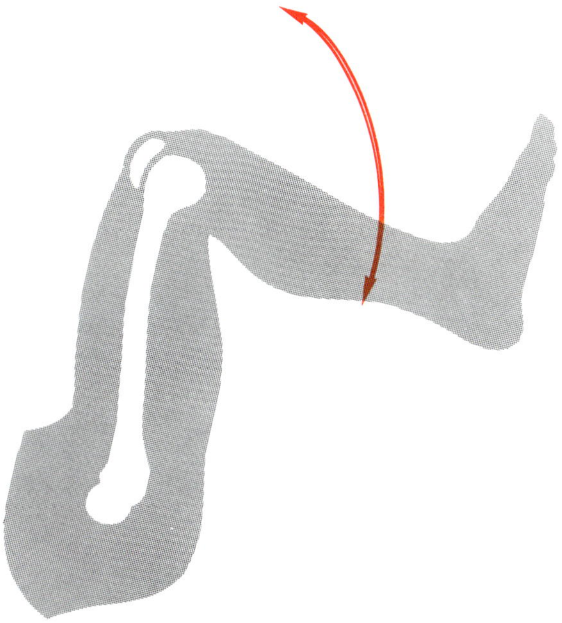

29

Prior to definitive ly tightening the fixing wire, the knee should be flexed and extended a number of times.

Postoperative care

No immobilizing dressing, no weightbearing for 6 weeks after surgery. Alternatively, an anterior plaster shell may be applied and weight bearing, with daily exercises without the shell, can be started after active mobility of 0-0-90 against gravity has been obtained.

13. Knee Joint

Anatomy

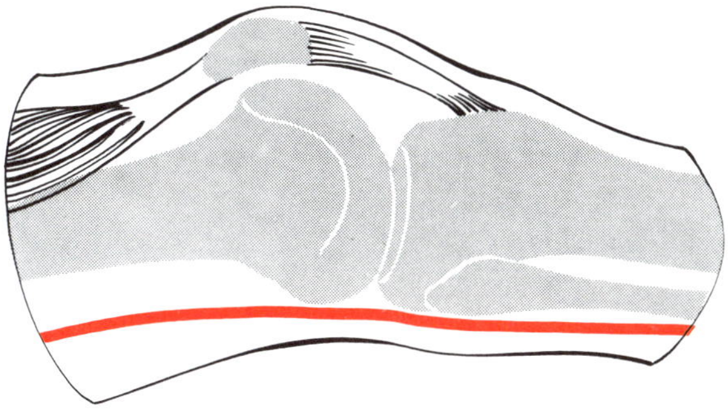

1
When the *knee is extended*, the popliteal vessels and nerves course close to the joint capsule.

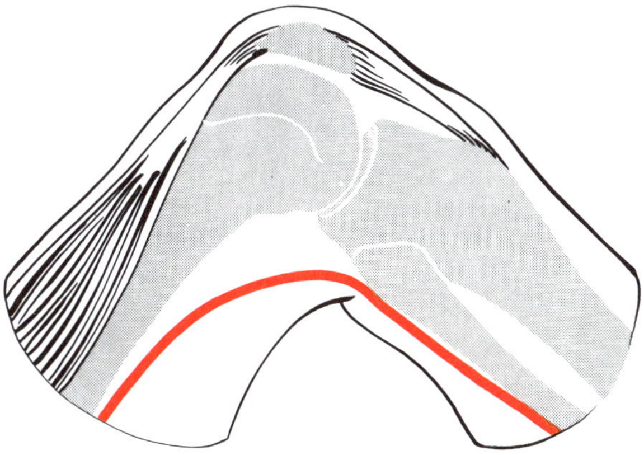

2
With the *knee flexed*, the distance increases to such an extent that injuries are virtually impossible when operating on the capsule.

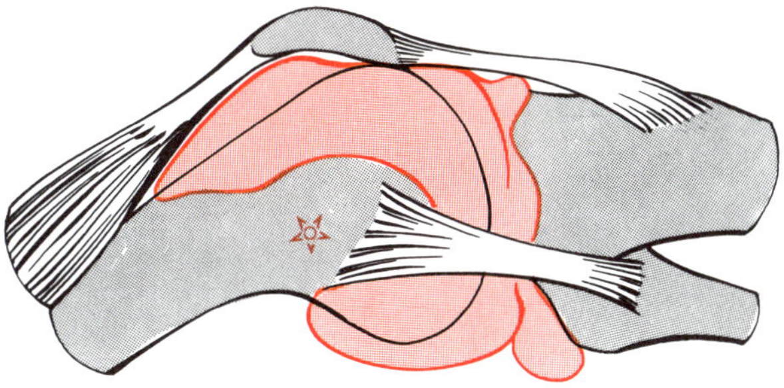

3
Line of attachment of the joint capsule (to be kept in mind, for instance, in instituting supracondylar extension). (See Fig. 193–1.)

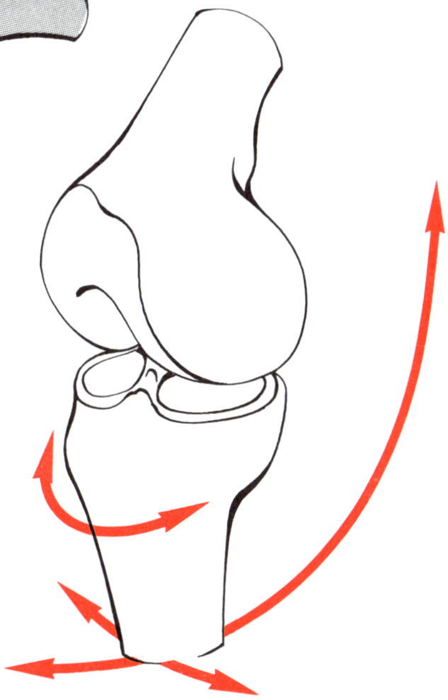

4
Direction of movements at the knee joint.

Ligaments

Types of injuries

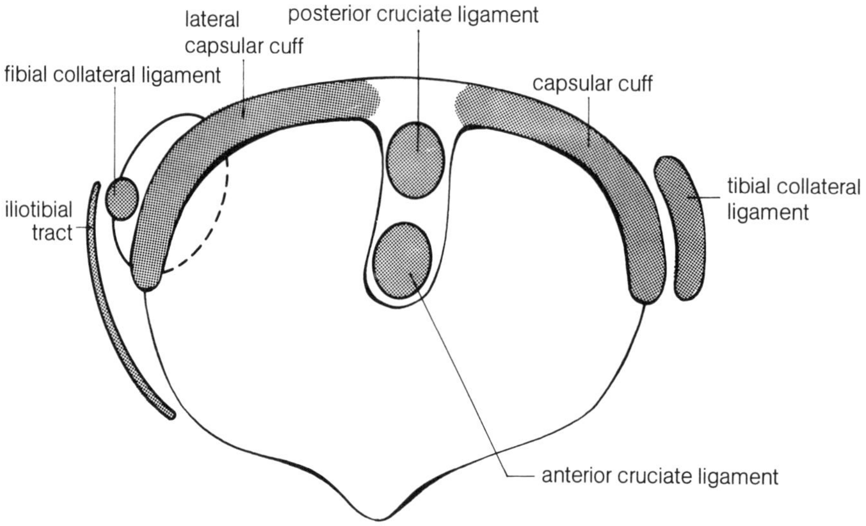

1

Isolated ligament injuries of the knee joint are rare. The following structures can be involved:

- tibial or fibial collateral ligament,
- anterior or posterior cruciate ligament,
- right or left posterior rotator cuff,
- right or left meniscus.

Isolated injuries

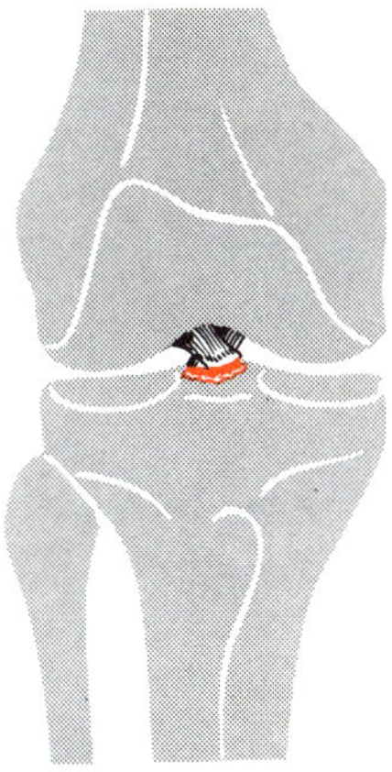

2

Cruciate ligament (infrequent): drawer sign not well-marked; not increased in the rotated position (See Fig. 244–2.).

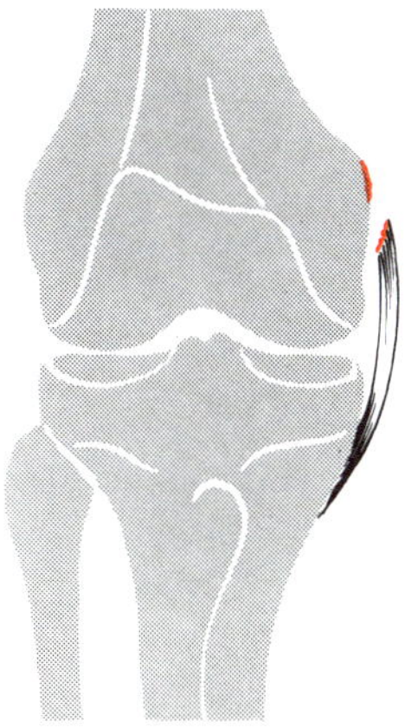

3

Collateral ligament (tibial ligament infrequent) at its insertion or…

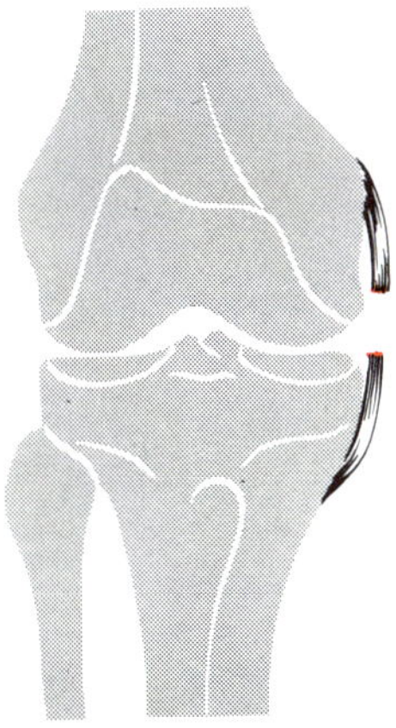

4

… in its middle: in the extended position, the joint surfaces cannot be separated, or only on the ipsilateral side. Drawer sign absent.
In 30° flexion, the joint surfaces can be separated to a certain extent (more on the injured than on the noninjured side).

Complex injuries

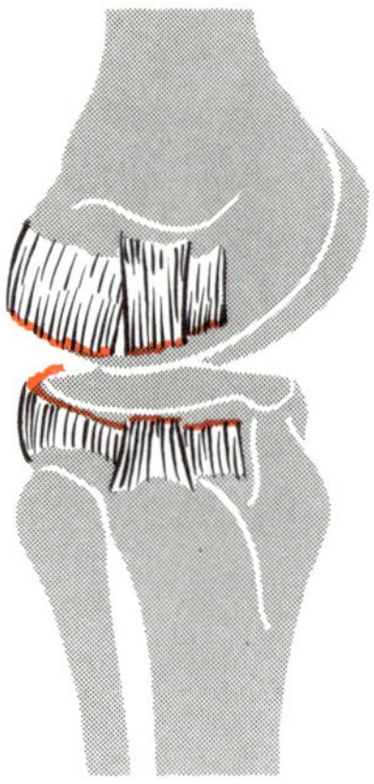

5

Collateral ligament and posterior capsular cuff: "false drawer sign" with the knee rotated to the uninjured side. No drawer sign with the knee rotated to the injured side.

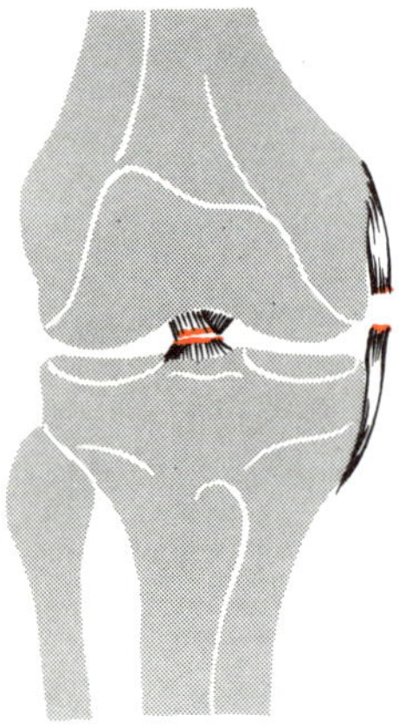

6

Collateral ligament and cruciate ligament: Joint surfaces distinctly separable laterally in 30° flexion, not in extension.

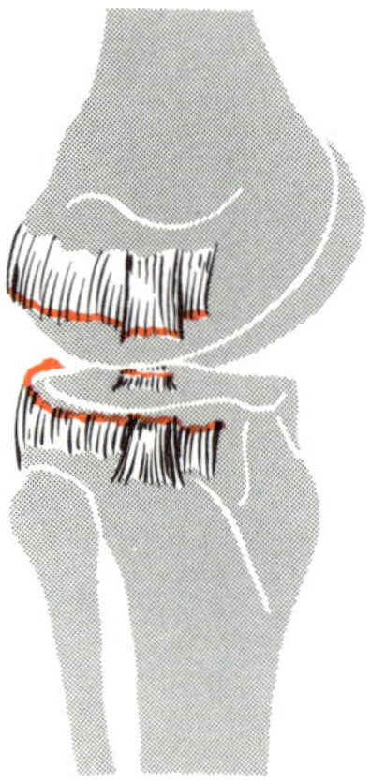

7

Collateral ligament plus cruciate ligament plus posterior capsular cuff: "genuine drawer sign", independent of internal or external rotation. In the extended position as well, the joint surfaces can be separated laterally.

Indication

Operation, when separation of the joint surfaces or the drawer sign *cannot be counterbalanced even by vigorous tensing of the musculature.*

Timing of the operation

Fresh injuries should be operated as soon as possible because, even after a few days, ligament stumps degenerate and suturing is no longer feasible.

Operative possibilities

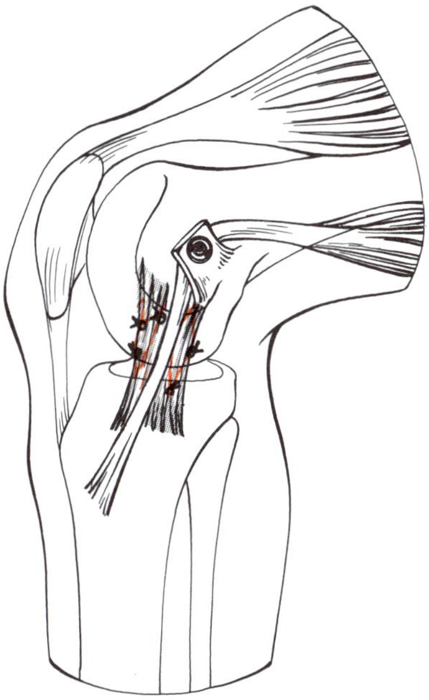

8
Massive fraying or defects of ligaments are additionally secured by functional, pedicle, or free grafts. (See pp. 236–9.)

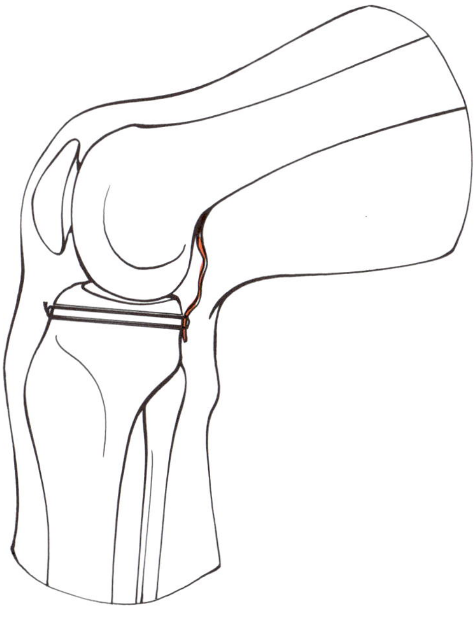

9
Transosseous reinsertion of the posterior capsular cuff (See Figs. 236–8 and 238–5 ff.).

Principle

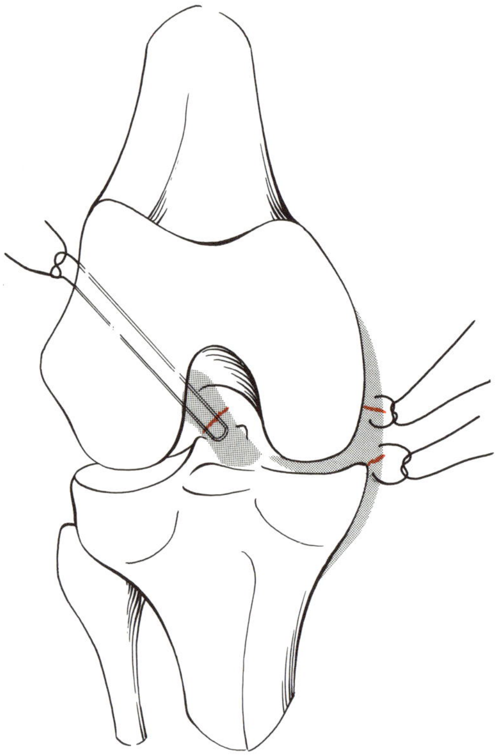

10
Interligamentous tears are reunited by suturing.

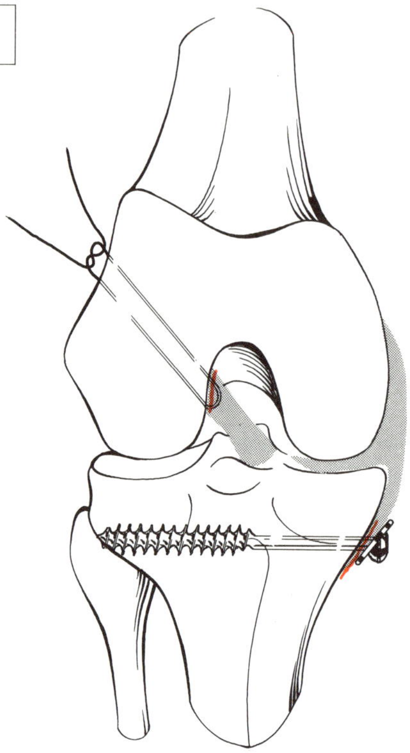

11
Avulsed fragments of bone are screwed on with use of toothed supporting disks (See Fig. 21–13). It is advantageous to prepare the bed for anchorage by removing the cortex and creating a cancellous surface.

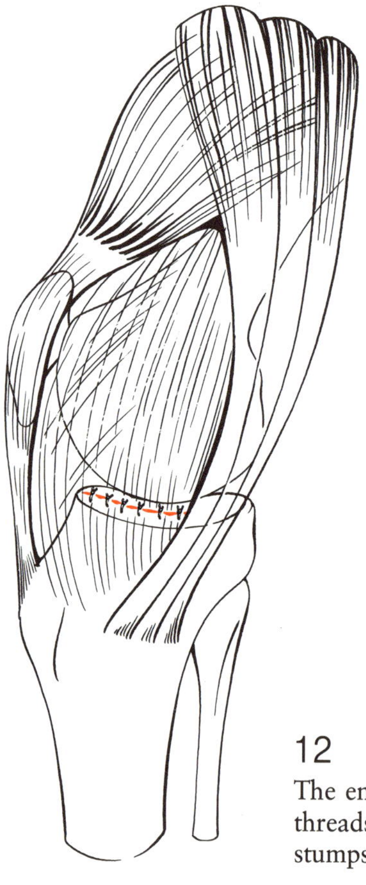

12
The end of the ligaments are not united in a stable manner by strong threads and many sutures, but only by accurately *approximating* the stumps with use of fine suture material.

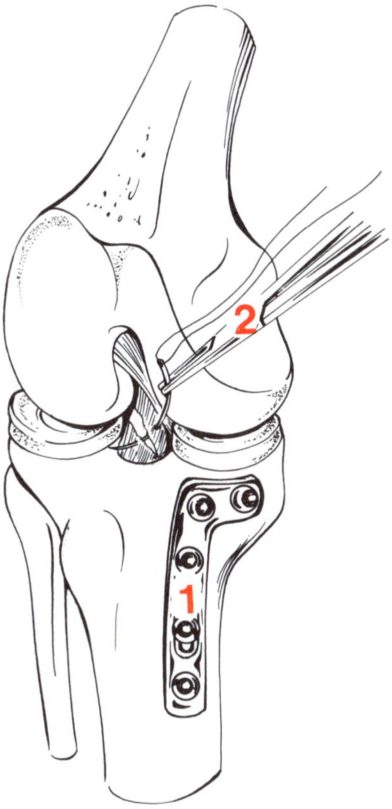

13
Osteosyntheses are performed prior to taking care of the ligaments.

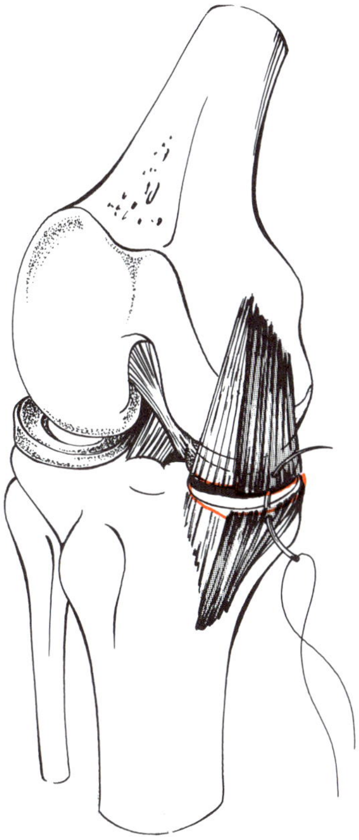

14
Meniscofemoral and meniscotibial connections are reinserted.

Postoperative care

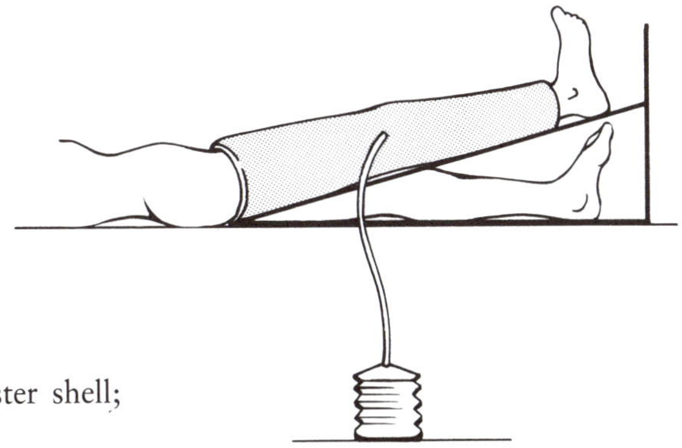

15
For the first days, plaster shell; later on, walking cast.

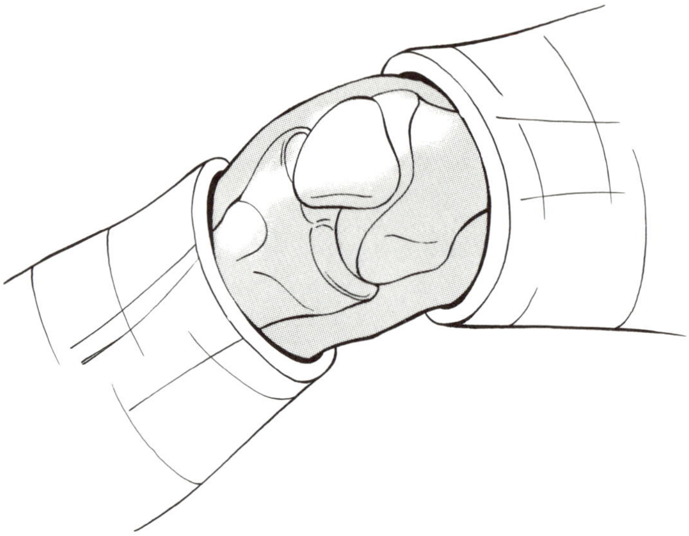

16

After applying the customary long-leg cast, a cylindrical piece 15 cm long is cut out over the knee joint.

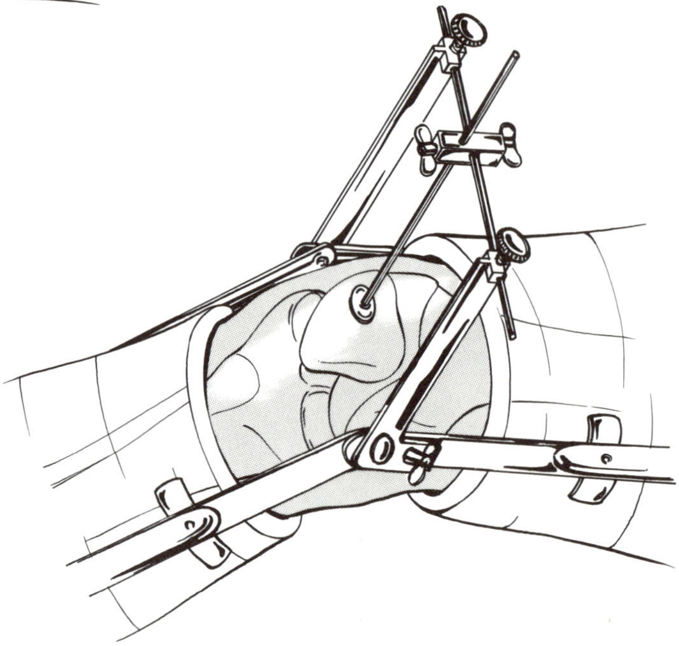

17

The articulated bars are fitted with use of a centering device.

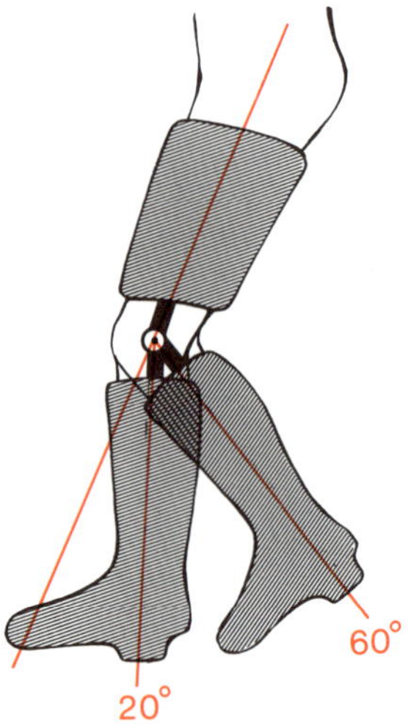

18

The articulated bars allow a mobility of 0-20-40 degrees.

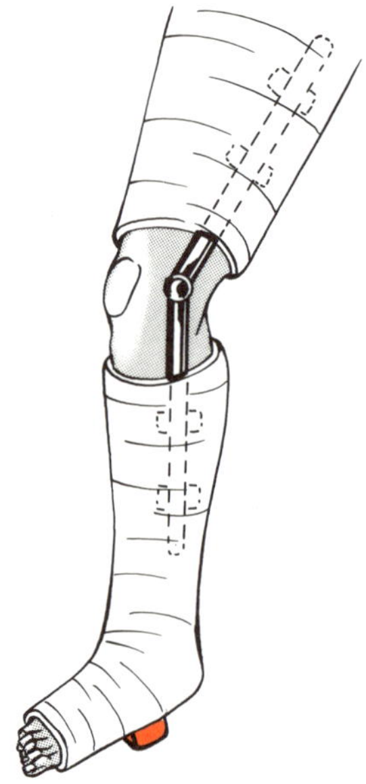

19

Even weightbearing is permissible with this kind of plaster cast.

Collateral ligaments

Diagnosis

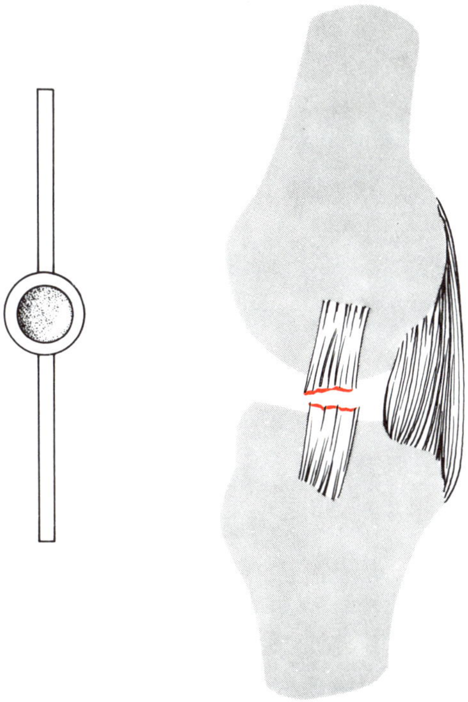

1

With the knee extended, an uninjured posterior capsular cuff can mimic stability of the collateral ligaments.

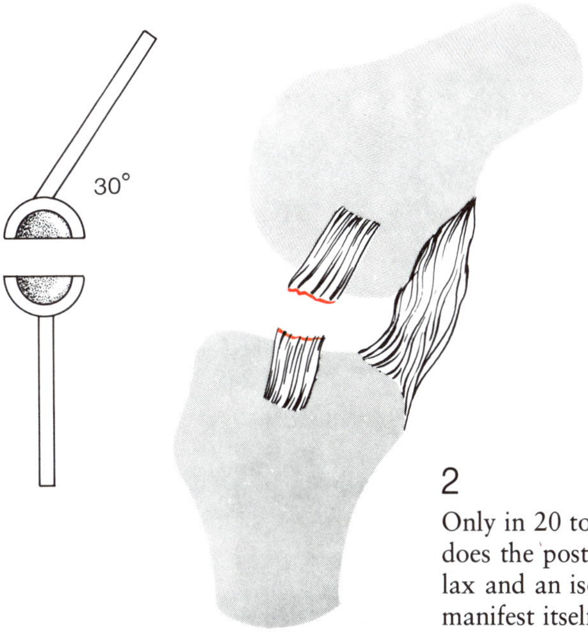

2

Only in 20 to 30 degrees of flexion does the posterior capsular cuff relax and an isolated ligament injury manifest itself.

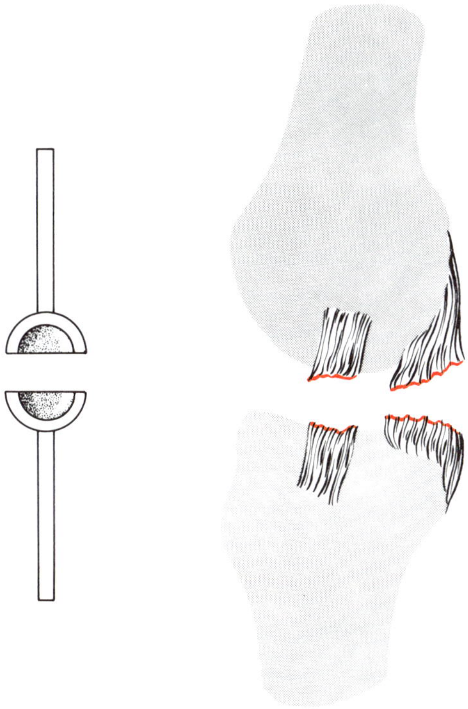

3

Separability of the articular surfaces with the knee joint extended gives evidence that more than an isolated injury of the collateral ligament is present.

Tibial collateral ligament

Diagnosis

1

Lateral separability of the joint surfaces: the tibial collateral ligament is injured about 15 to 20 times more often than the tibial ligament. Most frequently it is avulsed from its proximal (bony) insertion. In the majority of cases there exist additional injuries, such as tears of the capsule, the meniscofemoral or menisco-tibial connection, accompanied by hemorrhage into the joint. (See also Figs. 233–1 ff. for the differential diagnosis between isolated ligament injury and combination with injury of the posterior capsular cuff.)

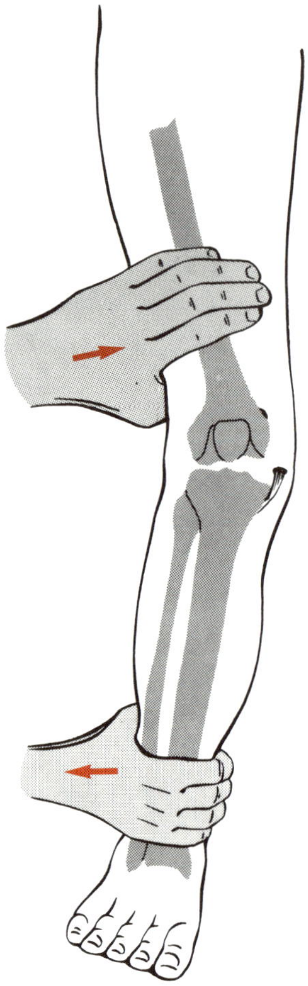

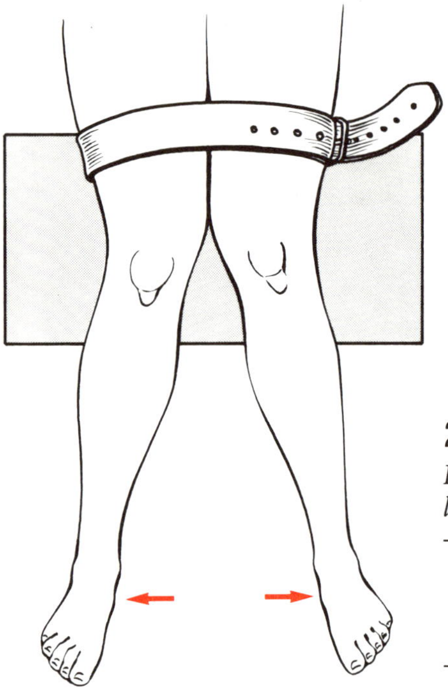

2

Roentgenogram with the lower leg slightly bent toward the side of the intact ligament.

- knee in 20° to 30° flexion. When the knee is extended an uninjured posterior capsular cuff can mimic stability of the collateral ligament. Only with flexion of 20° to 30° does the capsule relax and an isolated ligament injury become apparent.
- lower leg externally rotated.

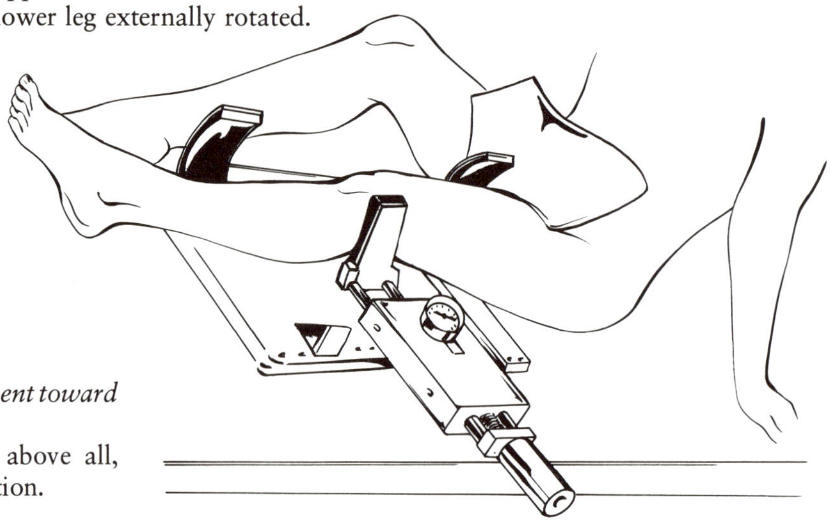

3

Roentgenogram with the lower leg slightly bent toward the side of the intact ligament.

A special device allows atraumatic and, above all, standardized examination and documentation.

Principle: See Figs. 230–10 ff.

Approach

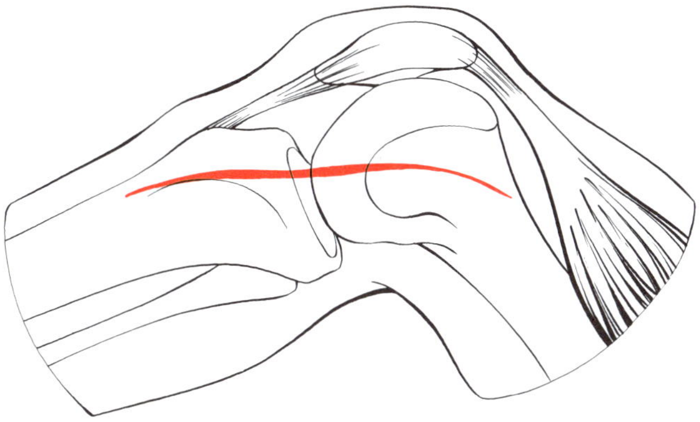

4
Skin incision, that also facilitates inspection of, and operation on, the posterior capsule.

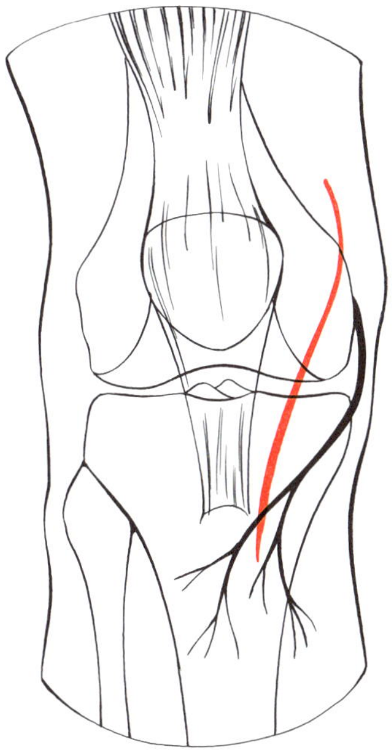

5
In performing the incision, one should take into account the course of the infrapatellar branch of the saphenus nerve.

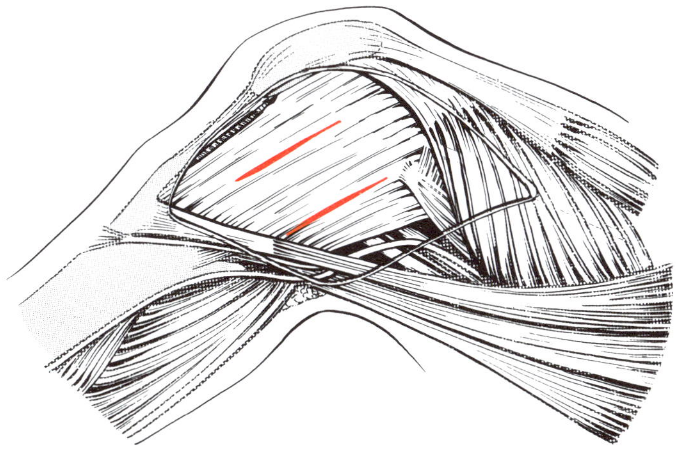

6
Exposing the tibial collateral ligament.

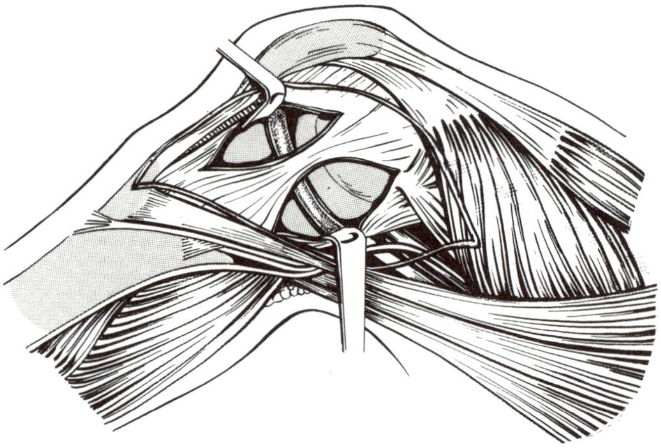

7
Inspection of the joint cavity.

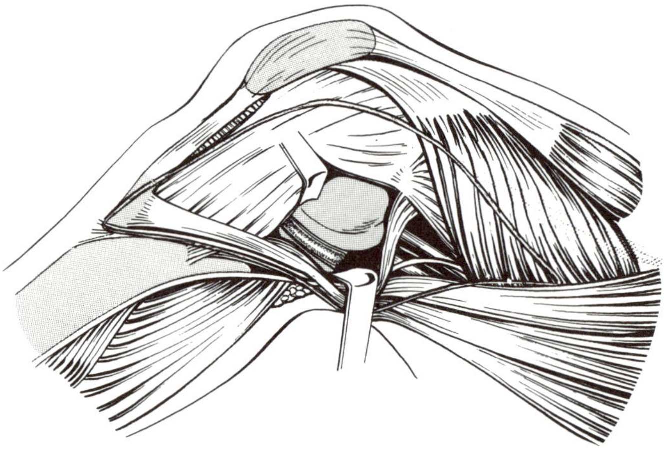

8
With disruption of the posterior capsular cuff, a suture is carried from the posterior to the anterior through drill holes across the head of the tibia (See Figs. 237–5 ff.).

Interligamentous tears are sutured; avulsions from bone are sutured and screwed on (See Fig. 21–13.).

Myoplasty of the gracilis muscle is often expedient for prophylactic reasons (See Fig. 236–9).

Postoperative care See Fig. 231–15.

Possibilities of reconstruction

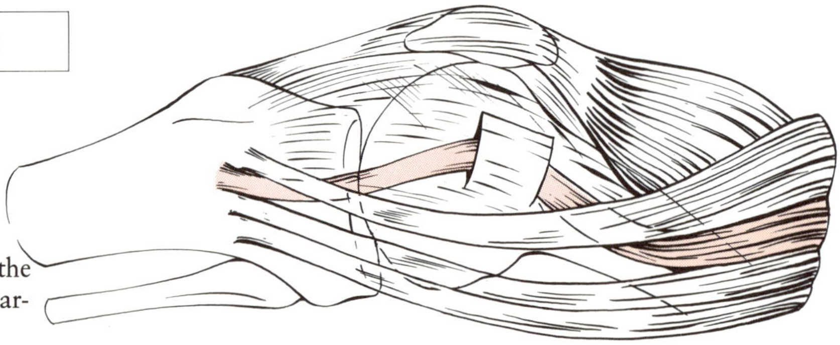

9
Dynamic or static plastic repair, using the tendon of the gracilis, semitendinosus or sartorius muscles.

Fibular collateral ligament

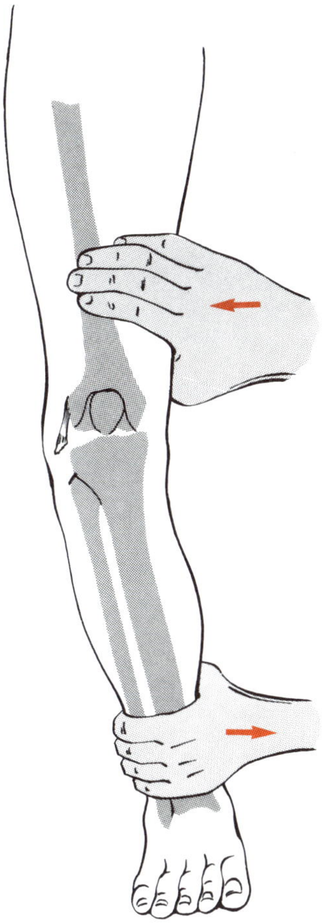

Diagnosis

1
Isolated rupture of the fibular ligament in particular is an infrequent event. It is often associated with avulsion from the head of the fibula. Hemarthrosis is absent since the ligament possesses no connection with the joint space.

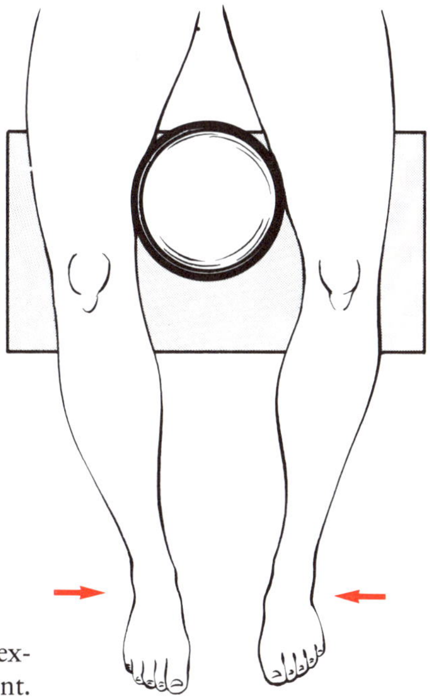

2
Radiographic study of the fibular ligament:
– knee in 20° to 30° flexion. Separability of the joint surfaces even with the knee extended proves that more than an isolated injury of the collateral ligament is present.

Principle: See Figs. 230–10 ff.

Approach

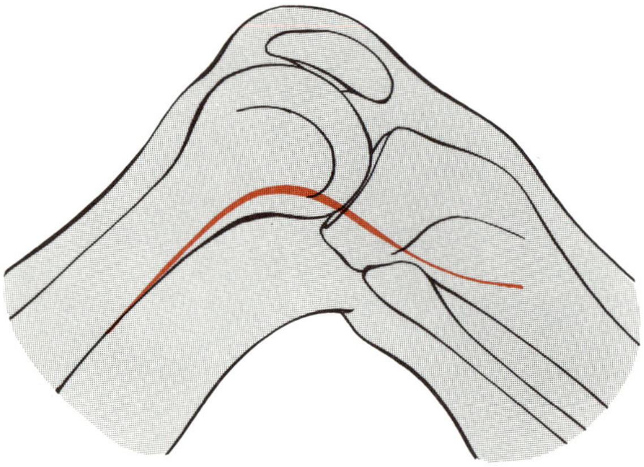

3
Skin incision.

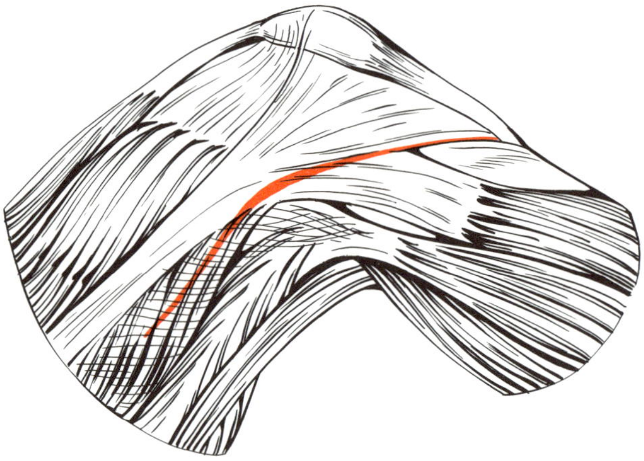

4
Splitting of the fascia.

Tactics

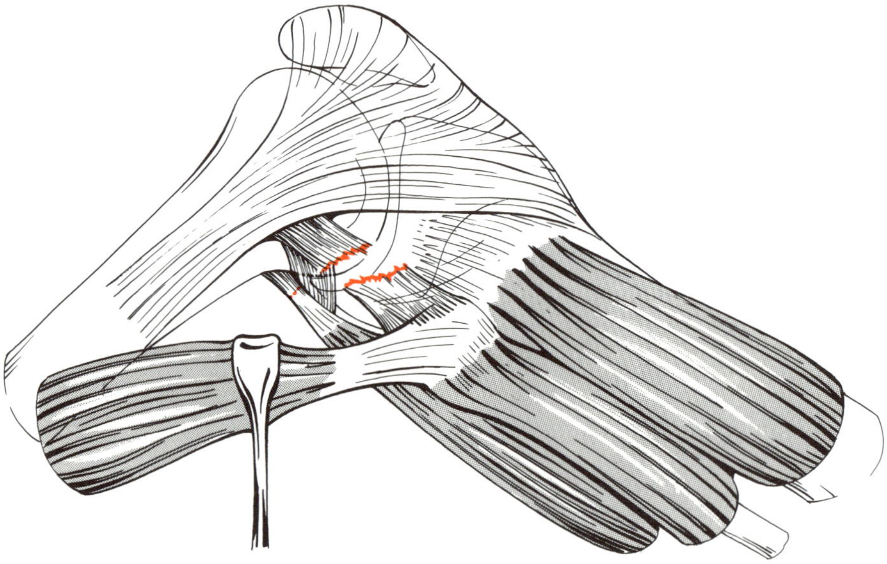

5
Interligamentous tear of the fibular collateral ligament. With a complex injury, the subjacent capsule is also torn away from the head of the tibia posteriorly. In this instance, the tendinous portion of the gastrocnemius muscle is divided in such a way that it can subsequently be reunited.

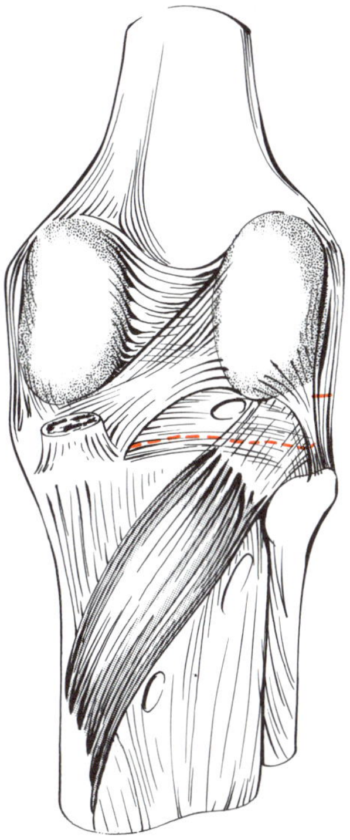

6

Knee joint viewed from behind. Avulsion of the posterior capsule from the head of the tibia.

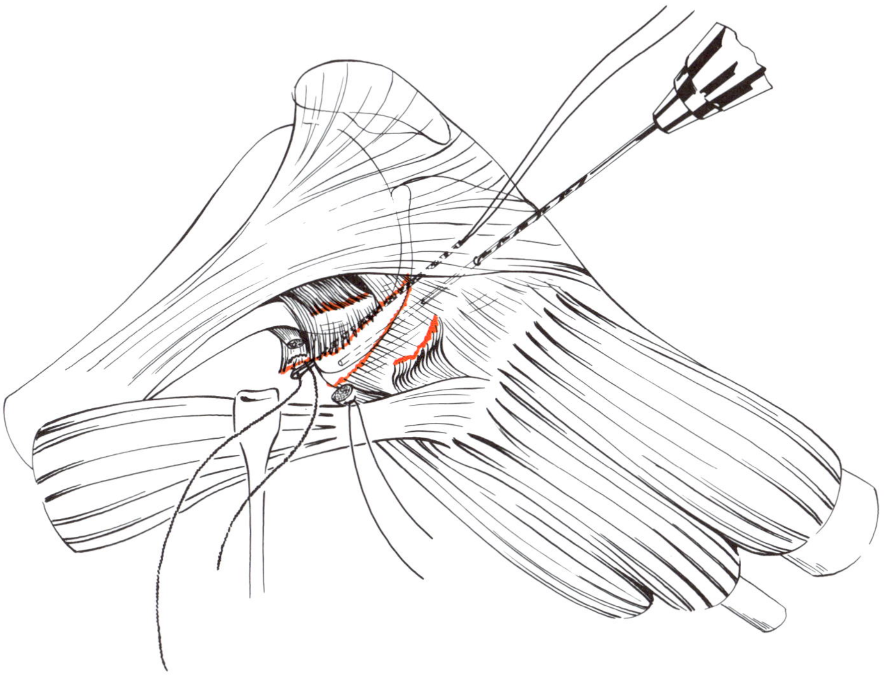

7

Drill holes 2mm wide are created. By use of a wire loop, the ends of the wire, fastened to the posterior capsule, are pulled, in an anterior direction, through the drill holes.

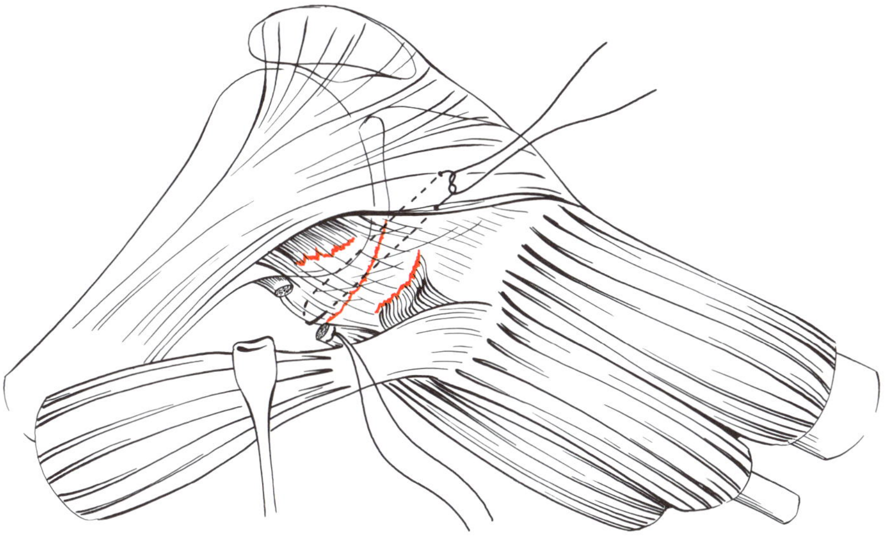

8

Following reinsertion of the torn-off posterior capsule the collateral ligament is sutured.

Postoperative care

See Figs. 231–15 ff.

Possibilities of reconstruction

Using the tendon of the biceps or sartorius muscle, as shown in Fig. 236–9.

Cruciate ligaments

Anatomy

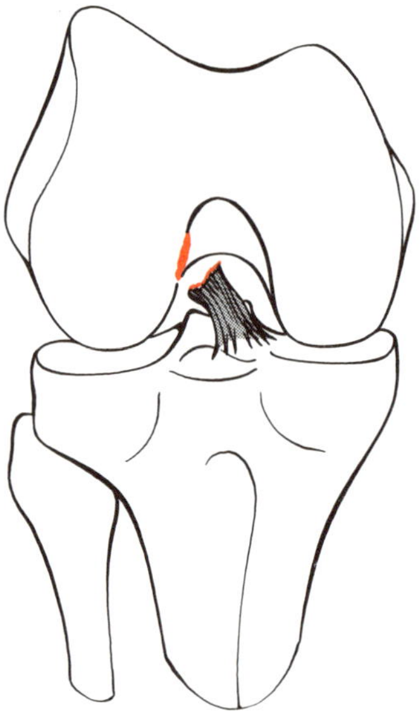

1

Proximal insertion of *anterior cruciate ligament.*

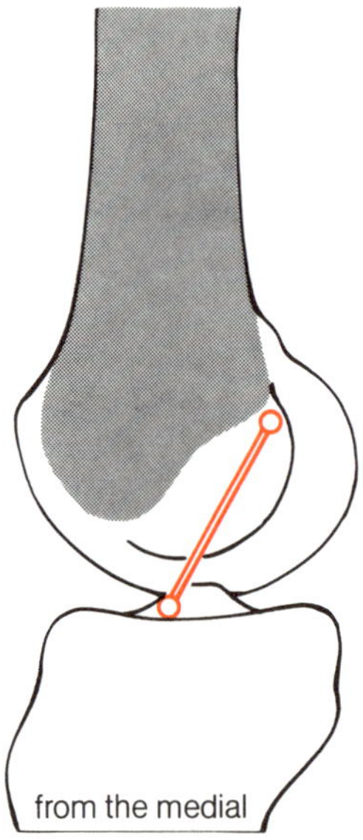

2

Only by accurately inserting the anterior cruciate ligament is it possible to avoid *extension* at the knee joint without slackening of the ligament and resultant instability.

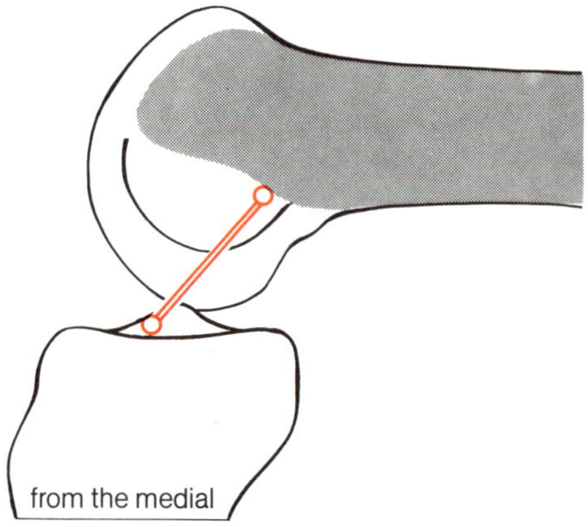

3

Similarly, only accurate insertion of the anterior cruciate ligament allows *flexion* at the knee joint without overstretching the ligament.

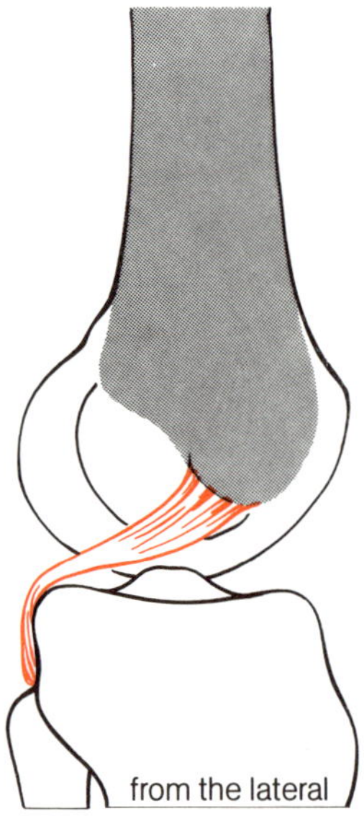

4

The site of insertion of the anterior cruciate ligament lies in the dorsal third of the lateral femoral condyle.

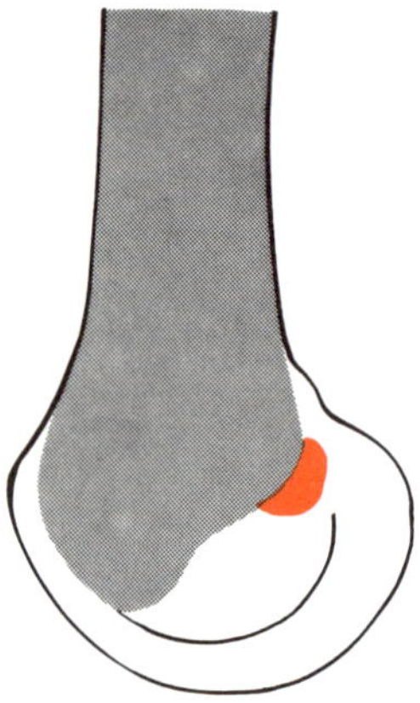

5

Sites of insertion of the *posterior cruciate ligament.*

Diagnosis

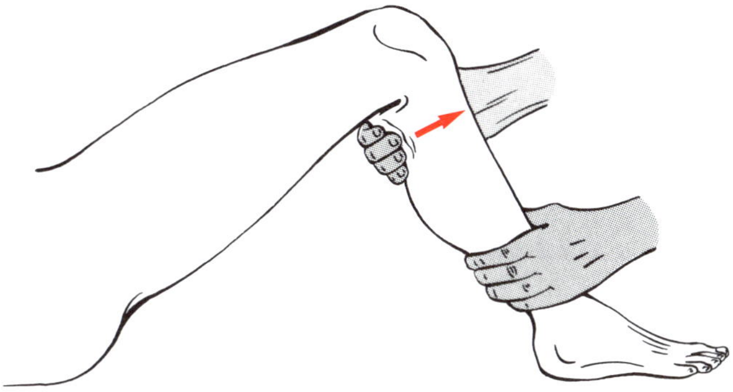

6

Drawer sign. Isolated disruption of the cruciate ligaments occurs infrequently; generally it is part of a complex injury (See p. 244 f.). Clinical and radiographic examination is done by eliciting the so-called drawer sign.

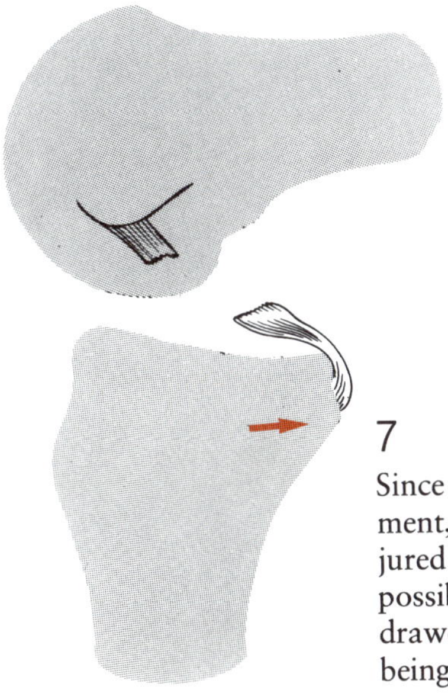

7

Since the posterior cruciate ligament, which is singularly seldom injured tenses on flexing the knee, the possible eliciting of a "posterior drawer sign" is a reliable proof of its being injured.

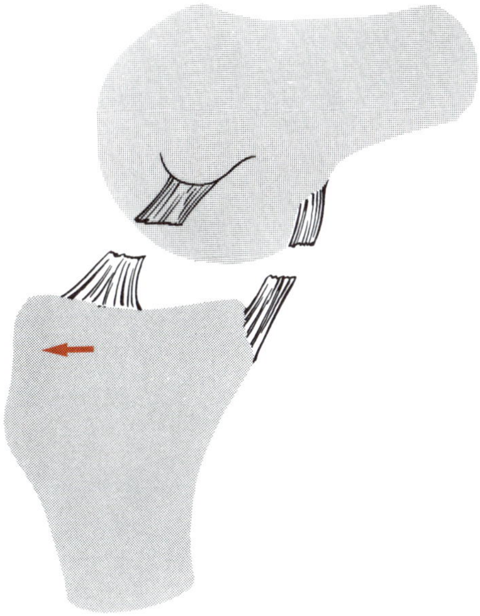

8

The anterior cruciate ligament, in contrast, tenses only on extending the knee. Without concomitant disruption of the posterior capsule, the drawer sign is but little marked.

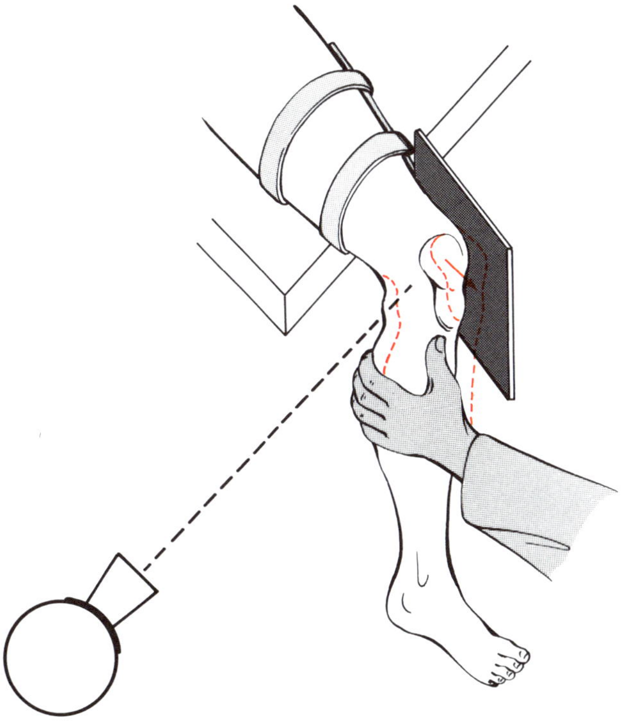

9

The cassette is doubly exposed: once in the normal position of the knee joint and once with the drawer sign elicited. Do not omit a comparative radiographic study of the uninjured side.

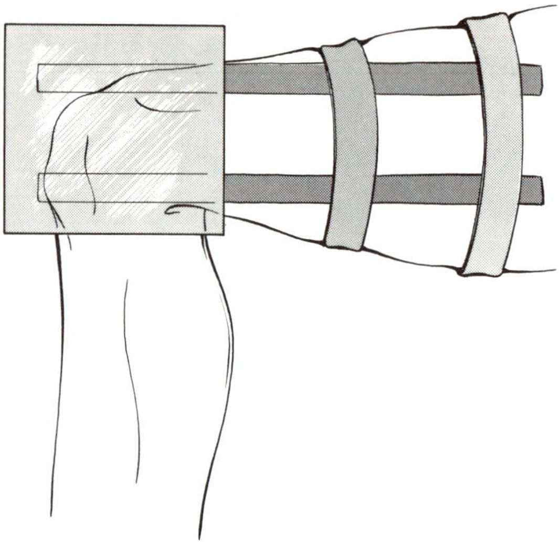

10

The cassette is fastened to the thigh with a wooden, radiolucent holding fixture so that it can move along with the thigh.

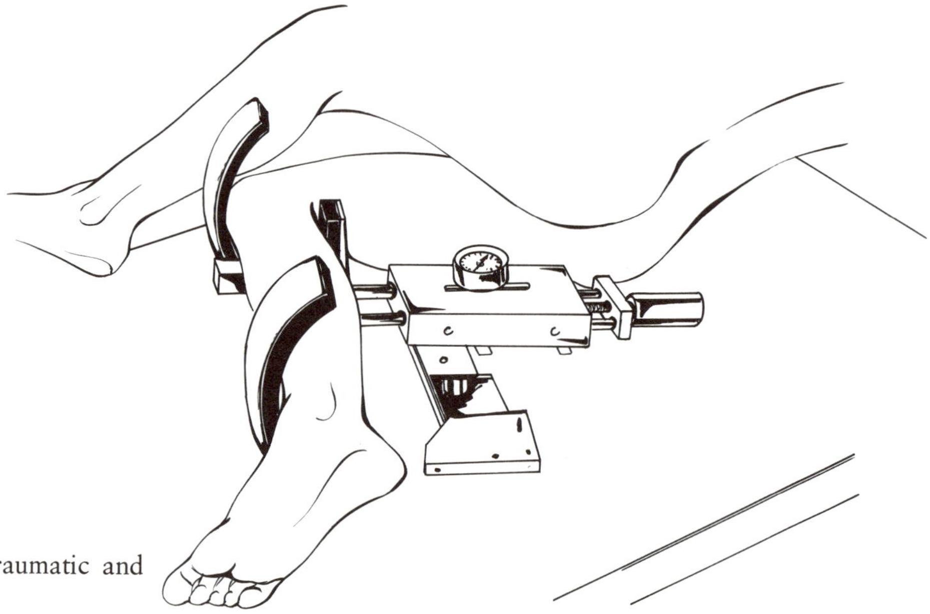

11

A special device allows more atraumatic and standardized roentgenograms.

Principle See Figs. 230–10ff.

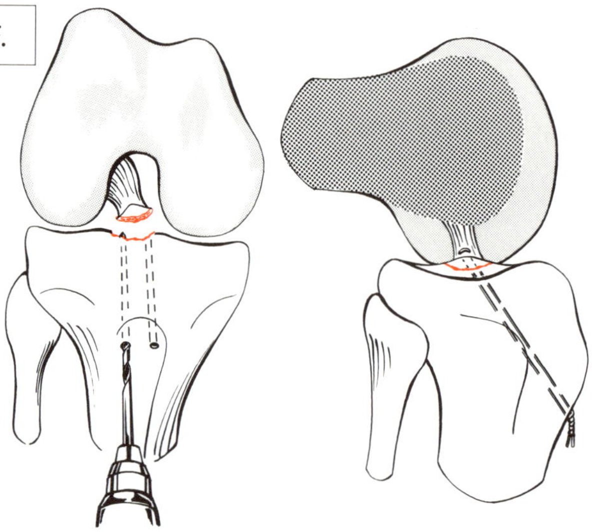

12

Transosseous fixation *distally*.

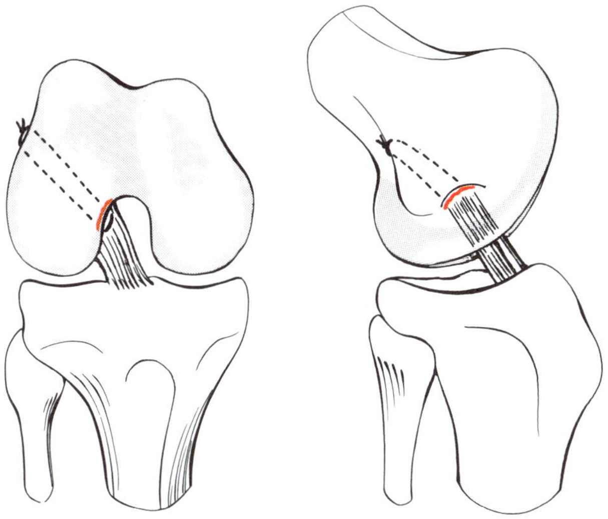

13
Transosseous fixation *proximally*.

Approach See Figs. 235–4 ff.

Postoperative care. See Figs. 231–15 ff.

Possibilities of reconstruction

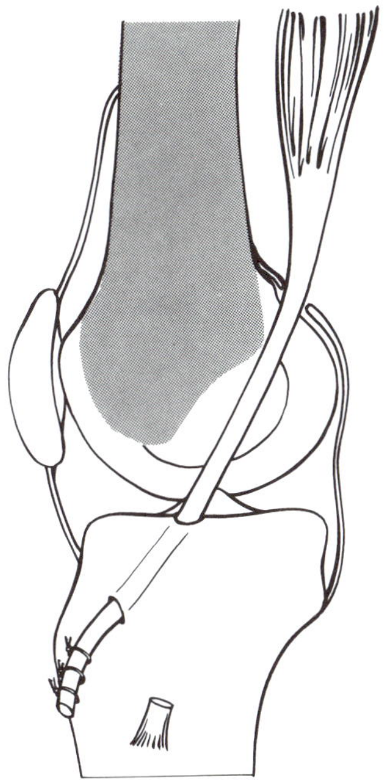

14
Anterior cruciate ligament: dynamic or static myoplasty using the gracilis or the semitendinosus muscle.

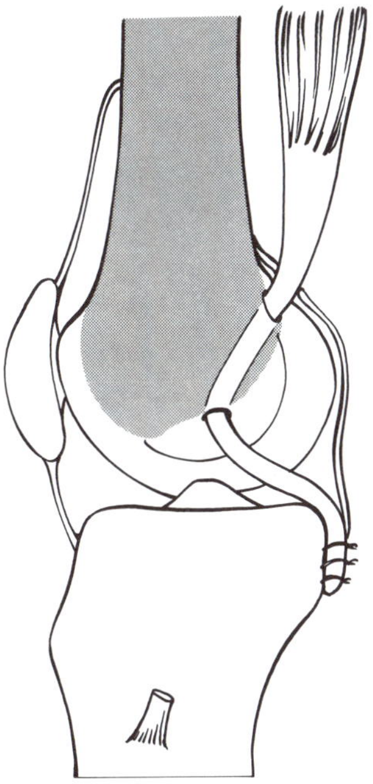

15
Posterior cruciate ligament: Similarly, dynamic or static myoplasty using the gracilis or the semitendinosus muscle.

Complex injury

Types of injuries See Figs. 228–5 ff.

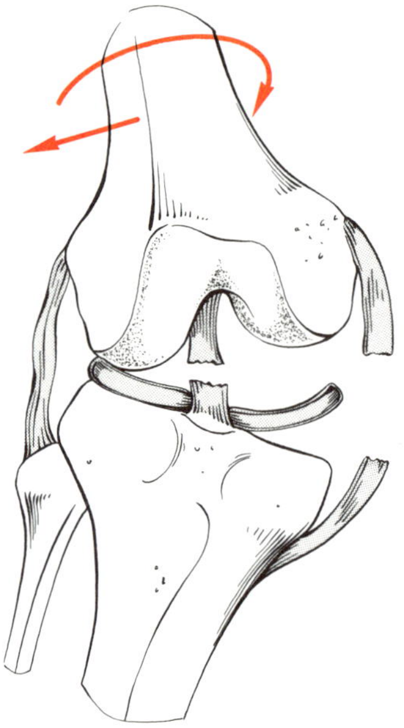

1

Very often one meniscus or both are involved in complex instabilities. A relatively frequent and typical combination is the "unlucky triad" which, as an anteromedial complex instability, comprises an injury of the anterior cruciate ligament, the tibial collateral ligament with the capsular cuff, and the medial meniscus.

Diagnosis

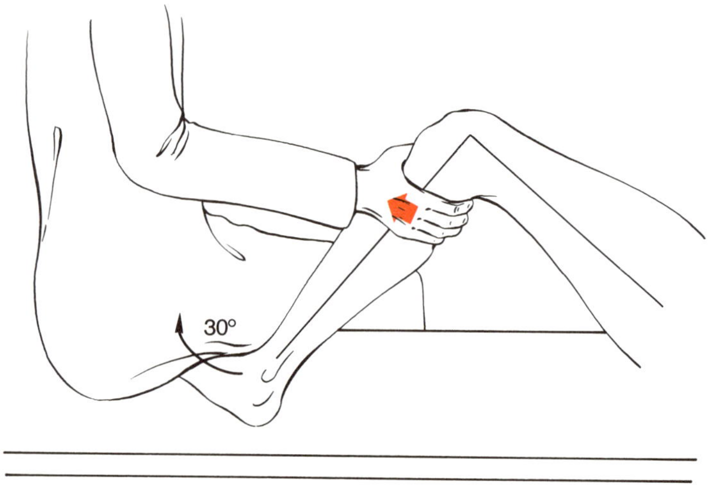

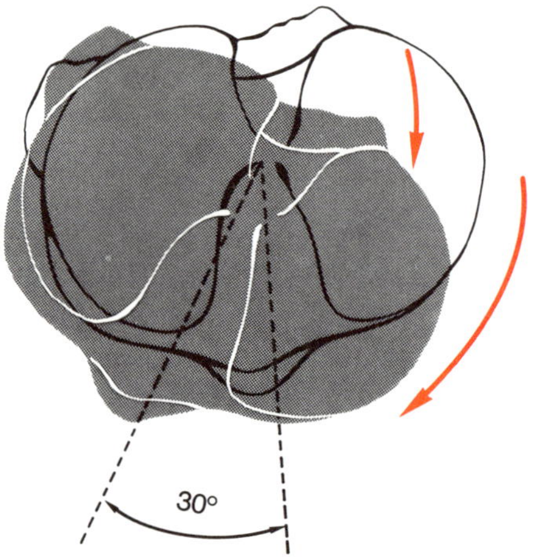

2

Complex instabilities: to ascertain whether – and what kind of – complex instability is present, proceed as follows:
Try to elicit the drawer sign, once in the intermediate position, once with the foot fixed in 30° external rotation (for injuries in the postero*lateral* region), and once with the foot fixed in 15° internal rotation (for injuries in the postero*medial* region).
In these rotary positions the respective compartments do not allow any drawer movement on their side, as long as they are uninjured.

3

In performing this examination, one tries to locate the pivot point; it migrates from the unstable compartment to the stable side. This phenomenon manifests itself by the fact that, with the corresponding rotation, the drawer sign is more distinct in the injured half of the joint than it is in the intermediate position or on rotation in the opposite direction.

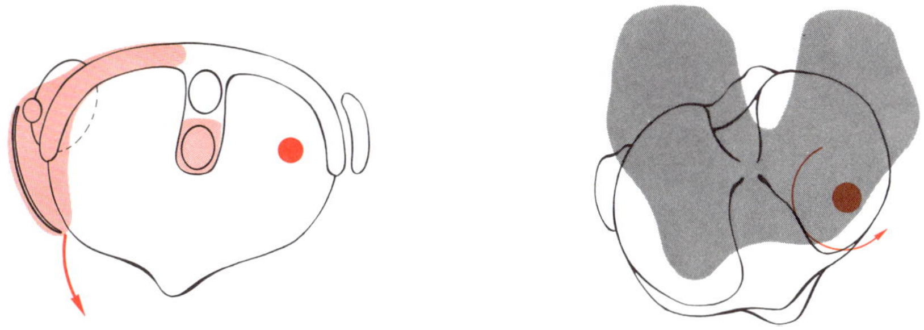

4
Findings in order of frequency: finding in *anteromedial* complex instability = anterior cruciate ligament plus tibial collateral ligament plus medial posterior capsular cuff. This combination if often associated with injury of the medial meniscus. (See Fig. 244–1, “unlucky triad”.)

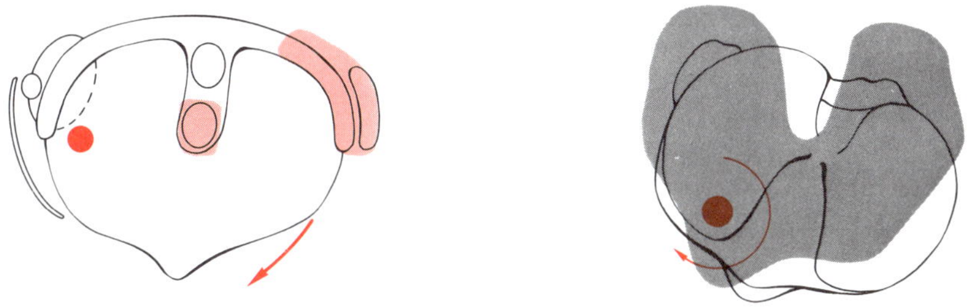

5
Finding in *anterolateral* complex instability = anterior cruciate ligament plus fibular collateral ligament plus lateral posterior capsular cuff. Association with injury of the lateral meniscus is possible.

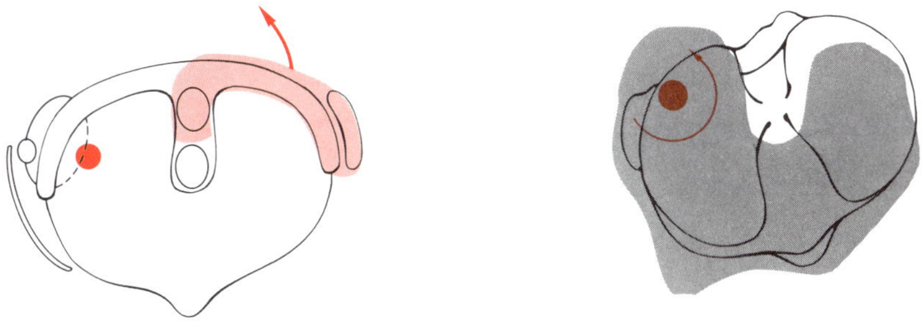

6
Finding in *posterolateral* complex instability = posterior cruciate ligament plus fibular collateral ligament plus lateral posterior capsular cuff.

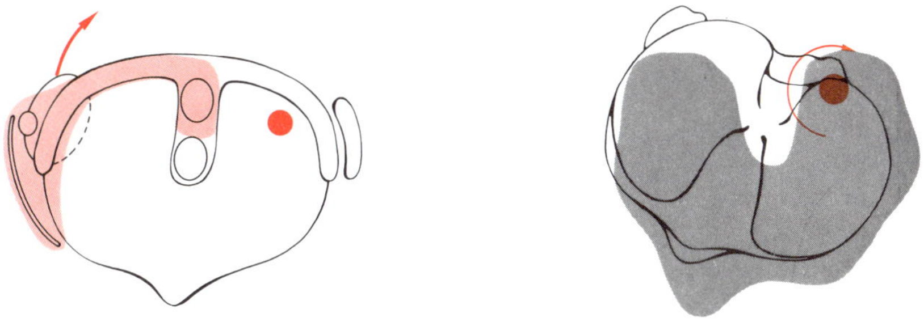

7
Finding in *posteromedial* complex instability = posterior cruciate ligament plus tibial collateral ligament plus medial posterior capsular cuff. Association with injury of either meniscus or both menisci is possible.

Operation

See Figs. 238–3 ff. (lateral injury) and Fig. 236–8 (medial injury).

Meniscus

Anatomy

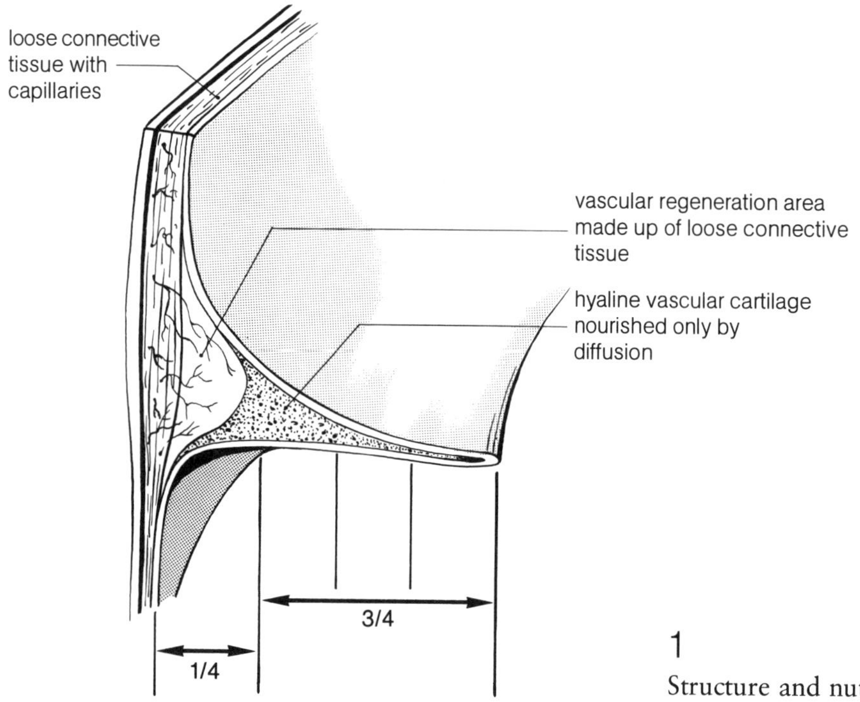

1
Structure and nutritional conditions of the meniscus.

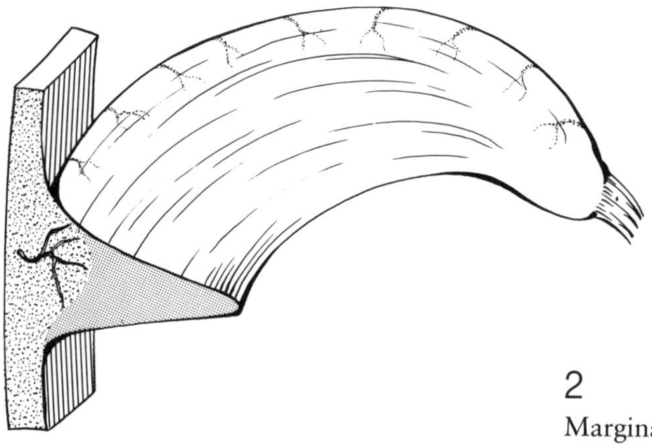

2
Marginal area nourished by blood vessels.

3

The pivot point of the knee joint lies eccentrically on the medial side of the joint. The femoral condyles in the diagram show a backward divergence (similar to the angular setting of the front wheels of an automobile to improve its directional stability).

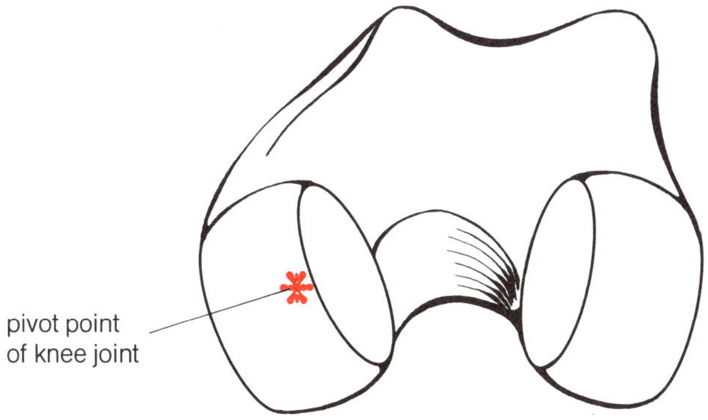

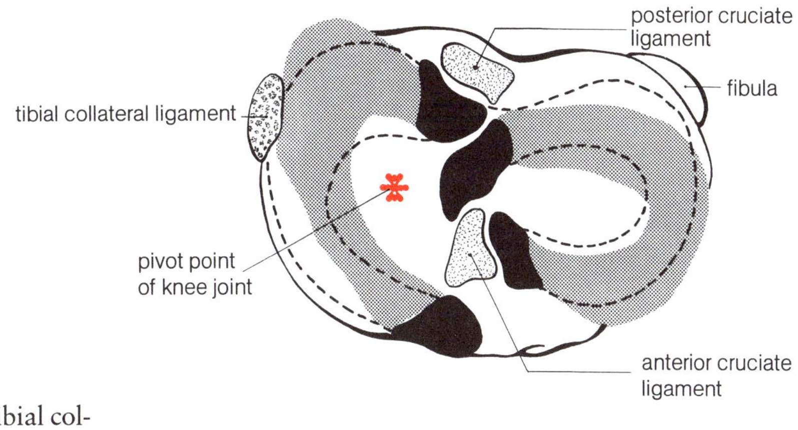

4

The medial meniscus is firmly attached to its tibial collateral ligament. Thus it is less movable and, with the varying positions of the knee joint, it undergoes stronger deformation than the lateral meniscus. That is why locking and injuries occur about ten times more frequently in the medial than in the lateral meniscus.

Types of injuries

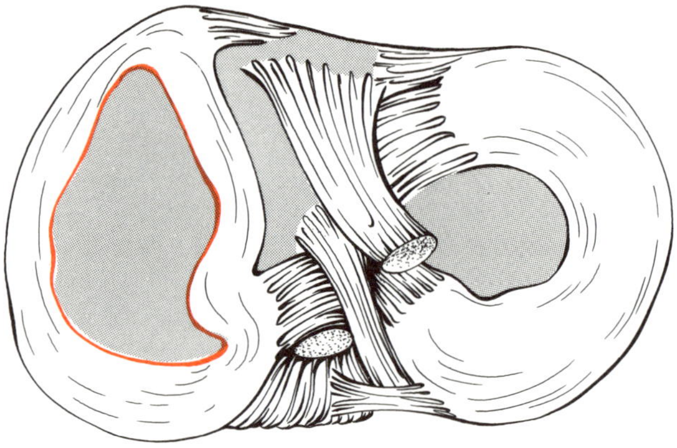

5

Most frequent type of meniscus injury: longitudinal or "bucket handle" tear (with the inner portion of the meniscus often being dislocated medialward between the condyles of femur and tibia) and...

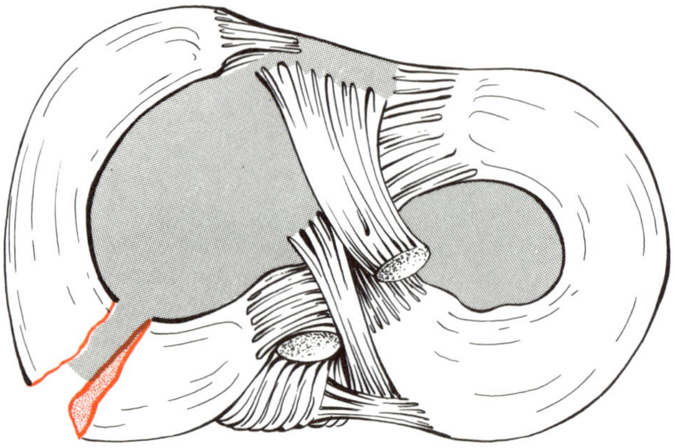

6

... transverse tear, which frequently lies posteriorly and is difficult of access. Occasionally the ruptured portion remains in place as "residual posterior meniscus" and gives rise to renewed discomfort.

Positioning See Fig. 219–6.

Approach

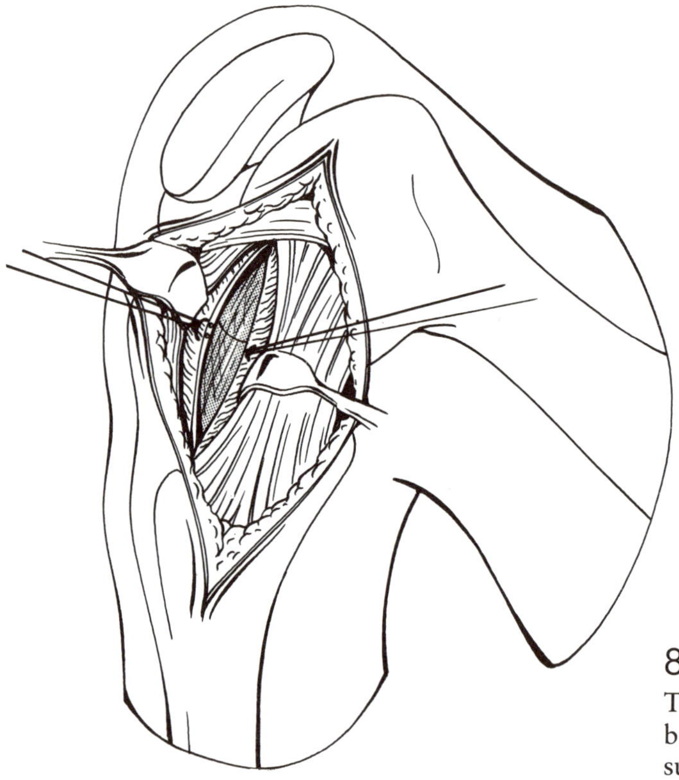

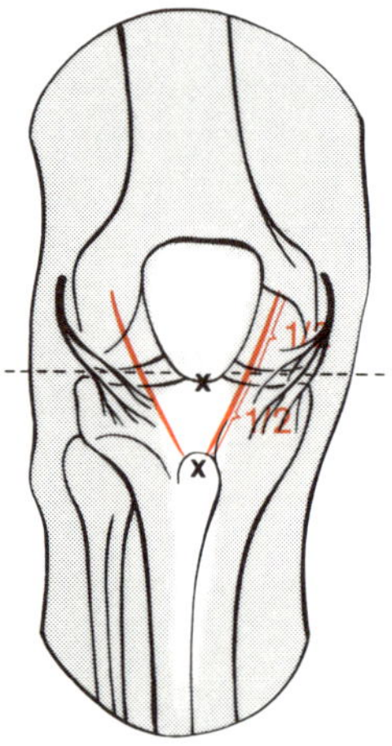

7

Skin incision about 6 to 7 cm long, lateral to the border of the patella and directed toward the tibial tubercle.

8

The anterior and inferior genicular vessels are undersewn before being divided and prior to opening the joint capsule.

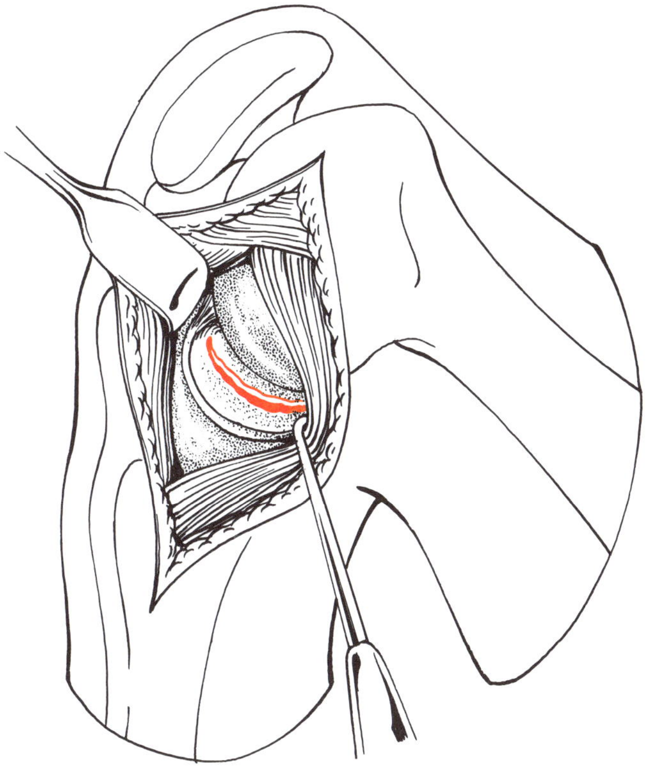

9

After opening the joint capsule the injured meniscus becomes visible.

Tactics

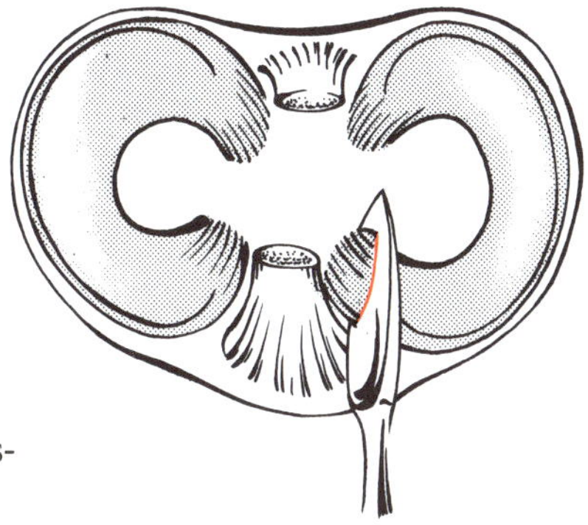

10

The anterior extremity and the anterior circumference of the meniscus are resected.

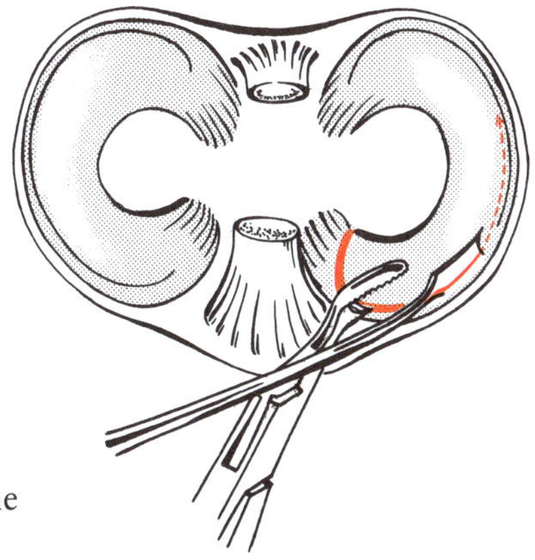

11

The anterior circumference is resected backward to beyond the collateral ligament under direct vision.

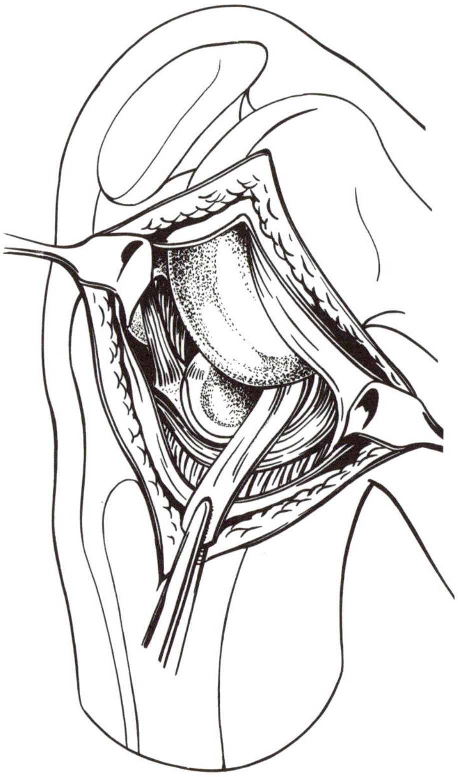

12

In doing so, particular caution should be exercised in the region of the tibial collateral ligament.

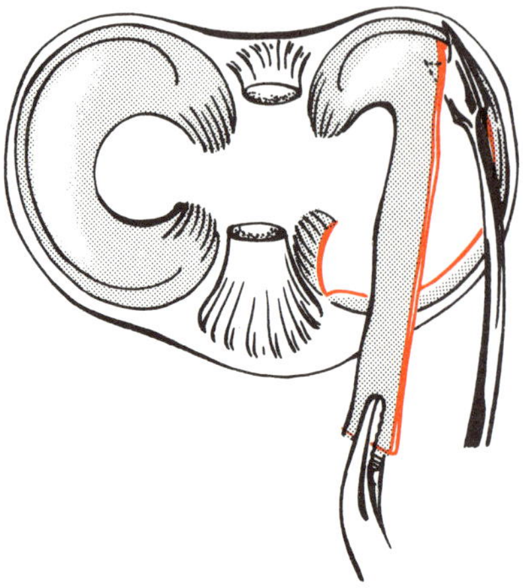

13

When the set of ligaments is not too tight, one can often succeed in removing the meniscus completely...

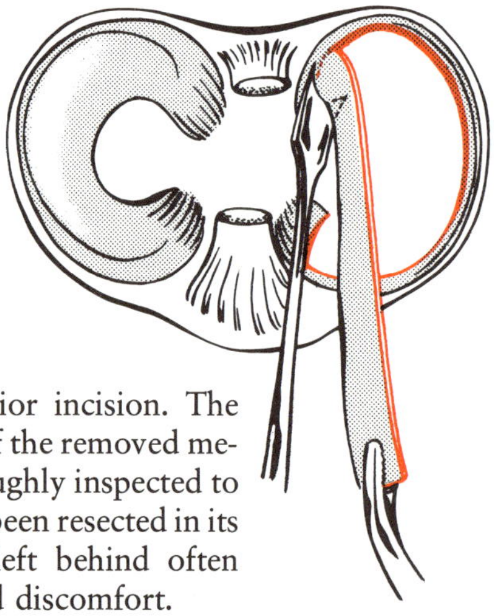

14

... through an anterior incision. The posterior extremity of the removed meniscus must be thoroughly inspected to be certain that it has been resected in its entirety. Remnants left behind often give rise to continued discomfort.

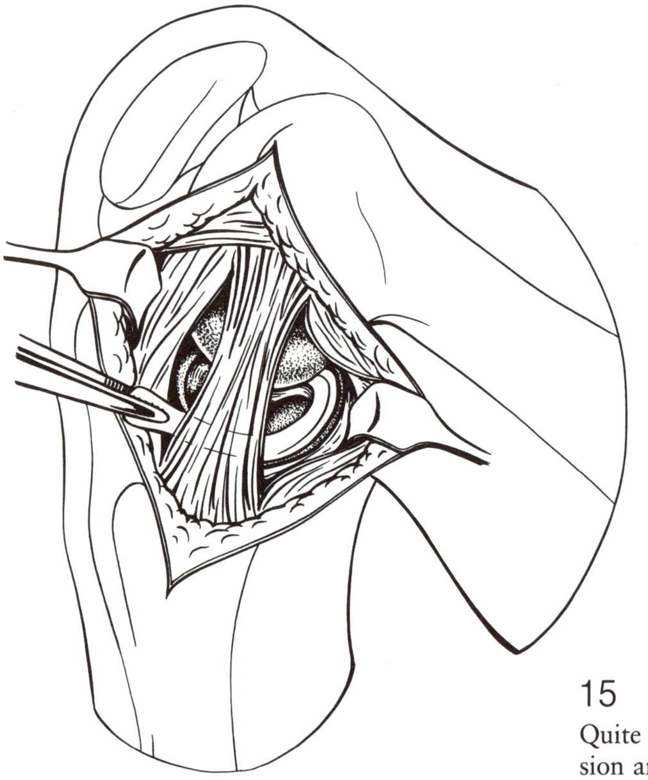

15

Quite frequently, however, the posterior extremity and its supension are not accessible through an anterior incision.

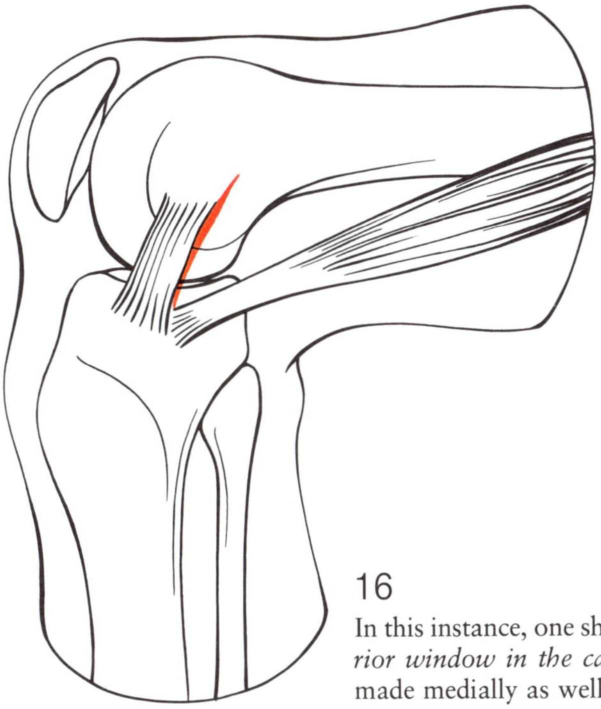

16

In this instance, one should not hesitate to create a *posterior window in the capsule.* To this end, an incision is made medially as well as...

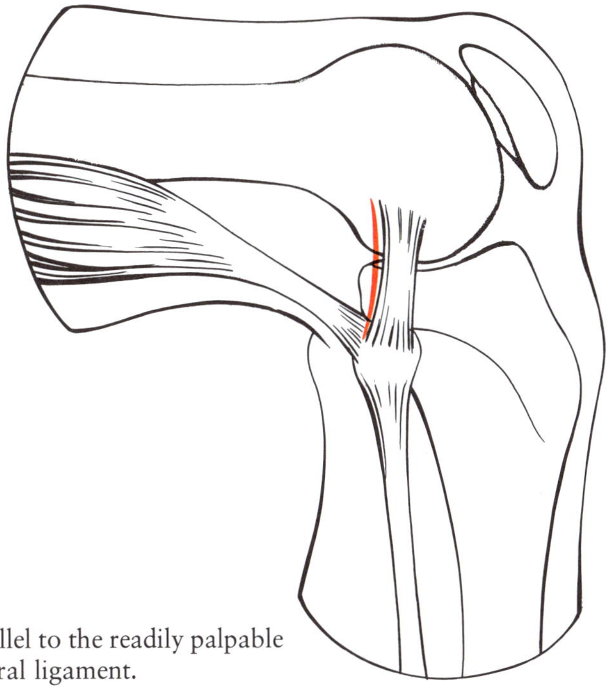

17

... laterally, posterior and parallel to the readily palpable posterior border of the collateral ligament.

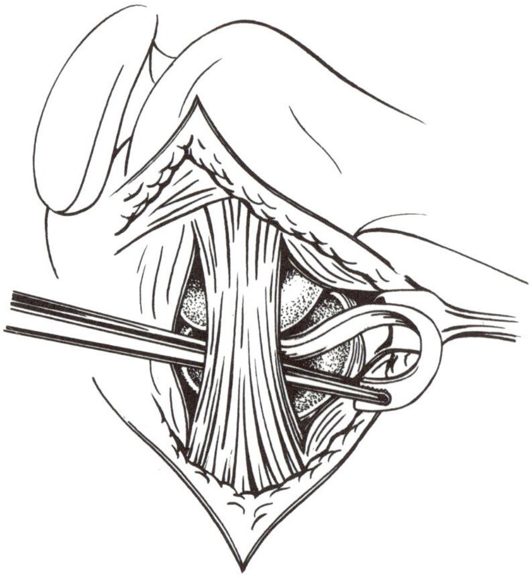

18

The meniscus is mobilized from the anterior to the posterior beyond the collateral ligament; then it is pushed dorsally underneath the collateral ligament into the posterior arthrotomy wound.

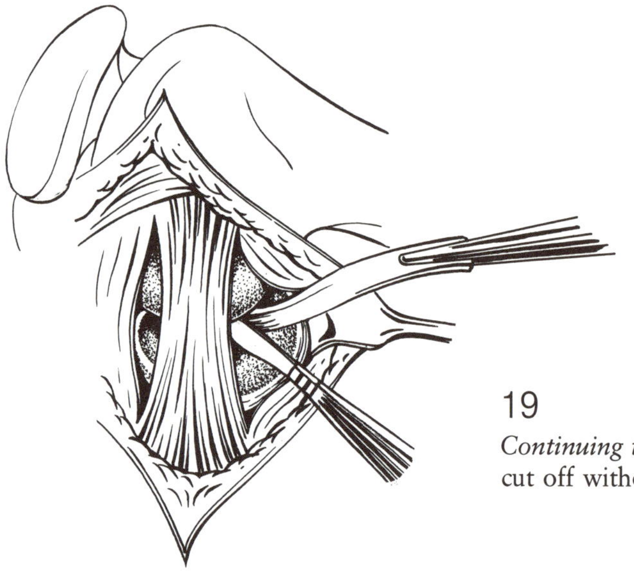

19

Continuing the procedure under direct vision, the meniscus can then be cut off without difficulty from its posterior attachment.

Closure of the wound

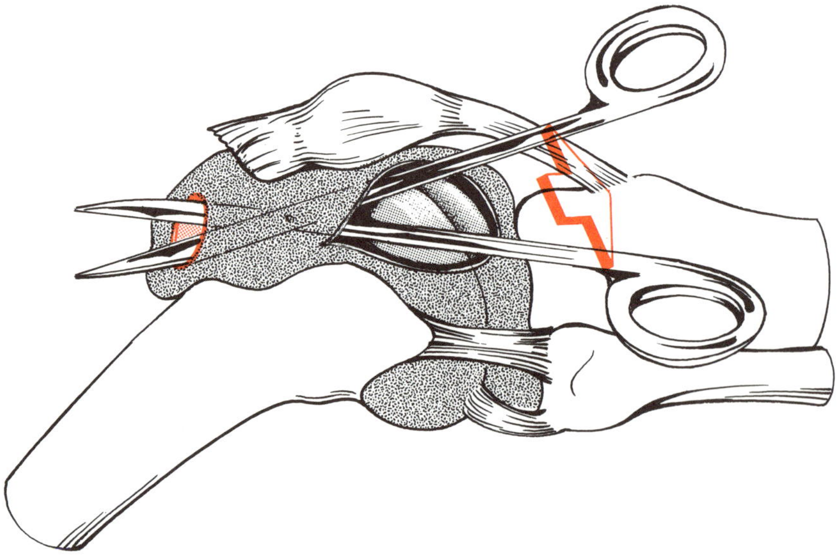

20

Creating a window in the suprapatellar pouch has proved helpful in avoiding a postoperative effusion into the joint. To this end, the pouch is pierced at its highest point with closed long scissors which are then opened and withdrawn. Following this, tight closure of the capsule in the region of the arthrotomy wound can be performed. In this way the synovial fluid is prevented from soaking the wound.

Head of tibia

Types of injuries

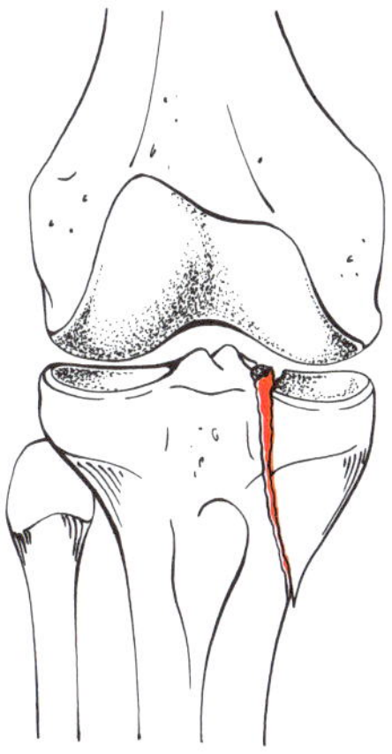

1

Cleanly broken-off fragments without comminuted areas can occasionally be fixed with sufficient stability by using two screws. Additional support with a plate is advisable, though.

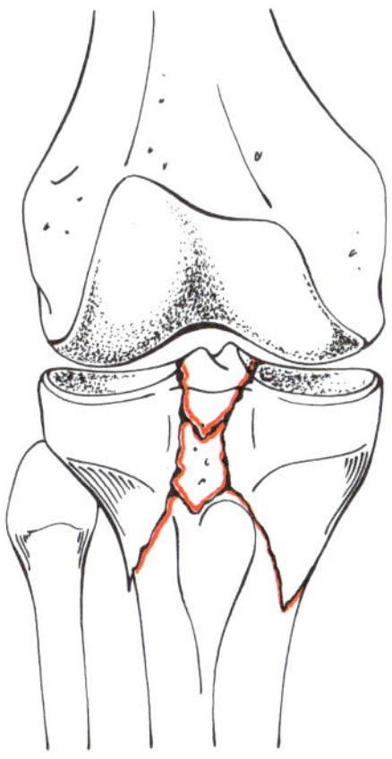

2

Bicondylar fractures always require support with a plate. Appropriate means for this purpose are half-tubular and T plates. Narrow plates, under the thin soft-tissue cover, often fill up the space too much.

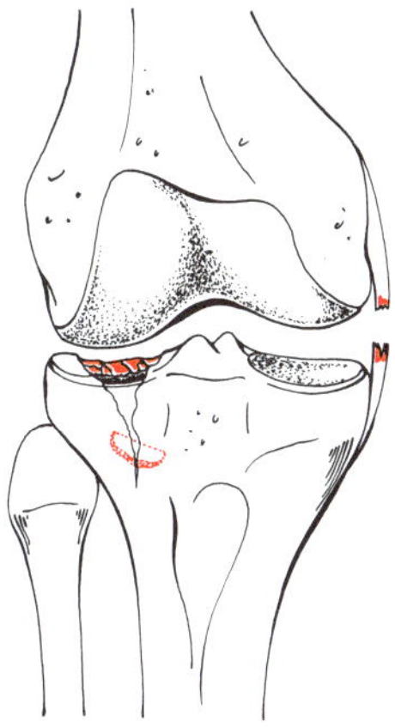

3

In depressed fractures, the depressed portions of the joint must be lifted and, in most cases, be lined with cancellous bone underneath.

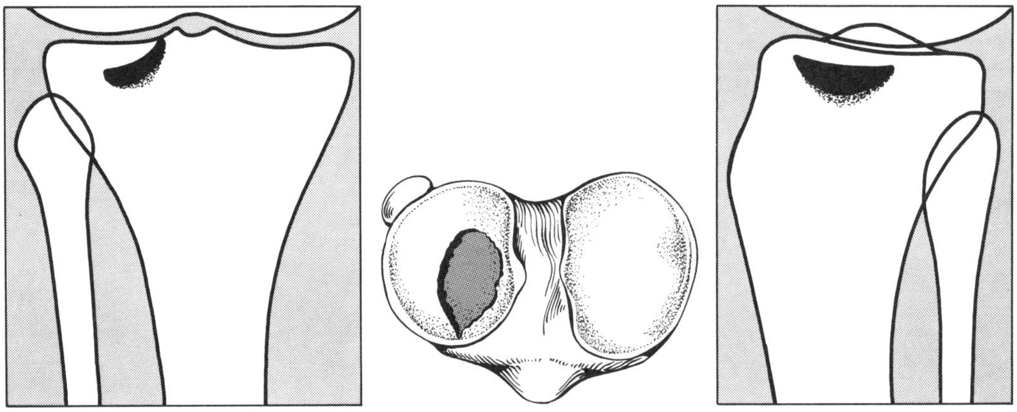

4

The operation plan must take into account the site of the depression. Routine roentgenograms are inconclusive in this respect and often mimic a central depression (See Fig. 255–7.).

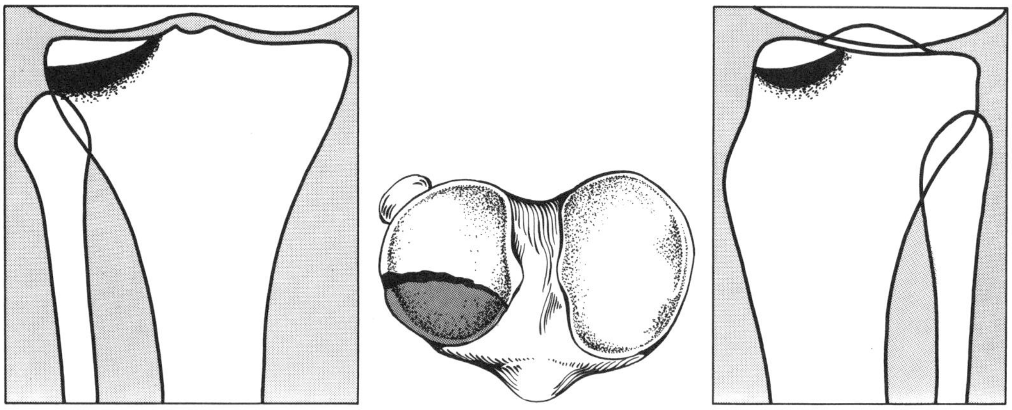

5

Frequently, however, only an anterior lesion is present; this can be corrected with relative ease.

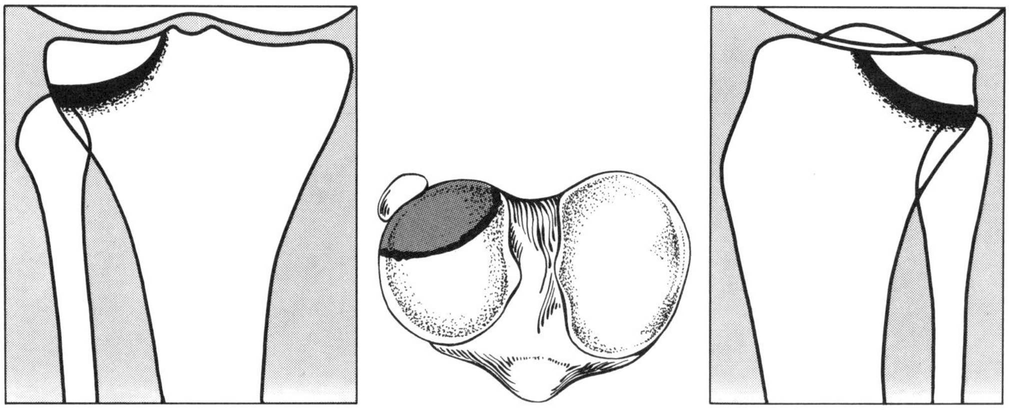

6

Very frequently parts of the posterior condyle are depressed. Elevating them, particularly in the lateral condyle, is rather difficult and therefore, insufficiently achieved as a rule.

DIAGNOSIS

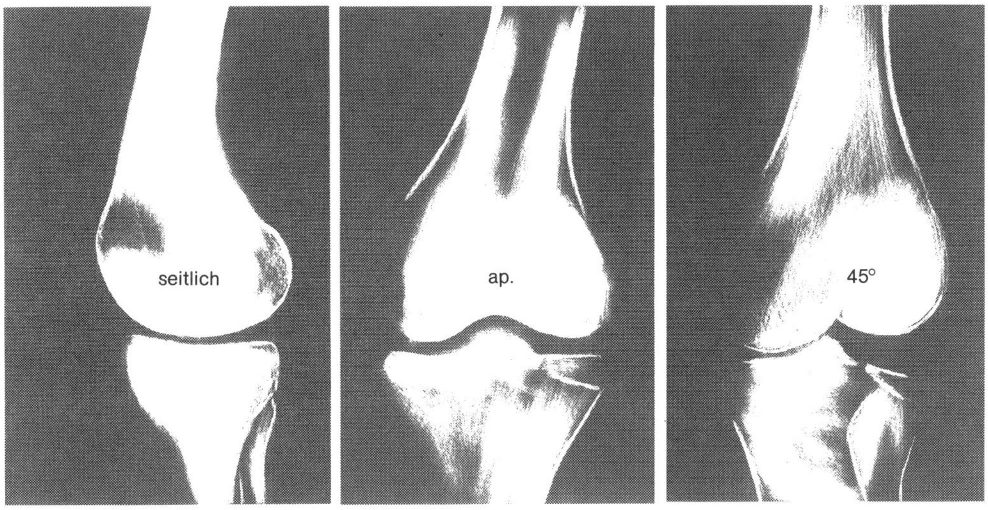

7

Oblique roentgenograms taken at a 45° angle of rotation generally settle the diagnosis and are, in fact, essential in drawing up the operation plan. Taken *after* the operation, these roentgenograms are generally very revealing.

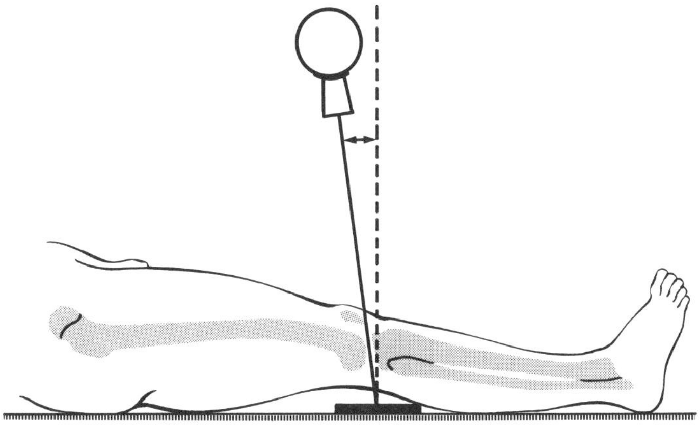

8

In making an anteroposterior roentgenogram, take into account that the plateau of the head of the tibia slopes dorsally by about 7 degrees. Accordingly, the central ray must be adjusted by the same amount from the cranial...

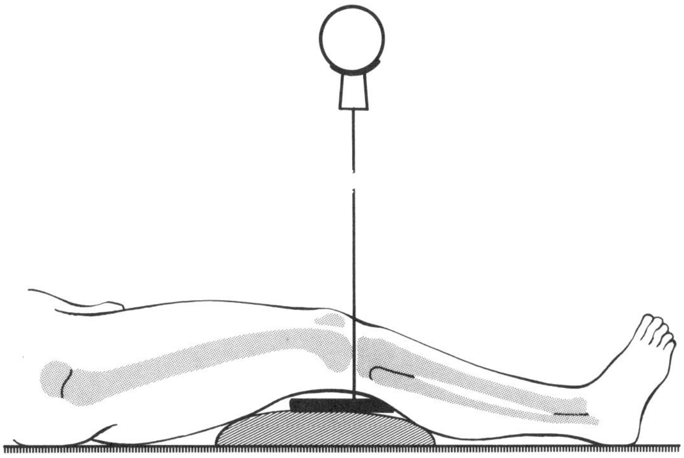

9

... or the knee joint must be slightly flexed.

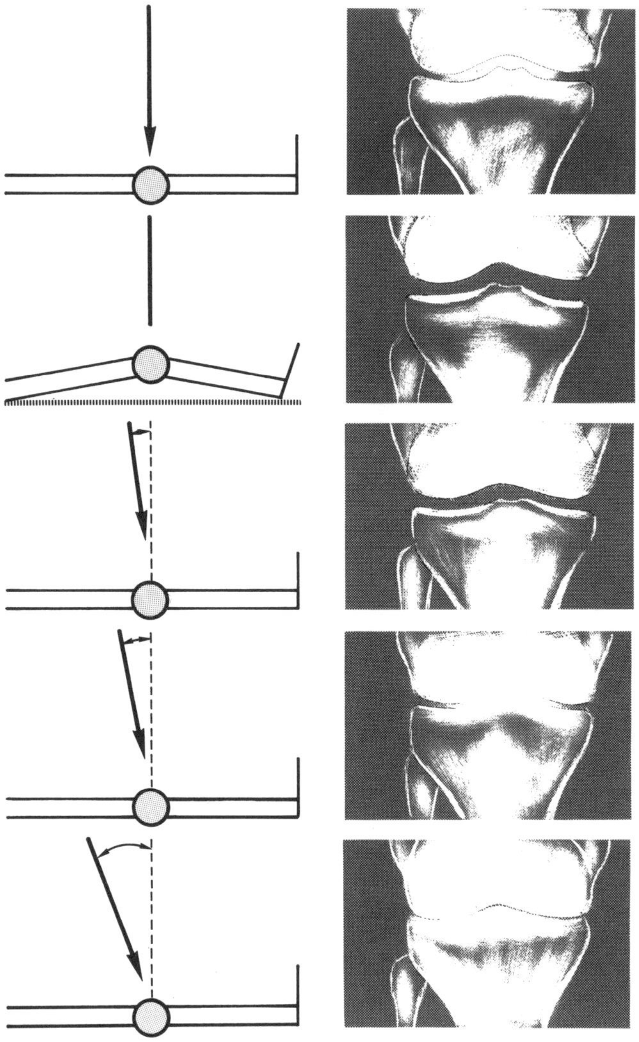

10

Comparative series of roentgenograms, showing the projection of the articular surface of the tibia with different modes of adjusting the central ray. The X-rays reveal the importance of an accurate radiographic technique for obtaining usable roentgenograms.

11

Teleroentgenograms of both knee joints with concomitant projection of the hip joint and the subtalar joint give information about the actual axes of the joints, independent of faulty projections. Such roentgenograms should be made (at the latest) after concluding treatment of a fracture of the tibial head or a subcondylar fracture.

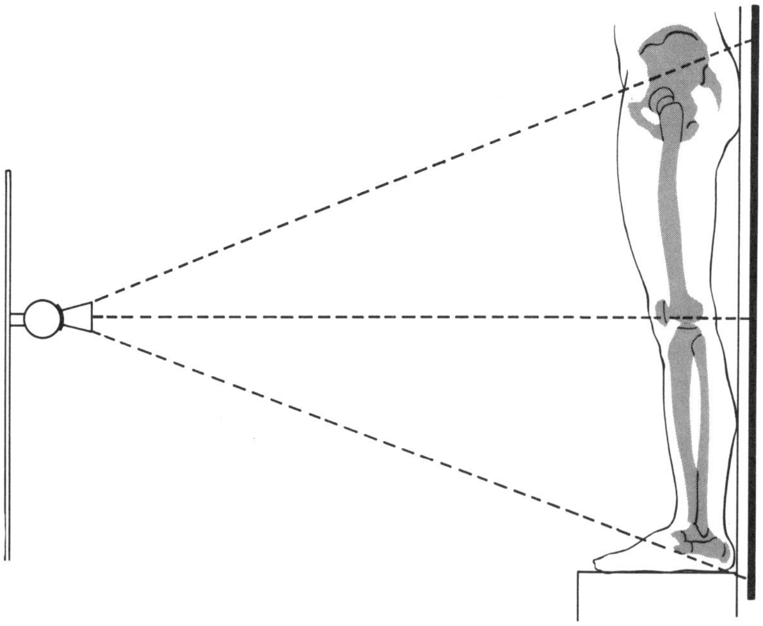

Operative possibilities

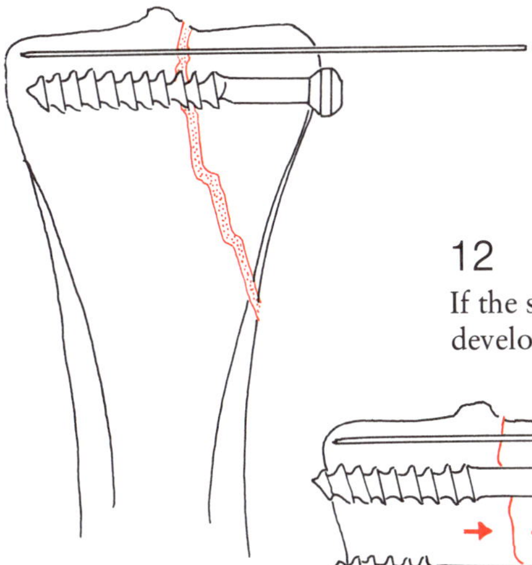

12
If the screw thread does not cross the cleft of the fracture, a blocking effect develops.

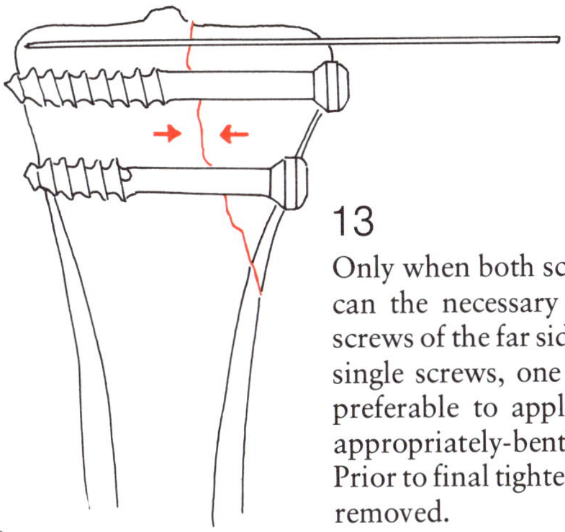

13
Only when both screw threads cross the fracture completely can the necessary interfragmental compression arise. The screws of the far side should grip the opposite cortex. In using single screws, one should insert at least two of them. It is preferable to apply, in additional, a supporting plate (an appropriately-bent half-tubular plate, a T or an L plate). Prior to final tightening of the screws, drilling wires should be removed.

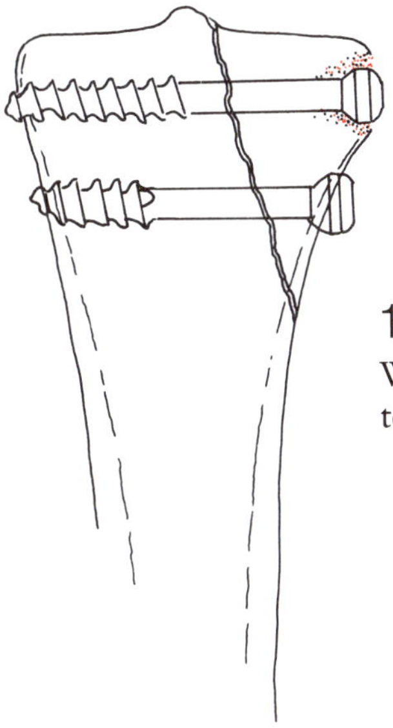

14
When the cortex is thin and the bone osteoporotic, heads of single screws tend to sink in.

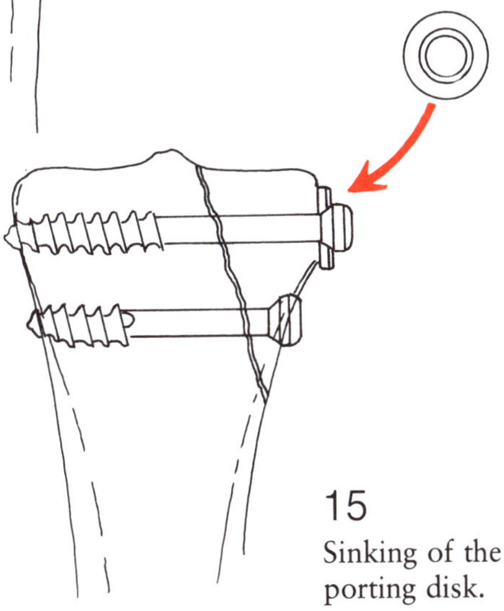

15
Sinking of the screwhead can be prevented by using a supporting disk.

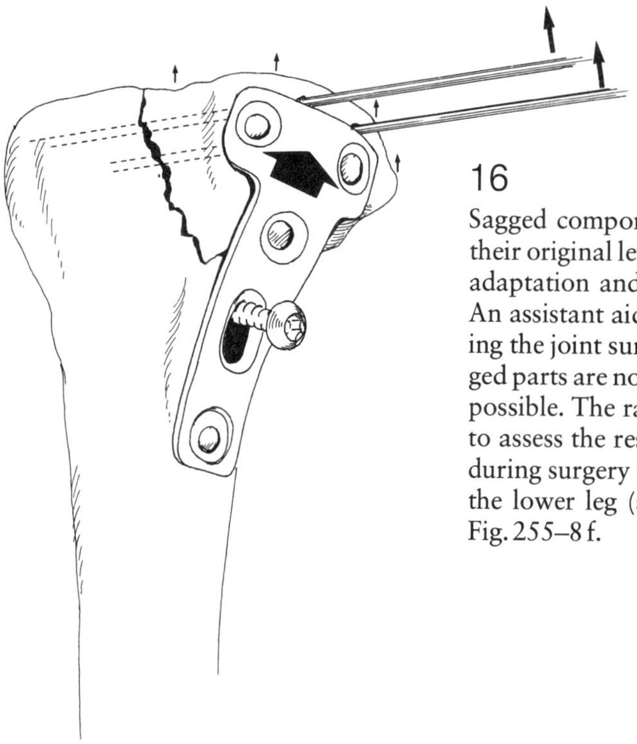

16

Sagged components of the joint must be lifted, at least, to their original level. Drilling wires help in maintaining an even adaptation and serve as abutment in pushing up the plate. An assistant aids in this maneuver by appropriately separating the joint surfaces at the same time. In most cases the sagged parts are not lifted high enough; excessive lifting is hardly possible. The radiographic image intensifier does not suffice to assess the result; a roentgenogram must usually be taken during surgery that includes a sufficient length of the axis of the lower leg (size 15 × 40 cm). As for the central ray, see Fig. 255–8 f.

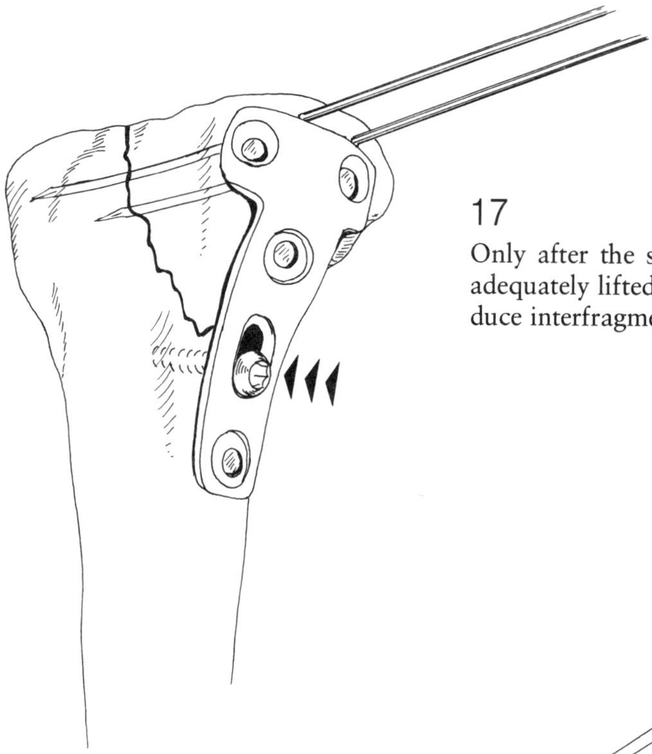

17

Only after the sagged components of the joint have been adequately lifted can the parts be secured by screws to produce interfragmental compression.

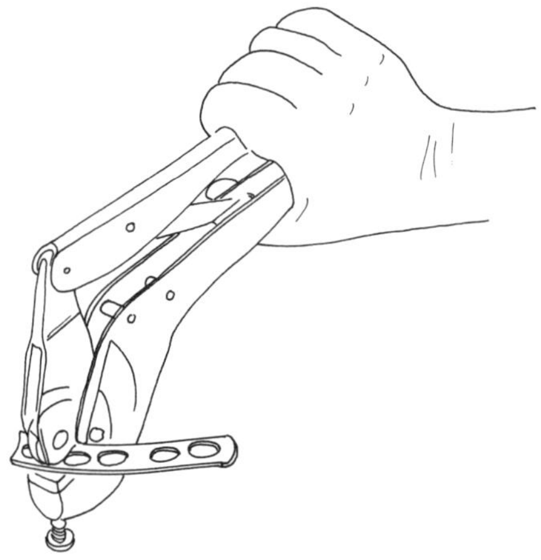

18

Half-tubular, T and L plates can very well be molded to the bone without excessively filling up the soft tissues. As pure support they are sufficiently strong here.

Positioning

See Figs. 192–6 and 207–9 ff.

Approach

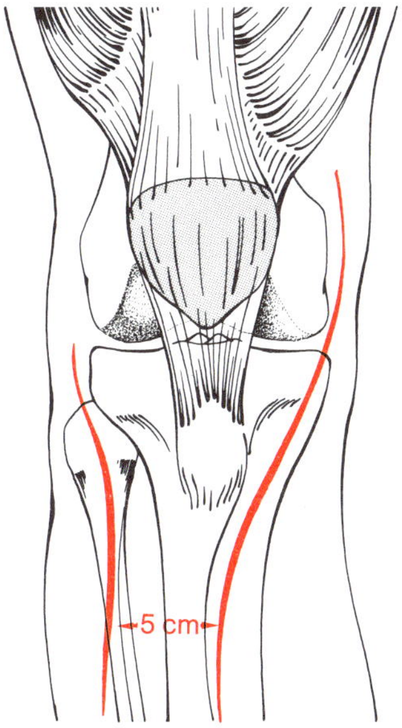

19

The triangular skin incision is unnecessary. A longitudinal incision allows the same exposure and affords greater ease in performing an osteosynthesis without extensive detachment of soft structures. Necrosis of the skin is not liable to occur here.

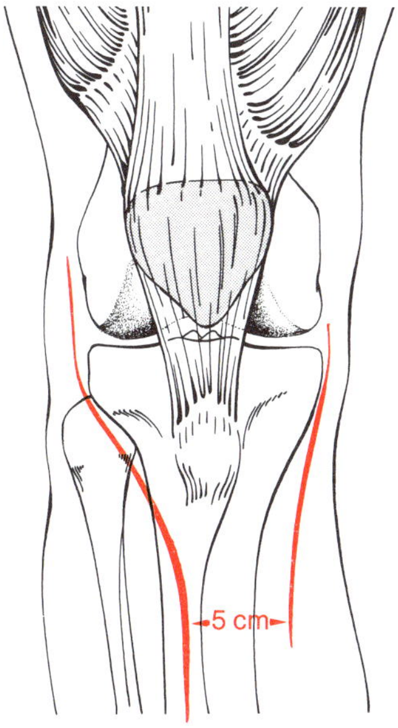

20

In making such a longitudinal incision, take care to place the second (straight) incision far enough posterior to the S-shaped incision (which is generally lateral) so that a wide bridge of skin and soft tissues remains anteriorly.

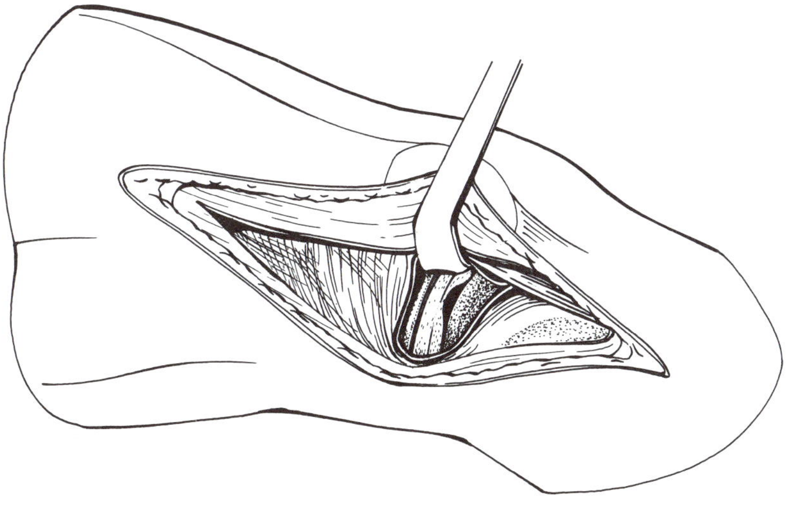

21

The fascia is split in the direction of its fibers. The joint is opened transversely underneath the meniscus. If the meniscus is uninjured, it should be preserved. It is pulled cranially with a fine hook and thus does not impede the operation. A narrow border of the meniscus attachment is left behind at the border of the head of the tibia. This facilitates the reinsertion of the meniscus after completion of the operation.

Tactics

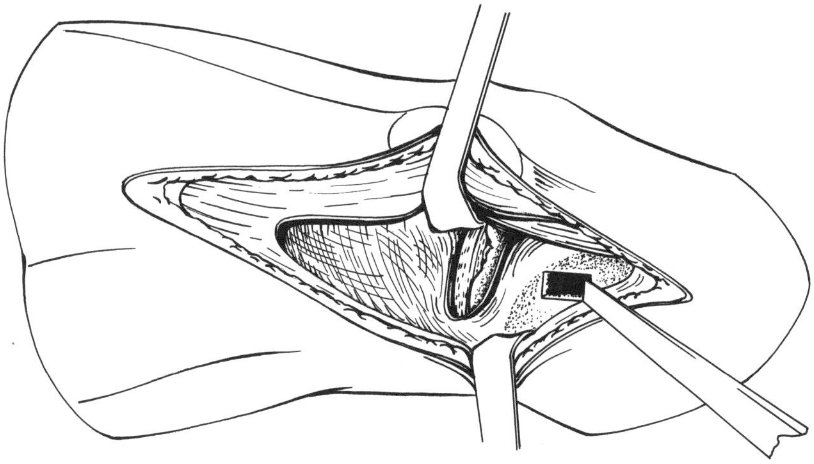

22
The fragments are best lifted through a small window in the cortex created distally.

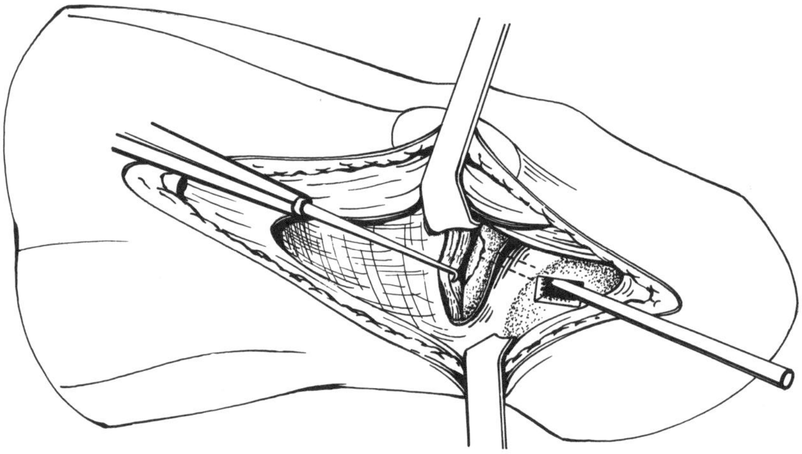

23
By means of this window, the fragments can be lifted under concomitant observation of the articular surface through the lateral aperture of the arthrotomy.

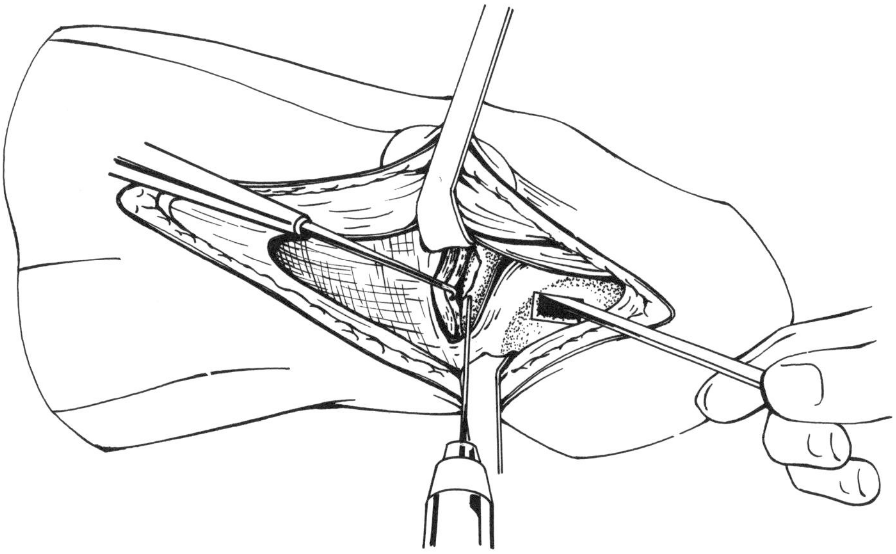

24
Following preliminary fixation, cancellous bone is underlaid until all the voids are packed.

25
Routine *splitting of the fascia* (See Figs. 283–4 ff.) is advised to prevent the rather frequent occurrence of the anterior tibial syndrome (anterior tibial compartment syndrome).

14. Lower Leg

Lower leg – proximal part

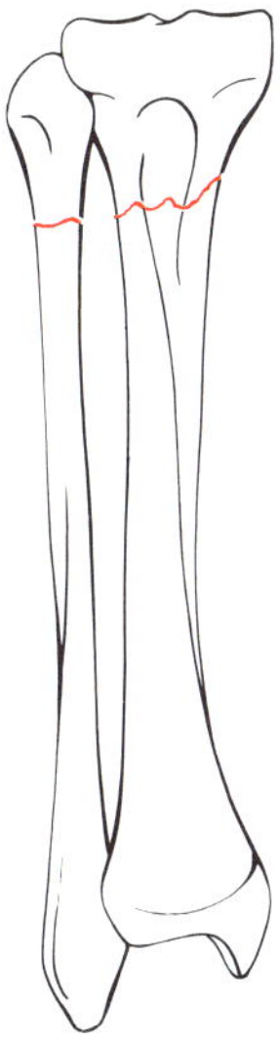

1
Transverse fracture.

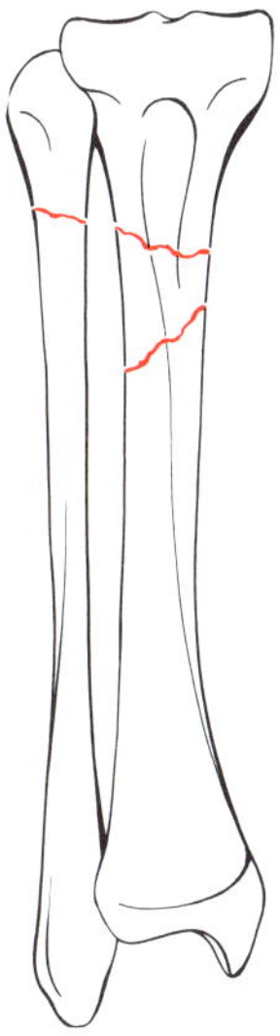

2
Comminuted fracture.

Closed: two plates. Exceptionally, intramedullary nailing with screw through the upper end of the nail.
Open: osteosynthesis with two plates.

Principle

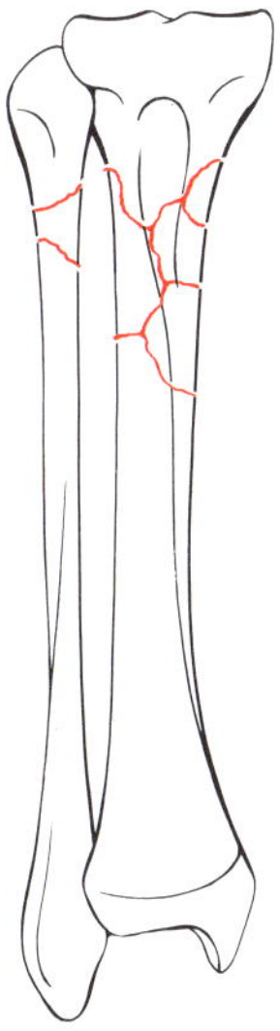

3
Multifragment fracture. Osteosynthesis with two plates.

Operative possibilities

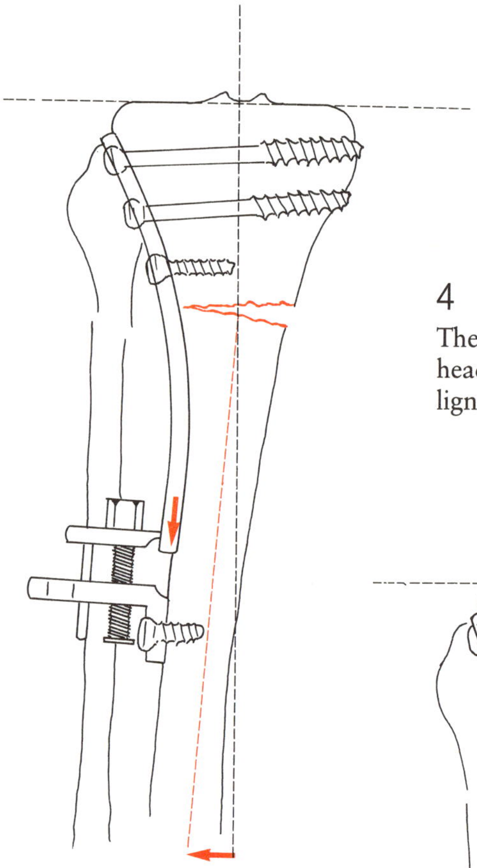

4

The operative procedure is similar to that employed for a fracture of the head of the tibia, yet without opening the joint. A great hazard is the malalignment that is apt to occur, principally on tightening the plate.

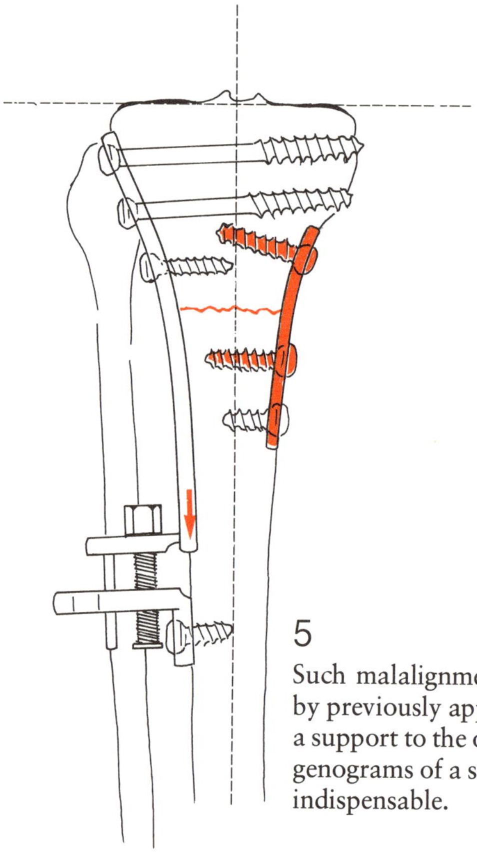

5

Such malalignment can be corrected or controlled by previously applying a small half-tubular plate as a support to the opposite side. Intraoperative roentgenograms of a sufficient length of the lower leg are indispensable.

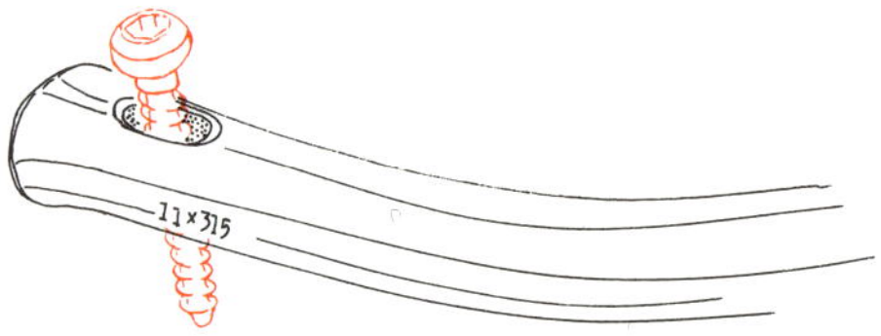

6

In the presence of a short proximal fragment, a screw inserted through the proximal holes in the nail…

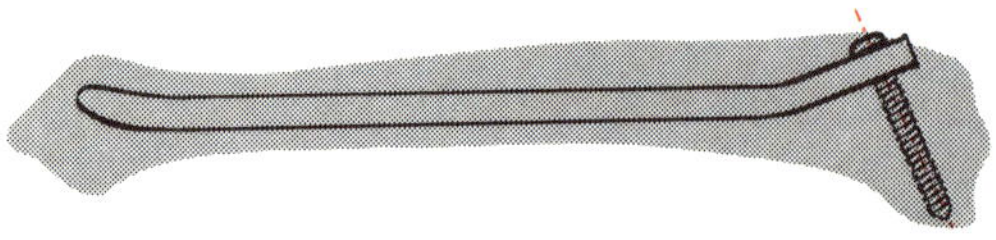

7

… can provide additional anchorage.

Lower leg – middle part

Principle

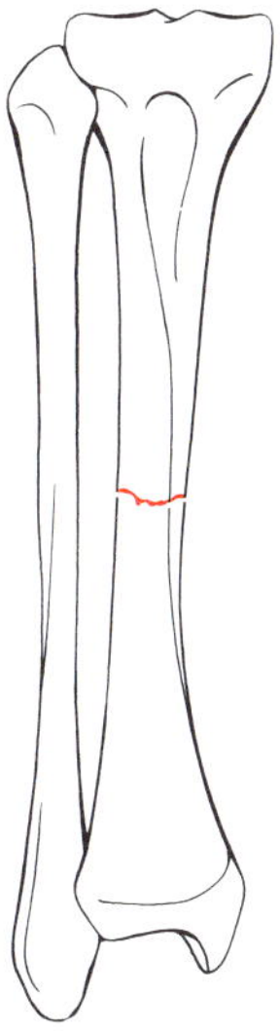

1
Transverse fracture.

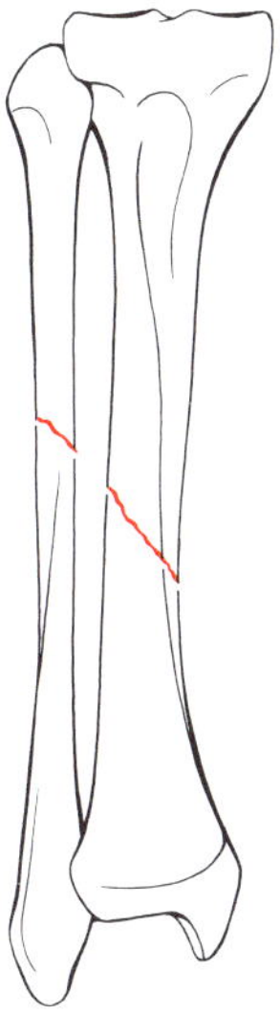

2
Short oblique fracture.

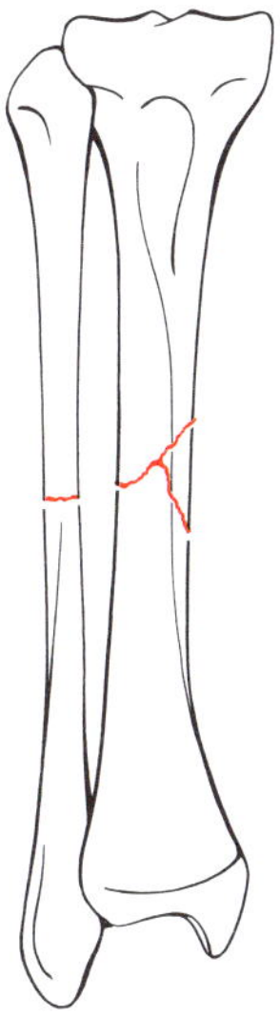

3
Fracture with short bent wedge.

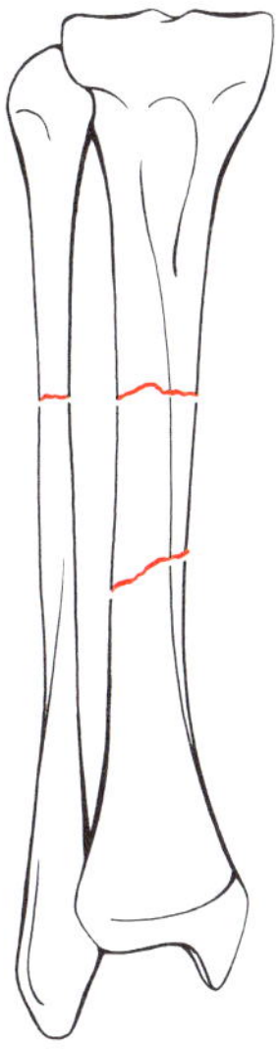

4
Comminuted fracture.

Closed fracture: intramedullary nailing (See p. 267 ff.).
Open fracture (only small perforation from the inside): intramedullary nailing (See p. 267 ff.) or plate fixation (See p. 277.).
Wide open fracture, hazard of infection, skin defect, primary closure of skin not possible: either stable osteosynthesis with use of tube tightener (preferable); or adaptation osteosynthesis using a thin nail without drilling (if desired, a thick Rush pin), combined with a minimal plaster cast or a plaster shell and, after the wound has healed, stable nailing after drilling.

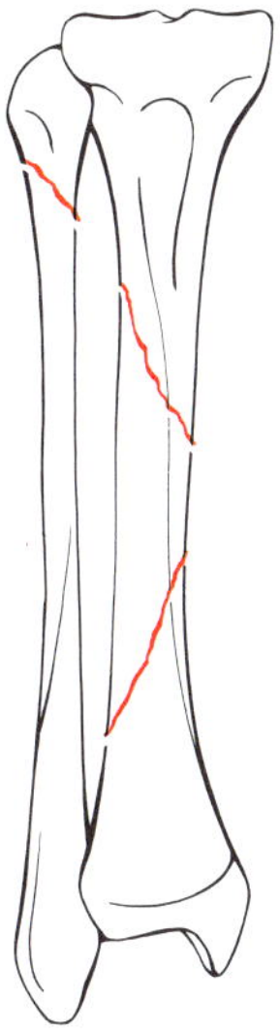

5
Long oblique and spiral fracture.

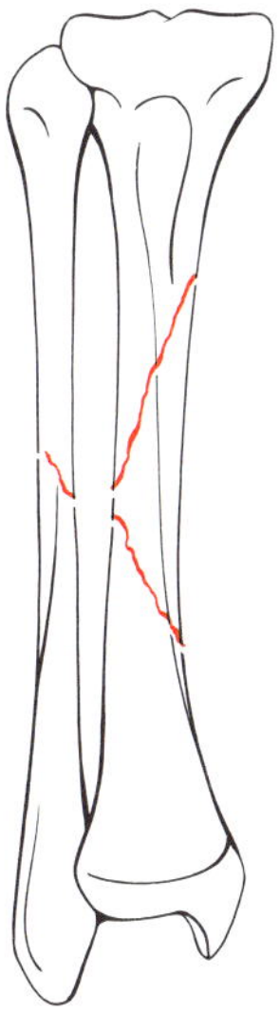

6
Long bent wedge.

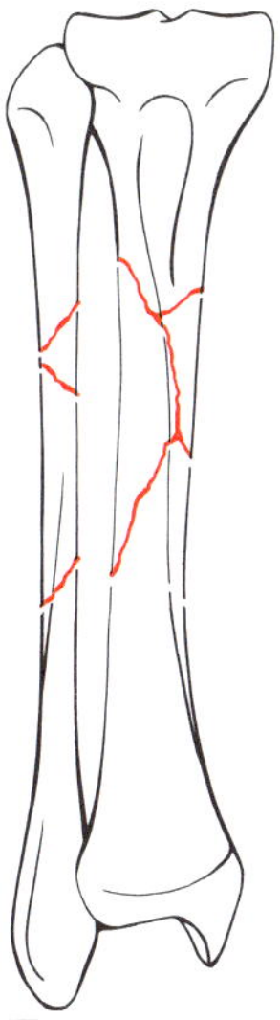

7
Fracture with more than one break.

Closed and open fractures: interfragmental compression through screw traction and plate fixation (See p. 277.).

Anterolateral approach

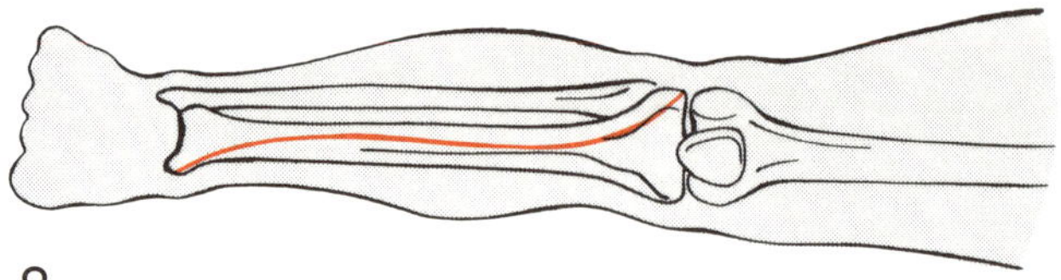

8

Skin incision a fingerbreadth lateral to the anterior edge of the tibia (Note also Figs. 282–2ff.)...

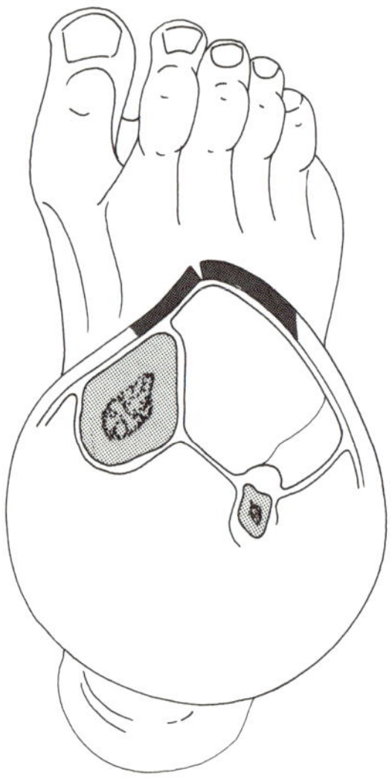

9

... and from there penetrating along the fascia toward the edge of the tibia.

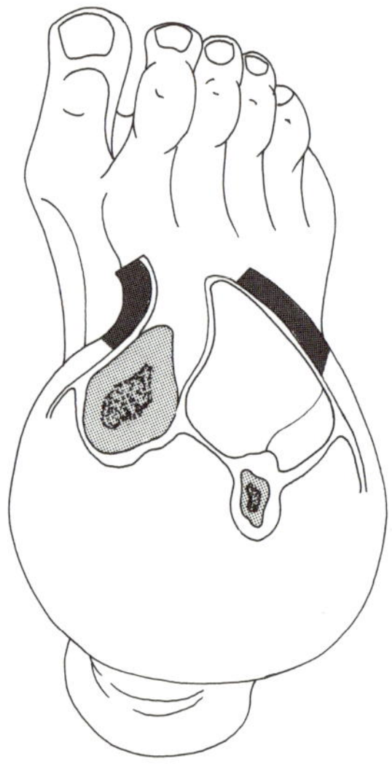

10

The muscles are first pushed only to the lateral side while medially they should as far as possible be left attached to the bone. Therefore, Hohmann elevators are unsuitable instruments here and retractors are preferable.

Medial approach

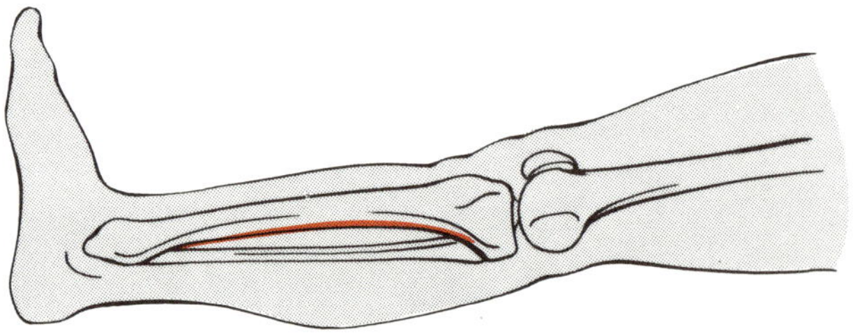

11

Skin incision a fingerbreadth posterior to the palpable medial edge of the tibia.

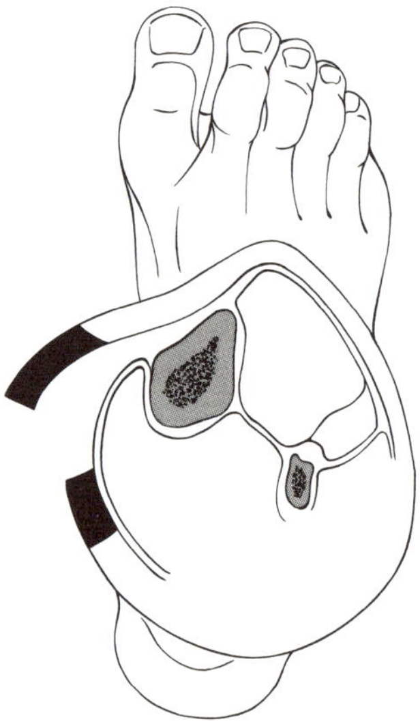

12

By so doing, the suture does not lie right above the implant when the wound is closed. Thus one avoids a shortened pathway for secondary invasion by pathogenic bacteria.

Lower leg – distal part

Principle

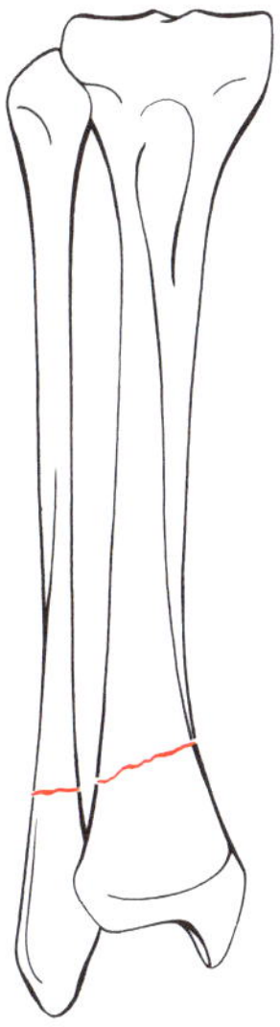

1
Transverse fracture.

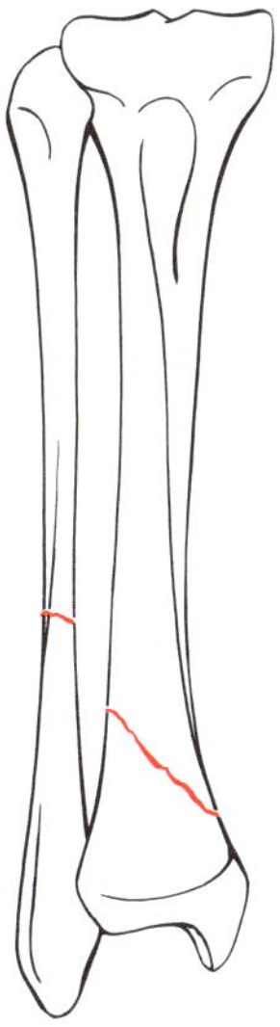

2
Short oblique fracture.

Closed fracture: plate fixation. In exceptional cases presenting poor soft-tissue conditions, intramedullary nail with detachable wires (relative indication!).
Open fracture: plate fixation and stabilization of the fibula.

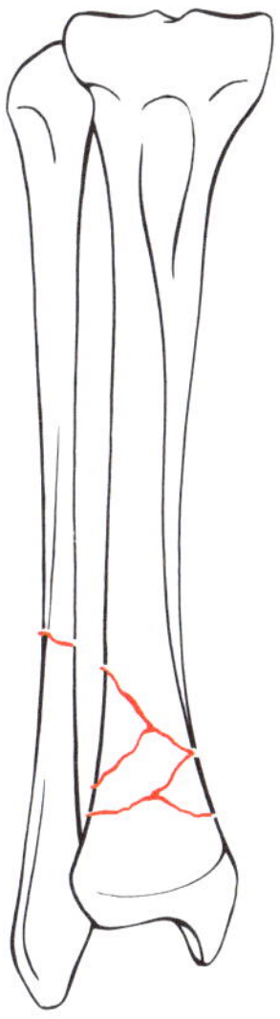

3
Fracture with more than one break.

Closed and open fracture: interfragmental compression through screw traction and plate fixation with stabilization of the fibula.

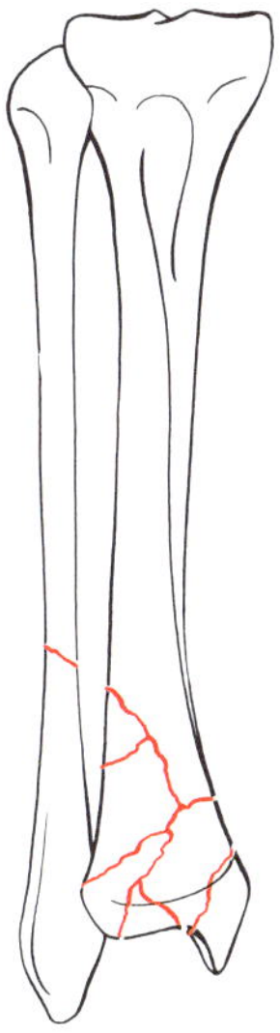

4
Multifragment fracture with involvement of the joint.

Closed and open fractures: plate fixation with the primary aim of obtaining a satisfactory articular surface and immediate stability that is resistant to exercise. Drilling wires should, if possible, be resorted to only temporarily during surgery.

1. Restoration of the normal length of the fibula
2. Reconstruction of the distal articular surface of the tibia.
3. Plate fixation.
4. Cancellous bone grafting (comminuted area!).

Plate fixation

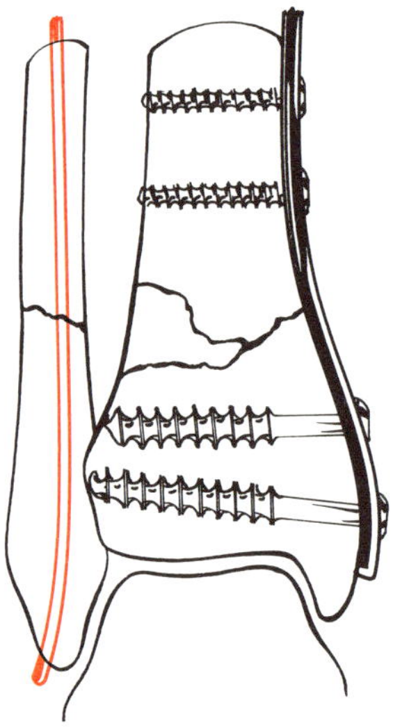

5

In distal fractures, including deep breaks of the fibula, this bone must, in principle, be stabilized. In most cases, however, excessive tension of the soft tissues does not allow one to undertake this procedure concomitantly with osteosynthesis of the tibia. So the second stage of the operation has to be postponed until, after about 10 to 14 days, the edema and the hematoma have receded. In an occasional case of transverse fracture of the tibia, closed reduction and stabilization with a Rush pin can save the patient a second operation.

Nail fixation

(For special cases, see Figs. 165–1 and 265–2.)

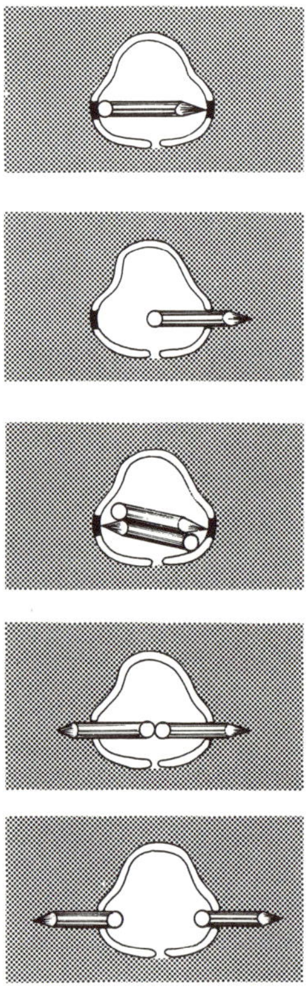

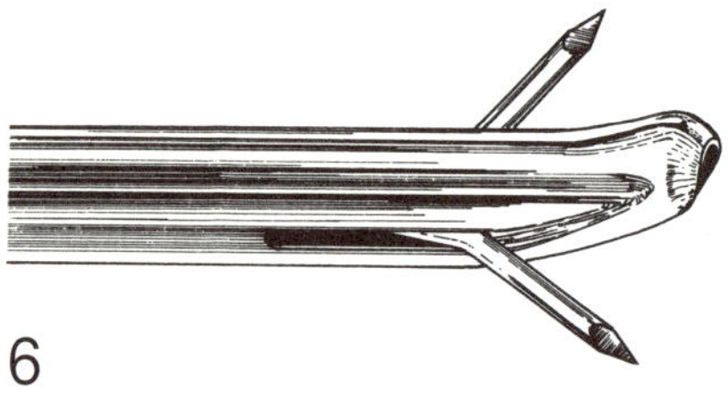

6

If the *distal* fragment is very short, additional anchorage can be secured by separable wires. Such anchorage serves primarily to prevent lateral angulation (varus or valgus position) than to increase rotary stability. Note the marked upward bend of the end of the nail, that is destined to improve the crossing of the fracture site by the nail.

7

The points of the detachable wires, the ends of which are angled, glide along the lateral grooves of the nail and thus are securely guided to the lateral exit slits. Before the first wire is definitively detached near its end, the point of the second wire should also be guided into its exit slit. Otherwise, the first wire becomes too easily diverted. A nail thickness of 10 mm or less will admit only a single separable wire.

Closed intramedullary nailing

Indication

Advantage: accurate determination of nail length. No additional damage to the bone through pushing away of soft tissues.
Disadvantage: Radiation exposure. However, one should be able to make do with 60 seconds of total exposure. This is certainly possible with a wellconsidered use of x-rays, particularly when a video recorder is available.

Principle

See Figs. 55–1 ff., 263–1 to 263–4, 261–1 f., 262–6 f., 265–1 f.

Positioning

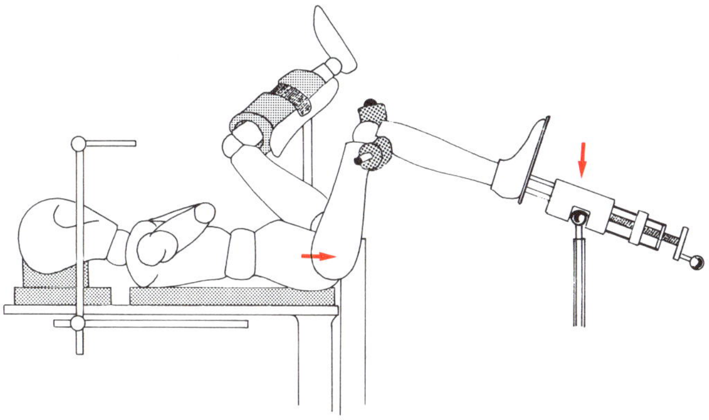

1
With the buttocks placed close to the crossbar, flexion at the knee is facilitated. Lowering the foot induces an angle of at least 90° to develop. This allows insertion of the nail without difficulty.

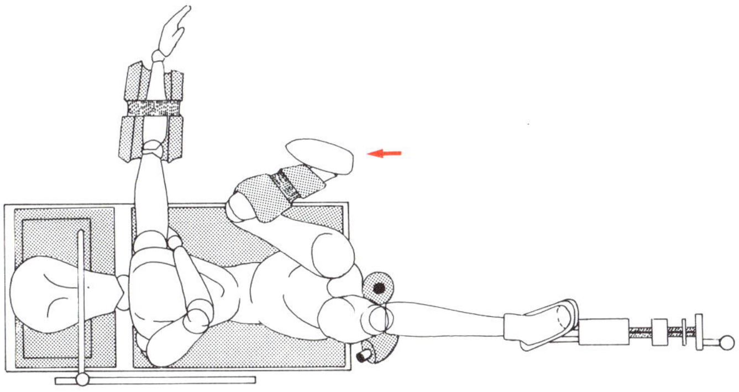

2
By abducting the uninjured leg and placing it as far cranially as possible, one insures sufficient space for the image intensifier.

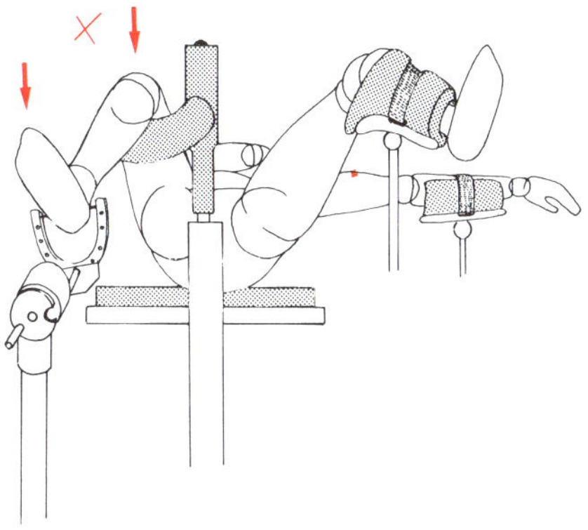

3
Note rotation of lower leg. Bearing line: center of the patella to the crease between great toe and second toe.

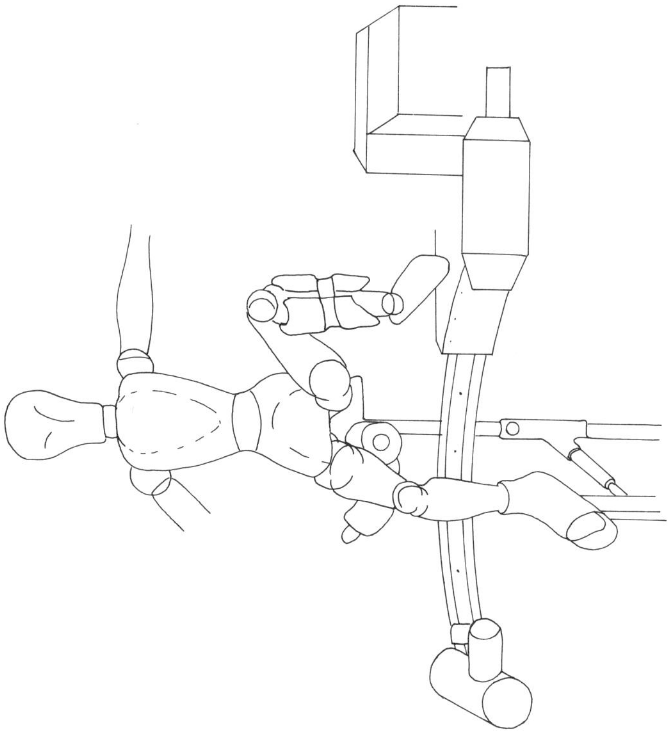

4
Setting up the image intensifier. Test it in both planes prior to sterile draping.

Sterile draping I

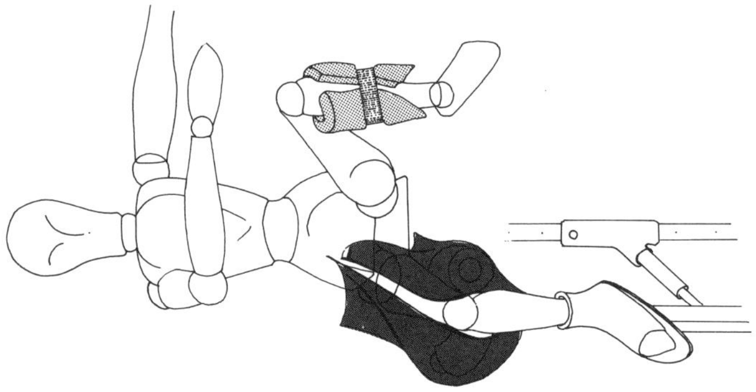

5
Drape size 3.

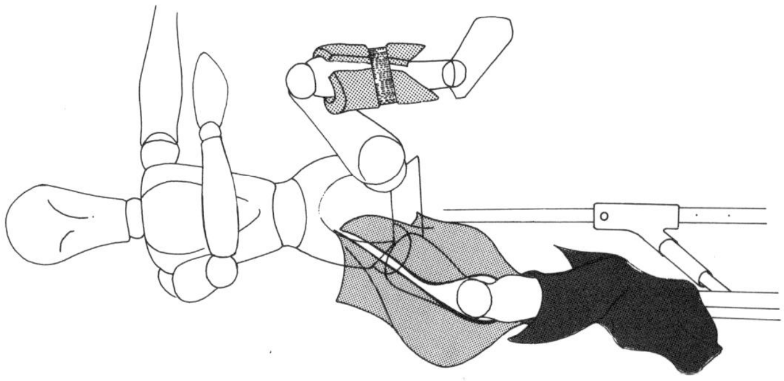

6
Drape size 4.

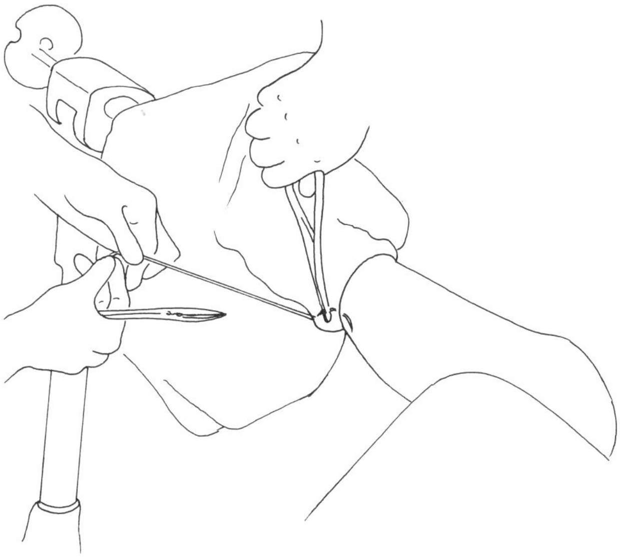

7
The drape is sewn on, since metal clips would interfere with the x-ray examination.

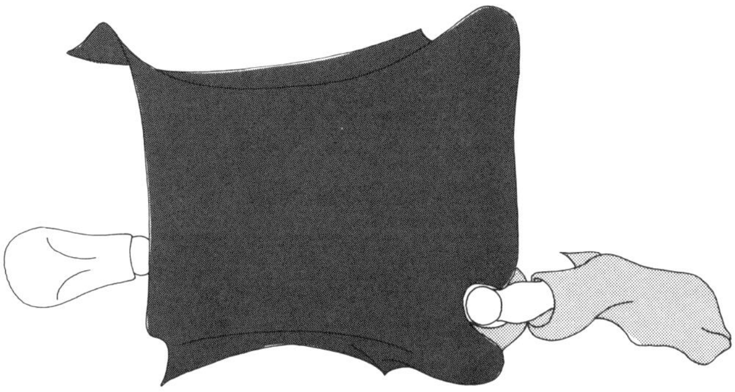

8
Drape size 1.

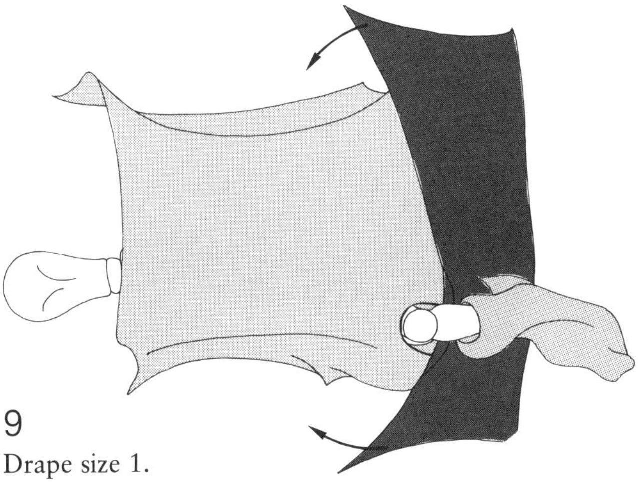

9
Drape size 1.

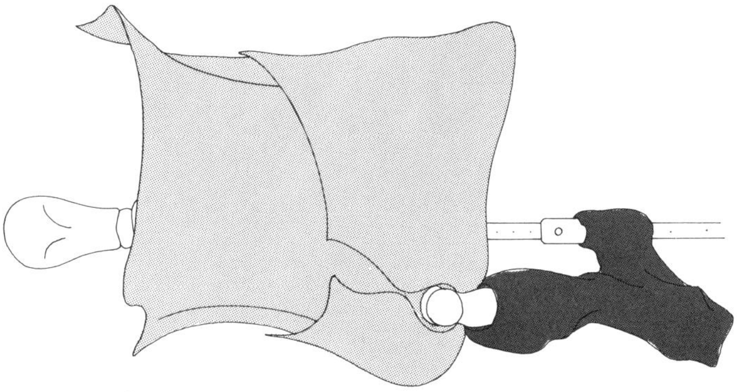

10
Drape size 1.

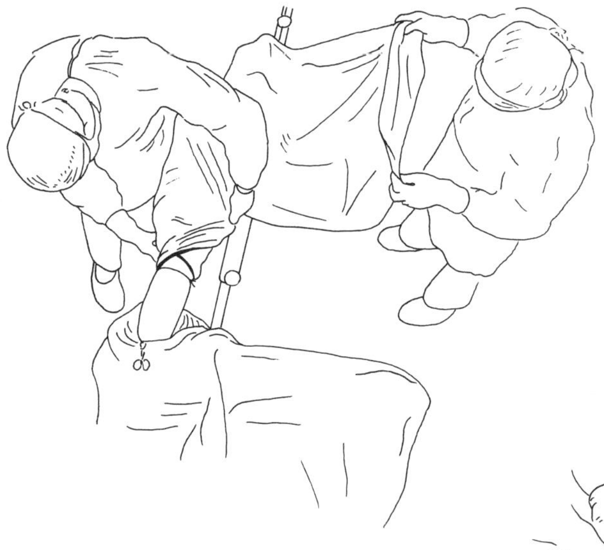

11
The drape should be applied snugly so that it does not hinder the movements of the image intensifier.

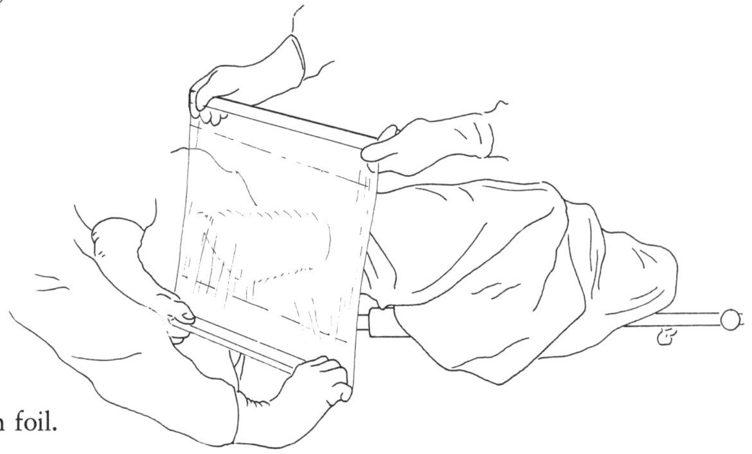

12
Draping with foil.

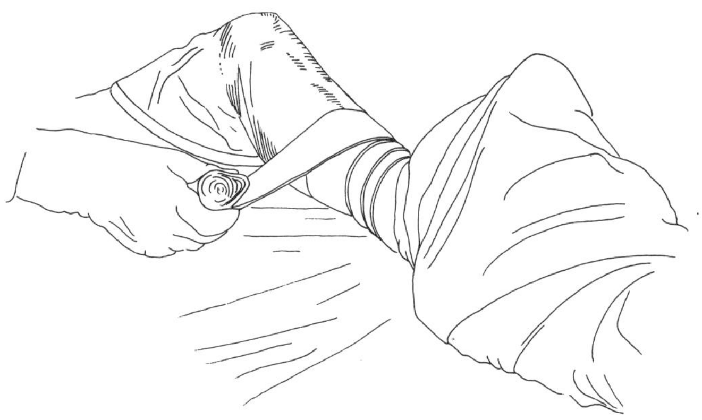

13
An elastic bandage applied to the lower leg produces a slight compression of the soft tissues and thereby a certain stabilization of the fragments, which greatly facilitates the procedure.

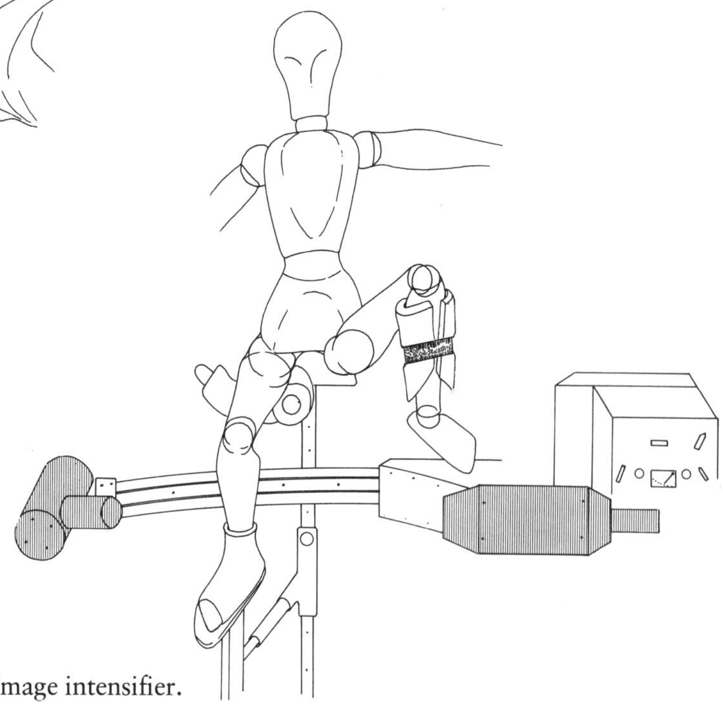

14
Sterile draping of the image intensifier.

Sterile draping II

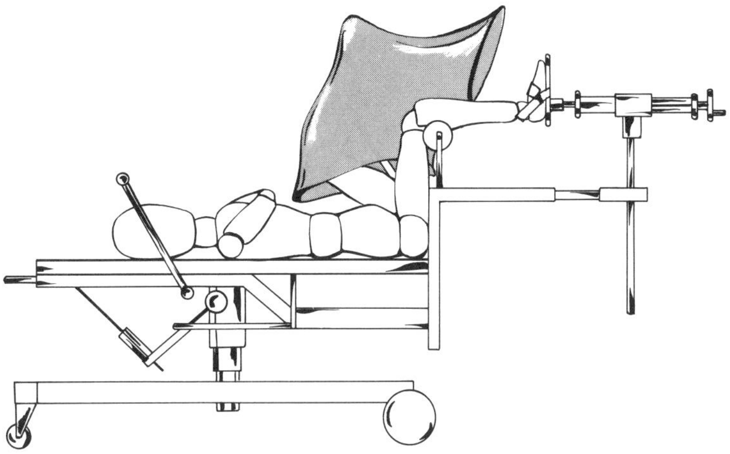

15
Drape size 5.

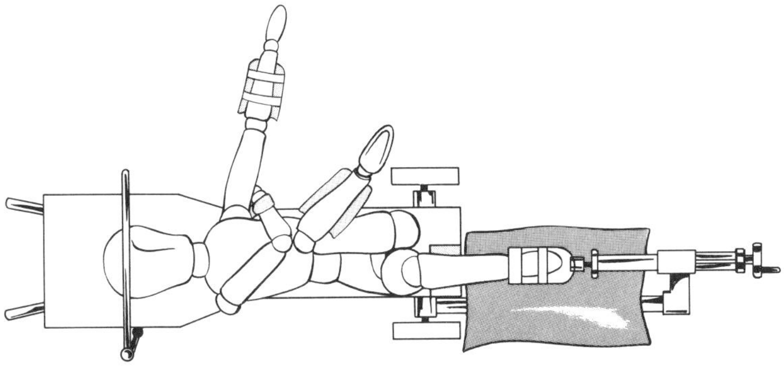

16
Drape size 4, lined underneath with a material impermeable to moisture.

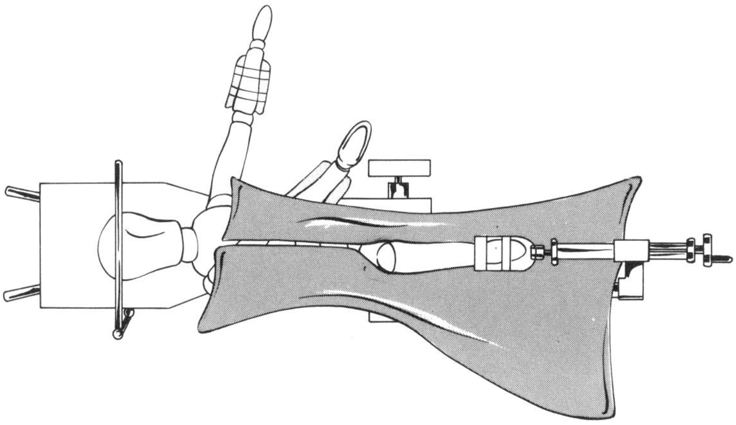

17
Drape size 2.

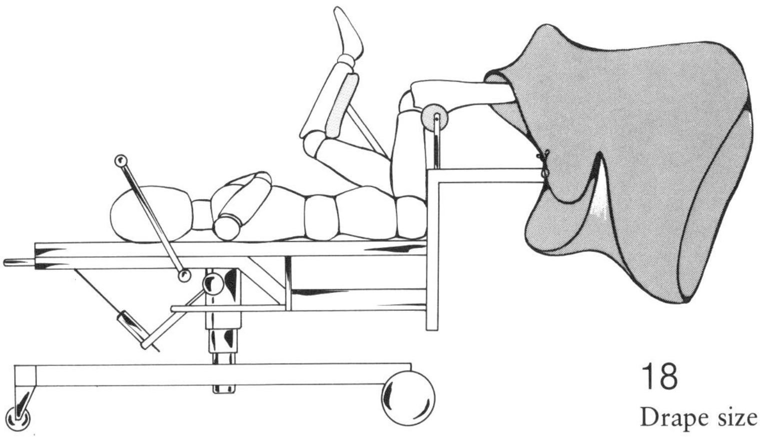

18
Drape size 5.

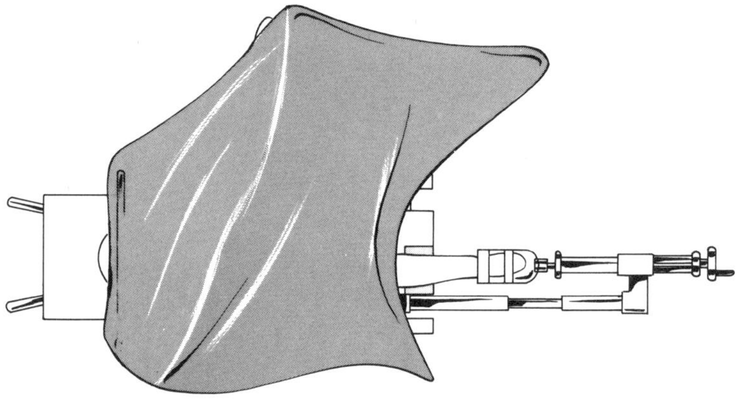

19
Drape size 1.

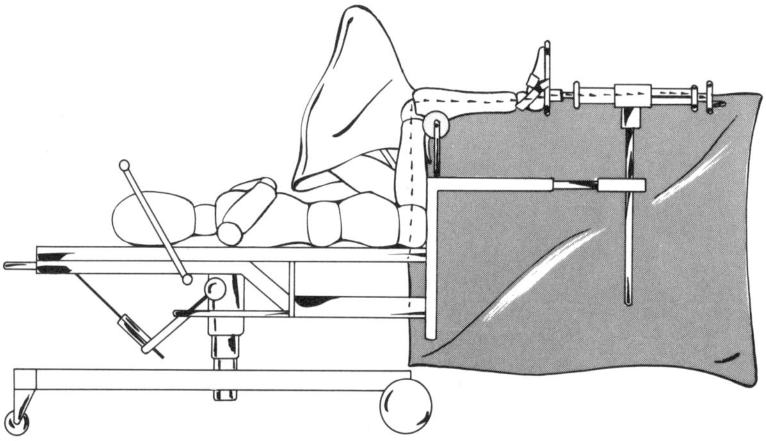

20
Drape size 1.

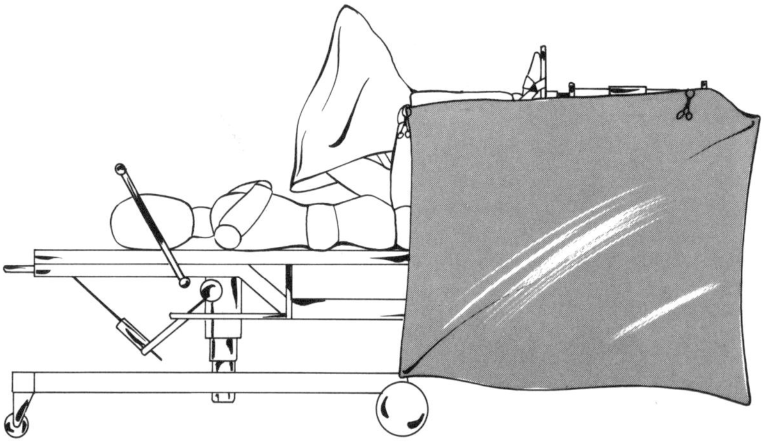

21
Drape size 1.

Approach

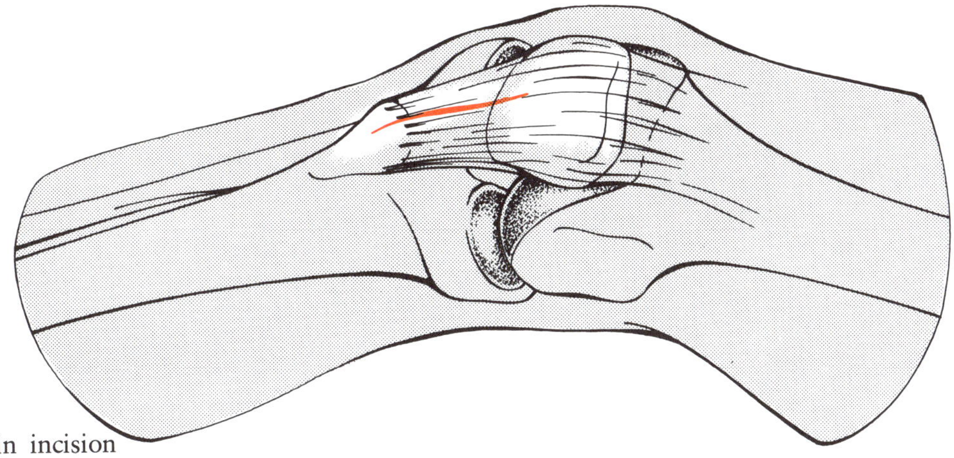

22
Longitudinal or transverse skin incision about 5 cm long.

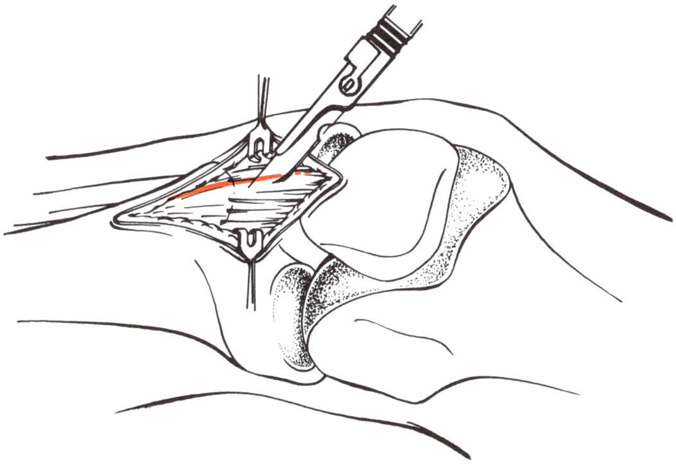

23
Longitudinal splitting of the fascia. In the proximal half of the wound, the incision must not be deeper than barely necessary for dividing the patellar tendon. Close underneath there are venous plexuses which bleed briskly and obstruct visibility.

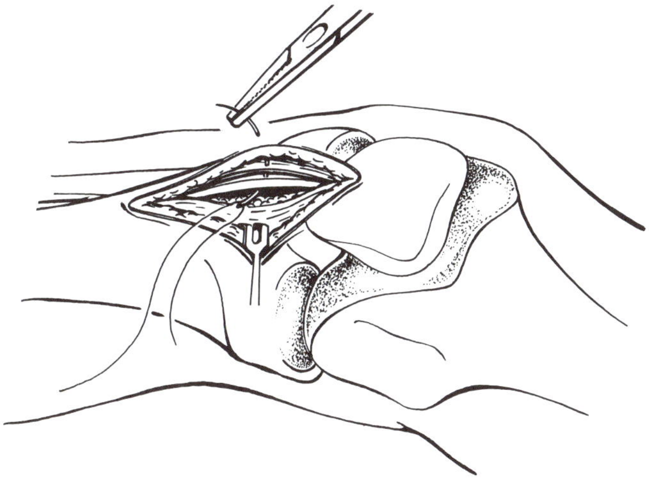

24
Retention sutures; these should grip only a small portion of the borders of the patellar ligament but a good deal of the skin. When the sutures are tied, the skin acts like a cover on the borders of the tendon.

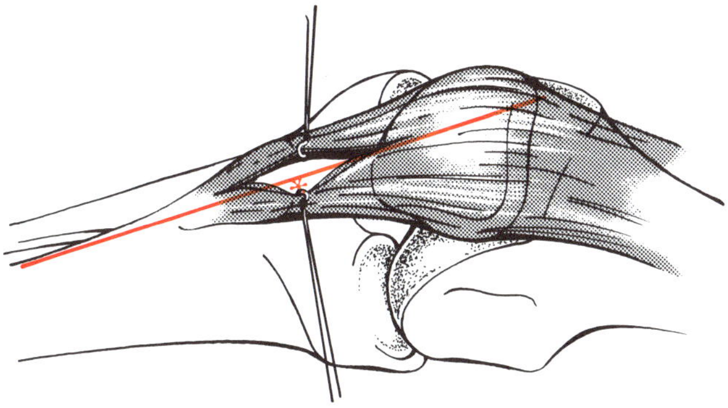

25
The site for inserting the nail should lie directly medial to the midline. Thus, on being knocked in, the nail receives a slight varus curvature which counteracts the tendency to the valgus position.

Tactics First see Figs. 56–6 to 57–13.

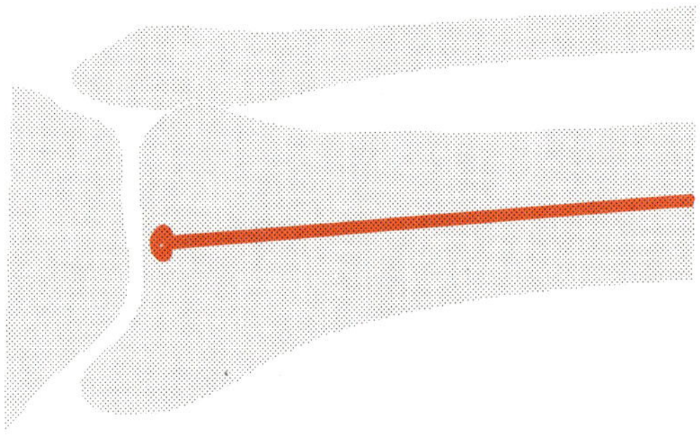

26

In the distal fragment, the tip of the drill pin *must* be kept in the midline, from the outset, particularly with respect to the anteroposterior plane of transillumination. Once the tip has taken a wrong direction, it is extremely difficult to correct.

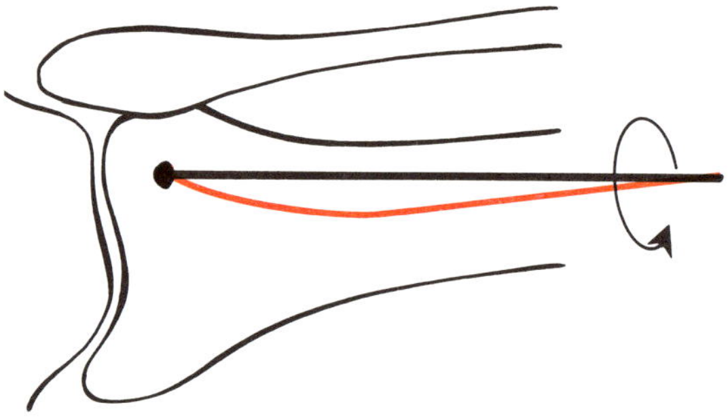

27

If, despite care, the tip of the pin has deviated (generally medialward), a slight rotation often can return its axis to the midline. The drilling is continued no further than just anteriorly to the curvature of the pin end, because otherwise the head of the drill would break off.

See Fig. 60–21.

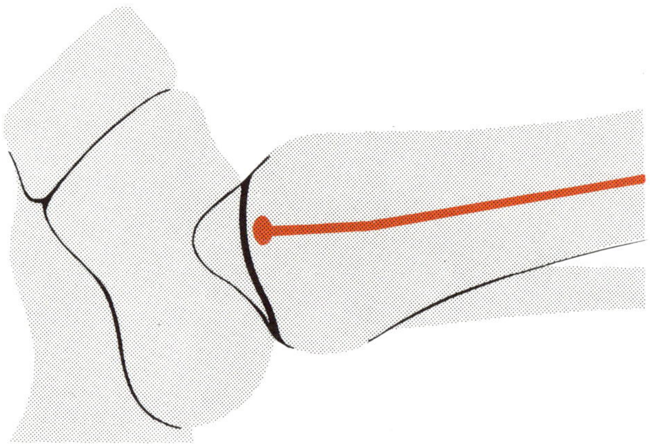

28

The tip of the drill pin, and later the guide rod as well, should advance until just above the articular surface. Check against the image intensifier.

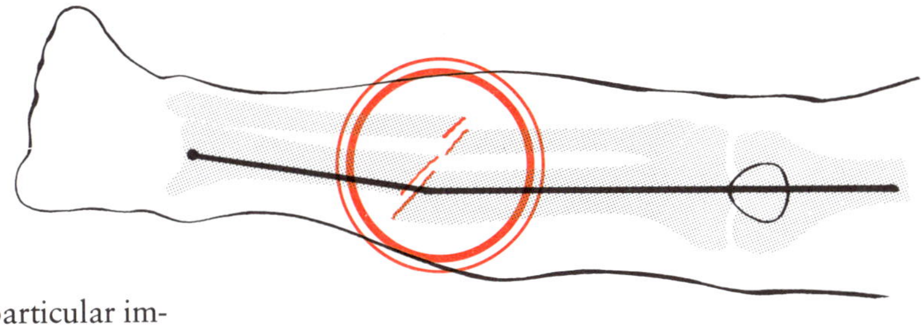

29

Prior to the first turn of the drill – which is of particular importance to the correct position of the nail – one must make allowance for the considerable tendency of the tibia to assume a valgus position. This tendency should be counteracted by holding the leg in the appropriate position while the nail is being inserted.

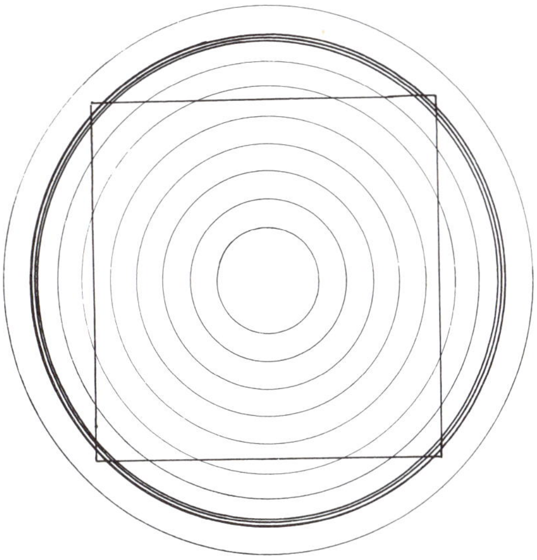

30

This valgus position is always underestimated, a phenomenon that is favored by the optical illusion produced by the rounded image of the image intensifier.

See also Figs. 57–14 to 63–32.

For *distal* fractures, see Fig. 266–6 f., for *proximal* fractures, see Fig. 262–6 f.

Closure of the wound

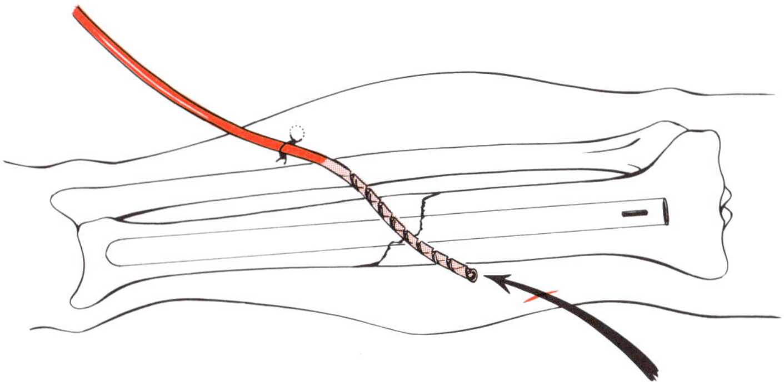

31

Transverse fractures and short oblique fractures that have been adequately reduced should invariably be provided with an installation for suction drainage. This is introduced transcutaneously and carried through the soft structures to the fracture site so as to prevent the development of a subcutaneous hematoma.

Open intramedullary nailing

Indication See p. 267.

Principle See Figs. 263–1 ff.

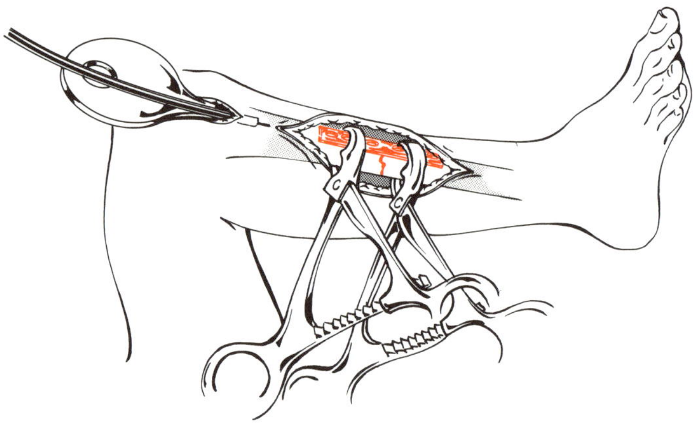

Exposure of the fracture and reduction.

1

Stabilizing the fracture with plate and Lambotte forceps.

Nailing: see Figs. 273–22 ff.

Plate

Types of injuries

See Figs. 261–1 ff., 263–1 ff. and 265–1 ff.

Indication

See Figs. 161–1 ff., 263–1 ff. and 265–1 ff.

Principle

See Figs. 27–2 ff. and 266–5.

Positioning

See Fig. 219–16 f. Supine or prone position.

Approach

Anterior approaches: see Fig. 259–19 (proximal) and Figs. 264–8 ff. (center).

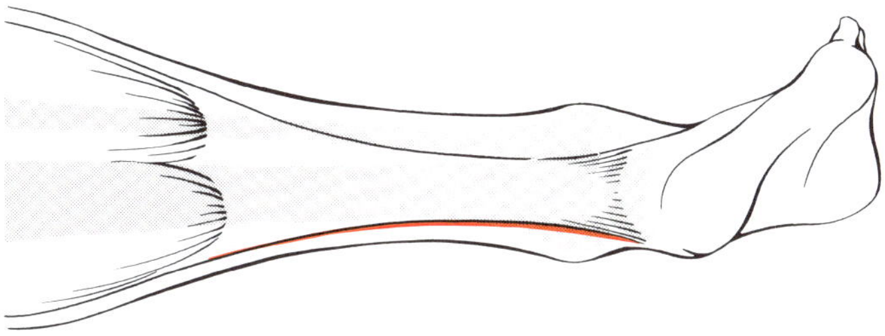

1
Posterior approach. Skin incision medial to the border of the Achilles tendon.

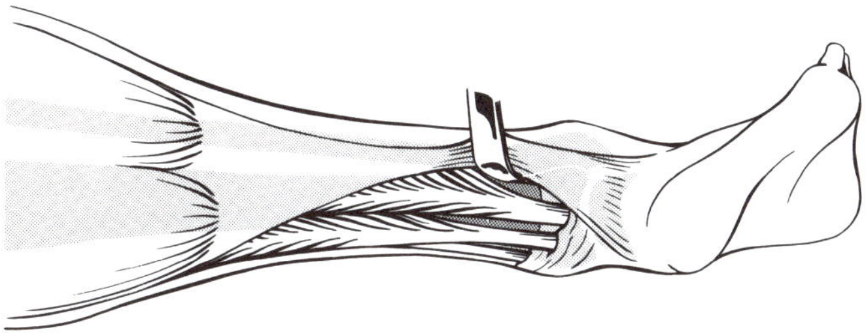

2
The fascia is divided between the flexor hallucis longus muscle (laterally) and the flexor digitorum longus muscle (medially).

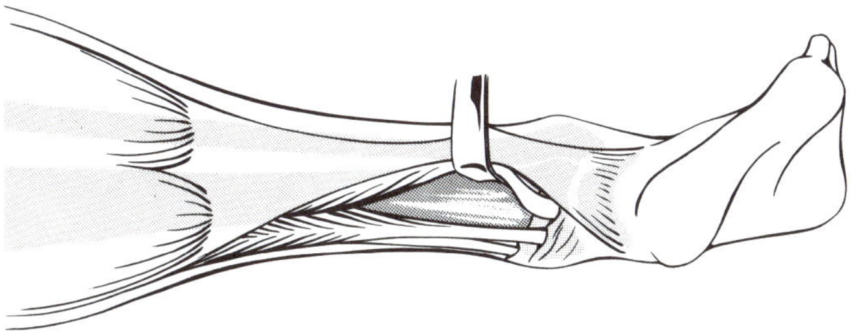

3
After insertion of the retractors, the posterior surface of the tibia is readily accessible. Deep sutures are not required to close the wound because no retinacula have been divided.

Tactics

See p. 27 ff.

Closure of the wound

Only backstitch suture of the skin, no suturing of fascia or subcutaneous tissues.
Splitting of the fascia as shown in Figs. 268–1 ff. should be omitted only in exceptional cases.

Achilles tendon

Positioning

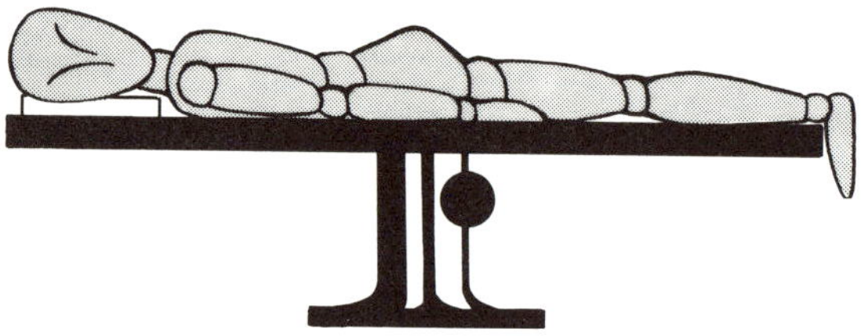

1
Prone position.

Approach

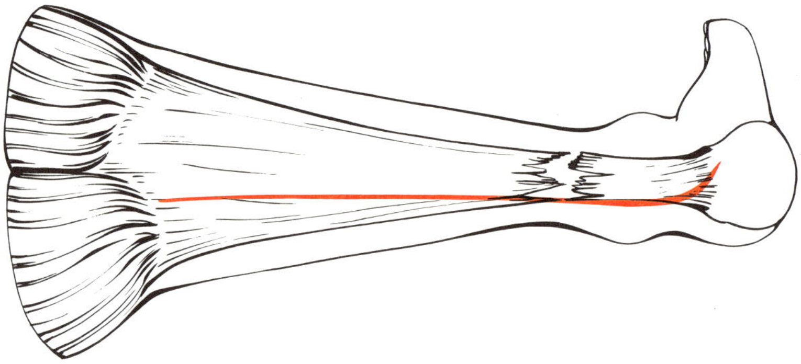

2
Skin incision.

Tactics

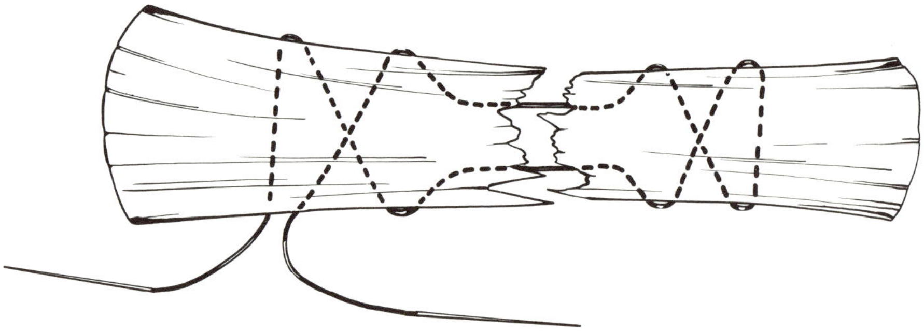

3
Bunnel suture with nonabsorbable thread. On tightening and tying the suture, the knee is flexed and the foot is brought into the equinus position.

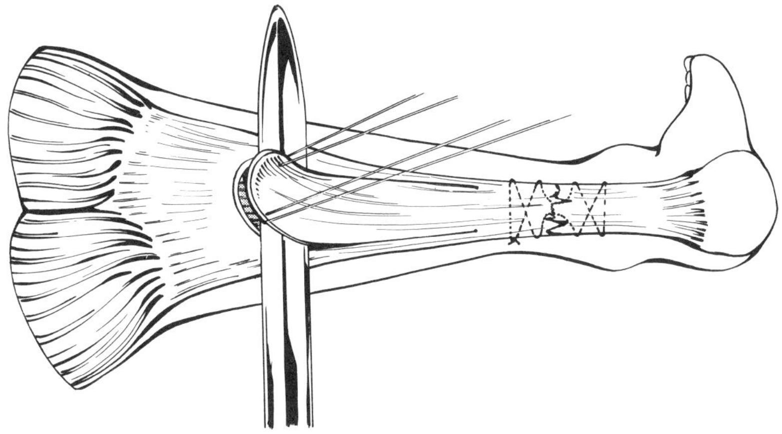

4

Following adequate adaptation of the tendon stumps with a number of additional fine interrupted sutures, a proximal pedicle flap is fashioned from the superficial leaf of the middle half of the tendon. (In most cases this can be done more easily before the Bunnel suture has been applied.)

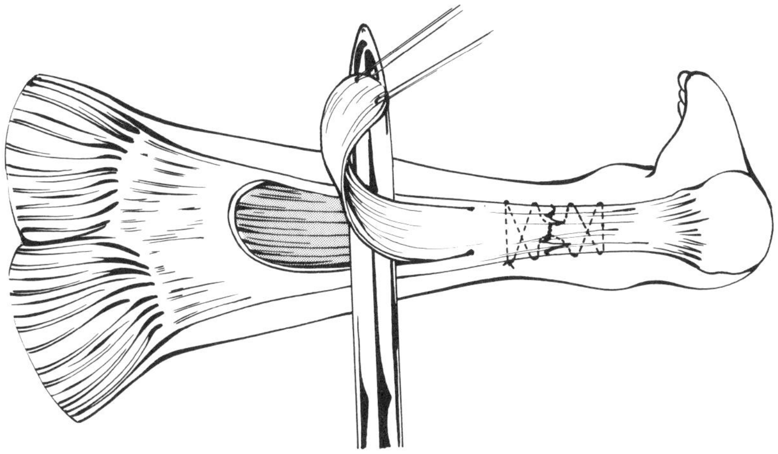

5

The fashioning must be undertaken with great care so that the flap may have sufficient breadth and remain in the superficial leaf. Furthermore, it is important that, proximally, at least half of the tendon fibers remain in place and that the incision be carried parallel to the tendon fibers.

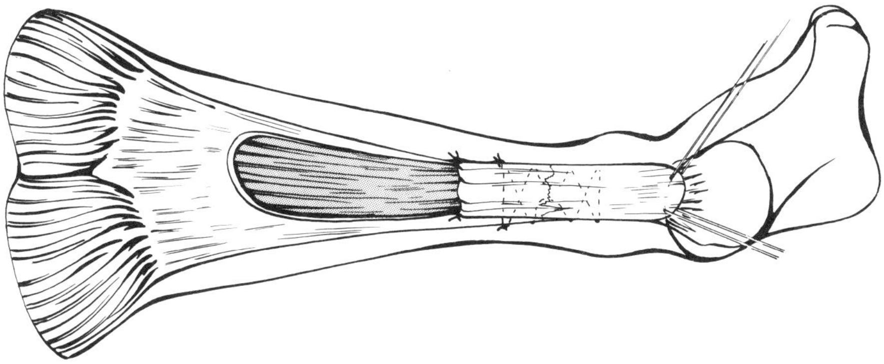

6

Distally the flap is fixed under slight tension with fine Dexon (equinus position!)...

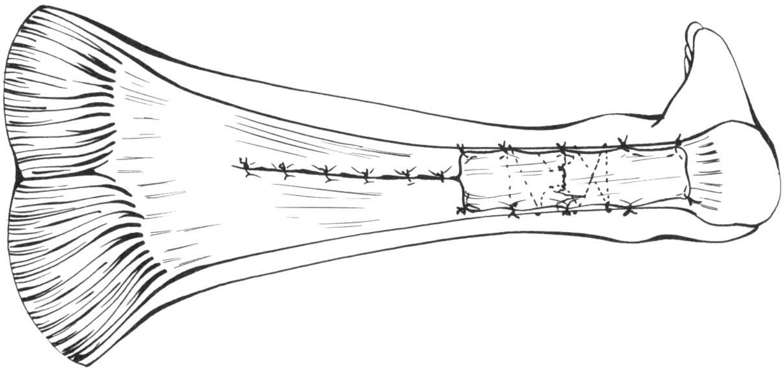

7

... and then the sutured site is stitched onto the tendon, enveloping it as completely as possible. The proximal cleft is closed.

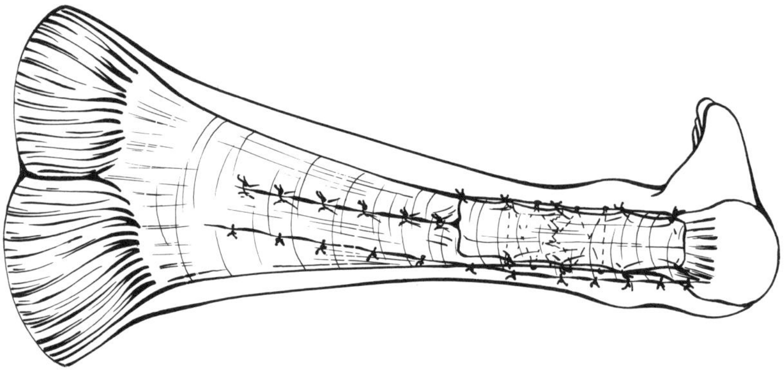

8

On closing the wound, the peritendinous gliding tissue is carefully reunited over the tendon, using extremely fine sutures. Skin closure.

Postoperative care

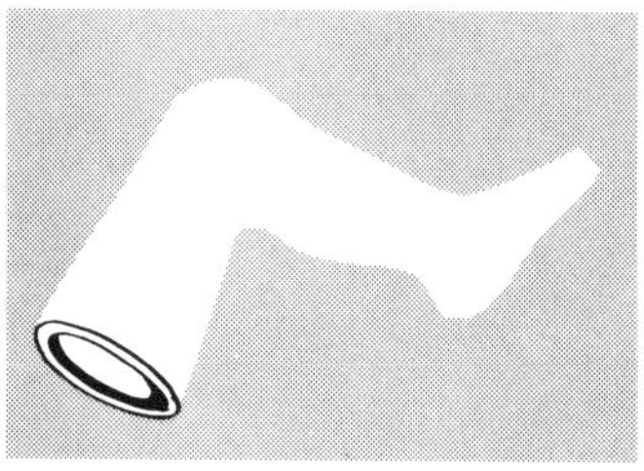

9

A long-leg plaster shell is applied with the knee flexed and the foot in the equinus position. The leg is elevated on a splint.

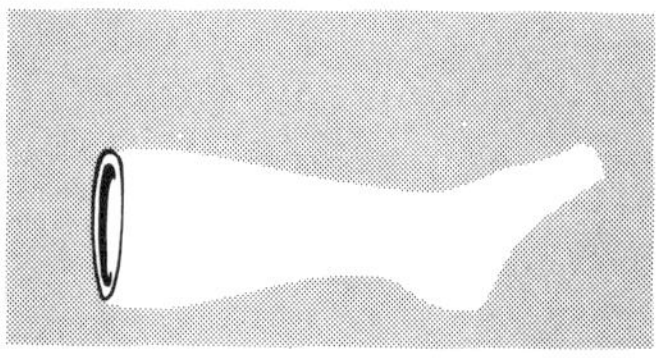

10

A below-knee plaster shell is applied for two weeks with the foot in the equinus position. The patient is permitted to become ambulatory on forearm crutches.

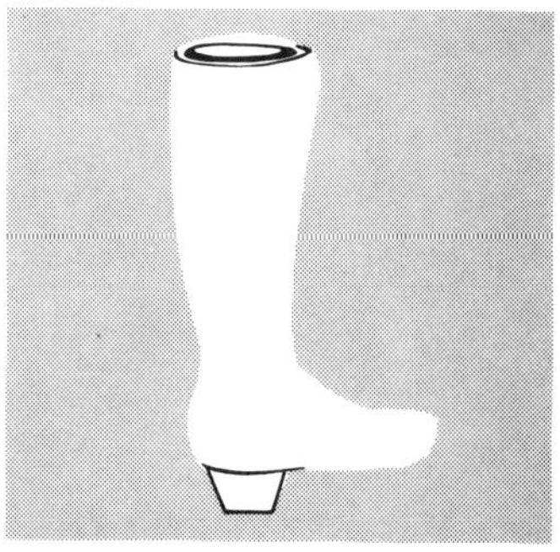

11

Walking cast for the lower leg with the foot in the intermediate position.

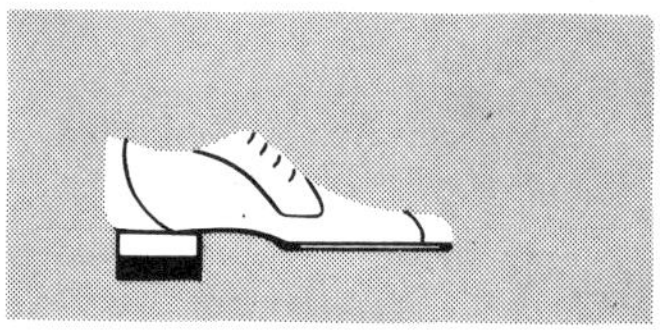

12

Both heels are raised by about 1 to 2 cm for 3 to 4 weeks.

Anterior tibial compartment syndrome

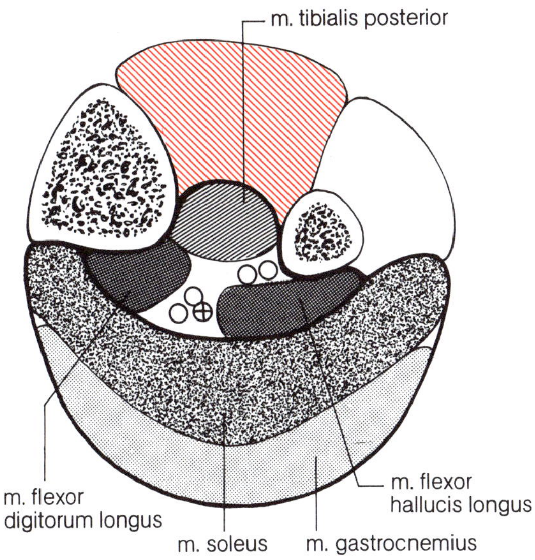

Anatomy

1

Reduction of venous return and self-strangulation of the musculature following fracture, contusion or operation affect, above all, the compartment of the tibialis anterior muscle.

Diagnosis

Anterior tibial syndrome: paralytic signs similar to paralysis of the common peroneal nerve (in abortive cases often the only sign), muscle compartment stony hard, unbearable spontaneous pain until the muscles have undergone necrosis.

Posterior muscle compartment: pain, equinus position, pain increases on dorsiflexion of the foot, posterior muscle compartment greatly distended or even stony hard. Initial symptoms *similar to deep phlebothrombosis*.

Operation, indication and timing

The indication for surgery should be established very liberally because possible complications are few and their incidence is extremely low. Anterior splitting of the compartment as a routine measure of prophylaxis, as for example in performing plate fixation in the lower leg or the head of the tibia (!), is not only justifiable but advisable.

Timing of the operation: as a prophylactic measure at the conclusion of an operation or – in an emergency – at the appearance of the first suspicious manifestations.

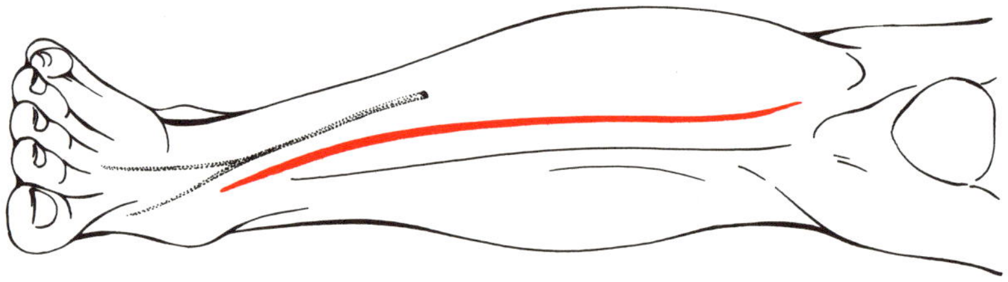

Principle

2

To be effective, splitting of the fascia must be done as extensively as possible, i.e., over a length of 25 cm at least.

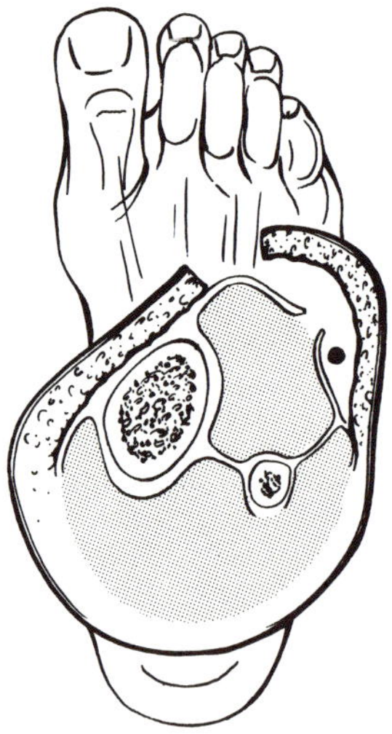

3

The fascia must be split as far laterally as possible (Beware of injuring the superficial peroneal nerve!).

Tactics

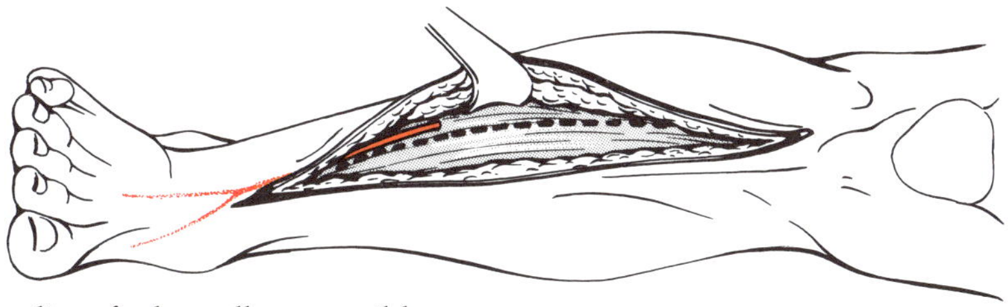

4

To relieve the *anterior compartment*, the fascia is split as far laterally as possible, but still medially to the point where the superficial peroneal nerve makes its exit.

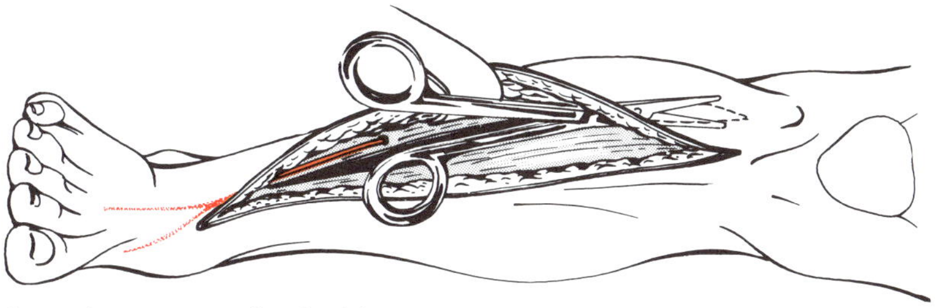

5

The fascia is exposed in its entire length by detaching the covering skin by blunt dissection until the superficial peroneal nerve becomes visible at its point of exit.

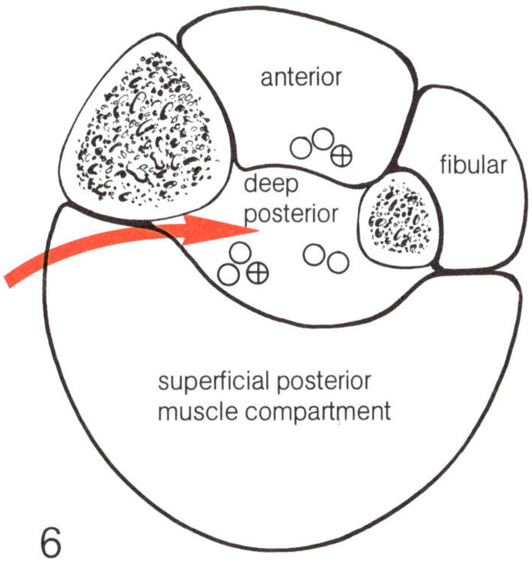

6

To relieve the *posterior compartment*, incise on the medial side (not in the midline). By so doing, one can penetrate toward the fascia of the deep compartment without major detachment of muscles.

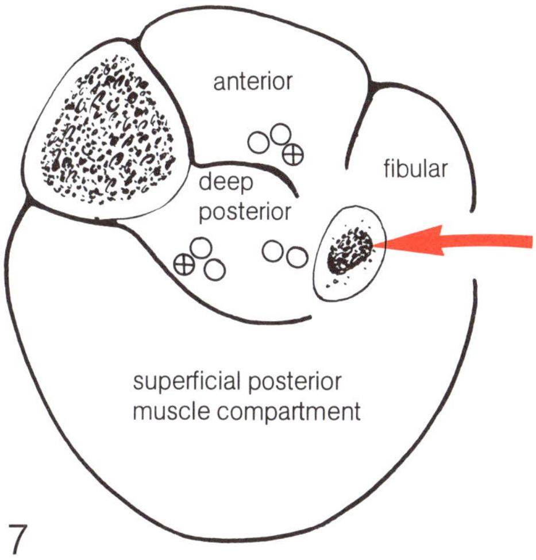

7

To relieve *all four compartments simultaneously*, fibulectomy is a possibility.

Postoperative care

The skin remains open. The leg is elevated on a splint. When the posterior fascia has been split the skin edges can be approximated with sterile strips. Secondary suturing can generally be done after 10 to 14 days.

Possibilities of reconstruction

Troublesome gaps in the fascia can be closed, for example, with Dura.

15. Talocrural Joint

Anatomy

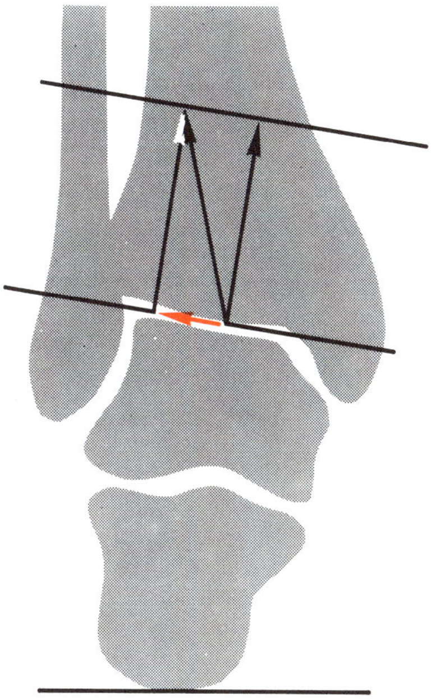

1

On weight bearing, strain is always directed toward the distal tibiofibular joint.

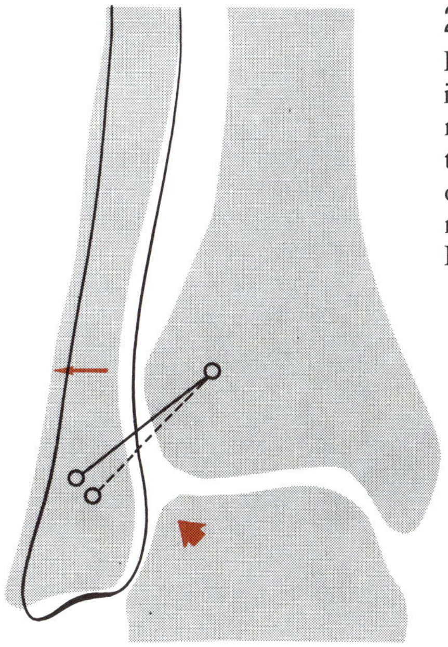

2

In spite of its inherent lack of extensibility, the syndesmosis allows a certain resilience of the external malleolus, due to the oblique course of the fibers. It is only this circumstance that allows any movement at the talocrural joint (See Fig. 305–1.).

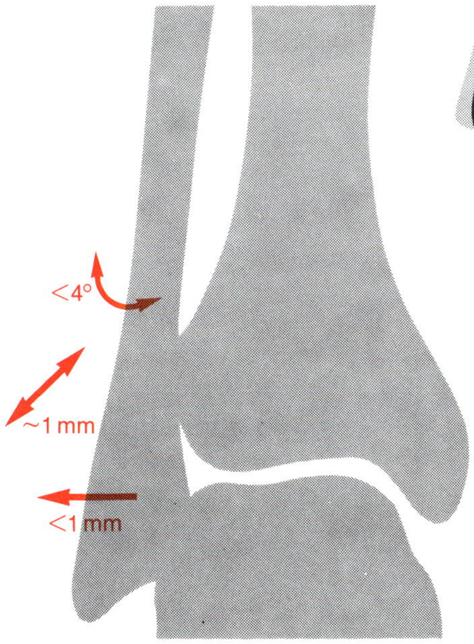

3

Excursions in the fibulotibial snydesmosis.

Types of injuries

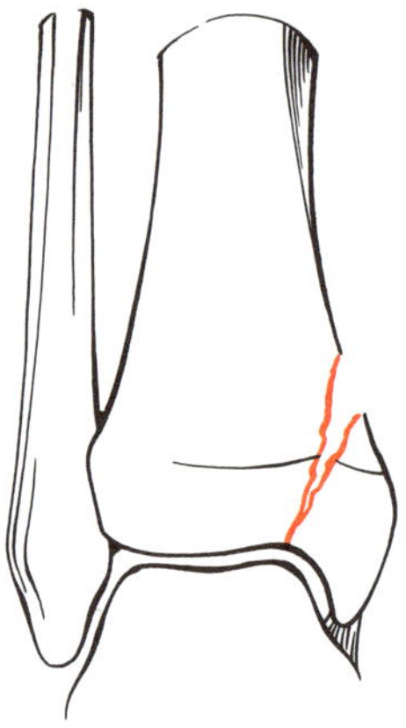

4

Medial ligament or *medial malleolus:*
Isolated fractures of the medial malleolus are very infrequently accompanied by subluxation of the tibiotalar joint, because the fibula alone affords sufficient support.

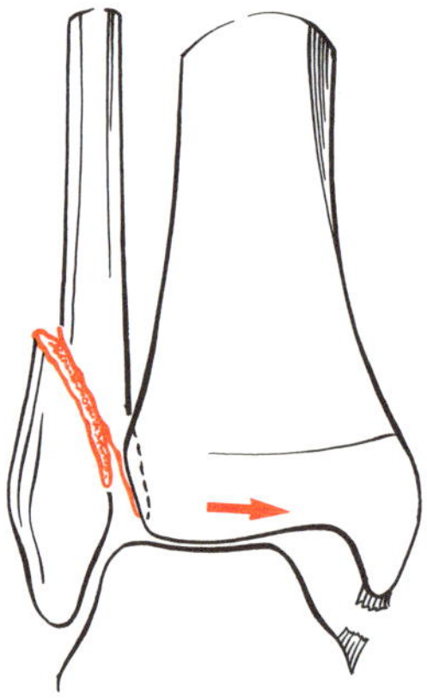

5

Lateral ligament of lateral malleolus: Isolated fractures of the lateral malleolus are almost regularly accompanied by subluxation of the tibiotalar joint. In most instances, however, the tibial collateral ligament also tears away and must be sutured.

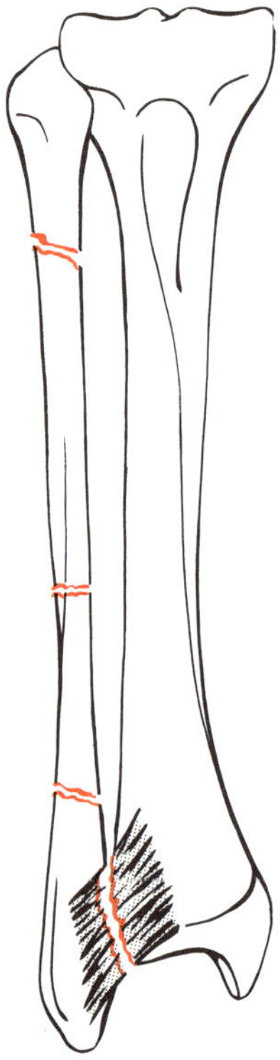

6

Rupture of the *anterior syndesmosis:* this injury is almost invariably associated with (high) fracture of the fibula. Injury to the syndesmosis can occur *without* fracture of the fibula as well as *with* fracture of the fibula of any localization above the syndesmosis. Therefore in every case it is necessary to search for an injury of the syndesmosis, i.e., this structure must be exposed during operation.

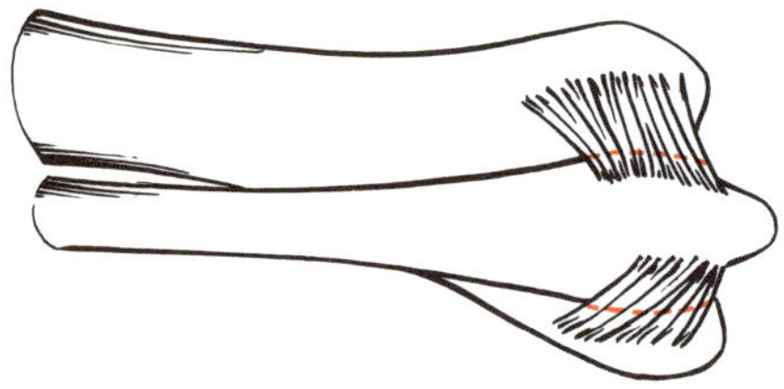

7

Injury of the *posterior syndesmosis:* this is almost always an associated injury. It does not need any treatment.

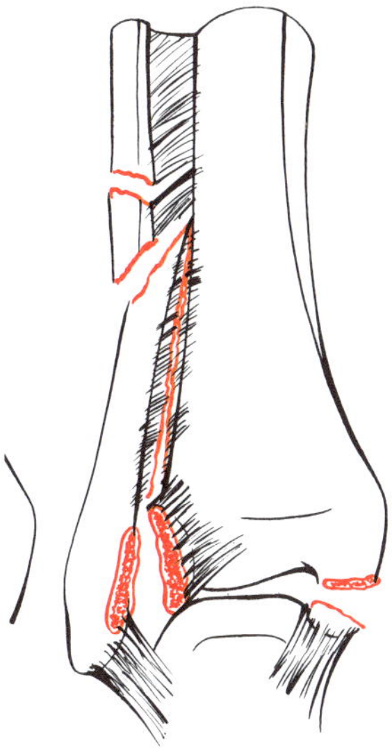

8
Rupture of the *interosseous membrane:* almost always associated with the injuries depicted in Figs. 264–4 and 286–5.

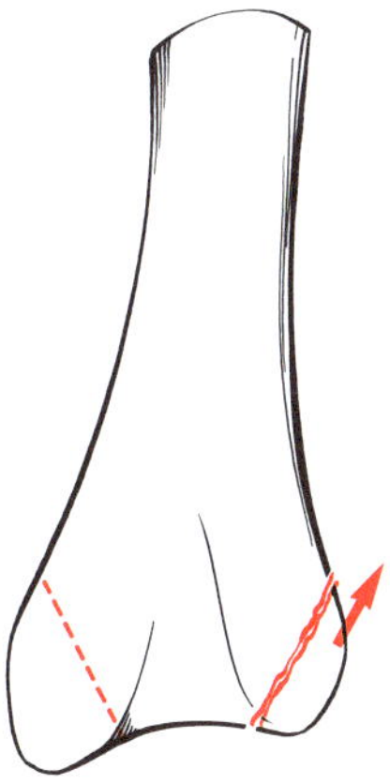

9
Posterior (Volkmann's triangle) or *anterior* breaking off of the edge of the tibia: almost invariably associated with one of the aforementioned injuries.

Diagnosis

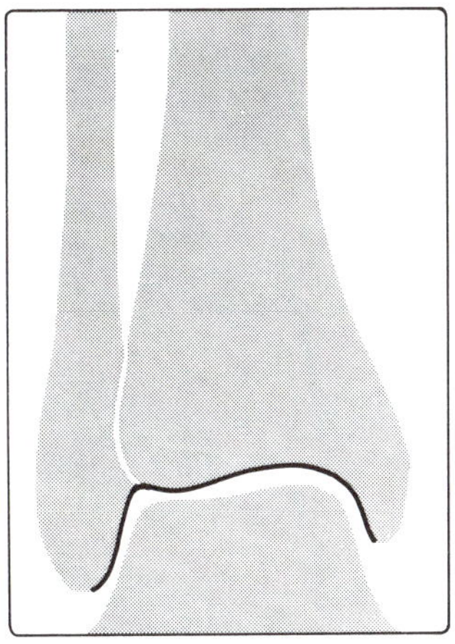

10
Diagnosis of shortening of the fibula: the anteroposterior roentgenogram provides an accurate picture of the fibulotibial joint space.
Joint line unbroken = normal closure of the ankle mortise, fibula not shortened.

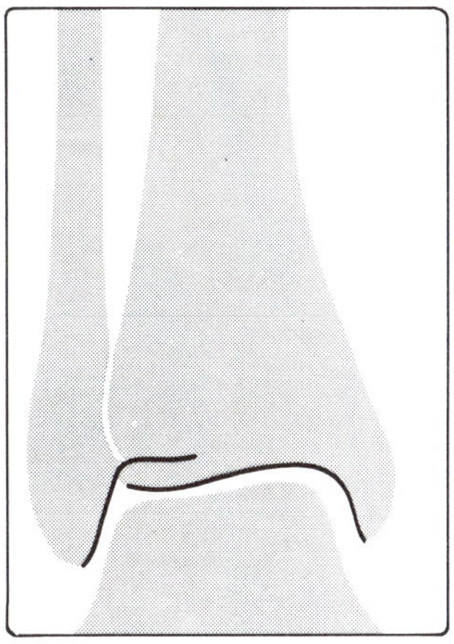

11
Broken joint line = in this instance: shortening of the fibula.

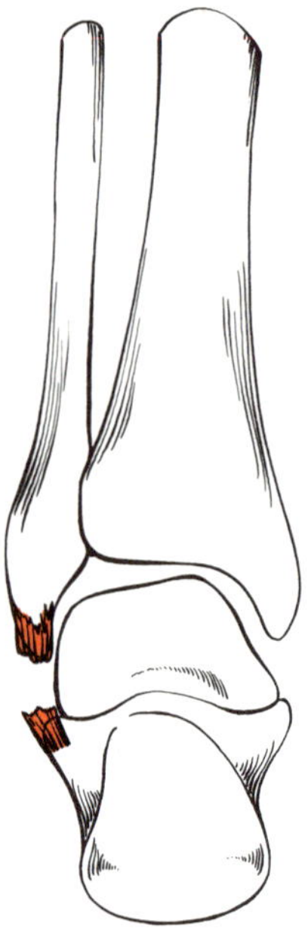

12

Roentgenogram with the lower leg slightly bent toward the side of the intact ligament...

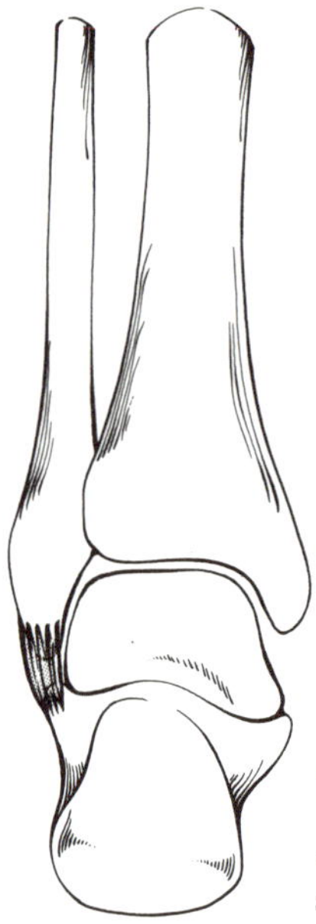

13

... always to be compared with the uninjured side.

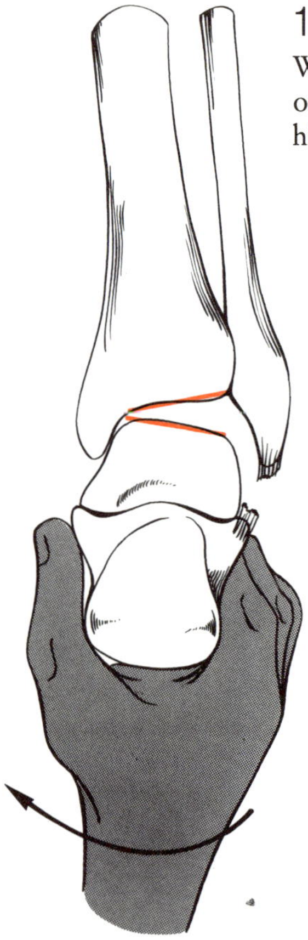

14

With this sort of roentgenogram it is of the greatest importance that the hindfoot be clasped and tilted...

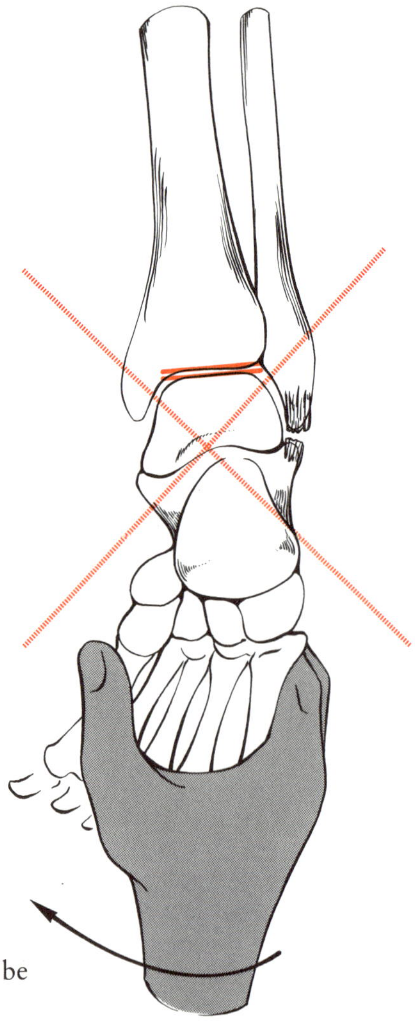

15

... and not only the forefoot be twisted.

16

Standardized roentgenograms can be obtained with the device indicated by Scheuba.

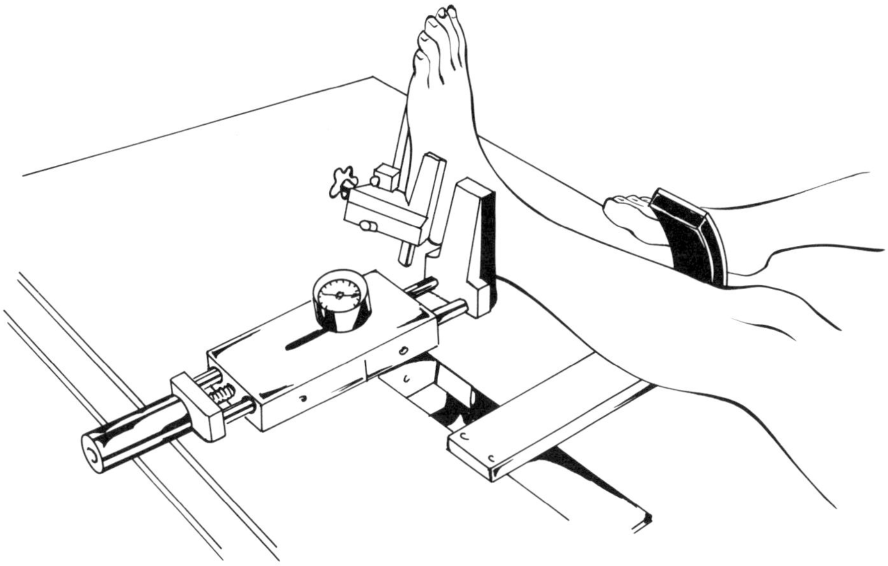

Indication

All ligament injuries – in which the roentgenograms taken with the lower leg bent toward the uninjured side show (and document) that the articular surfaces of the talocrural joint can be separated – and all injuries of the bones are an indication for operative management.

Timing of the operation

Within the first hours after the injury (before major swelling has developed). Prompt reduction and elevation of the leg (to more than 60°) prevent the occurrence of secondary necrosis of soft tissues through pressure from the inside by edges of fragments and rapid development of major swelling. Otherwise the operation is deferred for 5 to 8 days until the swelling has subsided. In the meantime: closed reduction and plaster immobilization.

Operative possibilities, principle

Injuries of the *collateral ligaments:* adapting suture, first applied laterally, then medially.

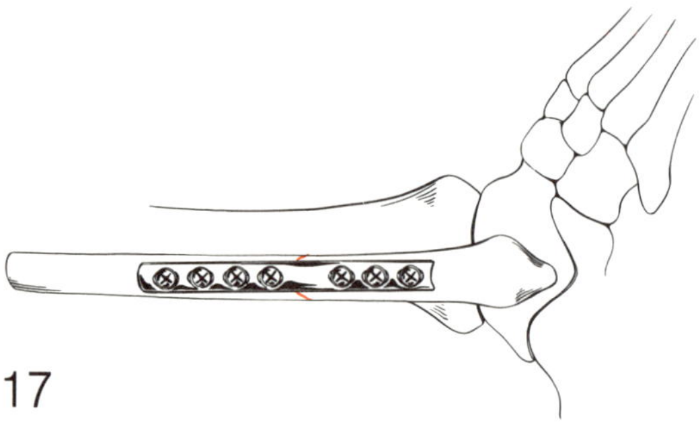

17
Lateral malleolus: one – third tubular plate.

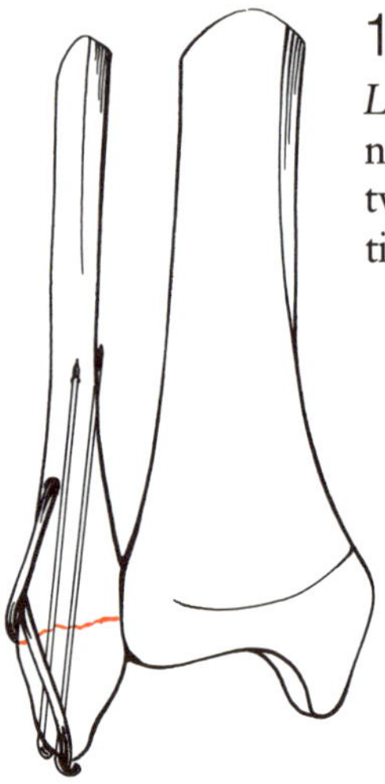

18
Lateral malleolus, transverse fracture underneath the syndesmosis: external fixation over two parallel drilling wires for the purpose of traction.

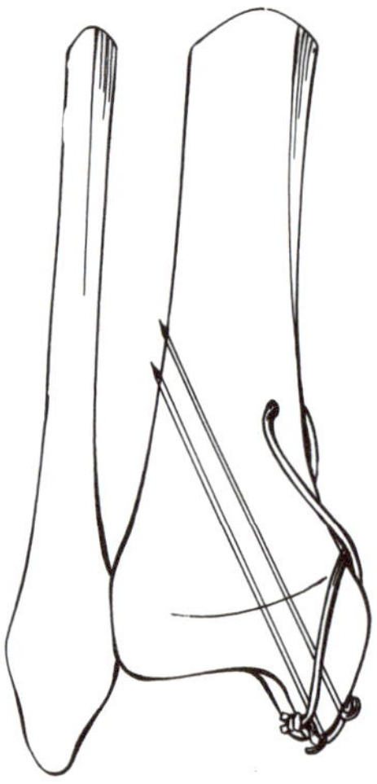

19
Medial malleolus: traction fixation over two parallel drilling wires.

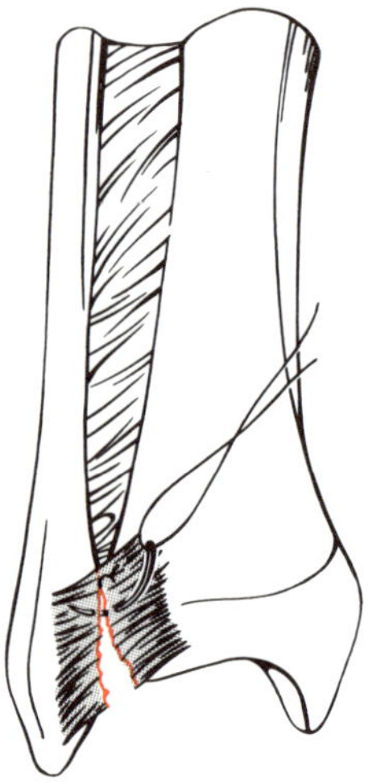

20
Syndesmosis: suture.

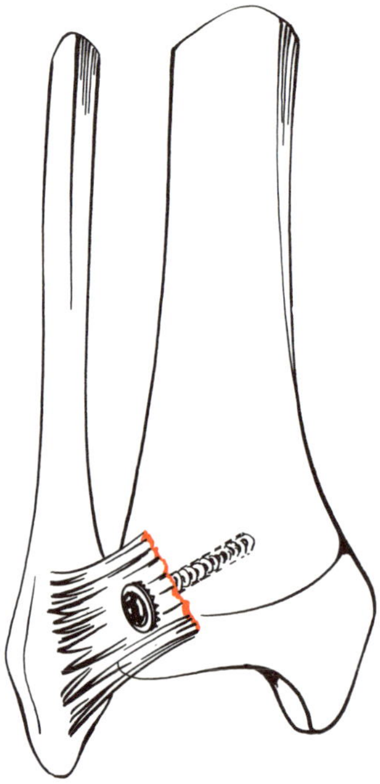

21
Syndesmosis, avulsions from bone: screw with toothed supporting disk.

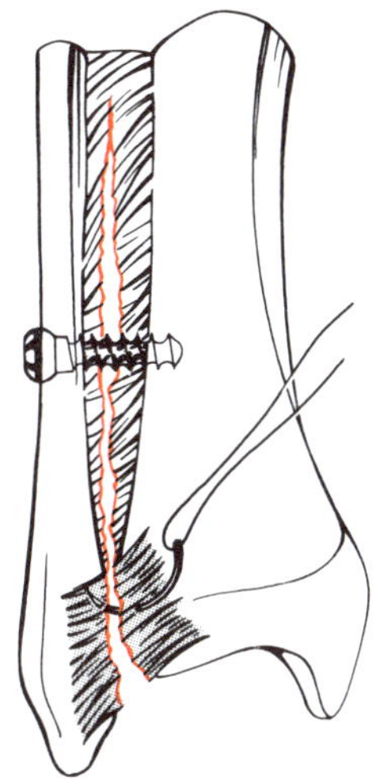

22

Interosseous membrane: short adjusting screw. An adjusting screw is always employed when the crural interosseous membrane is concomitantly ruptured to such an extent that, despite stable reconstruction of the fibula in the distal tibiofibular joint, there remains the tendency to displacement (subluxation of the talocrural joint).

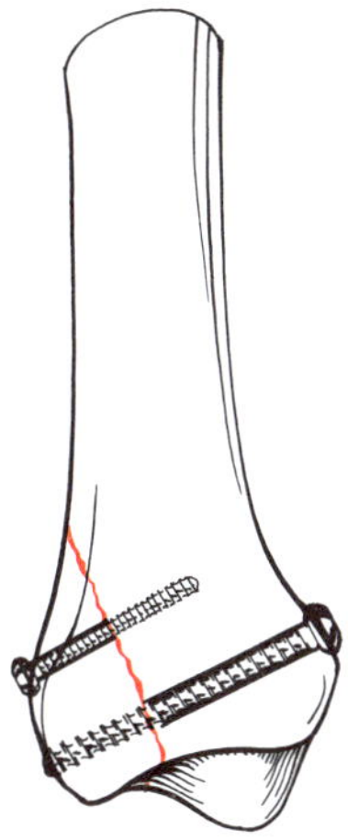

23

Volkmann's triangle: traction screw plus small-fragment screw.

Postoperative care

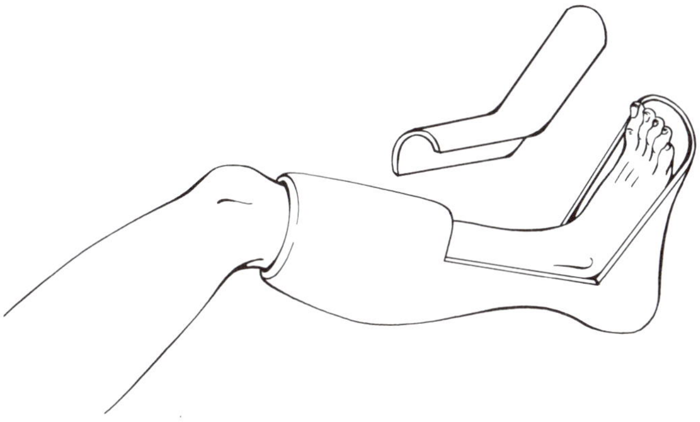

24

Postoperatively, a well-padded, closed, below-knee plaster cast is applied and the leg is elevated on a splint. When the drainage is removed and the dressing is changed on the first or second day after operation, a plaster shell is applied as shown in the figure.

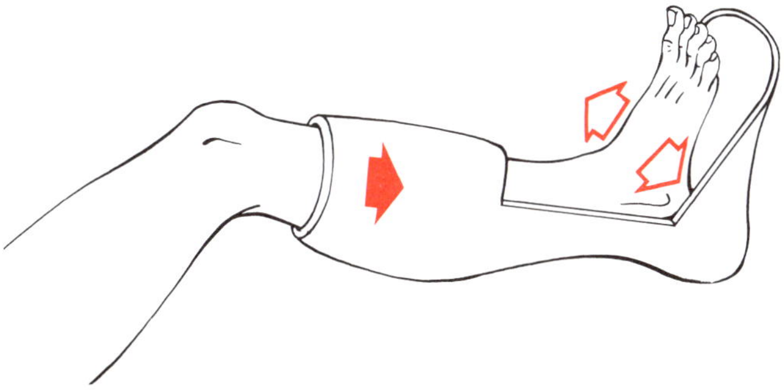

25

The patient is thus enabled to perform guided movements, starting with dorsiflexion. Later on the plaster shell can be pushed down and plantar flexion be exercised in addition.

Talocrural joint – medial compartment

Anatomy See Figs. 285–1 ff.

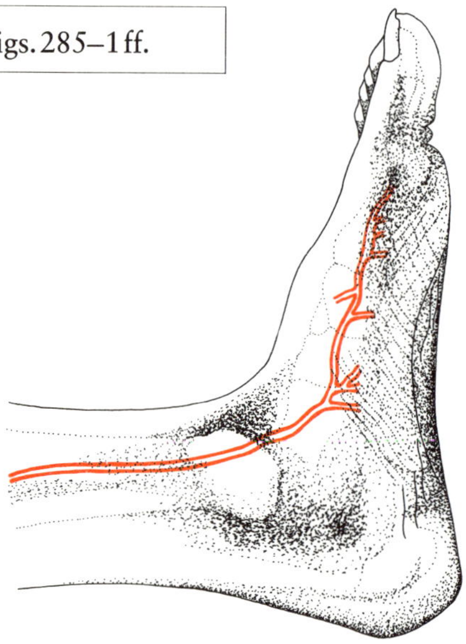

1
The great saphenous vein and the v. saphena marginalis medialis can be pulled away anteriorly.

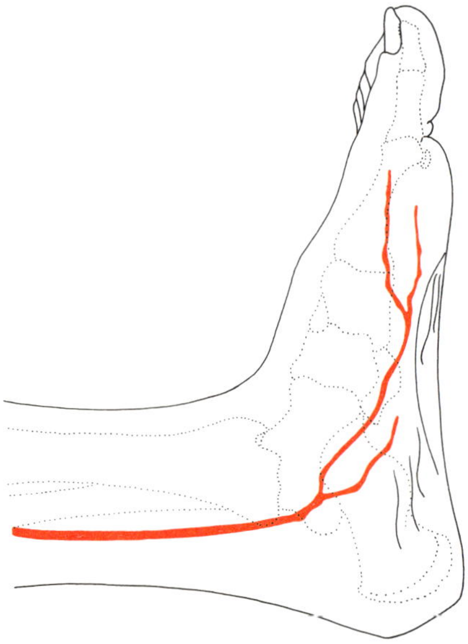

2
The tibialis posterior artery, though not greatly endangered, should be borne in mind.

Diagnosis See Figs. 287–10 ff.

Operative indication and timing

See p. 289.

Principle See Fig. 290–19

Positioning See Fig. 219–16 f.

Approach

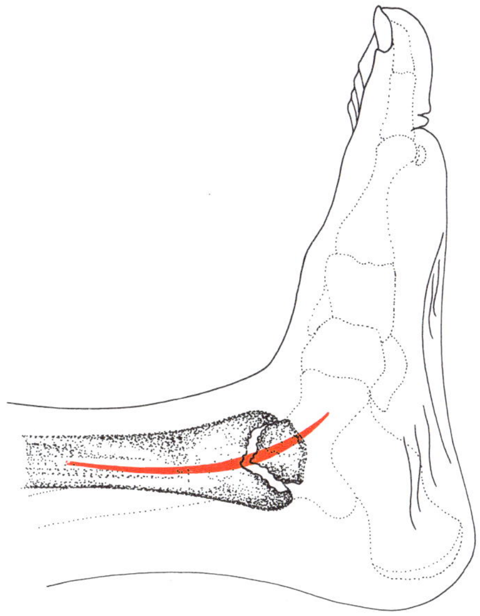

3
Skin incision.

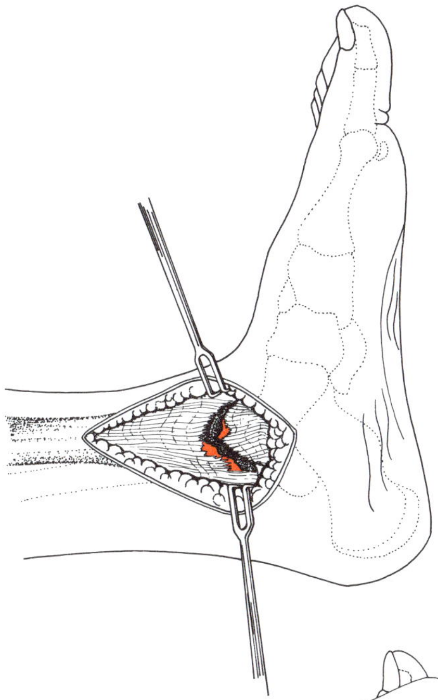

4
The incision is carried down to the bone; the fracture becomes visible.

Tactics

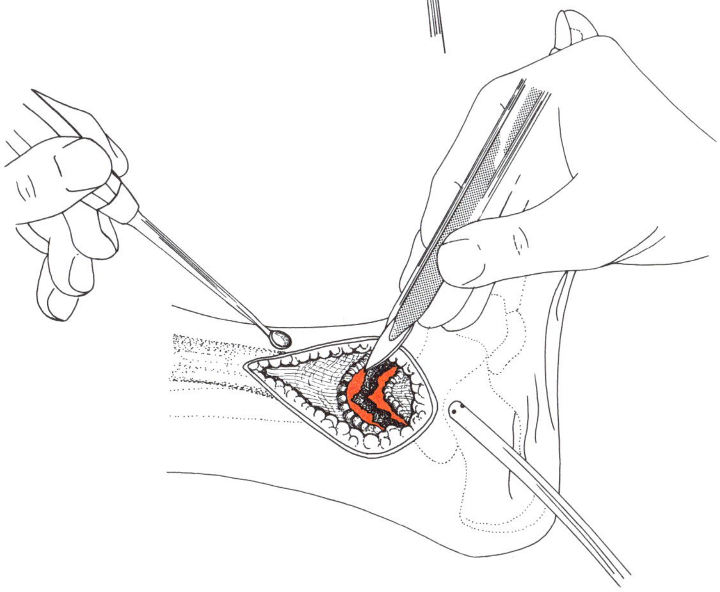

5
By sharp dissection, the periosteum is cautiously pushed 1–2 mm away from the borders of the fracture. Thus one can expose edges of the fracture which are important for the reduction; these edges could be too easily destroyed with a raspatory. The surfaces of the fracture are cleared of coagula and infolded shreds of periosteum by means of a spoon and a suction device.

6

Reduction with use of a single-pronged hook. Two strong drilling wires are inserted, ...

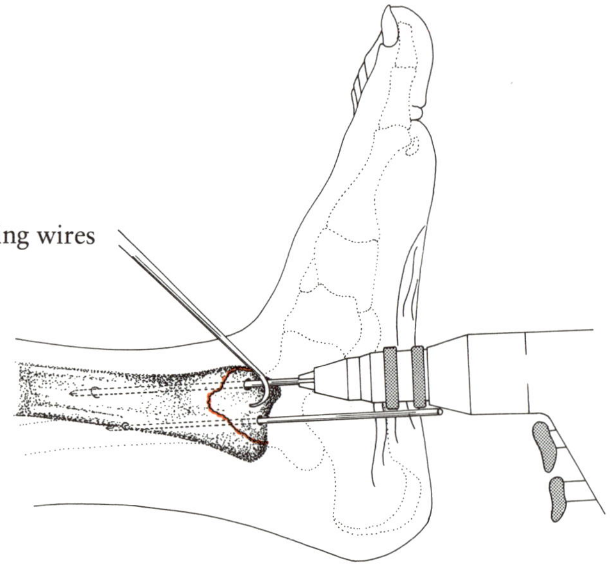

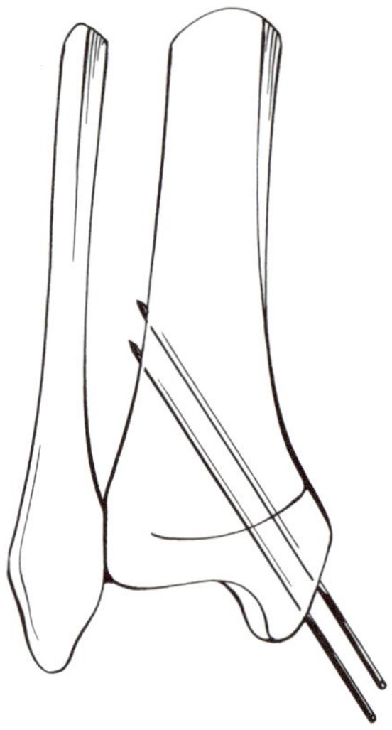

7

...the points of which should take purchase in the opposite cortex. The right direction is found more easily by keeping in mind that the location of the medial malleolus in the tibia is not exactly lateral but slightly anterior.

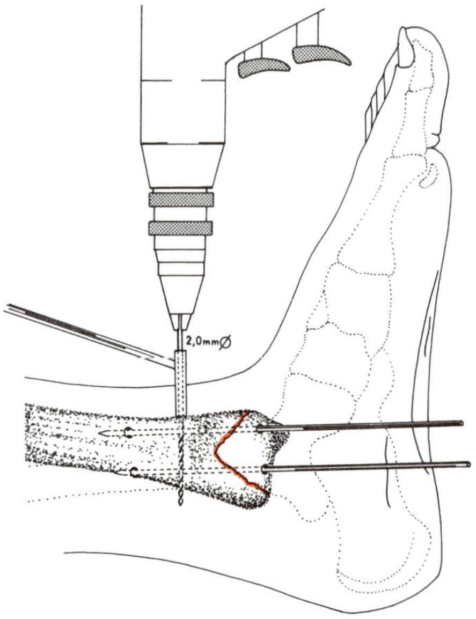

8

Stabilization by external traction wire. Transverse drill hole with 2.0 mm drill.

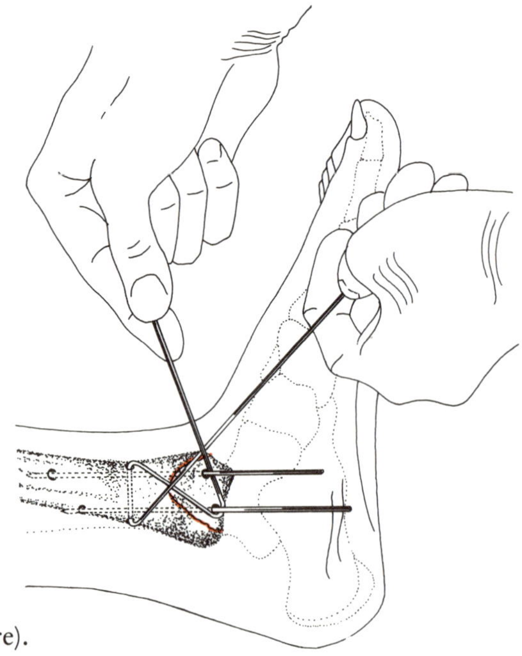

9

Applying the traction wiring (soft 1 mm wire).

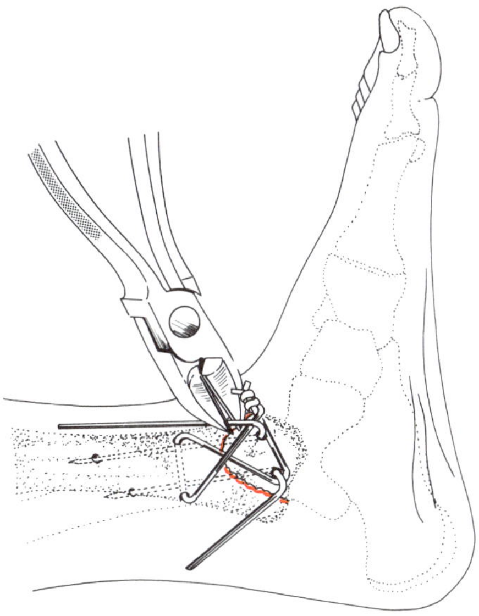

10
The wires are bent, one after the other, toward the fracture and then nipped off.

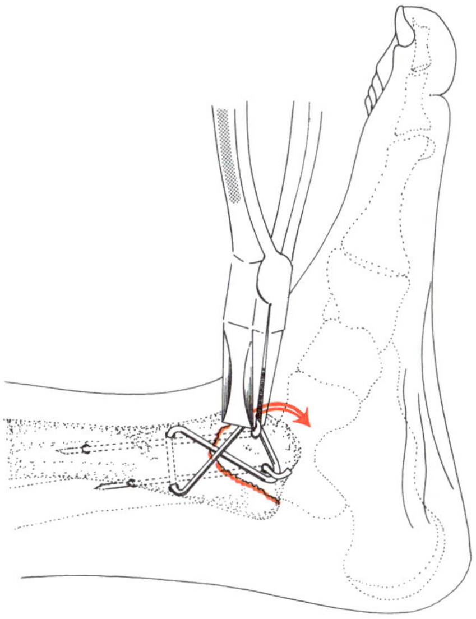

11
Once nipped, the wires are twisted distalward so that their ends are buried in the soft structures. The hooks should not be made too small since they constitute an additional hold that prevents the wires from slipping out.

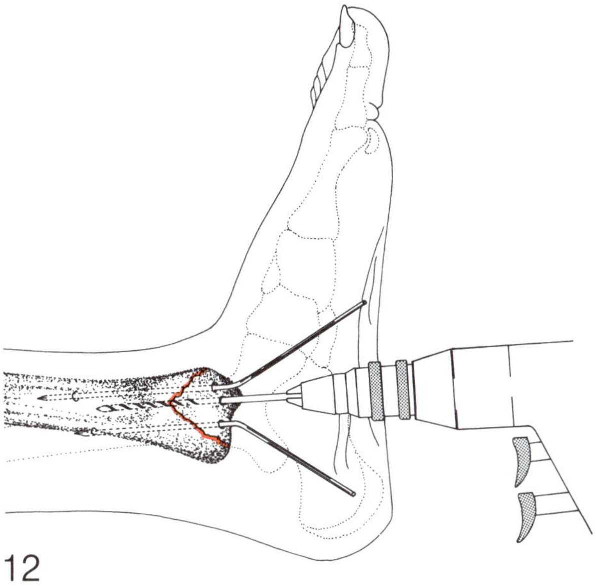

12
When the fixation is to be effected by a malleolar screw, a drill hole is made with the 3.2 mm drill. The required lengths of the screws are then determined.

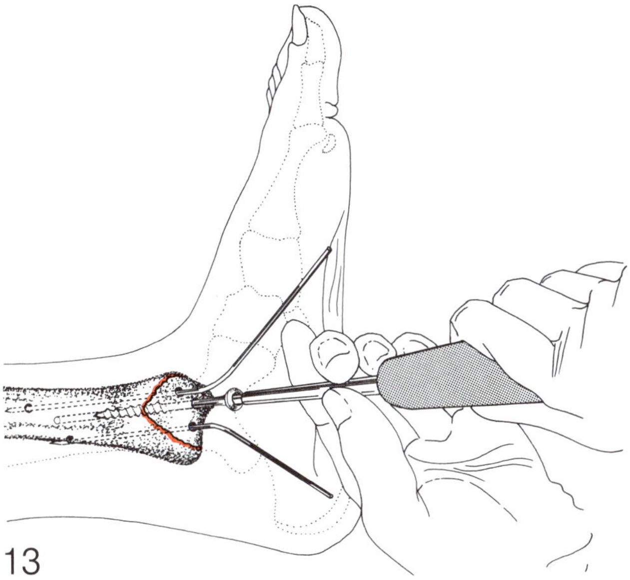

13
After tightening the screws, the drilling wires are removed. If there is a tendency for the fragment to rotate, an additional navicular screw can be inserted. External traction wiring is preferable.

Closure of the wound

The wound is rinsed with Ringer's solution and suction drainage is instituted. Only backstitch suture for the skin, no buried sutures.

Postoperative care See Fig. 292–24 f.

Talocrural joint – lateral compartment

Anatomy

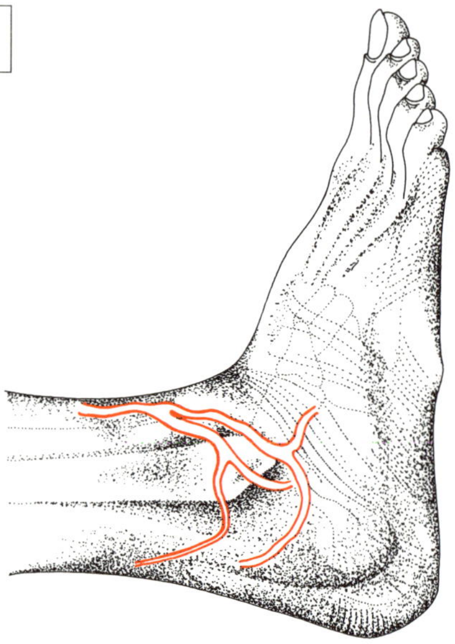

1

Venous plexuses at the lateral malleolus. Here, ligation is required.

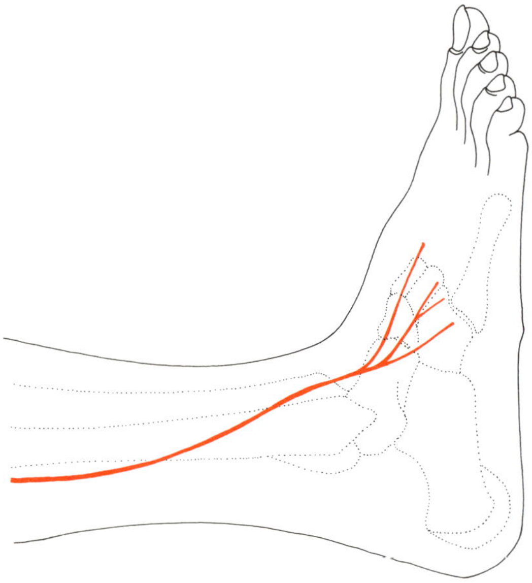

2

Superficial (fibular) peroneal nerve. This nerve must not be injured. It is best pulled away anteriorly.

Diagnosis See Figs. 287–10 ff.

Operative indication and timing See p. 289

Principle See Fig. 290–17 f.

Operative possibilities

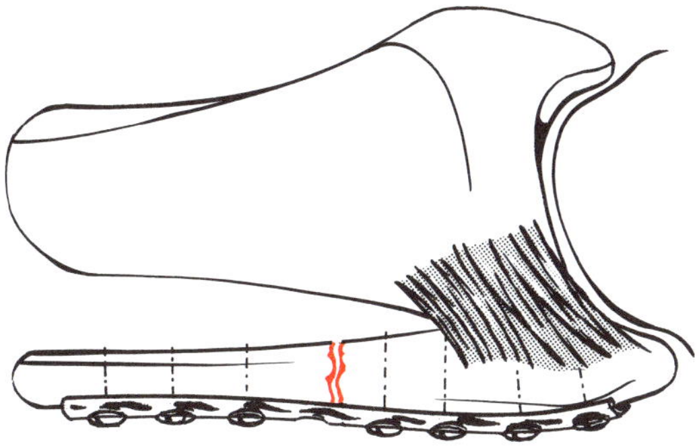

3
Of greatest importance is the restoration of the original length of the lateral malleolus. Only then will there be no subluxation when at rest and on weight bearing.
Virtually all fractures can be stabilized with a one – third tubular plate.

4
Interfragmental compression can often be obtained with use of a traction screw (3.5 mm). On no account, however, must a navicular or cancellous screw be used for this purpose, only a cortical screw.

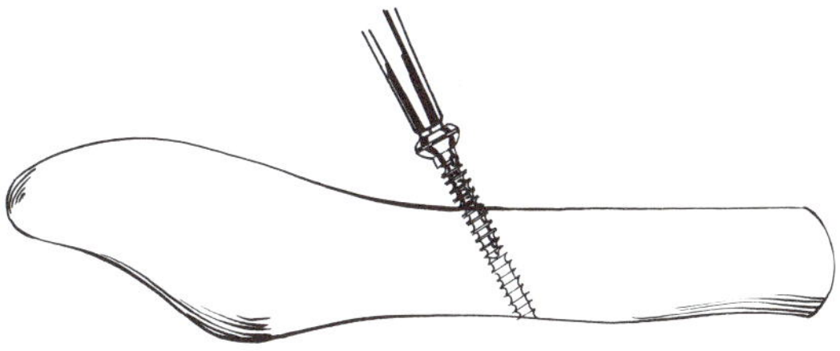

5
A navicular or a cancellous screw is very apt to break off when being removed.

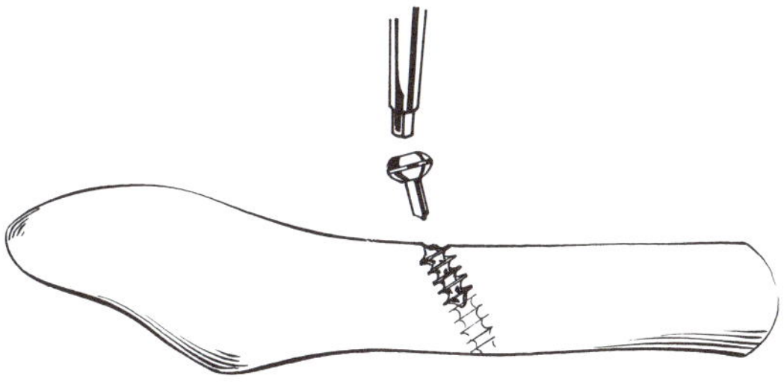

6
Transverse fractures below the syndesmosis can also be cared for by applying an external wire for traction. Other methods such as a Rush pin or a single screw frequently offer technical difficulties and can easily lead to displacement of the fragment.

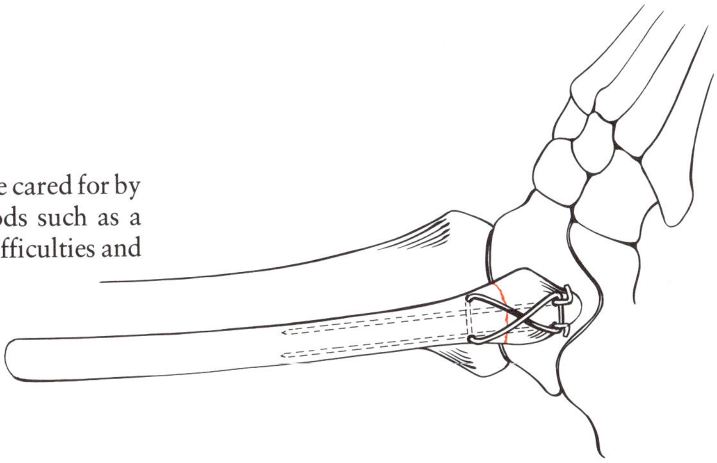

7
By using drilling wires of adequate thickness, one can safely anchor their points in the cortex. Only when placed within the marrow cavity are the wires liable to move backward.

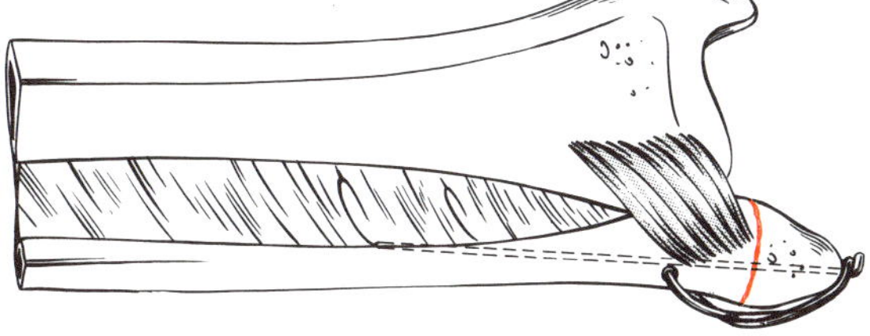

Positioning See Fig. 219–16f.

Approach

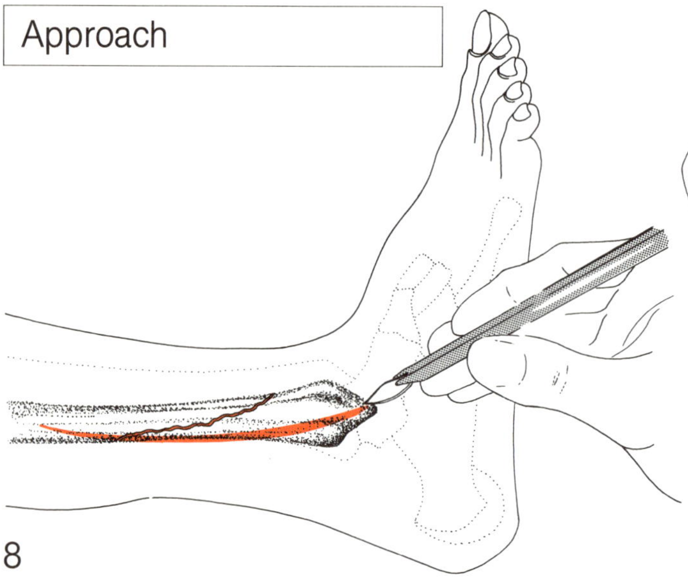

8
Skin incision as usual. When injury of the syndesmosis is suspected, the incision can also be carried from the anterior around the tip of the lateral malleolus. This procedure, however, involves greater danger of injuring the superficial peroneal nerve, whereas the customary skin incision, if of sufficient length, will allow adequate exposure.

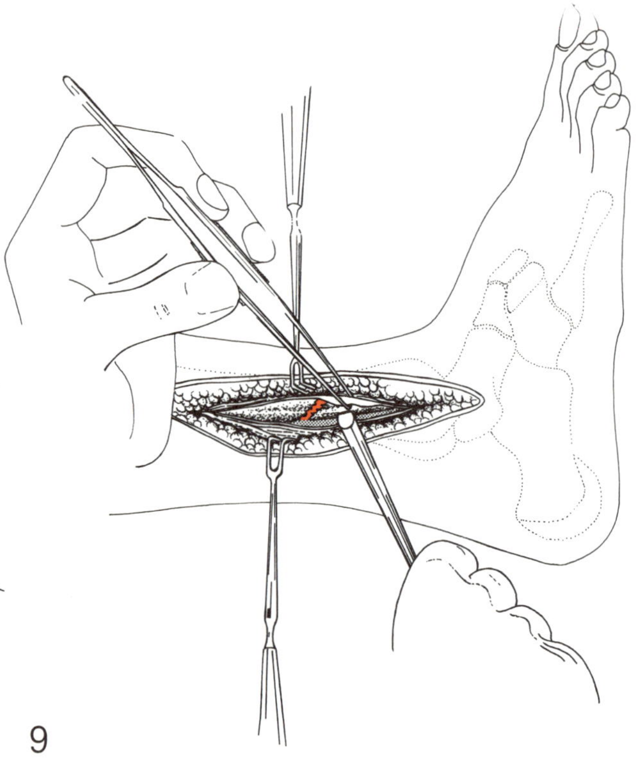

9
The tissues are divided by scalpel down to the bone so that no lateral pouches or fissures are produced. The soft structures are pushed away from the bone with a raspatory.

Tactics

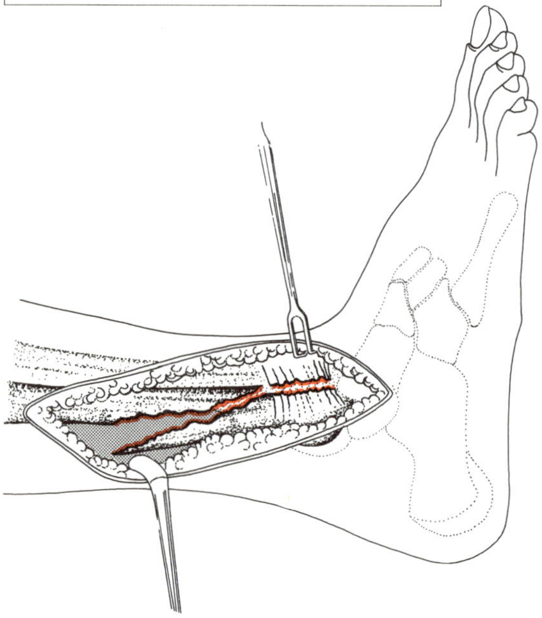

10
The syndesmosis is exposed and examined; above all, the proximal tip of the fragment is exposed.

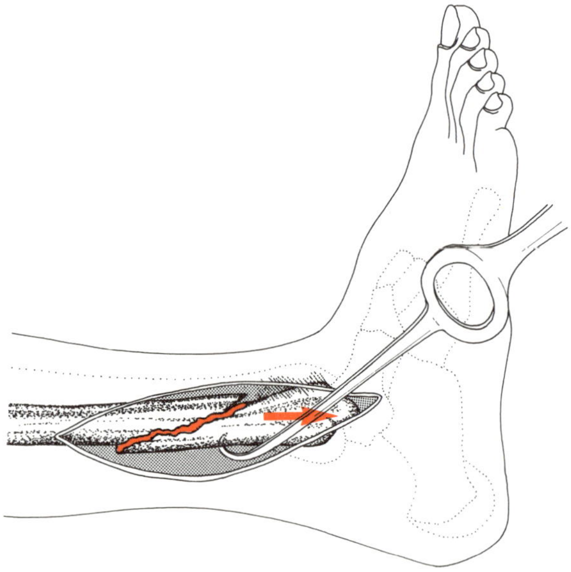

11
Reduction with use of a large single-pronged hook.

12

Preliminary fixation with small repositioning forceps. Following this, application of screw traction and plate fixation, using a one-third tubular plate with 7 or 8 holes.

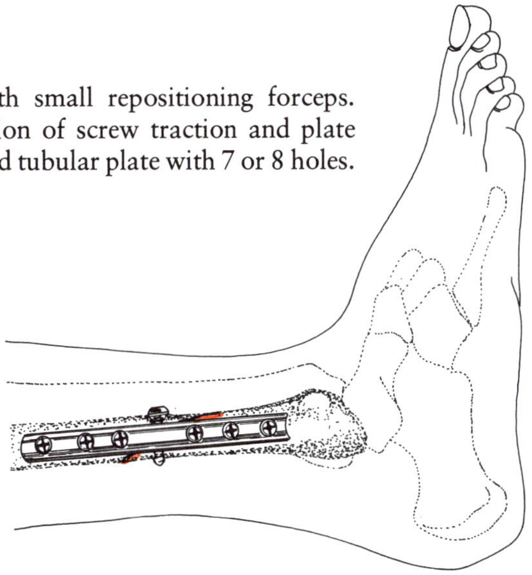

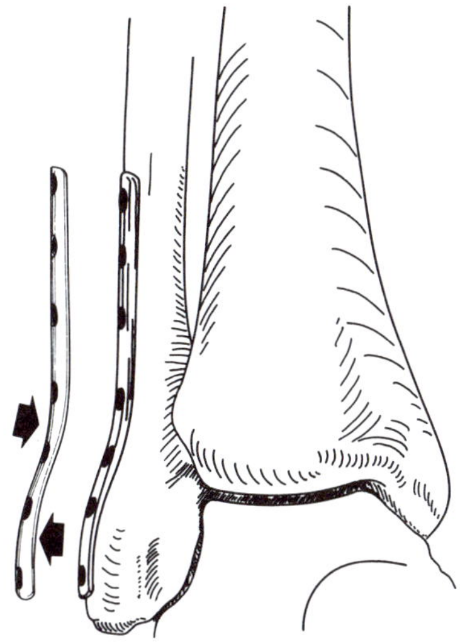

13

The third-tubular plate must be adjusted to the shape of the lateral malleolus so as not to force it into an adducted position.

14

This can be done easily and precisely with the use of two strong, flat pliers applied transversely to the plate. Be careful to avoid kinking the plate.

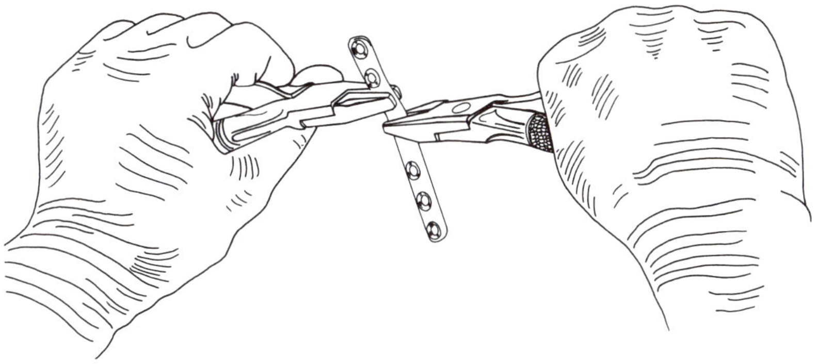

Closure of the wound See p. 295.

Postoperative care See p. 292.

Possibilities for reconstruction

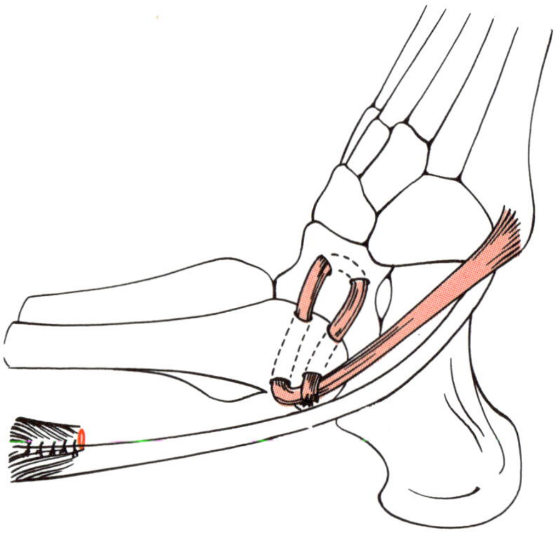

15

Plastic reconstruction of the ligaments is done by the Watson-Jones technique, using the tendon of the peroneus brevis muscle or a part of it.

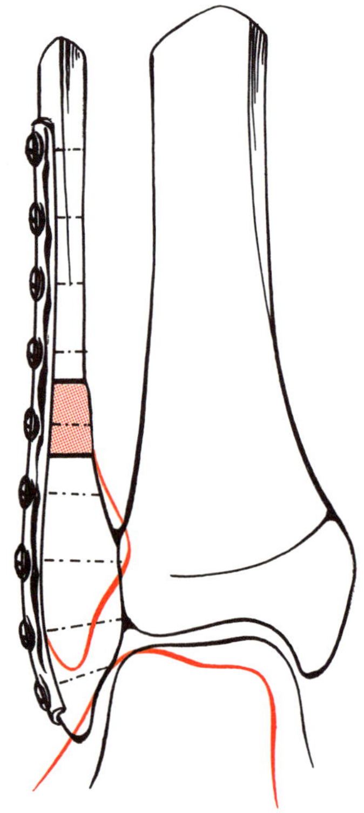

16

Lengthening osteotomy of fibula.

Adjusting screw

Indication See p. 289.

Tactics

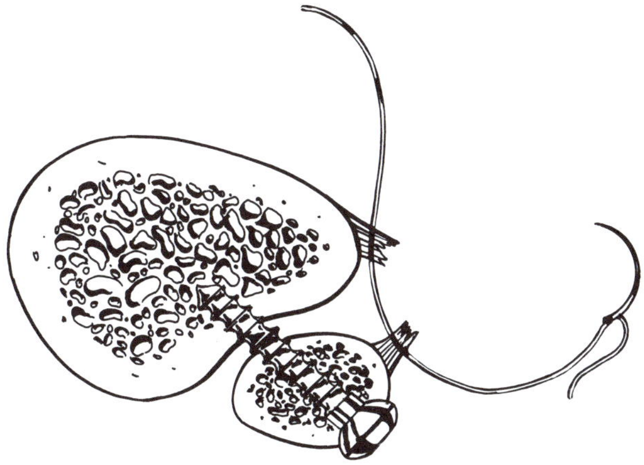

1
An injured syndesmosis is sutured. When the interosseous membrane has been concomitantly ruptured, the appropriate distance is first created and then maintained with an adjusting screw. In the tibia, the adjusting screw engages only one cortex.

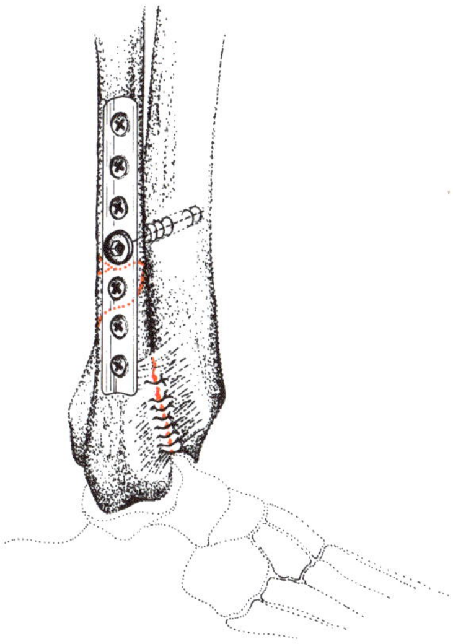

2
An adjusting screw (or a 4.5 mm cortical screw) can also be inserted through a one-third tubular plate.

Inferior edge of the tibia

Indication

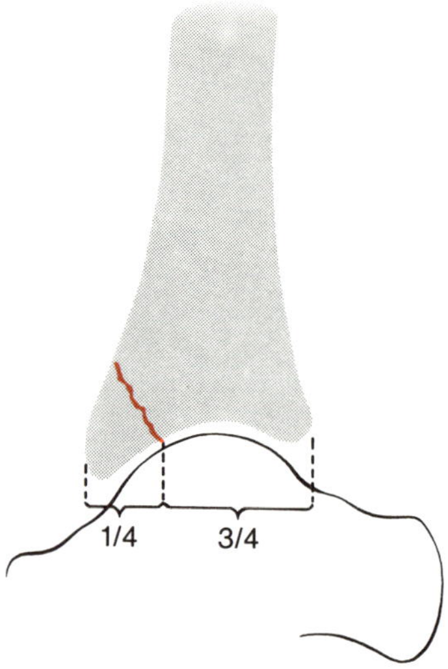

1

Operation is indicated when more than a quarter of the fracture involves the joint.

Approach

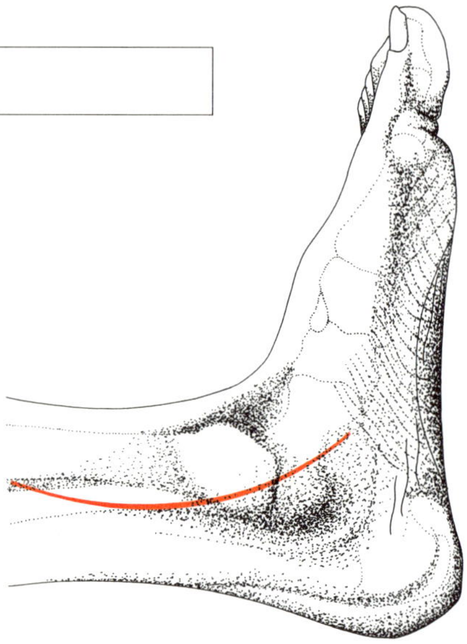

2

Skin incision posterior to the medial malleolus. The incision is carried right down to the bone and from there it advances dorsally.

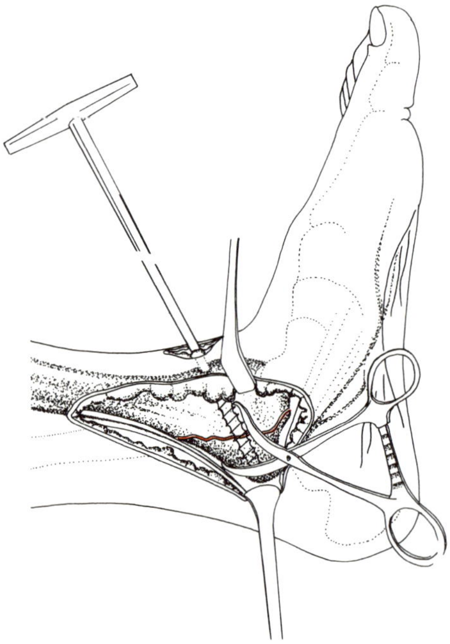

3

Reduction is facilitated by taking care to expose the proximal edge of the fracture adequately from the outset. Following reduction, fixation is undertaken through a separate small incision. (Caution: spare the dorsalis pedis artery!)

Tactics

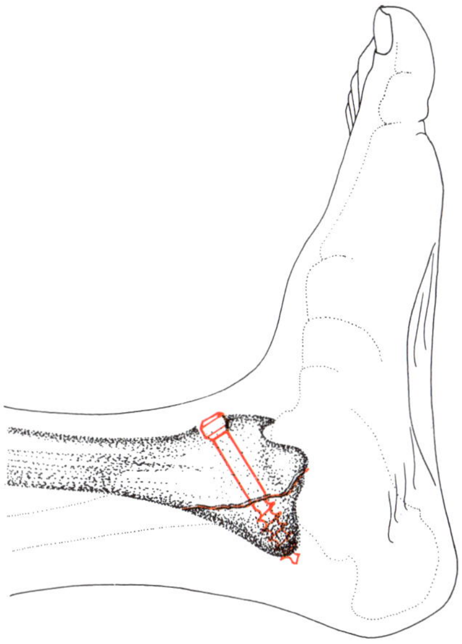

4

Compression osteosynthesis using a cancellous screw with a short thread (See p. 24.) or, preferably, a traction screw (See p. 22.). For small fragments, even the short thread of the cancellous screw is too long. One does better to allow the thread to project posteriorly so that it is certain to traverse the cleft of the fracture. Cancellous screws are often difficult to remove later. (See p. 297.) It is most often possible to insert the screw from a dorsal direction. Rotation is prevented by a second (small-fragment) screw. (See Fig. 291–23.)

16. Foot

Talus

Anatomy

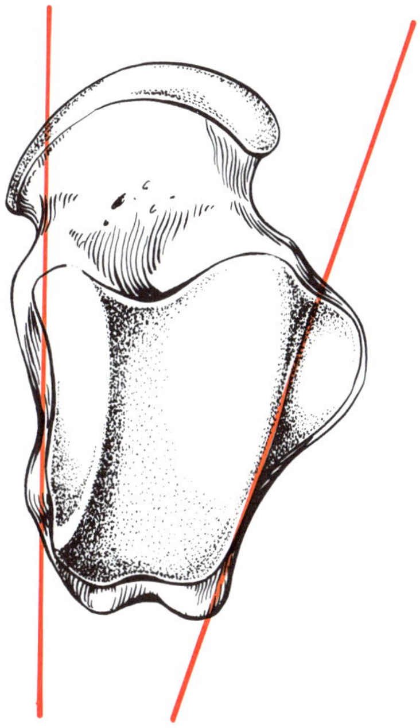

1
Top view of talus: articular surface wedge-shaped.

2
Bottom view of tibia and fibula: corresponding wedge shape of the distal ends of both bones of the lower leg.

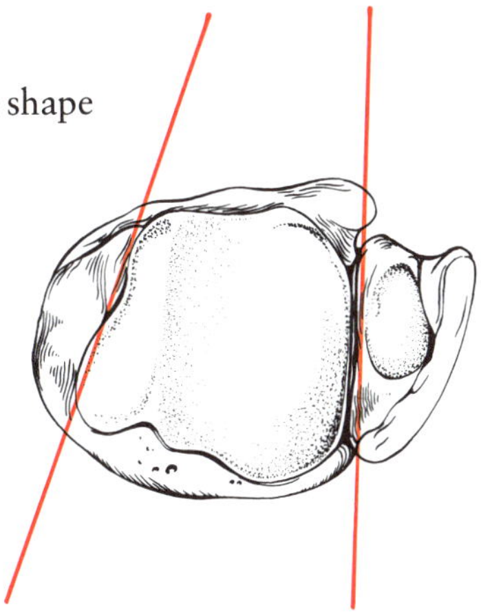

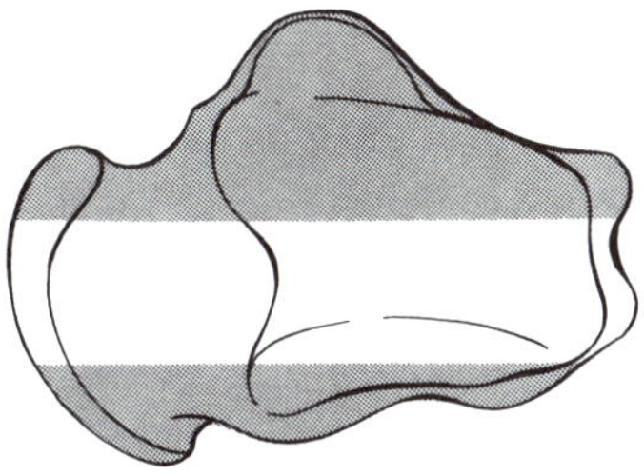

3
Blood supply to talus. In the top view, three zones can be distinguished.

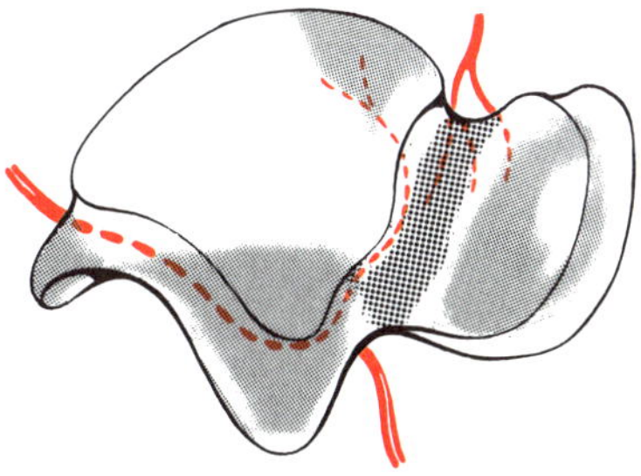

4
The blood supply to the chief articular surfaces of the talus is derived from the anterior tibial artery, the branches of which enter the neck of the talus from the cranial and from the caudal. Fractures of the neck of the talus cut off the interosseous connecting pathway to the body of the talus. The aim of treatment is to further the *revitalization* which starts from that site by rapid and adequate interfragmental stabilization.

Approach

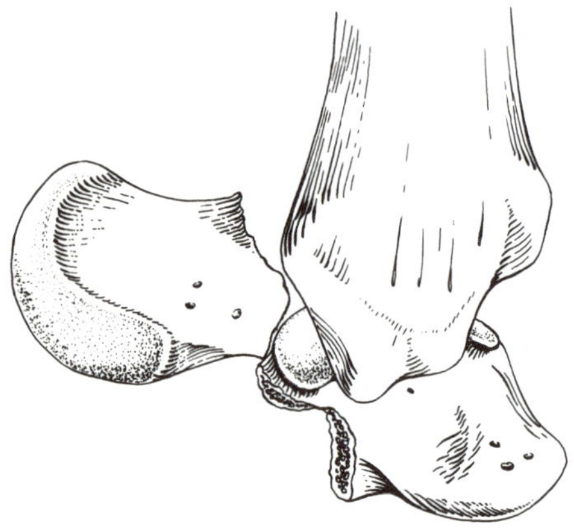

5

The anterior approach is suitable for fractures of the neck of the talus and for *fractures in the anterior region* of the body of the talus.

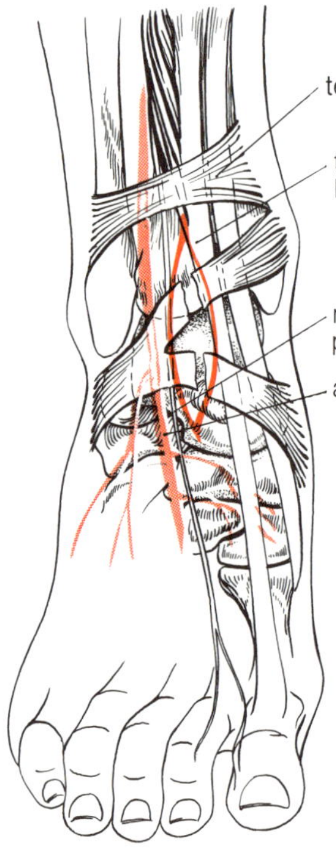

6

Longitudinal incision over the instep in continuation of the second digit cranially. Caution: spare the dorsalis pedis artery.

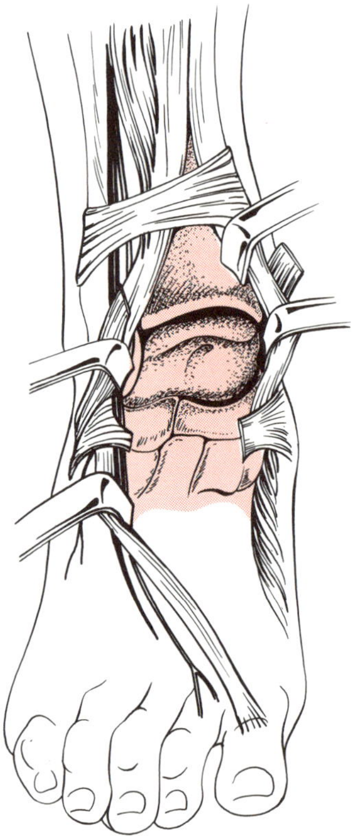

7

After opening the talocrural joint, large parts of the talus can be brought into view by plantar flexion of the foot.

For approach through the soft tissues in fractures of the *mesial and dorsal region,* see Fig. 292–1f.

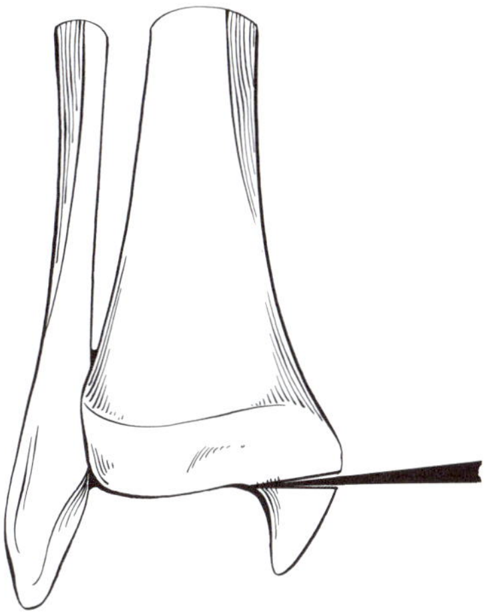

8

For the localizations of the fracture shown in the figure – subtalar dislocation, flake fractures of the edge of the talus – osteomy and folding down of the medial malleolus afford the best exposure. To this end, a wide incision must generally be made in the posterior capsule.

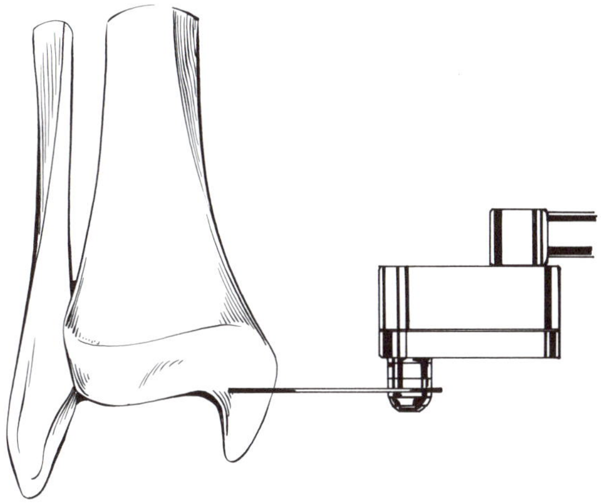

9

The innermost layer of bone and the cartilage are best sectioned with the chisel. Thus, reposition for definite union by external traction wiring over two parallel drill wires is performed more easily than when making a clean cut with the saw that would involve a loss of substance.

Tactics

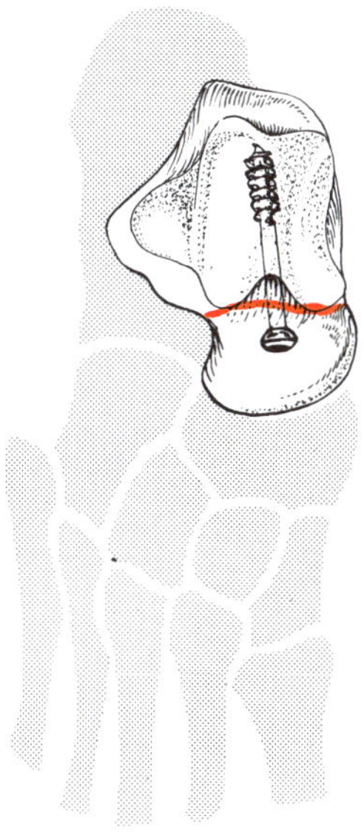

10

Fixation by means of a cancellous screw or...

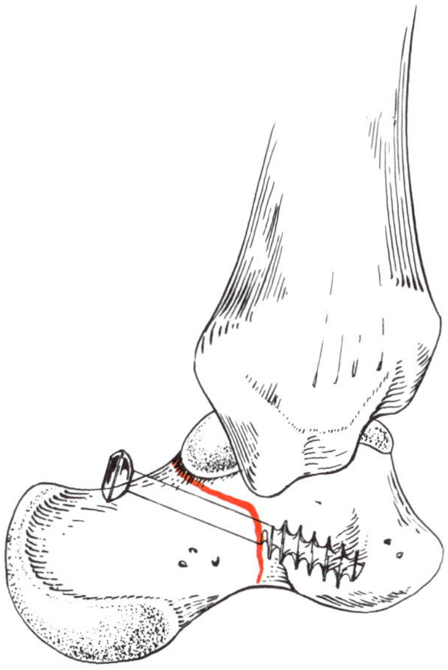

11

...two to three small-fragment screws.

Metatarsals

Principle

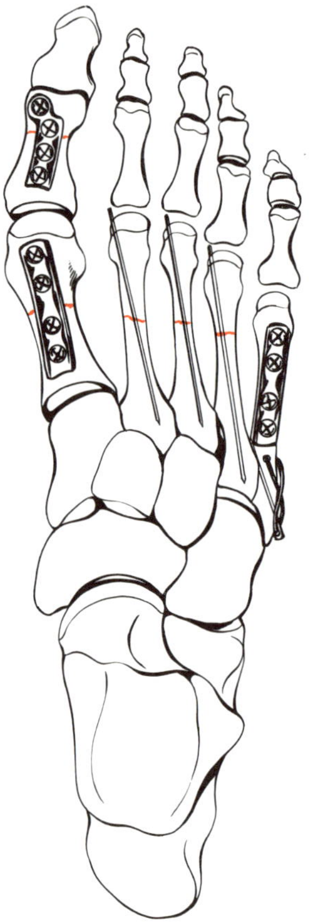

1
The first and the fifth digits should be stabilized in every case because they form the pillars of the plantar arch. The middle metatarsals can be fixed by (closed) osteosynthesis with use of drilling wires.

Approach

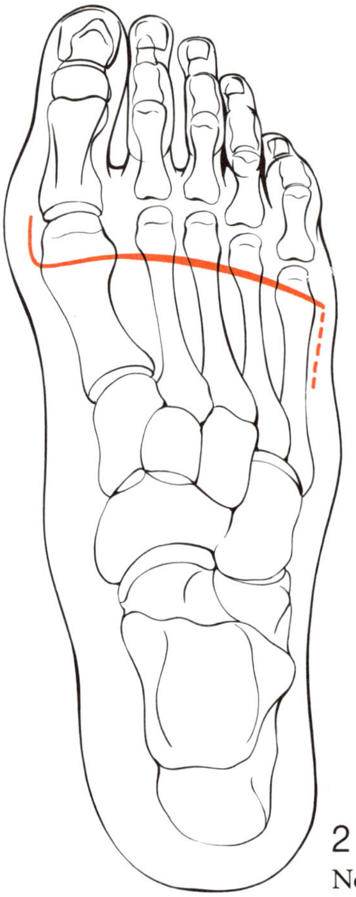

2
No plantar incision!

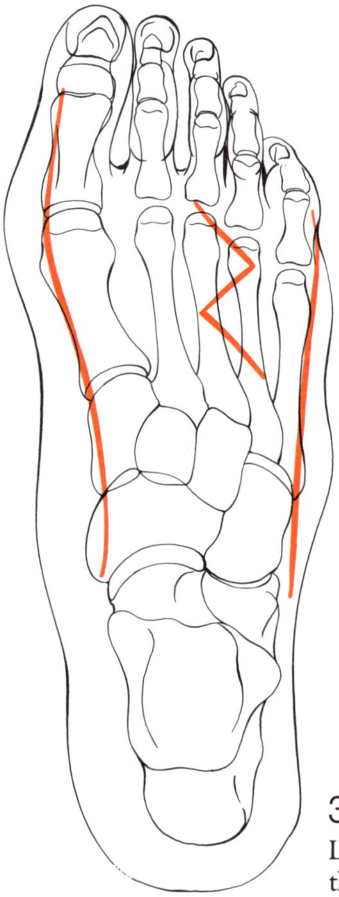

3
Lateral longitudinal incisions through the dorsum.

Tactics

Metatarsals I and V: set of flat, small-fragment instruments.

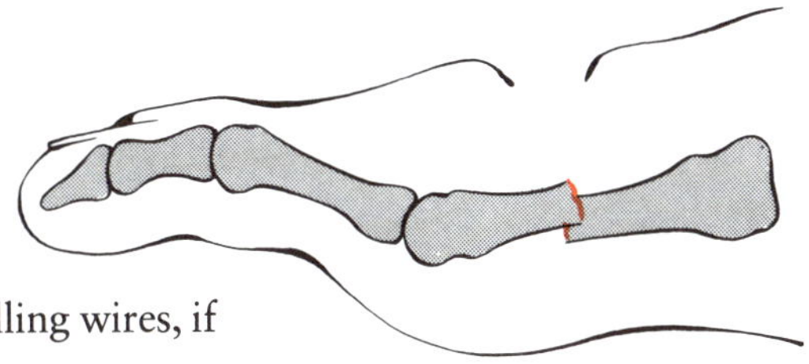

4
Metatarsals II to IV: Osteosynthesis with drilling wires, if necessary following open reduction.

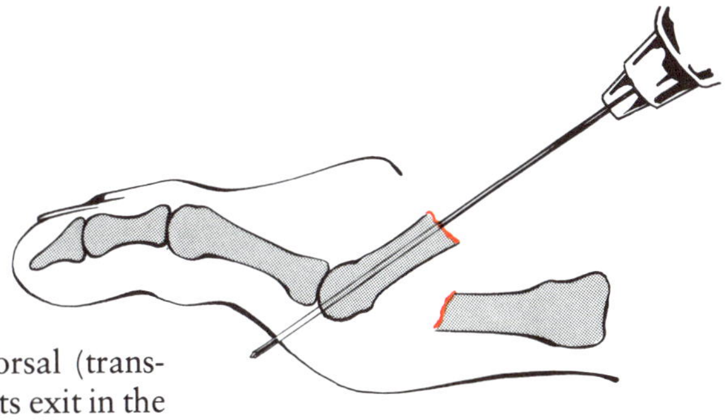

5
The distal fragment is threaded from the dorsal (transcutaneously) and transfixed; the wire makes its exit in the sole of the foot.

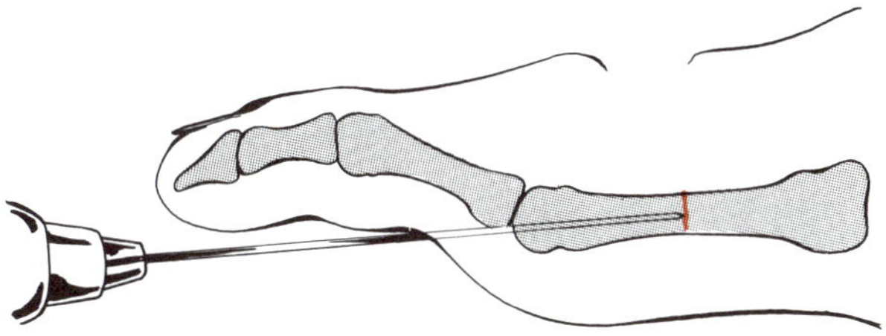

6
Resetting of the drill jig, reduction of the fracture, insertion of the wire into the proximal fragment, similar to retrograde nailing.

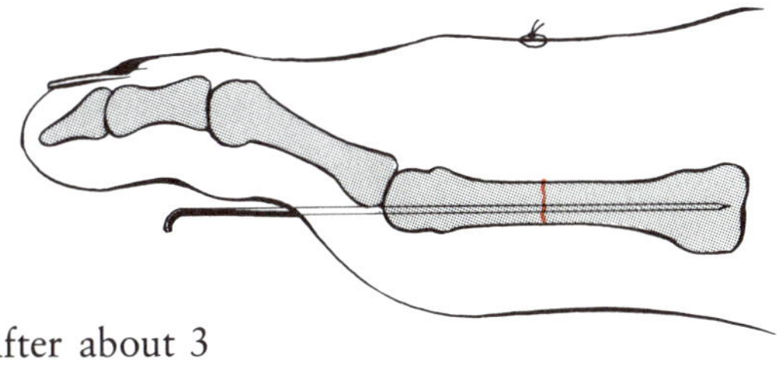

7
The distal end of the wire is not buried. After about 3 weeks the wire can be removed without anesthesia.

Avulsion of the fifth metatarsal

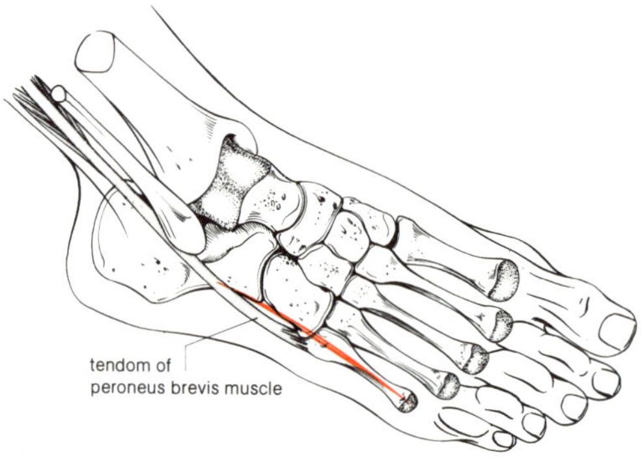

1
Skin incision.

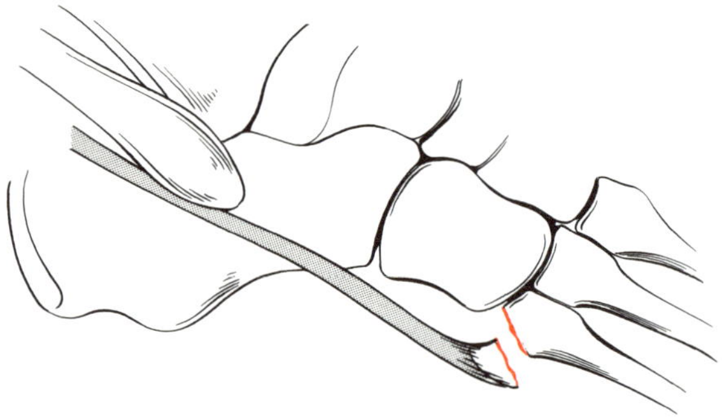

2
Displaced fragment.

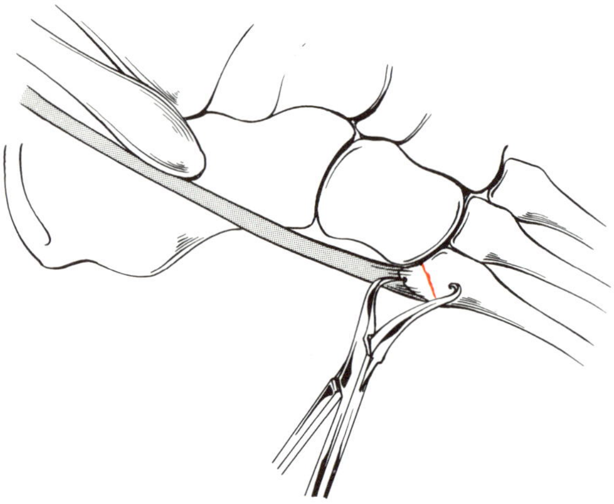

3
Creation of a transverse drill hole with a 2 mm drill through the main fragment. Reposition of the fragment.

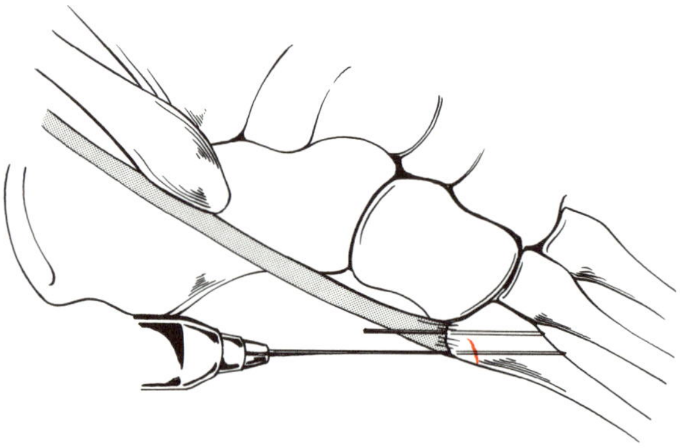

4
Two parallel drilling wires.

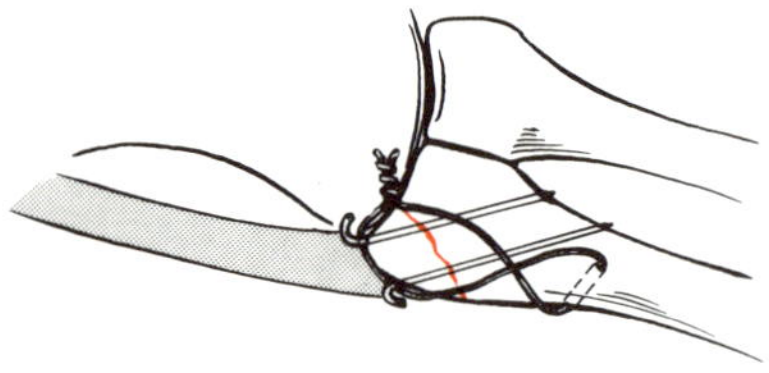

5
Wiring for external fixation.

Subject index